SIXTH EDITION

NASM ESSENTIALS OF
PERSONAL FITNESS TRAINING

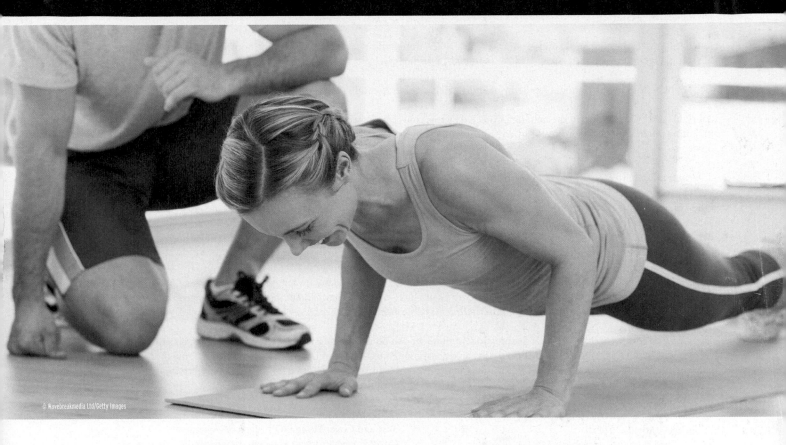

© Wavebreakmedia Ltd/Getty Images

EDITORS (listed in alphabetical order)

Micheal A. Clark, DPT, MS, CES, PES

Scott C. Lucett, MS, NASM-CPT, CES, PES

Erin McGill, MA, NASM-CPT, CES, PES, FNS

Ian Montel, NASM-CPT, CES, PES

Brian Sutton, MS, MA, NASM-CPT, CES, PES

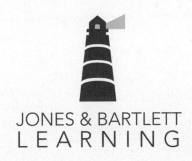

JONES & BARTLETT
LEARNING

World Headquarters
Jones & Bartlett Learning
5 Wall Street
Burlington, MA 01803
978-443-5000
info@jblearning.com
www.jblearning.com

National Academy of Sports Medicine
1750 East Northrop Boulevard
Suite 200
Chandler, Arizona 85286
800-460-6276
www.nasm.org

Jones & Bartlett Learning books and products are available through most bookstores and online booksellers. To contact Jones & Bartlett Learning directly, call 800-832-0034, fax 978-443-8000, or visit our website, www.jblearning.com.

Production Credits

VP, Executive Publisher: David D. Cella
Publisher: Cathy L. Esperti
Acquisitions Editor: Sean Fabery
VP, Manufacturing and Inventory Control: Therese Connell
Director of Marketing: Andrea DeFronzo
Director of Vendor Management: Amy Rose
Production Assistant: Brooke Haley

Composition: S4Carlisle Publishing Services
Text and Cover Design: Off Madison Avenue
Cover Image: Front: © Wavebreakmedia Ltd/Getty Images;
   Back: © Jacob Lund Photography/Creative Market
Printing and Binding: LSC Communications
Cover Printing: LSC Communications

To order this product, use ISBN: 978-1-284-16008-6

Library of Congress Cataloging-in-Publication Data unavailable at time of printing.

6048

Printed in the United States of America
22 21 20   10 9 8 7

Table of Contents

National Academy of Sports Medicine Code of Professional Conduct

The following code of professional conduct is designed to assist certified and noncertified members of the National Academy of Sports Medicine (NASM) to uphold (both as individuals and as an industry) the highest levels of professional and ethical conduct. This Code of Professional Conduct reflects the level of commitment and integrity necessary to ensure that all NASM members provide the highest level of service and respect for all colleagues, allied professionals, and the general public.

Professionalism

Each certified or noncertified member must provide optimal professional service and demonstrate excellent client care in his or her practice. Each member shall:

1. Abide fully by the NASM Code of Professional Conduct.
2. Conduct themselves in a manner that merits the respect of the public, other colleagues, and NASM.
3. Treat each colleague and client with the utmost respect and dignity.
4. Not make false or derogatory assumptions concerning the practices of colleagues and clients.
5. Use appropriate professional communication in all verbal, nonverbal, and written transactions.
6. Provide and maintain an environment that ensures client safety that, at a minimum, requires that the certified or noncertified member:
   a. Shall not diagnose or treat illness or injury (except for basic first aid) unless the certified or noncertified member is legally licensed to do so and is working in that capacity at that time.
   b. Shall not train clients with a diagnosed health condition unless the certified or noncertified member has been specifically trained to do so, is following procedures prescribed and supervised by a valid licensed medical professional, or is legally licensed to do so and is working in that capacity at that time.
   c. Shall not begin to train a client before receiving and reviewing a current health history questionnaire signed by the client.
   d. Shall hold a CPR and AED certification at all times.
7. Refer the client to the appropriate medical practitioner when, at a minimum, the certified or noncertified member:
   a. Becomes aware of any change in the client's health status or medication.
   b. Becomes aware of an undiagnosed illness, injury, or risk factor.
   c. Becomes aware of any unusual client pain or discomfort during the course of the training session that warrants professional care after the session has been discontinued and assessed.
8. Refer the client to other healthcare professionals when nutritional and supplemental advice is requested unless the certified or noncertified member has

been specifically trained to do so or holds a credential to do so and is acting in that capacity at the time.

9. Maintain a level of personal hygiene appropriate for a health and fitness setting.
10. Wear clothing that is clean, modest, and professional.
11. Remain in good standing and maintain current certification status by acquiring all necessary continuing-education requirements (see NASM CPT Certification Candidate Handbook).

Confidentiality

Each certified and noncertified member shall respect the confidentiality of all client information. In his or her professional role, the certified or noncertified member should:

1. Protect the client's confidentiality in conversations, advertisements, and any other arena, unless otherwise agreed to by the client in writing, or as a result of medical or legal necessity.
2. Protect the interest of clients who are minors by law, or who are unable to give voluntary consent by securing the legal permission of the appropriate third party or guardian.
3. Store and dispose of client records in secure manner.

Legal and Ethical

Each certified or noncertified member must comply with all legal requirements within the applicable jurisdiction. In his or her professional role, the certified or noncertified member must:

1. Obey all local, state, provincial, or federal laws.
2. Accept complete responsibility for his or her actions.
3. Maintain accurate and truthful records.
4. Respect and uphold all existing publishing and copyright laws.

Business Practice

Each certified or noncertified member must practice with honesty, integrity, and lawfulness. In his or her professional role, the certified or noncertified member shall:

1. Maintain adequate liability insurance.
2. Maintain adequate and truthful progress notes for each client.
3. Accurately and truthfully inform the public of services rendered.
4. Honestly and truthfully represent all professional qualifications and affiliations.
5. Advertise in a manner that is honest, dignified, and representative of services that can be delivered without the use of provocative or sexual language or pictures.
6. Maintain accurate financial, contract, appointment, and tax records including original receipts for a minimum of four years.
7. Comply with all local, state, federal, or providence laws regarding sexual harassment.

NASM expects each member to uphold the Code of Professional Conduct in its entirety. Failure to comply with the NASM Code of Professional Conduct may result in disciplinary actions including but not limited to, suspension or termination of membership and certification. All members are obligated to report any unethical behavior or violation of the Code of Professional Conduct by other NASM members.

Letter from NASM

We applaud you on your dedication and commitment to helping others live healthier lives and thank you for entrusting the National Academy of Sports Medicine (NASM) with your education. By following the techniques presented in this textbook you will gain the information, insight, and inspiration you need to change the world as a health and fitness professional.

For more than 25 years, NASM has been the leading authority in certification, continuing education, and career development for health and fitness professionals. As the world's foremost resource for fitness and sports medicine information, NASM continues to elevate industry standards by providing outstanding educational programs and quality certification courses for our members.

Scientific research and techniques also continue to evolve, and, as a result, you must remain on the cutting edge to remain competitive. Designed exclusively by NASM, the Optimum Performance Training™ (OPT™) model is the industry's first evidence-based training system founded on the scientific rationale of human movement science. Now, more than ever, it is imperative that health and fitness professionals fully understand all components of exercise programming. OPT is your solution. With OPT you'll successfully train any client toward any goal. It's proven. It's easy to use.

We look forward to working with you to help shape the future of fitness. Welcome to the NASM family!

User's Guide

NASM Essentials of Personal Fitness Training, Sixth Edition, helps you to master goal-specific program design, accurate assessment, and development and modification of exercise in a safe and effective manner. Please take a few moments to look through this user's guide, which will introduce you to the tools and features that will enhance your learning experience.

Objectives open each chapter and present learning goals to help you focus on and retain the crucial topics discussed.

The Scientific Rationale for Integrated Training

OBJECTIVES

After studying this chapter, you should be able to:

- ✔ Explain the history of the profession of personal training.
- ✔ Identify common characteristics of personal training clients.
- ✔ Demonstrate an understanding of the principles of integrated exercise program design.
- ✔ Describe the Optimum Performance Training™ (OPT™) model.

Sidebars, set in the margins, highlight the definitions of key terms that are presented in the chapter. The key terms are bolded throughout the chapter for easy reference.

Current Training Programs

For the majority of sedentary adults, low- to moderate-intensity exercise is extremely safe and can be very effective. However, if the training intensity is too high initially, then the individual will experience excessive overload, which may lead to injury (31). In the first 6 weeks of one study that focused on training sedentary adults, there was a 50% to 90% injury rate (32). Overtraining injuries can occur even though exercise training programs are specifically designed to minimize the risk of injury.

It is important to note that **deconditioned** does not simply mean a person is out of breath when climbing a flight of stairs or that they are overweight. It is a state in which a person may have muscle imbalances, decreased flexibility, or a lack of core and joint stability. All of these conditions can greatly affect the ability of the human body to produce proper movement and can eventually lead to injury.

Most training programs do not emphasize multiplanar movements (or movements in all directions) through the full muscle action spectrum (concentric acceleration, eccentric deceleration, and isometric stabilization) in an environment that enriches proprioception. A **proprioceptively enriched environment** is one that challenges internal balance and stabilization mechanisms of the body. Examples of this include performing a Stability Ball Dumbbell Chest Press or Single-leg Squat versus the traditional Bench Press and Barbell Squat exercises. It is important to note, the National Academy of Sports Medicine (NASM) only recommends training in a proprioceptive environment that can be *safely* controlled based on the client's movement capabilities and overall conditioning level. Exercises must be regressed if the client cannot perform an exercise with ideal posture and technique.

Deconditioned A state of lost physical fitness, which may include muscle imbalances, decreased flexibility, and a lack of core and joint stability.

Proprioception The cumulative sensory input to the central nervous system from all mechanoreceptors that sense body position and limb movement.

Proprioceptively enriched environment An unstable (yet controllable) physical situation in which exercises are performed that causes the body to use its internal balance and stabilization mechanisms.

STRETCH Your Knowledge

Evidence to Support the Use of Plyometric Training for Injury Prevention and Performance Enhancement

- Chimera et al. (2004) in a pretest and posttest with control group design using 20 healthy Division I female athletes found that a 6-week plyometric training program improved hip abductor and adductor coactivation ratios to help control varus (bowlegged) and valgus (knock-knees) moments at the knee during landing (1).
- Wilkerson et al. (2004) in a quasi-experimental design with 19 female basketball players demonstrated that a 6-week plyometric training program improved hamstring to quadriceps ratio, which has been shown to enhance dynamic knee stability during the eccentric deceleration phase of landing (2). This is one of the factors contributing to the high incidence of anterior cruciate ligament (ACL) injuries in female athletes.
- Luebbers et al. (2003) in a randomized controlled trial with 19 subjects demonstrated that 4-and 7-week plyometric training programs enhanced anaerobic power and vertical jump height (3).
- Hewett et al. (1996) in a prospective study demonstrated decreased peak landing forces, enhanced muscle-balance ratio between the quadriceps and hamstrings, and decreased rate of anterior cruciate ligament injuries in female soccer, basketball, and volleyball players who incorporated plyometric training into their program (4).

REFERENCES

1. Chimera NJ, Swanik KA, Swanik CB, Straub SJ. Effects of plyometric training on muscle-activation strategies and performance in female athletes. *J Athl Train.* 2004;39(1):24–31.
2. Wilkerson GB, Colston MA, Short NI, Neal KL, Hoewischer PE, Pixley JJ. Neuromuscular changes in female collegiate athletes resulting from a plyometric jump training program. *J Athl Train.* 2004;39(1):17–23.
3. Luebbers PE, Potteiger JA, Hulver MW, Thyfault JP, Carper MJ, Lockwood RH. Effects of plyometric training and recovery on vertical jump performance and anaerobic power. *J Strength Cond Res.* 2003;17(4):704–709.
4. Hewett TE, Stroupe AL, Nance TA, Noyes FR. Plyometric training in female athletes. Decreased impact forces and increased hamstring torques. *Am J Sports Med.* 1996;24(6):765–773.

Stretch Your Knowledge boxes emphasize key concepts and findings from current research.

Memory Joggers call out core concepts and program design instructions

Memory Jogger

It is important to understand the function of the muscle spindles and GTOs as they play an integral part in flexibility training.

Exercise sections discuss the purpose and procedures of various techniques that can be used with clients. Tips for proper Technique and Safety are also highlighted.

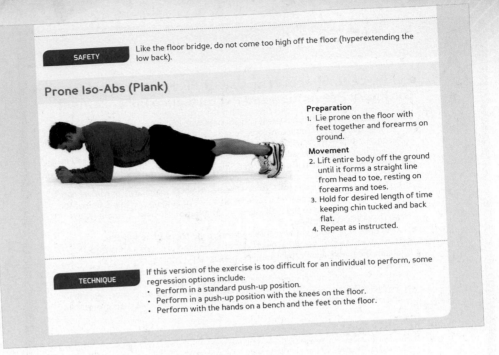

SAFETY   Like the floor bridge, do not come too high off the floor (hyperextending the low back).

Prone Iso-Abs (Plank)

Preparation
1. Lie prone on the floor with feet together and forearms on ground.

Movement
2. Lift entire body off the ground until it forms a straight line from head to toe, resting on forearms and toes.
3. Hold for desired length of time keeping chin tucked and back flat.
4. Repeat as instructed.

TECHNIQUE   If this version of the exercise is too difficult for an individual to perform, some regression options include:
- Perform in a standard push-up position.
- Perform in a push-up position with the knees on the floor.
- Perform with the hands on a bench and the feet on the floor.

High-quality, four-color photographs and artwork throughout the text help to draw attention to important concepts in a visually stimulating and intriguing manner. They help to clarify the text and are particularly helpful for visual learners.

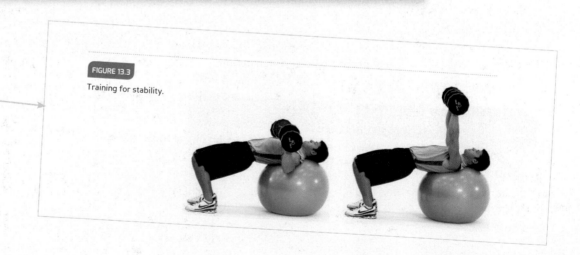

FIGURE 13.3

Training for stability.

Acknowledgments

Contributors

Donald A. Chu, PhD, PT, ATC, CSCS
Castro Valley, CA

Micheal Clark, DPT, MS, CES, PES

Michelle Cleere, PhD
Bay Area, CA

Lindsay J. DiStefano, PhD, ATC, PES
Storrs, CT

Christopher Frankel, MS
San Francisco, CA

Susan J, Hewlings, PhD, RD
Cudjoe Key, FL

Chris Hoffmann, MS, ART, AKC, RKC, NASM-CPT, CES, PES

Lisa-Michelle Hoffmann, NASM-CPT, CES, PES

Adam Horak, MBA, BS, NASM-CPT, CES, PES
Houston, TX

Karen Jashinsky, MBA, NASM-CPT

Douglas S. Kalman, PhD, RD, FISSN, FACN
Miami, FL

Donald T. Kirkendall, PhD
Durham, NC

Brett Klika, CSCS
San Diego, CA

Craig Liebenson, DC
Los Angeles, CA

Erin McGill, MA, NASM-CPT, CES, PES, FNS
Scottsdale, AZ

Scott Lucett, MS, NASM-CPT, CES, PES
Oxnard, CA

Pete McCall, MS, NASM-CPT, PES
San Diego, CA

Melanie L. McGrath, PhD, ATC
Omaha, NE

Marty Miller, DHSc, ATC, NASM-CPT, CES, PES, MMACS
Palm Beach Gardens, FL

Ian Montel, NASM-CPT, CES, PES
Gilbert, AZ

Darin A. Padua, PhD, ATC
Chapel Hill, NC

Matthew Rhea, PhD, CES, PEX, CSCS*D
St. George, UT

Richard Richey, MS, LMT, NASM-CPT, CES, PES
New York, NY

Gay Riley, MS, RD, CCN, NASM-CPT

Paul Robbins, MS
Phoenix, AZ

Scott O. Roberts, PhD, FACSM
Chico, CA

Mabel J. Robles, MS, NASM-CPT, CES, PES, FNS, WFS, WLS
Gilbert, AZ

Kyle Stull, DHSc, MS, LMT, NASM-CPT, CES, PES
Austin, TX

Brian G. Sutton, MS, MA, NASM-CPT, CES, PES
Chandler, AZ

C. Alan Titchenal, PhD, CNS
Honolulu, HI

Craig Valency, MA, CSCS
San Diego, CA

Robert Weinberg, PhD, CC-AASP
Cincinnati, OH

Edzard Zeinstra, PE, MSc

Reviewers

Brian Sutton, MS, MS, PES, CES, NASM-CPT

Scott O. Roberts, PhD, FACSM

Scott Lucett, MS, PES, CES, NASM-CPT

Photography

Ben Bercovici
President
In Sync Productions
Calabasas, CA

Anton Polygalov
Photographer
In Sync Productions
Calabasas, CA

Roy Ramsay
Director Educational Technology
Assessment Technologies Institute

Jason Shadrick
Media Design Specialist
Assessment Technologies Institute

Morgan Smith
Media Developer
Assessment Technologies Institute

MODELS

A special acknowledgement goes out to our models, who made all of these exercises look easy: Christine Silva, Steven McDougal, Joey Metz, Rian Chab, Jessica Kern, Geoff Etherson, Monica Munson, Harold Spencer, Alexis Weatherspoon, Golden Goodwin, Sean Brown, Monica Carlson, Allie Shira, Mel Mueller, Cameron Klippsten, Mike Chapin, and Ric Miller.

Fundamentals of Human Movement Science

The Scientific Rationale for Integrated Training

OBJECTIVES

After studying this chapter, you will be able to:

✔ Explain the history of the profession of personal training.

✔ Identify common characteristics of personal training clients.

✔ Demonstrate an understanding of the principles of integrated exercise program design.

✔ Describe the Optimum Performance Training™ (OPT™) model.

Overview of the Personal Training Industry

There has never been a better time than the present to consider a career in personal training. According to the US Department of Labor, the demand for personal trainers is expected to increase faster than the average for all occupations (1). The increasing demand for personal trainers is due in part to the escalation of obesity, diabetes, and various chronic diseases, and to the advancing age of Americans. Another factor related to the rise in demand for personal trainers is that health clubs rely on them for their largest source of non-dues revenue (2). In addition to traditional health club markets, some of the fastest growing areas of growth for personal trainers are in corporate, medical, and wellness settings.

A Brief History of Fitness and Personal Training in America

1950 to 1960—Health clubs, or "gyms," as they were called back in the 1950s, were a male-dominated environment in which men trained with free weights to increase size (body builders), strength (power lifters), explosive strength (Olympic lifters), or a combination of all of these goals (athletes). In 1951 Jack LaLanne began hosting

America's first television fitness show called The Jack LaLanne Show, which aired until 1984. Jack's workouts consisted mainly of calisthenics intermixed with tips on counting calories, weight training, and nutrition. What most people don't know about Jack LaLanne is that, in addition to his pioneering TV show, in 1936 at the age of 21 he opened up his first health club in Oakland, Calif., and was the inventor of the cable pulley weight training system and the Smith weight lifting machine, both of which are still used in virtually every gym around the world.

1960 to 1970—In the 1960s women's fitness centers or "figure salons" became a popular trend. Unlike male-oriented gyms where the focus was on developing muscle size and strength, women's fitness centers typically focused on weight loss and spot reduction. And instead of barbells and dumbbells, most of the exercise machines in women's fitness centers were passive; for example, a rolling machine was used to roll away fat, and an electronic vibrating belt supposedly helped jiggle the fat from the thighs. In the early 1960s President John F. Kennedy changed the name of the President's Council on Youth Fitness to the President's Council on Physical Fitness to address not only children but adults as well. President Kennedy's public support of fitness and exercise had a significant impact on generating greater awareness of health and spawned a tremendous interest in jogging, or running as it was called back then. In 1966 Bill Bowerman, the head track coach for the University of Oregon, published a book titled *Jogging*, which helped launch the jogging/running boom in the United States.

In 1965 Joe Gold opened the first Gold's Gym in Venice Beach, Calif. The original Gold's Gym was the backdrop for the movie *Pumping Iron* starring Arnold Schwarzenegger and remains a shrine for serious bodybuilders and weightlifters. In 1970 Joe sold the chain, but the Gold's Gym Empire went on to become one of the largest chains of coed gyms in the world with more than 650 to date worldwide.

1970 to 1980—By the 1970s joining a health club or exercising outdoors was becoming more socially acceptable, and soon men and women of all ages were exercising side by side. Joining a health club provided a way of achieving social interaction and health simultaneously. Health clubs began offering an alternative to participating in team sports or activities, which often involve some, and in some cases high, levels of skill and endurance before the activity can be enjoyed. Health clubs became an outlet for men and women of all ages, regardless of physical ability, that could be used year-round day or night. The growth in popularity of health clubs was a sign that members of society at the time were becoming conscious of their appearance and that physical appearance could be improved by changing physical characteristics through exercise.

As the popularity and growth in new health clubs steadily increased throughout the 1970s, they became the desired location for people seeking information on ways to improve their health and ways to get started on an exercise program. By default, the expert of the 1970s was the person working in a health club who had been training the longest, looked the most fit, or was the strongest. Unfortunately, physical appearance does not always have anything to do with knowledge of exercise science or training principles. Despite the lack of qualified staff during the early days of the health club industry, the majority of new members would often seek out advice from a perceived expert and offer that person money in exchange for their training knowledge and guidance. Thus, the personal training profession was born.

Although anyone with some basic experience and knowledge of training could potentially provide adequate information on training principles such as loads, sets, reps, etc., their understanding and application of human movement science (functional

Muscle imbalance
Alteration of muscle length surrounding a joint.

anatomy, functional biomechanics, and motor behavior) is something very different. In the early days of fitness training it was not common practice to assess a new client for past medical conditions, training risk factors, **muscle imbalances**, and goals. This resulted in training programs that simply mimicked those of the current fitness professional or instructor. Programs were rarely designed to meet an individual client's goals, needs, and abilities.

The Present: The Rise of Chronic Disease

Chronic diseases, such as asthma, cancer, diabetes, and heart disease, are widespread and rising dramatically in the United States. Largely preventable factors such as poor lifestyle choices and lack of access or emphasis on preventive care have led to dramatic increases in chronic disease rates within the past three decades. Not surprisingly, chronic diseases have become the leading cause of death and disability in the United States, accounting for 70% of deaths in the United States. The impact of chronic disease affects nearly every American, directly or indirectly, to some degree. Chronic disease is associated with worsening health and quality of life, eventual permanent disability with time, and a reduced life span. Indirectly, chronic disease takes a toll on the nation's economy by lowering productivity and slowing economic growth as a result of escalating corporate health-care costs and the fact that 75 cents of every dollar spent on health care, or about $1.7 trillion annually, goes toward treating chronic illness.

Chronic disease is defined as an incurable illness or health condition that persists for a year or more, resulting in functional limitations and the need for ongoing medical care. Despite widespread knowledge that most chronic diseases are preventable and manageable through early detection, treatment, and healthy living, chronic disease usually leads to some degree of permanent physical or mental impairment that significantly limits one or more activities of daily living (ADL) in at least 25% of those diagnosed with a chronic health condition.

The US Centers for Disease Control and Prevention reported that seven of the top ten causes of death are caused by chronic diseases (2). The top two leading causes of death in the United States are cardiovascular disease and cancer, and a large majority of those deaths could have been prevented if a healthy lifestyle was followed (3). Recent estimates indicate the cost of cardiovascular disease is approximately $555 billion (4).

Another chronic condition often associated with cardiovascular disease is obesity, which is currently a worldwide problem. **Obesity** is the condition of being considerably overweight, and refers to a person with a body mass index (BMI) of 30 or greater, or who is at least 30 pounds over the recommended weight for their height (5). A desirable BMI for adults 20 years and older is between 18.5 and 24.9. The calculations for determining BMI are noted in **Figure 1.1**. At present 66% of Americans older than age 20 are overweight. Approximately 34% of Americans are obese, which equates to approximately 72 million Americans (6). The same trend is occurring among youth (ages 2–19) as more than nine million young people are overweight or obese (7). Nearly one in five children and adolescents in the United States has obesity (8). **Overweight** is defined as a person with a BMI of 25 to 29.9, or who is between 25 to 30 pounds over the recommended weight for their height (5). Excessive body weight is associated with a myriad of health risks including cardiovascular disease, type 2 diabetes, high cholesterol, osteoarthritis, some types of cancer, pregnancy complications, shortened life expectancy, and decreased quality of life.

Obesity The condition of being considerably overweight, and refers to a person with a body mass index of 30 or greater, or who is at least 30 pounds over the recommended weight for their height.

Overweight Refers to a person with a body mass index of 25 to 29.9, or who is between 25 to 30 pounds over the recommended weight for their height.

$$BMI = 703 \times \frac{weight\ (lb)}{height^2\ (in^2)}$$

$$BMI = \frac{weight\ (kg)}{height^2\ (m^2)}$$

© ilolab/ShutterStock, Inc.

FIGURE 1.1

Equations used to calculate body mass index.

Cholesterol has received much attention because of its direct relationship with cardiovascular disease and obesity. **Blood lipids**, also known as cholesterol and triglycerides, are carried in the bloodstream by protein molecules known as high-density lipoproteins, or "good cholesterol," and low-density lipoproteins, or "bad cholesterol." A healthy total cholesterol level is less than 200 mg/dL. A borderline high cholesterol level is between 200 and 239 mg/dL, and a high-risk level is more than 240 mg/dL. Alarmingly, more than 50% of adults have total cholesterol values of 200 mg/dL or higher (9).

Another condition affecting nearly 23 million Americans is diabetes (10). **Diabetes mellitus** is a condition in which blood glucose or "blood sugar" is unable to enter cells either because the pancreas is unable to produce insulin or the cells have become insulin resistant. Type 1 diabetes, often referred to as juvenile diabetes because symptoms of the disease typically first appear in childhood, is the result of the pancreas not producing insulin. As a result, blood sugar is not optimally delivered into the cells, resulting in "hyperglycemia" or high blood sugar.

Type 2 diabetes is associated with obesity, particularly abdominal obesity, and accounts for 90 to 95% of all diabetes (10). Patients with type 2 diabetes usually produce adequate amounts of insulin; however, their cells are resistant and do not allow insulin to bring adequate amounts of blood sugar (glucose) into the cell. Not surprisingly, more than 80% of all patients with type 2 diabetes are overweight or have a history of excessive weight. If diabetes is not properly managed, high blood sugar can lead to a host of problems including nerve damage, vision loss, kidney damage, sexual dysfunction, and decreased immune function. Once limited to overweight adults, type 2 diabetes now accounts for almost half of the new cases diagnosed in children (11).

Americans are living longer. The US Census Bureau reported that the proportion of the population older than 65 is projected to increase from 12.4% in 2000 to 19.6% in 2030. The number of individuals older than 80 is expected to increase from 9.3 million in 2000 to 19.5 million in 2030. This influences to the number of individuals developing chronic diseases and disability. In the United States, approximately 80% of all persons older than 65 have at least one chronic condition, and 50% have at least two. One in five adults report having doctor-diagnosed arthritis, and this is a leading cause of disability (12).

In 2002, the World Health Organization recognized lack of physical activity as a significant contributor to the risk factors for several chronic diseases, but unfortunately, few adults achieve the minimum recommended 30 or more minutes of moderate physical activity on 5 or more days per week (13). Physical activity has been proven to reduce the risk of chronic diseases and disorders that are related to lifestyle, such as increased triglycerides and cholesterol levels, obesity, glucose intolerance, high blood pressure, coronary heart disease, and strokes (14). More importantly, some research indicates that discontinuing (or significantly decreasing) physical activity can actually lead to a higher risk of chronic diseases that are related to lifestyle (15).

Blood lipids Also known as cholesterol and triglycerides, blood lipids are carried in the bloodstream by protein molecules known as high-density lipoproteins (HDL) and low-density lipoproteins (LDL).

Diabetes mellitus Chronic metabolic disorder caused by insulin deficiency, which impairs carbohydrate usage and enhances usage of fats and proteins.

Meanwhile, daily activity levels continue to decline (16). People are less active and are no longer spending as much of their free time engaged in physical activity. This is related in part to lack of physical activity in leisure time, but is even more likely the result of people spending increasing amounts of time in sedentary behaviors such as watching television and using computers, and excessive use of passive modes of transportation (cars, buses, and motorcycles). Physical education and after-school sports programs are also being cut from school budgets, further decreasing the amount of physical activity in children's lives. This new environment is producing more inactive, unhealthy, and nonfunctional people (17).

In 2008, the federal government issued its most comprehensive set of guidelines on physical activity to date. The guidelines are designed to provide information and guidance on the types and amounts of physical activity that provide substantial health benefits (to those who are apparently healthy as well as those with one or more chronic health conditions). These were the first set of physical activity guidelines that addressed the quality and quantity of exercise needed to improve health and prevent disease for not only adults but also children, seniors, and those individuals living with chronic disease.

Evidence of Muscular Dysfunction and Increased Injury

Research suggests that musculoskeletal pain is more common now than it was 40 years ago (18). One of the primary causes of muscular dysfunction is attributable to physical inactivity.

Low-Back Pain

Low-back pain is a primary cause of musculoskeletal degeneration seen in the adult population, affecting nearly 80% of all adults (19,20). Research has shown low-back pain to be predominant among workers in enclosed workspaces (such as offices) (21,22), as well as people engaged in manual labor (farming) (23). Low-back pain is also seen in people who sit for periods of time greater than 3 hours (22) and in individuals who have altered lumbar lordosis (curve in the lumbar spine) (24).

Knee Injuries

An estimated 80,000 to 100,000 anterior cruciate ligament (ACL) injuries occur annually in the general US population. Approximately 70% of these are noncontact injuries (25). In addition, ACL injuries have a strong correlation to acquiring arthritis in the affected knee (26). Most ACL injuries occur between 15 and 25 years of age (25). This comes as no surprise when considering the lack of activity and increased obesity occurring in this age group. US teenagers have an abundance of automation and technology, combined with a lack of mandatory physical education in schools (17). Fortunately, research suggests that enhancing neuromuscular stabilization (or body control) may alleviate the high incidence of noncontact injuries (27).

Musculoskeletal Injuries

In 2003, musculoskeletal symptoms were the number two reason for physician visits. Approximately 31 million visits were made to physicians' offices because of back problems in 2003, including more than 10 million visits for low-back problems. Approximately 19 million visits in 2003 were made because of knee problems, 14 million for shoulder problems, and 11 million for foot and ankle problems (28).

Unnatural posture, caused by improper sitting, results in increased neck, mid- and lower back, shoulder, and leg pain. Of work-related injuries, more than 40% are sprains (injured ligaments) and strains (injured tendons or muscles). More than one third of all work-related injuries involve the trunk, and of these, more than 60% involve the low back. These work-related injuries cost workers approximately 9 days per back episode or, combined, more than 39 million days of restricted activity. The monetary value of lost work time as a result of these musculoskeletal injuries was estimated to be approximately $120 billion in 2005 and continues to rise (29).

Exercise training programs need to address all of the components of health-related physical fitness using safe and effective training principles. Unfortunately, many training programs and fitness equipment used to condition the musculoskeletal system are often based on unsound training principles and guidelines. Vital to safe and effective exercise training programs is to train essential areas of the body, such as the stabilizing muscles of the hips, upper and lower back, and neck, and to use a proper progression of acute variables (i.e., sets, repetitions, and rest periods). The extent to which exercise training programs develop the musculoskeletal system is directly influenced by the potential risk of injury. The less conditioned our musculoskeletal systems are, the higher the risk of injury (30).

Current Training Programs

For the majority of sedentary adults, low- to moderate-intensity exercise is extremely safe and can be very effective. However, if the training intensity is too high initially, then the individual will experience excessive overload, which may lead to injury (31). In the first 6 weeks of one study that focused on training sedentary adults, there was a 50% to 90% injury rate (32). Overtraining injuries can occur even though exercise training programs are specifically designed to minimize the risk of injury.

It is important to note that **deconditioned** does not simply mean a person is out of breath when climbing a flight of stairs or that they are overweight. It is a state in which a person may have muscle imbalances, decreased flexibility, or a lack of core and joint stability. All of these conditions can greatly affect the ability of the human body to produce proper movement and can eventually lead to injury.

Most training programs do not emphasize multiplanar movements (or movements in all directions) through the full muscle action spectrum (concentric acceleration, eccentric deceleration, and isometric stabilization) in an environment that enriches **proprioception**. A **proprioceptively enriched environment** is one that challenges the internal balance and stabilization mechanisms of the body. Examples of this include performing a stability ball dumbbell chest press or single-leg squat versus the traditional bench press and barbell squat exercises. It is important to note, the National Academy of Sports Medicine (NASM) only recommends training in a proprioceptive environment that can be *safely* controlled based on the client's movement capabilities and overall conditioning level. Exercises must be regressed if the client cannot perform an exercise with ideal posture and technique.

Deconditioned A state of lost physical fitness, which may include muscle imbalances, decreased flexibility, and a lack of core and joint stability.

Proprioception The cumulative sensory input to the central nervous system from all mechanoreceptors that sense body position and limb movement.

Proprioceptively enriched environment An unstable (yet controllable) physical situation in which exercises are performed that causes the body to use its internal balance and stabilization mechanisms.

The Future

The personal training industry is growing dramatically, especially in regard to personal trainers' abilities to work with individuals with one or more chronic health conditions or musculoskeletal impairments. The majority of clients who seek out personal training services are physically inactive and have poor overall functional capacities. A decrease in everyday activity has contributed to many of the postural deficiencies seen in people (33).

Today's client is not ready to begin physical activity at the same level that a typical client could 20 or 30 years ago. Therefore, today's training programs cannot stay the same as programs of the past.

The new mindset in fitness should cater to creating programs that address functional capacity, as part of a safe program designed especially for each individual person. In other words, training programs must consider an individual's goals, needs, and abilities in a safe and systematic fashion. This is best achieved by introducing an integrated approach to program design. It is on this premise that NASM presents the rationale for integrated training and the OPT model.

SUMMARY

The typical gym members of the 1950s were mainly athletes, and, in the 1970s, those involved in recreational sports. The first fitness professionals were physically fit individuals who did not necessarily have education in human movement science or exercise physiology. They did not design programs to meet the specific goals, needs, and abilities of their clients.

Today, more people work in offices, have longer work hours, use better technology and automation, and are required to move less on a daily basis. This new environment produces more sedentary people, and leads to dysfunction and increased incidents of injury including chronic disease, low-back pain, knee injuries, and other musculoskeletal injuries.

In working with today's typical client, who is likely to be deconditioned, the fitness professional must use special consideration when designing fitness programs. An integrated approach should be used to create safe programs that consider functional capacity for each individual person. These programs must address factors such as appropriate forms of flexibility, increasing strength and endurance, and training in different types of environments. These factors are the basis for NASM's OPT model.

Integrated Training and the OPT Model

Integrated training is a concept that incorporates all forms of training in an integrated fashion as part of a progressive system. These forms of training include flexibility training; cardiorespiratory training; core training; balance training; plyometric (reactive) training; speed, agility, and quickness training; and resistance training.

What Is the OPT Model?

The OPT model was conceptualized as a training program for a society that has more structural imbalances and susceptibility to injury than ever before. It is a process of programming that systematically progresses any client to any goal. The OPT model **Figure 1.2** is built on a foundation of principles that progressively and systematically allows any client to achieve optimal levels of physiologic, physical, and performance adaptations, including:

Physiologic Benefits
- Improves cardiorespiratory efficiency
- Enhances beneficial endocrine (hormone) and serum lipid (cholesterol) adaptations
- Increases metabolic efficiency (metabolism)
- Increases bone density

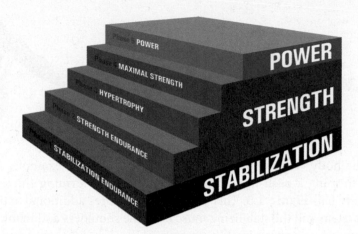

FIGURE 1.2

OPT model.

Physical Benefits

◆ Decreases body fat
◆ Increases lean body mass (muscle)
◆ Increases tissue tensile strength (tendons, ligaments, muscles)

Performance Benefits

◆ Strength
◆ Power
◆ Endurance
◆ Flexibility
◆ Speed
◆ Agility
◆ Balance

The OPT model is based on the scientific rationale of human movement science. Each stage has a designated purpose that provides the client with a systematic approach for progressing toward his or her individual goals, as well as addressing his or her specific needs. Now, more than ever, it is imperative that health and fitness professionals fully understand all components of programming as well as the right order in which those components must be addressed to help their clients achieve success.

Phases of Training

The OPT model is divided into three different levels of training—stabilization, strength, and power (Figure 1.2). Each level contains specific **phases of training**. It is imperative that the health and fitness professional understands the scientific rationale behind each level and each individual phase of training to properly use the OPT model.

Stabilization Level

The Stabilization Level consists of one phase of training—Phase 1: Stabilization Endurance Training. The main focus of this form of training is to increase **muscular endurance** and stability while developing optimal **neuromuscular efficiency** (coordination).

The progression for this level of training is proprioceptively based. This means that difficulty is increased by introducing a greater challenge to the balance and stabilization

Phases of training
Smaller divisions of training progressions that fall within the three building blocks of training.

Muscular endurance
A muscle's ability to contract for an extended period.

Neuromuscular efficiency The ability of the neuromuscular system to enable all muscles to efficiently work together in all planes of motion.

FIGURE 1.3

Proprioceptive push-up progression.

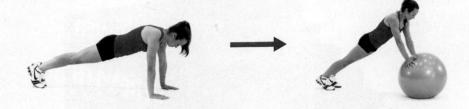

systems of the body (versus simply increasing the load). For example, a client may begin by performing a push-up and then progress by performing the same exercise using a stability ball **Figure 1.3**. This progression requires additional activation from the nervous system and the stabilizing muscles of the shoulders and trunk to maintain optimal posture while performing the exercise.

Stabilization and neuromuscular efficiency can only be obtained by having the appropriate combination of proper alignment (posture) of the human movement system (kinetic chain) and the stabilization strength necessary to maintain that alignment (34–36). Stabilization training provides the needed stimuli to acquire stabilization and neuromuscular efficiency through the use of proprioceptively enriched exercises and progressions. The goal is to increase the client's ability to stabilize the joints and maintain optimal posture.

It must be noted that stabilization training must be done before strength and power training. Research has shown that inefficient stabilization can negatively affect the way force is produced by the muscles, increase stress at the joints, overload the soft tissues, and, eventually, cause injury (30,37–39).

Stabilization Endurance Training not only addresses the existing structural deficiencies, it may also provide a superior way to alter body composition (reduce body fat) because all the exercises are typically performed in a circuit fashion (short rest periods) with a high number of repetitions (see Chapter 15 for more details) (40–42). By performing exercises in a proprioceptively enriched environment (controlled, unstable), the body is forced to recruit more muscles to stabilize itself. In doing so, more calories are potentially expended (40,41).

Goals and Strategies of Stabilization Level Training

PHASE 1: STABILIZATION ENDURANCE TRAINING

◆ Goals
  » Improve muscular endurance
  » Enhance joint stability
  » Increase flexibility
  » Enhance control of posture
  » Improve neuromuscular efficiency (balance, stabilization, muscular coordination)
◆ Training Strategies
  » Training in unstable, yet controllable environments (proprioceptively enriched)
  » Low loads, high repetitions

Strength Level

Prime mover The muscle that acts as the initial and main source of motive power.

The Strength Level of training follows the successful completion of stabilization training. The emphasis is to maintain stabilization endurance while increasing **prime mover** strength. This is also the level of training an individual will progress to if his or her goals are *hypertrophy* (increasing muscle size) or *maximal strength* (lifting heavy loads). The Strength Level in the OPT model consists of three phases.

In Phase 2: Strength Endurance Training, the goal is to enhance stabilization endurance while increasing prime mover strength. These two adaptations are accomplished by performing two exercises in a **superset** sequence (or back-to-back without rest) with similar joint dynamics **Table 1.1**. The first exercise is a traditional strength exercise performed in a stable environment (such as a bench press), whereas the second exercise is a stabilization exercise performed in a less stable (yet controllable) environment (such as a stability ball push-up). The principle behind this method is to work the prime movers predominantly in the first exercise to elicit prime mover strength. Then, immediately follow with an exercise that challenges the stabilization muscles. This produces an increased ability to maintain postural stabilization and dynamic joint stabilization.

Phase 3: Hypertrophy Training is designed for individuals who have the goal of maximal muscle growth (such as bodybuilders). Phase 4: Maximal Strength Training works toward the goal of maximal prime mover strength by lifting heavy loads. These two phases of training can be used as special forms of training and as progressions within Strength Level Training.

Superset Set of two exercises that are performed back-to-back, without any rest time between them.

Goals and Strategies of Strength Level Training

PHASE 2: STRENGTH ENDURANCE TRAINING

◆ Goals
  » Improve stabilization endurance and increase prime mover strength
  » Improve overall work capacity
  » Enhance joint stabilization
  » Increase lean body mass
◆ Training Strategies
  » Moderate loads and repetitions (8–12)
  » Superset: one traditional strength exercise and one stabilization exercise per body part in the resistance training portion of the program

PHASE 3: HYPERTROPHY TRAINING
(optional phase, depending on client's goals)

◆ Goal
  » Achieve optimal levels of muscular hypertrophy (increase muscle size)
◆ Training Strategies
  » High volume, moderate to high loads, moderate or low repetitions (6–12)

TABLE 1.1	Phase 2 Example Supersets	
Body Part	**Strength Exercise**	**Stabilization Exercise**
Chest	Barbell bench press	Stability ball push-up
Back	Seated cable row	Stability ball dumbbell row
Shoulders	Shoulder press machine	Single-leg dumbbell press
Legs	Leg press	Single-leg squat

PHASE 4: MAXIMUM STRENGTH TRAINING
(optional phase, depending on client's goals)

- ◆ Goals
  - » Increase motor unit recruitment
  - » Increase frequency of motor unit recruitment
  - » Improve peak force
- ◆ Training Strategies
  - » High loads, low repetitions (1–5), longer rest periods

Power Level

The Power Level of training should only be entered after successful completion of the Stabilization and Strength Levels. This level of training emphasizes the development of speed and power. This is achieved through one phase of training simply named Phase 5: Power Training.

The premise behind this phase of training is the execution of a traditional strength exercise (with a heavy load) superset with a power exercise (with a light load performed as fast as possible) of similar joint dynamics. This is to enhance prime mover strength while also improving the **rate of force production Table 1.2**.

Rate of force production Ability of muscles to exert maximal force output in a minimal amount of time.

Goals and Strategies of Power Level Training

PHASE 5: POWER TRAINING

- ◆ Goals
  - » Enhance neuromuscular efficiency
  - » Enhance prime mover strength
  - » Increase rate of force production
- ◆ Training Strategies
  - » Superset: one strength and one power exercise per body part in the resistance training portion of the program
  - » Perform all power exercises as fast as can be controlled

The Program Template

The uniqueness of the OPT model is that it packages scientific principles into an applicable form of programming. This is a direct result of research conducted at the NASM Research Institute in partnership with the University of North Carolina, Chapel Hill, and within NASM's clinical setting, used on actual clients. NASM has developed a template that provides health and fitness professionals with specific guidelines for creating an individualized program **Figure 1.4**.

TABLE 1.2   **Phase 5 Example Supersets**

Body Part	Strength Exercise	Power Exercise
Chest	Incline dumbbell press	Medicine ball chest pass
Back	Lat pulldown machine	Soccer throw
Shoulders	Overhead dumbbell press	Front medicine ball oblique throw
Legs	Barbell squat	Squat jump

Professional's Name:

NASM
NATIONAL ACADEMY OF SPORTS MEDICINE

CLIENT'S NAME:	DATE:

GOAL:	PHASE:

WARM-UP

Exercise:	Sets	Duration	Coaching Tip

CORE / BALANCE / PLYOMETRIC

Exercise:	Sets	Reps	Tempo	Rest	Coaching Tip

SPEED, AGILITY, QUICKNESS

Exercise:	Sets	Reps	Tempo	Rest	Coaching Tip

RESISTANCE

Exercise:	Sets	Reps	Tempo	Rest	Coaching Tip

COOL-DOWN

Exercise:	Sets	Duration	Coaching Tip

Coaching Tips:

National Academy of Sports Medicine

FIGURE 1.4 NASM program template.

How to Use the OPT Model

Chapters later in this text will be specifically dedicated to explaining how to use the OPT model in the fitness environment and detail the necessary components of an integrated training program. They include:

- Fitness assessments
- Flexibility training
- Cardiorespiratory training
- Core training
- Balance training
- Plyometric (reactive) training
- Speed, agility, and quickness training
- Resistance training
- Program design
- Exercise modalities

Each of these chapters explains how each component specifically fits into the OPT model and how to realistically apply the information given. Because the OPT model is based on the science of integrated training, all five phases within the OPT model often use all forms of exercise listed above. This is a far cry from traditional workouts that only incorporate generalized stretching, cardiovascular, and resistance exercise. Other chapters in this textbook review:

- Exercise science and physiology
- Nutrition
- Supplementation
- Chronic health conditions
- Lifestyle modification and behavioral coaching
- Professional development

All of this combined information should provide any individual with all of the tools necessary to become a skilled and well-rounded fitness professional.

SUMMARY

The OPT model provides a system for properly and safely progressing any client to his or her goals, by using integrated training methods. It consists of three levels—stabilization, strength, and power.

The Stabilization Level addresses muscular imbalances and attempts to improve the stabilization of joints and overall posture. This is a component that most training programs leave out even though it is arguably the most important to ensure proper neuromuscular functioning. This training level has one phase of training—Phase 1: Stabilization Endurance Training.

The Strength Level has three phases—Phase 2: Strength Endurance Training, Phase 3: Hypertrophy Training, and Phase 4: Maximum Strength Training. The Strength Level focuses on enhancing stabilization endurance and prime mover strength simultaneously (Phase 2), while also increasing muscle size (Phase 3) or maximal strength (Phase 4). Most traditional programs typically begin at this point and, as a result, often lead to injury. The Power Level is designed to target specific forms of training that are necessary for maximal force production. This level has one phase of training—Phase 5: Power Training.

All of these phases of training have been specifically designed to follow biomechanical, physiologic, and functional principles of the human movement system. They should provide an easy-to-follow systematic progression that minimizes injury and maximizes results. To help ensure proper organization and structure, NASM has developed a program template that guides health and fitness professionals through the process.

REFERENCES

1. Bureau of Labor Statistics US Department of Labor. Occupational Outlook Handbook, 2010-11 Edition. http://www.bls.gov/oco/ocos296.htm. Accessed May 14, 2010.
2. Centers for Disease Control and Prevention. 2017 Jun 28. Chronic Disease Overview. https://www.cdc.gov/chronicdisease/overview/index.htm. Accessed May 30, 2018.
3. Centers for Disease Control and Prevention. 2017 May 3. Deaths and Mortality. https://www.cdc.gov/nchs/fastats/deaths.htm. Accessed May 30, 2018.
4. American Heart Association. Cardiovascular Disease: A Costly Burden for America. Projections through 2035. https://healthmetrics.heart.org/wp-content/uploads/2017/10/Cardiovascular-Disease-A-Costly-Burden.pdf. Accessed May 30, 2018.
5. Must A, Spadano J, Coakley EH, Field AE, Colditz G, Dietz WH. The disease burden associated with overweight and obesity. *JAMA*. 1999;282(16):1523-1529.
6. Ogden CL, Carroll MD, McDowell MA, Flegal KM. Obesity Among Adults in the United States—No Statistically Significant Change Since 2003–2004. NCHS data brief no 1. Hyattsville, MD: National Center for Health Statistics; 2007.
7. Ogden CL, Carroll MD, Curtin LR, McDowell MA, Tabak CJ, Flegal KM. Prevalence of overweight and obesity in the United States, 1999–2004. *JAMA*. 2006;295(13):1549-1555.
8. Hales CM, Carroll MD, Fryar CD, Ogden CL. Prevalence of obesity among adults and youth: United States, 2015–2016. NCHS Data Brief. 2017;288:1-8.
9. American Heart Association. *Heart Disease and Stroke Statistics—2005 update*. Dallas, TX; 2004.
10. American Diabetes Association. 2007 National Diabetes Fact Sheet. http://www.diabetes.org/diabetes-basics/diabetes-statistics/. Accessed May 21, 2010.
11. Centers for Disease Control and Prevention. National Diabetes Fact Sheet: National Estimates and General Information on Diabetes in the United States, Revised Edition. Atlanta, GA; 1998.
12. Centers for Disease Control and Prevention. Summary health statistics for US adults: National Health Interview Survey, 2002. *Vital Health Stat 10*. 2004;10(222). http://www.cdc.gov/nchs/data/series/sr_10/sr10_222.pdf 11-15. Accessed Feb 8, 2006:11-15.
13. American College of Sports Medicine AHA. *Physical Activity and Public Health: Updated Recommendation for Adults from the American College of Sports Medicine and the American Heart Association*; 2007.
14. Pedersen BK, Saltin B. Evidence for prescribing exercise as therapy in chronic disease. *Scand J Med Sci Sports*. 2006;16(Suppl 1):3-63.
15. Sherman SE, Agostino RBD, Silbershatz H, Kannel WB. Comparison of past versus recent physical activity in the prevention of premature death and coronary artery disease. *Am Heart J*. 1999;138:900-907.
16. Centers for Disease Control and Prevention. Prevalence of physical activity, including lifestyle activities among adults—United States, 2000-2001. *MMWR Morb Mortal Wkly Rep*. 2003;52(32):764-769.
17. Zack MM, Moriarty DG, Stroup DF, Ford ES, Mokdad AH. Worsening trends in adult health-related quality of life and self-rated health—United States, 1993-2001. *Public Health Rep*. 2004;119(5):493-505.
18. Harkness EF, Macfarlane GJ, Silman AJ, McBeth J. Is musculoskeletal pain more common now than 40 years ago? Two population-based cross-sectional studies. *Rheumatology (Oxford)*. 2005;44(7):890-895.
19. Walker BF, Muller R, Grant WD. Low back pain in Australian adults: prevalence and associated disability. *J Manipulative Physiol Ther*. 2004;27(4):238-244.
20. Cassidy JD, Carroll LJ, Cote P. The Saskatchewan Health and Back Pain Survey. The prevalence of low back pain and related disability in Saskatchewan adults. *Spine*. 1998;23(17):1860-1866.
21. Volinn E. The epidemiology of low back pain in the rest of the world. A review of surveys in low- and middle-income countries. *Spine*. 1997;22(15):1747-1754.
22. Omokhodion FO, Sanya AO. Risk factors for low back pain among office workers in Ibadan, Southwest Nigeria. *Occup Med (Lond)*. 2003;53(4):287-289.
23. Omokhodion FO. Low back pain in a rural community in South West Nigeria. *West Afr J Med*. 2002;21(2):87-90.
24. Tsuji T, Matsuyama Y, Sato K, Hasegawa Y, Yimin Y, Iwata H. Epidemiology of low back pain in the elderly: correlation with lumbar lordosis. *J Orthop Sci*. 2001;6(4):307-311.
25. Griffin LY, Agel J, Albohm MJ, et al. Noncontact anterior cruciate ligament injuries: risk factors and prevention strategies. *J Am Acad Orthop Surg*. 2000;8(3):141-150.
26. Hill CL, Seo GS, Gale D, Totterman S, Gale ME, Felson DT. Cruciate ligament integrity in osteoarthritis of the knee. *Arthritis Rheum*. 2005;52:3:794-799.
27. Mandelbaum BR, Silvers HJ, Watanabe DS, et al. Effectiveness of a neuromuscular and proprioceptive training program

in preventing anterior cruciate ligament injuries in female athletes: 2-year follow-up. *Am J Sports Med.* 2005;33(7): 1003-1010.

28. Centers for Disease Control and Prevention. Ambulatory care visits to physician offices, hospital outpatient departments, and emergency departments: United States, 2001–02. *Vital Health Stat 13.* 2006;13(159):3-8. http://www.cdc.gov/nchs/data/series/sr_13/sr13_159.pdf. Accessed February 8, 2006.

29. Bureau of Labor Statistics. 2005 Dec 15. Workplace injuries and illnesses in 2004. News release. http://www.bls.gov/iif/home.htm. Accessed Feb 8, 2006.

30. Barr KP, Griggs M, Cadby T. Lumbar stabilization: core concepts and current literature, Part 1. *Am J Phys Med Rehabil.* 2005;84(6):473-480.

31. Watkins J. *Structure and Function of the Musculoskeletal System.* Champaign, IL: Human Kinetics, 1999.

32. Jones BH, Cowan DN, Knapik J. Exercise, training, and injuries. *Sports Med.* 1994;18(3):202-214.

33. Hammer WI. Muscle imbalance and postfacilitation stretch. In: Hammer WI, ed. *Functional Soft Tissue Examination and Treatment by Manual Methods.* 2nd ed. Gaithersburg, MD: Aspen Publishers; 1999:429-9.

34. Powers CM. The influence of altered lower-extremity kinematics on patellofemoral joint dysfunction: a theoretical perspective. *J Orthop Sports Phys Ther.* 2003;33(11):639-646.

35. Comerford MJ, Mottram SL. Movement and stability dysfunction—contemporary developments. *Man Ther.* 2001; 6(1):15-26.

36. Panjabi MM. The stabilizing system of the spine. Part I: Function, dysfunction, adaptation, and enhancement. *J Spinal Disord.* 1992;5(4):383-389.

37. Paterno MV, Myer GD, Ford KR, Hewett TE. Neuromuscular training improves single-limb stability in young female athletes. *J Orthop Sports Phys Ther.* 2004;34(6):305-316.

38. Hungerford B; Gilleard W, Hodges P. Evidence of altered lumbopelvic muscle recruitment in the presence of sacroiliac joint pain. *Spine.* 2003;28(14):1593-1600.

39. Edgerton VR, Wolf S, Roy RR. Theoretical basis for patterning EMG amplitudes to assess muscle dysfunction. *Med Sci Sports Exerc.* 1996;28(6)744-751.

40. Williford HN, Olson MS, Gauger S, Duey WJ, Blessing DL. Cardiovascular and metabolic costs of forward, backward, and lateral motion. *Med Sci Sports Exerc.* 1998;30(9):1419-1423.

41. Ogita F, Stam RP, Tazawa HO, Toussaint HM, Hollander AP. Oxygen uptake in one-legged and two-legged exercise. *Med Sci Sports Exerc.* 2000;32(10):1737-1742.

42. Lagally KM, Cordero J, Good J, Brown DD, McCaw ST. Physiologic and metabolic responses to a continuous functional resistance exercise workout. *J Strength Cond Res.* 2009;23(2): 373-379.

Basic Exercise Science

After studying this chapter, you will be able to:

✔ Define the components of the human movement system (kinetic chain).

✔ Explain the basic structure and function of:

- the nervous system
- the skeletal system
- the muscular system
- the endocrine system

✔ Describe how these systems respond and adapt to exercise.

Introduction to Human Movement

Human movement is accomplished through the functional integration of three systems within the human body, the nervous, skeletal, and muscular systems (1). The nerves, muscles, and joints must work together, or be linked (chain) to produce motion (kinetic) or human movement. The three systems responsible for human movement are also referred to as the kinetic chain (2,3). All components of the **human movement system** must work together to produce movement. If one component of the human movement system is not working properly, it will affect the other systems and ultimately affect movement (4–7). Therefore, it is important that personal trainers understand the systems involved in human movement and how they work together, forming a kinetic chain to produce efficient movement.

Human movement system The combination and interrelation of the nervous, muscular, and skeletal systems.

The Nervous System

Nervous system
A conglomeration of billions of cells specifically designed to provide a communication network within the human body.

The **nervous system** is one of the main organ systems of the body and consists of a network of specialized cells called neurons that transmit and coordinate signals, providing a communication network within the human body. The nervous system is divided into two parts, the central and peripheral nervous systems. The central nervous system (CNS) is composed of the brain and spinal cord. The peripheral nervous system (PNS) contains only nerves and connects the brain and spinal cord (CNS) to the rest of the body (8–11).

Sensory function The ability of the nervous system to sense changes in either the internal or external environment.

The three primary functions of the nervous system include sensory, integrative, and motor functions (8–10). **Sensory function** is the ability of the nervous system to sense changes in either the internal or external environment, such as a stretch placed on a muscle (internal) or the change from walking on the sidewalk to walking on sand (external). **Integrative function** is the ability of the nervous system to analyze and interpret the sensory information to allow for proper decision making, which produces an appropriate response. **Motor function** is the neuromuscular (or nervous and muscular systems) response to the sensory information, such as causing a muscle to contract when stretched too far, or changing one's walking pattern when walking in the sand as opposed to the sidewalk (8–10).

Integrative function
The ability of the nervous system to analyze and interpret sensory information to allow for proper decision making, which produces the appropriate response.

Motor function
The neuromuscular response to the sensory information.

Proprioception
The cumulative sensory input to the central nervous system from all mechanoreceptors that sense body position and limb movement.

The nervous system is responsible for the recruitment of muscles, learned patterns of movement, and the functioning of every organ in the human body. **Proprioception** is the body's ability to sense the relative position of adjacent parts of the body. For example, when we walk or run our feet give us proprioceptive feedback about the type of surface or terrain we are on. Training the body's proprioceptive abilities will improve balance, coordination, and posture, and enable the body to adapt to its surroundings without consciously thinking about what movement is most appropriate for any given situation. Thus, it becomes important to train the nervous system efficiently to ensure that proper movement patterns are being developed, which enhances performance and decreases the risk of injury (8,10,12).

Anatomy of the Nervous System

The Neuron

Neuron
The functional unit of the nervous system.

The functional unit of the nervous system is known as the **neuron Figure 2.1** (8). Billions of neurons make up the complex structure of the nervous system and provide it with the ability to communicate internally with itself, as well as externally with the outside environment. A neuron is a specialized cell that processes and transmits information through both electrical and chemical signals. Neurons form the core of the nervous system, which includes the brain, spinal cord, and peripheral ganglia. Collectively, the merging of many neurons together forms the nerves of the body. Neurons are composed of three main parts: the cell body, axon, and dendrites (8–10,13).

Sensory (afferent) neurons Transmit nerve impulses from effector sites (such as muscles and organs) via receptors to the brain and spinal cord.

The cell body (or soma) of a neuron contains a nucleus and other organelles, including lysosomes, mitochondria, and a Golgi complex. The axon is a cylindrical projection from the cell body that transmits nervous impulses to other neurons or effector sites (muscles, organs). The axon is the part of the neuron that provides communication from the brain and spinal cord to other parts of the body. The dendrites gather information from other structures and transmit it back into the neuron (8–10,13).

There are three main functional classifications of neurons that are determined by the direction of their nerve impulses. **Sensory (afferent) neurons** respond to touch,

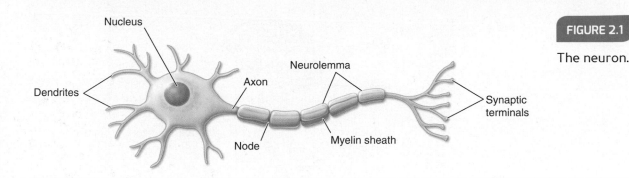

Nucleus

Neurolemma

Dendrites

Axon

Synaptic terminals

Node

Myelin sheath

FIGURE 2.1

The neuron.

sound, light, and other stimuli and transmit nerve impulses from effector sites (such as muscles and organs) to the brain and spinal cord. **Interneurons** transmit nerve impulses from one neuron to another **Motor (efferent) neurons** transmit nerve impulses from the brain and spinal cord to the effector sites such as muscles or glands (9,13).

A classic example of how these three neurons work together to produce a given response can be seen in the example of a person touching a hot object. The sensory (afferent) neurons send a signal from the hand to the brain telling the brain that the object is hot. This signal makes its way to the brain by traveling from one neuron to another via the interneurons. Once the signal has made it to the brain, the brain then interprets the information sent from the sensory neurons (the object is hot) and sends the appropriate signals down to the muscles of the hand and arm via the motor neurons, telling the muscles to contract to pull the hand away from the hot object, protecting the hand from injury.

The Central and Peripheral Nervous Systems

The nervous system is composed of two interdependent divisions, the central nervous system (CNS) and the peripheral nervous system (PNS) (1,8–10,13). The **central nervous system** consists of the brain and the spinal cord, and its primary function is to coordinate the activity of all parts of the body **Figure 2.2** (1,8–10,13).

The **peripheral nervous system** (PNS) consists of nerves that connect the CNS to the rest of the body and the external environment. The nerves of the PNS are how the CNS receives sensory input and initiates responses. The peripheral nervous system consists of 12 cranial nerves, 31 pairs of spinal nerves (which branch out from the brain and spinal cord), and sensory receptors **Figure 2.3** (8–10,13). These peripheral nerves serve two main functions. First, they provide a connection for the nervous system to activate different effector sites, such as muscles (motor function). Second, peripheral nerves relay information from the effector sites back to the brain via sensory receptors (sensory function), thus providing a constant update on the relation between the body and the environment (8–11,13).

Two further subdivisions of the PNS include the somatic and autonomic nervous systems **Figure 2.4**. The somatic nervous system consists of nerves that serve the outer areas of the body and skeletal muscle, and are largely responsible for the voluntary control of movement. The autonomic nervous system supplies neural input to the involuntary systems of the body (e.g., heart, digestive systems, and endocrine glands) (9,13).

The autonomic system is further divided into the sympathetic and parasympathetic nervous systems. During exercise, both systems serve to increase levels of activation in

Interneurons Transmit nerve impulses from one neuron to another.

Motor (efferent) neurons Transmit nerve impulses from the brain and spinal cord to effector sites.

Central nervous system The portion of the nervous system that consists of the brain and spinal cord.

Peripheral nervous system Cranial and spinal nerves that spread throughout the body.

FIGURE 2.2

The central nervous system.

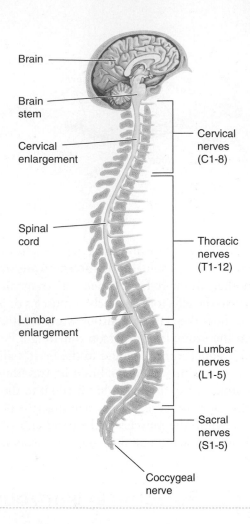

- Brain
- Brain stem
- Cervical enlargement
- Spinal cord
- Lumbar enlargement
- Cervical nerves (C1-8)
- Thoracic nerves (T1-12)
- Lumbar nerves (L1-5)
- Sacral nerves (S1-5)
- Coccygeal nerve

preparation for activity (sympathetic) or serve to decrease levels of activation during rest and recovery (parasympathetic) (9,13).

Sensory receptors are specialized structures located throughout the body that convert environmental stimuli (heat, light, sound, taste, motion) into sensory information that the brain and spinal cord use to produce a response. These receptors are subdivided into four categories: mechanoreceptors, nociceptors, chemoreceptors, and photoreceptors. Mechanoreceptors respond to mechanical forces (touch and pressure), nociceptors respond to pain (pain receptors), chemoreceptors respond to chemical interaction (smell and taste), and photoreceptors respond to light (vision) (10,13). This chapter only addresses mechanoreceptors inasmuch as these receptors are the most important ones for personal trainers to be familiar with because they primarily pertain to human movement.

Mechanoreceptors are specialized structures that respond to mechanical pressure within tissues and then transmit signals through sensory nerves (14–19). Mechanoreceptors respond to outside forces such as touch, pressure, stretching, sound waves, and motion, and transmit impulses through sensory nerves, which, in turn, enable us to detect touch, sounds, and the motion of the body and to monitor the position of our muscles, bones, and joints (proprioception). Mechanoreceptors are located in muscles, tendons, ligaments, and joint capsules and include muscle spindles, Golgi tendon organs, and joint receptors (17,18,20–24).

Mechanoreceptors
Sensory receptors responsible for sensing distortion in body tissues.

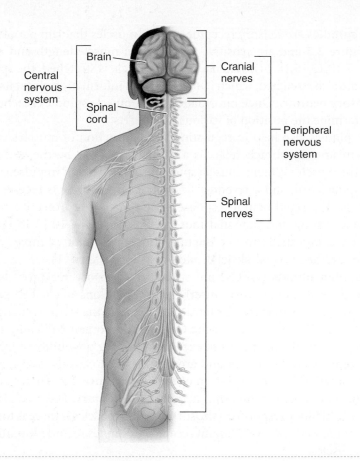

Brain

Central
nervous
system

Spinal
cord

Cranial
nerves

Peripheral
nervous
system

Spinal
nerves

FIGURE 2.3

The peripheral nervous
system.

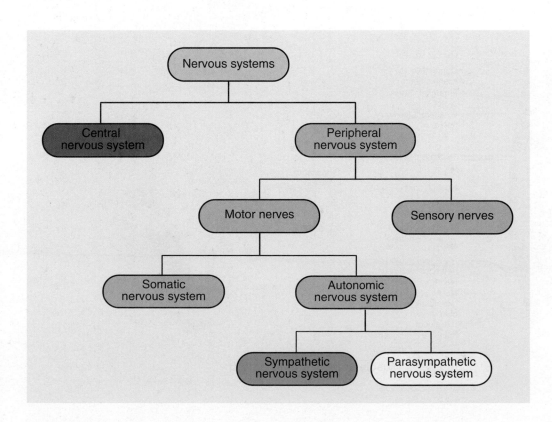

Nervous systems

Central
nervous system

Peripheral
nervous system

Motor nerves

Sensory nerves

Somatic
nervous system

Autonomic
nervous system

Sympathetic
nervous system

Parasympathetic
nervous system

FIGURE 2.4

Nervous system
structure.

Muscle spindles
Receptors sensitive to change in length of the muscle and the rate of that change.

Golgi tendon organs Receptors sensitive to change in tension of the muscle and the rate of that change.

Joint receptors
Receptors surrounding a joint that respond to pressure, acceleration, and deceleration of the joint.

Muscle spindles are sensory receptors within muscles that run parallel to the muscle fibers **Figure 2.5** and are sensitive to change in muscle length and rate of length change (1,5–7,10,13,15,18,24). When a specific muscle is stretched, the spindles within that muscle are also stretched, which in turn conveys information about its length to the CNS via sensory neurons. Once information from muscle spindles reaches the brain it can then determine the position of various body parts.

Muscle spindles also help in regulating the contraction of muscles via the stretch reflex mechanism. The stretch reflex is a normal response by the body to a stretch stimulus in the muscle. When a muscle spindle is stretched, an impulse is immediately sent to the spinal cord, and a response to contract the muscle is received within 1 to 2 milliseconds. The rapid neural response is designed as a protective mechanism to prevent overstretching and potential muscle damage (1,5–7,10,13,15,18,24). Human movement is accomplished through the functional integration of three systems within the human body, the nervous, skeletal, and muscular systems (1).

Golgi tendon organs (GTOs) are specialized sensory receptors located at the point where skeletal muscle fibers insert into the tendons of skeletal muscle. GTOs are sensitive to changes in muscular tension and rate of the tension change **Figure 2.6** (1,5–7,10,13,15,18,24). Activation of the Golgi tendon organ will cause the muscle to relax, which prevents the muscle from excessive stress or possibility of injury.

Joint receptors are located in and around the joint capsule, and they respond to pressure, acceleration, and deceleration of the joint **Figure 2.7**. These receptors act to signal extreme joint positions and thus help to prevent injury. They can also act to initiate a reflexive inhibitory response in the surrounding muscles if there is too much stress placed on that joint (17,18,25–27). Joint receptor examples include Ruffini endings and Pacinian corpuscles.

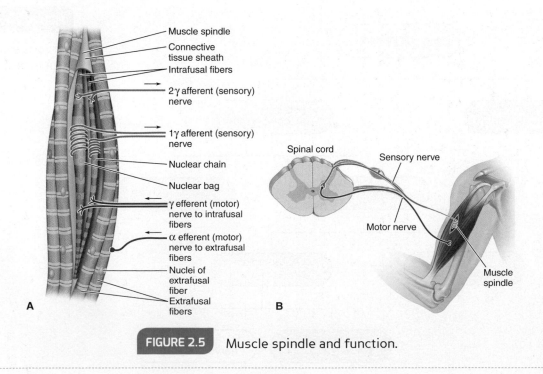

FIGURE 2.5   Muscle spindle and function.

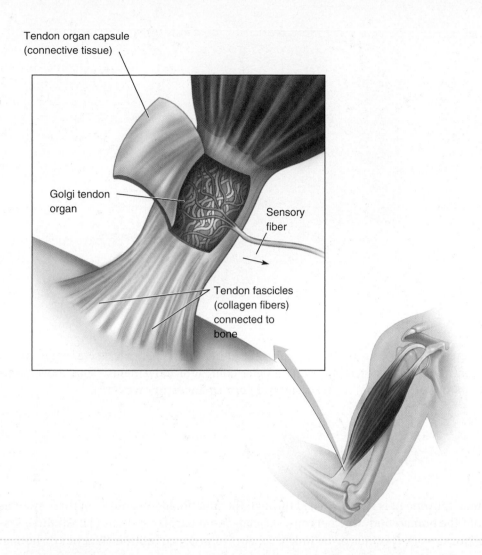

Tendon organ capsule
(connective tissue)

Golgi tendon
organ

Sensory
fiber

Tendon fascicles
(collagen fibers)
connected to
bone

FIGURE 2.6

Golgi tendon organ.

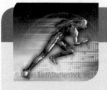

Memory Jogger

It is important to understand the function of the muscle spindles and GTOs as they play an integral part in flexibility training.

Physical Activity and the Nervous System

In the early stages of training the majority of performance improvements likely result from changes in the way the central nervous system controls and coordinates movement. This appears to be particularly so for resistance training (15). When we perform an activity, our senses provide constant feedback regarding limb position, force generation, and the performance outcome (i.e., was the movement successful?). Unsuccessful or poor performances can be cross-referenced with other sensory input, and a new

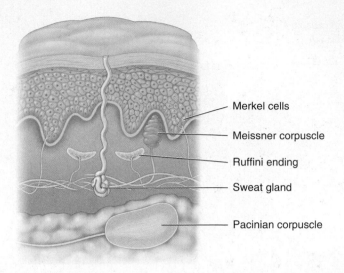

FIGURE 2.7

Joint receptors.

Merkel cells

Meissner corpuscle

Ruffini ending

Sweat gland

Pacinian corpuscle

movement strategy can be tried. Regular training and practice cause adaptations in the central nervous system, allowing greater control of movements. Thus movements become smoother and more accurate, and performance improves (15).

SUMMARY

Human movement is accomplished through the functional integration of three systems within the human body, the nervous, skeletal, and muscular systems (1). All three systems must work together or be linked (chain) to produce motion (kinetic) or human movement. The three systems responsible for human movement are also referred to as the kinetic chain.

The nervous system is composed of billions of neurons that transfer information throughout the body, through two interdependent systems: the central nervous system (brain and spinal cord) and the peripheral nervous system (nerves that branch out from the brain and spinal cord). The nervous system gathers information about our external and internal environments, processes that information, and then responds to it. It has three major functions, which are sensory (recognizes changes), integrative (combines information and interprets it), and motor (produces a neuromuscular response).

Skeletal System

Skeletal system
The body's framework, composed of bones and joints.

The **skeletal system** serves many important functions; it provides the shape and form for our bodies in addition to supporting, protecting, allowing bodily movement, producing blood for the body, and storing minerals **Figure 2.8** (9,28,29). It is important to note that the growth, maturation, and functionality of the skeletal system are

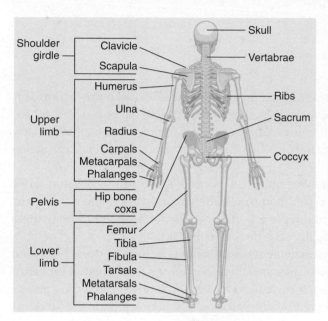
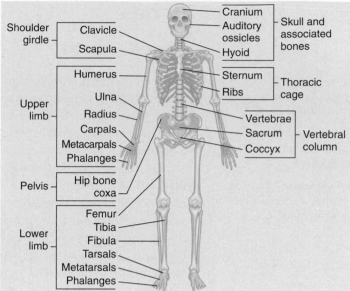

FIGURE 2.8   The skeletal system.

greatly affected by posture, physical activity, and nutrition status (28). For example, poor nutrition and physical inactivity contribute to osteoporosis, which has a negative effect on skeletal health and human movement. The skeletal system is a vital part of human movement via the interaction of the muscular and skeletal systems. Muscles are connected to bones by tendons. **Bones** form junctions that are connected by muscles and connective tissue. These junctions are known as **joints** (30). Joints are the sites where movement occurs as a result of muscle contraction (30,31).

Bones Provide a resting ground for muscles and protection of vital organs.

Joints Junctions of bones, muscles, and connective tissue at which movement occurs. Also known as an articulation.

Divisions of the Skeletal System

The skeletal system is divided into two divisions: the axial and appendicular skeletal systems (9,30). The **axial skeleton** is made up of the skull, the rib cage, and the vertebral column. There are approximately 80 bones in the axial skeleton (9). The **appendicular skeleton** is made up of the upper and lower extremities as well as the shoulder and pelvic girdles (9). The pelvic girdle is often considered a component of either the axial or appendicular system and is actually a link between the two systems (30). The appendicular skeleton encompasses approximately 126 bones.

There are 206 bones in the skeletal system, of which approximately 177 are used in voluntary movement (9,29,30). The bones in the human body form more than 300 joints (29).

Bones serve two vital functions in movement. The first is leverage. Bones act and perform as levers when acted on by muscles (28,30). The second primary function of bones relative to movement is to provide support (28). This translates into posture, which is necessary for the efficient distribution of forces acting on the body (28,31–34).

Axial skeleton Portion of the skeletal system that consists of the skull, rib cage, and vertebral column.

Appendicular skeleton Portion of the skeletal system that includes the upper and lower extremities.

Bones

Bone Growth

Remodeling The process of resorption and formation of bone.

Osteoclasts A type of bone cell that removes bone tissue.

Osteoblasts A type of cell that is responsible for bone formation.

Throughout life, bone is constantly renewed through a process called **remodeling**. This process consists of resorption and formation. During resorption, old bone tissue is broken down and removed by special cells called **osteoclasts**. During bone formation, new bone tissue is laid down to replace the old. This task is performed by special cells called **osteoblasts**.

During childhood through adolescence, new bone is added to the skeleton faster than old bone is removed. As a result, bones become larger, heavier, and denser. For most people, bone formation continues at a faster pace than removal until bone mass peaks usually by the time individuals reach their thirties (35).

It is also worth noting that remodeling tends to follow the lines of stress placed on the bone (29). Exercise and habitual posture, therefore, have a fundamental influence on the health of the skeletal system. Incorrect exercise technique, coupled with a generally poor alignment, will lead to a remodeling process that may reinforce the predominating bad posture.

Types of Bones

There are five major types of bones in the skeletal system **Table 2.1** (9). Their shape, size, and proportion of bone tissue determine their classification (28). The categories include long bones, short bones, flat bones, irregular bones, and sesamoid bones (9,28).

Long Bones

Long bones are characterized by their long cylindrical body (shaft), with irregular or widened bony ends (9,28,30). They are shaped much like a beam and exhibit a slight curvature that is necessary for efficient force distribution **Figure 2.9** (9,28). Long bones are composed predominantly of compact bone tissue to ensure strength and stiffness

---

TABLE 2.1   Types of Bone

Bone Type	Characteristic	Example
Long	Long, cylindrical shaft and irregular or widened ends	Humerus, femur
Short	Similar in length and width and appear somewhat cubical in shape	Carpals of hand, tarsals of feet
Flat	Thin, protective	Scapulae, patella
Irregular	Unique shape and function	Vertebrae
Sesamoid	Small often round bones embedded in a joint capsule or found in locations where a tendon passes over a joint	Patella

(9,28). However, they do have considerable amounts of spongy bone tissue for shock absorption (9,28). The long bones of the upper body include the clavicle, humerus, radius, ulna, metacarpals, and phalanges, whereas in the lower body there are the femur, tibia, fibula, metatarsals, and phalanges.

ANATOMIC FEATURES OF A LONG BONE

A detailed analysis of a long bone is useful in helping to highlight some of the properties and functions of the skeletal system. **Figure 2.10** shows a cross section of a typical long bone (in this case the humerus).

Epiphysis (epiphyses) is the end of long bones, which is mainly composed of cancellous bone, and houses much of the red marrow involved in red blood cell production. They are also one of the primary sites for bone growth, and during growth periods can be vulnerable to injury.

Diaphysis is the shaft portion of a long bone, and in comparison to the bone ends is predominantly compact bone (although the inside of the shaft is hollow). The principal role of the diaphysis is support.

Epiphyseal plate is the region of long bone connecting the diaphysis to the epiphysis. It is a layer of subdividing cartilaginous cells in which growth in length of the diaphysis occurs. Multiplying cartilaginous cells are arranged like columns of coins (29), which move toward the diaphysis, becoming more calcified as they go. Osteoblasts will eventually complete the process of bone formation. When adults stop growing the plates will harden and fuse so no further growth takes place. Epiphyseal plate damage

Epiphysis The end of long bones, which is mainly composed of cancellous bone, and house much of the red marrow involved in red blood cell production. They are also one of the primary sites for bone growth.

Diaphysis The shaft portion of a long bone.

Epiphyseal plate The region of long bone connecting the diaphysis to the epiphysis. It is a layer of subdividing cartilaginous cells in which growth in length of the diaphysis occurs.

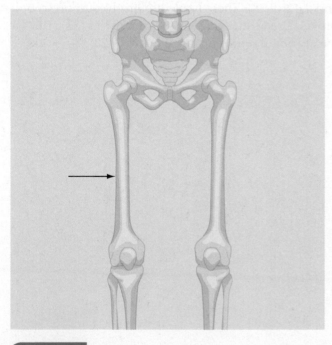

FIGURE 2.9   Long bones.

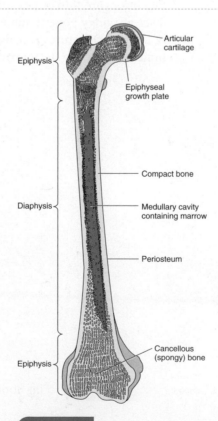

FIGURE 2.10   Anatomic features of a long bone.

before cessation of growth could result in a shorter bone; however, there is little evidence to suggest that exercise has any effect on bone length in children. Instead, exercise is likely to lead to broader, stronger bones (provided it is accompanied with appropriate diet).

Periosteum forms a tough fibrous membrane that coats the bone. It contains nerves, blood vessels, and bone-producing cells. Its inner surface provides the materials for nutrition repair and facilitates growth in the diameter of the bone. It also plays a fundamental role in movement by providing the point of attachment for tendons.

Medullary cavity is a space that runs down through the center of the diaphysis and contains fatty yellow marrow that is predominantly composed of adipose tissue and serves as a useful energy reserve.

Articular (hyaline) cartilage covers the ends of articulating bones. It is a hard, white, shiny tissue that, along with synovial fluid, helps reduce friction in freely movable (synovial joints). It is fundamental for smooth joint action.

Short Bones

Short bones are similar in length and width and appear somewhat cubical in shape **Figure 2.11** (9,30). They consist predominantly of spongy bone tissue to maximize shock absorption (9,28,30). The carpals of the hands and tarsals of the feet fit this category (9,28,30).

Flat Bones

Flat bones are thin bones comprising two layers of compact bone tissue surrounding a layer a spongy bone tissue **Figure 2.12** (9,28). These bones are involved in protection of internal structures and also provide broad attachment sites for muscles (28). The flat bones include the sternum, scapulae, ribs, ilium, and cranial bones (9,28,30).

Periosteum A dense membrane composed of fibrous connective tissue that closely wraps (invests) all bone, except that of the articulating surfaces in joints, which are covered by a synovial membrane.

Medullar cavity The central cavity of bone shafts where marrow is stored.

Articular (hyaline) cartilage Cartilage that covers the articular surfaces of bones.

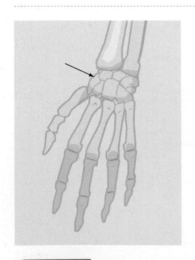

FIGURE 2.11 Short bones.

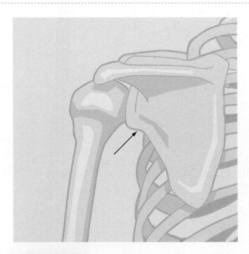

FIGURE 2.12 Flat bones.

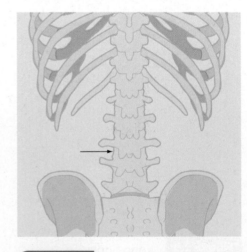

FIGURE 2.13 Irregular bones.

Irregular Bones

Irregular bones are bones of unique shape and function that do not fit the characteristics of the other categories **Figure 2.13** (9,28,30). These include the vertebrae, pelvic bones, and certain facial bones (9,28,30).

Sesamoid Bones

Sesamoid bones are small bones embedded in a joint capsule or found in locations where a tendon passes over a joint. Sesamoid bones develop within particular tendons at a site of considerable friction or tension. They serve to improve leverage and protect the joint from damage.

Bone Markings

The majority of all bones have specific distinguishing structures known as surface markings (9). These structures are necessary for increasing the stability in joints as well as providing attachment sites for muscles (9). Some of the more prominent and important ones will be discussed here. These surface markings can be divided into two simple categories: depressions and processes (9).

Depressions

Depressions are simply flattened or indented portions of the bone (9). A common depression is called a fossa. An example is the supraspinous or infraspinous fossa located on the scapulae (shoulder blades) **Figure 2.14**. These are attachment sites for the supraspinatus and infraspinatus muscles, respectively (9).

    Another form of a depression is known as a sulcus. This is simply a groove in a bone that allows soft tissue (i.e., tendons) to pass through (9). An example of this is the intertubercular sulcus located between the greater and lesser tubercles of the humerus (upper arm bone) **Figure 2.15** (9). This is commonly known as the groove for the biceps tendon.

Depressions Flattened or indented portions of bone, which can be muscle attachment sites.

Processes

Processes are projections protruding from the bone to which muscles, tendons, and ligaments can attach (9). Some of the more common processes are called process, condyle, epicondyle, tubercle, and trochanter (9). Examples of processes include the spinous processes found on the vertebrae and the acromion and coracoid processes found on the scapulae **Figure 2.16**.

    Condyles are located on the inner and outer portions at the bottom of the femur (thigh bone) and top of the tibia (shin bone) to form the knee joint **Figure 2.17**. Epicondyles are located on the inner and outer portions of the humerus to help form the elbow joint **Figure 2.18**.

    The tubercles are located at the top of the humerus at the glenohumeral (shoulder) joint **Figure 2.19**. There are the greater and lesser tubercles, which are attachment sites for shoulder musculature.

Processes Projections protruding from the bone where muscles, tendons, and ligaments can attach.

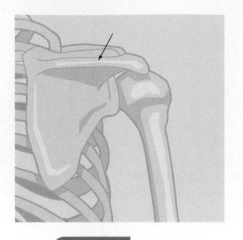

FIGURE 2.14 Fossa.

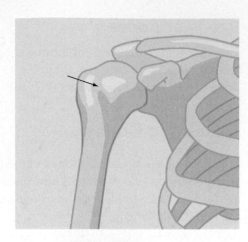

FIGURE 2.15 Sulcus.

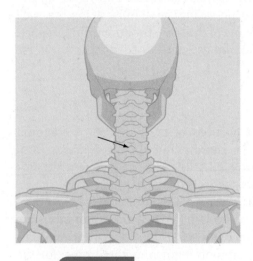

FIGURE 2.16 Process.

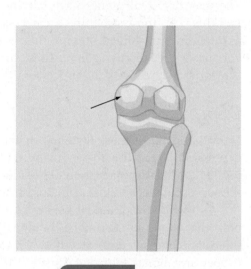

FIGURE 2.17 Condyle.

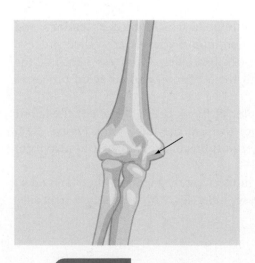

FIGURE 2.18 Epicondyle.

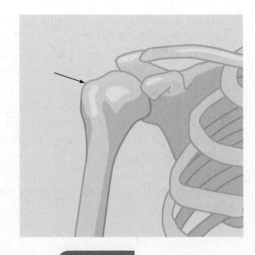

FIGURE 2.19 Tubercle.

Finally, the trochanters are located at the top of the femur and are attachment sites for the hip musculature **Figure 2.20** (9). The greater trochanter is commonly called the hipbone.

Vertebral Column

The **vertebral column** (also called the backbone, or spinal column) consists of a series of irregularly shaped bones, called vertebrae **Figure 2.21**. These bones are divided into five different categories depending on where they are located in the backbone **Table 2.2** (36).

The first seven vertebrae starting at the top of the spinal column are called the cervical vertebrae (cervical spine, C1–C7). These bones form a flexible framework and provide support and motion for the head.

The next 12 vertebrae located in the upper and middle back are called the thoracic vertebrae (thoracic spine, T1–T12). These bones move with the ribs to form the rear anchor of the rib cage. Thoracic vertebrae are larger than cervical vertebrae and increase in size from top to bottom.

Below the thoracic spine are the five vertebrae comprising the lumbar vertebrae (lumbar spine, L1–L5). These bones are the largest in the spinal column. These vertebrae support most of the body's weight and are attached to many of the back muscles. The lumbar spine is often a location of pain for individuals because these vertebrae carry the most amount of body weight and are subject to the largest forces and stresses along the spine.

The sacrum is a triangular bone located just below the lumbar vertebrae. It consists of four or five sacral vertebrae in a child, which become fused into a single bone during adulthood.

The bottom of the spinal column is called the coccyx or tailbone. It consists of three to five bones that are fused together in an adult. Many muscles connect to the coccyx.

In between the vertebrae are intervertebral discs made of fibrous cartilage that act as shock absorbers and allow the back to move. In addition to allowing humans to stand upright and maintain their balance, the vertebral column serves several other important functions. It helps to support the head and arms, while permitting freedom

Vertebral column
A series of irregularly shaped bones called vertebrae that houses the spinal cord.

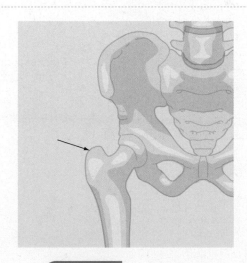

FIGURE 2.20 Trochanter.

FIGURE 2.21

Vertebral column.

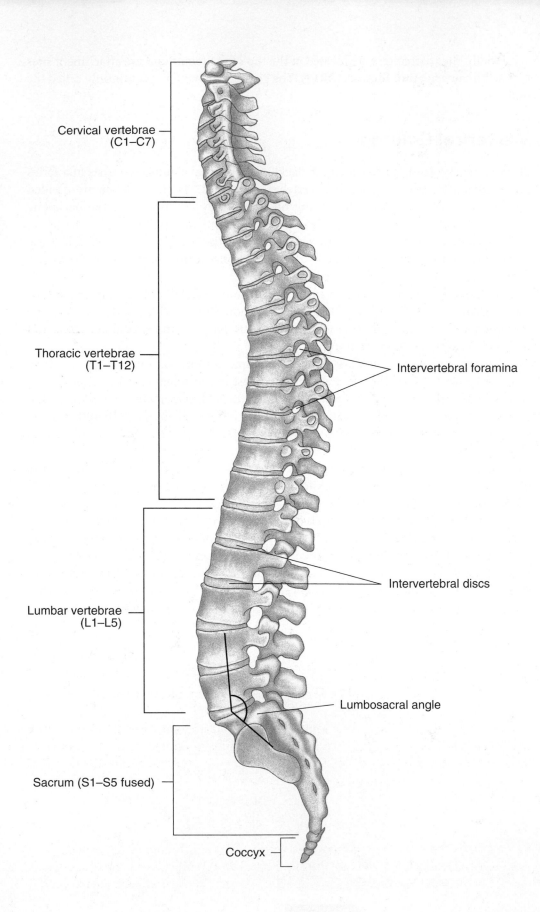

Cervical vertebrae
(C1–C7)

Thoracic vertebrae
(T1–T12)

Intervertebral foramina

Intervertebral discs

Lumbar vertebrae
(L1–L5)

Lumbosacral angle

Sacrum (S1–S5 fused)

Coccyx

TABLE 2.2	Vertebral Column
Cervical spine (C1–C7)	1st seven vertebrae starting at the top of the spinal column
Thoracic spine (T1–T12)	Twelve vertebrae located in the upper/middle back behind the ribs
Lumbar spine (L1–L5)	Five vertebrae of the low back below the thoracic spine
Sacrum	Triangular bone located below the lumbar spine
Coccyx	Located below the sacrum, more commonly known as the tailbone

of movement. It also provides attachment for many muscles, the ribs, and some of the organs and protects the spinal cord, which controls most bodily functions (36).

The optimal arrangement of curves is referred to as a neutral spine and represents a position in which the vertebrae and associated structures are under the least amount of load. The adult human spine has three major curvatures:

- a posterior cervical curvature—a posterior concavity of the cervical spine
- an anterior thoracic curvature—a posterior convexity of the thoracic spine
- a posterior lumbar curvature—a posterior concavity of the lumbar spine

Joints

Joints are formed by one bone that articulates with another bone (9). Joints can be categorized by both their structure and their function (or the way they move) (9,29,31). Joint motion is referred to as **arthrokinematics**, with the three major motion types being roll, slide, and spin (7,31,37). It is important to note that motions rarely occur, if ever, as an isolated, true motion. As is the case with the human body, variations and combinations of these joint motions take place during functional movement (37).

Arthrokinematics Joint motion.

In a rolling movement, one joint rolls across the surface of another much like the tire of a bicycle rolls on the street **Figure 2.22**. An example of roll in the body is the femoral condyles moving (rolling) over the tibial condyles during a squat.

In a sliding movement, one joint's surface slides across another much like the tire of a bicycle skidding across the street **Figure 2.23**. An example of slide in the human body is the tibial condyles moving (sliding) across the femoral condyles during a knee extension.

In a spinning movement, one joint surface rotates on another much like twisting the lid off of a jar **Figure 2.24**. An example of a spin movement in the human body is the head of the radius (a bone of the forearm) rotating on the end of the humerus during pronation and supination of the forearm.

Classification of Joints

Synovial joints are the most common joints associated with human movement. They comprise approximately 80% of all the joints in the body and have the greatest capacity for motion (9,28,29,31). Synovial joints all have a synovial capsule (collagenous structure)

Synovial joints Joints that are held together by a joint capsule and ligaments and are most associated with movement in the body.

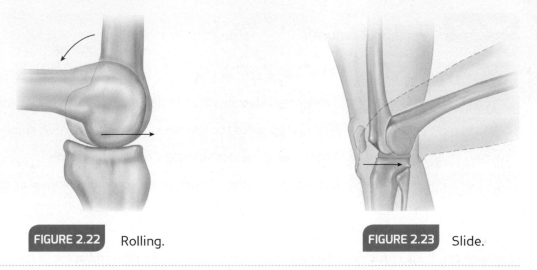

FIGURE 2.22 Rolling.

FIGURE 2.23 Slide.

surrounding the entire joint, a synovial membrane (the inner layer of the capsule) and hyaline cartilage which pads the ends of the articulating bones. This design gives synovial joints their increased mobility (31). Synovial joints also have another unique quality in that they produce synovial fluid. Synovial fluid resembles egg whites and works much like engine oil. It is secreted within the joint capsule from the synovial membrane and is essential for lubricating the joint surfaces to reduce excessive wear and to nourish the cartilage cells that line the joint (9,28,29,31).

There are several types of synovial joints in the body. They include gliding (plane), condyloid (condylar or ellipsoidal), hinge, saddle, pivot, and ball-and-socket joints (9,28,29).

A gliding (plane) joint is a nonaxial joint that has the simplest movement of all joints (9,28). It moves either back and forth or side to side. An example is the joint between the navicular bone and the second and third cuneiform bones in the foot or the carpals of the hand and in the facet (spine) joints **Figure 2.25** (9,28,29).

Condyloid (condylar or ellipsoidal) joints are termed so because the condyle of one bone fits into the elliptical cavity of another bone to form the joint (9). Movement predominantly occurs in one plane (flexion and extension in the sagittal plane) with minimal movement in the others (rotation in the transverse plane; adduction and abduction in the frontal plane). Examples of condyloid joints are seen in the wrist between the radius and carpals and in the joints of the fingers (metacarpophalangeal) **Figure 2.26** (28).

The hinge joint is a uniaxial joint allowing movement predominantly in only one plane of motion, the sagittal plane. Joints such as the elbow, interphalangeal (toe), and ankle are considered hinge joints **Figure 2.27** (9,28).

The saddle joint is named after its appearance. One bone looks like a saddle with the articulating bone straddling it like a rider. This joint is only found in the carpometacarpal joint in the thumb (9,28). It allows movement predominantly in two planes of motion (flexion and extension in the sagittal plane; adduction and abduction in the frontal plane) with some rotation to produce circumduction (circular motion) **Figure 2.28** (9,28).

Pivot joints allow movement in predominantly one plane of motion (rotation, pronation, and supination in the transverse plane). These joints are found in the atlantoaxial joint at the base of the skull (top of spine) and the proximal radioulnar joint at the elbow **Figure 2.29** (9,28).

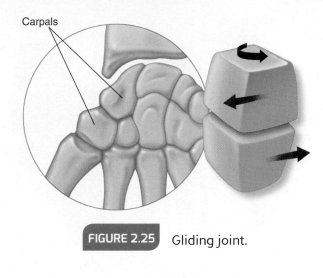

FIGURE 2.25   Gliding joint.

Carpals

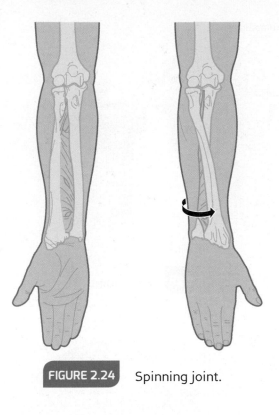

FIGURE 2.24   Spinning joint.

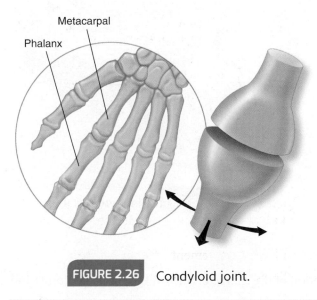

Phalanx

Metacarpal

FIGURE 2.26   Condyloid joint.

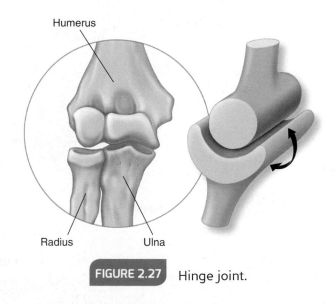

Humerus

Radius   Ulna

FIGURE 2.27   Hinge joint.

Ball-and-socket joints are the most mobile of the joints. They allow movement in all three planes. Examples of these joints are the shoulder and hip **Figure 2.30** (9,28).

Nonsynovial joints are named as such because they have no joint cavity, fibrous connective tissue, or cartilage in the uniting structure. These joints exhibit little to no movement. Examples of this joint type are seen in the sutures of the skull, the distal joint of the tibia and fibula, and the symphysis pubis (pubic bones) **Figure 2.31** (9,31).

Nonsynovial joints
Joints that do not have a joint cavity, connective tissue, or cartilage.

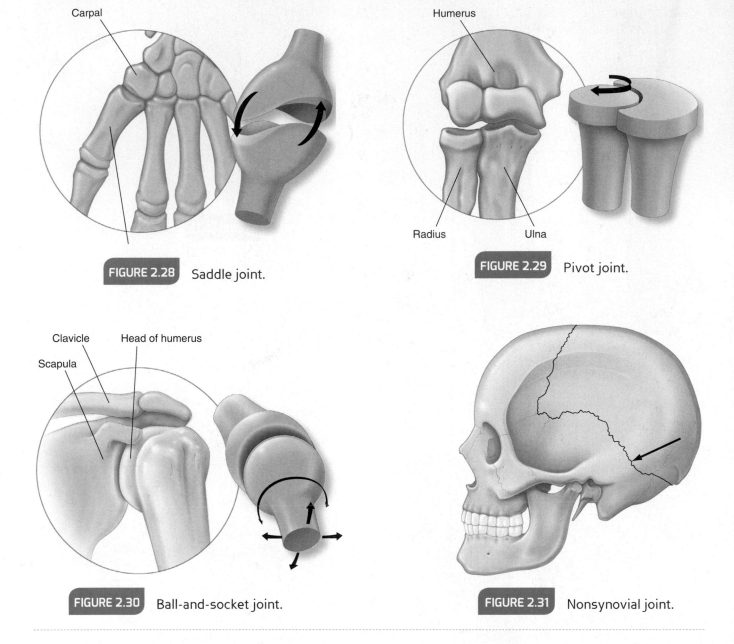

FIGURE 2.28   Saddle joint.

FIGURE 2.29   Pivot joint.

FIGURE 2.30   Ball-and-socket joint.

FIGURE 2.31   Nonsynovial joint.

See Table 2.3 for a full description of the characteristics of these types of joints and examples of each.

Function of Joints

Joints serve numerous functional requirements of the musculoskeletal system; most importantly, joints allow for motion and thus movement (30,31). Joints also provide stability, allowing for movement to take place without unwanted movement.

All joints in the human body are linked together, which implies that movement of one joint directly affects the motion of others (7,31). This is an essential concept for personal trainers to understand because it creates an awareness of how the body functionally operates and is the premise behind kinetic chain movement (7,31).

TABLE 2.3	Types of Joints	
Joint	**Characteristic**	**Example**
Nonsynovial	No joint cavity and fibrous connective tissue; little or no movement	Sutures of the skull
Synovial	Produces synovial fluid, has a joint cavity and fibrous connective tissue	Knee
Gliding	No axis of rotation; moves by sliding side-to-side or back and forth	Carpals of the hand
Condyloid	Formed by the fitting of condyles of one bone into elliptical cavities of another; moves predominantly in one plane	Knee
Hinge	Uniaxial; moves predominantly in one plane of motion (sagittal)	Elbow
Saddle	One bone fits like a saddle on another bone; moves predominantly in two planes (sagittal, joint of thumb frontal)	Only: carpometacarpal
Pivot	Only one axis; moves predominantly in one plane of motion (transverse)	Radioulnar
Ball-and-socket	Most mobile of joints; moves in all three planes of motion	Shoulder

The concept of kinetic chain movement is easy to demonstrate. First, start by standing with both feet firmly on the ground and then roll your feet inward and outward. Notice what your knee and hips are doing. Next, keep your feet stationary and rotate your hips, notice what your knees and feet are doing. Moving one of these joints will inevitably move the others. If you understand this concept, then you understand what true kinetic chain movement is. It should also be easy to see that if one joint is not working properly, it will affect other joints (7).

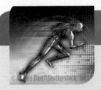

Memory Jogger

This is an extremely important concept to understand when performing movement assessments, designing programs, and monitoring exercise technique, all of which will be covered in later chapters.

Joint Connective Tissue

Ligaments are fibrous connective tissues that connect bone to bone and provide static and dynamic stability as well as input to the nervous system (proprioception) **Figure 2.32** (38,39). Ligaments are primarily made up of a protein called collagen with varying amounts of a second protein called elastin. Collagen fibers are situated in a more parallel fashion to the forces that are typically placed on the ligament. Thus, they provide the ligament with the ability to withstand tension (tensile strength).

Ligament Primary connective tissue that connects bones together and provides stability, input to the nervous system, guidance, and the limitation of improper joint movement.

Elastin gives a ligament some flexibility or elastic recoil to withstand the bending and twisting it may have to endure. Not all ligaments will have the same amount of elastin; for example, the anterior cruciate ligament of the knee contains very little elastin and is predominantly composed of collagen. Because of this, it is much better suited for resisting strong forces and makes a good stabilizing structure of the knee (38,39). Finally, it is important to note that ligaments are characterized by having poor vascularity (or blood supply), meaning that ligaments do not heal or repair very well and may be slower to adapt to stresses placed on the body, such as stress caused by exercise (38–41).

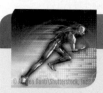

Memory Jogger

The slow repairing capabilities of ligaments will be important to remember when considering the number of days' rest taken and the structure of your daily exercise programming plan when performing high-intensity exercise. This will be discussed in Chapter 15, Program Design.

Exercise and Its Effect on Bone Mass

Like muscle, bone is living tissue that responds to exercise by becoming stronger. Individuals who exercise regularly generally achieve greater peak bone mass (maximal bone density and strength) than those who do not. Exercising allows us to maintain muscle strength, coordination, and balance, which in turn help to prevent falls and related fractures. This is especially important for older adults and people who have been diagnosed with osteoporosis.

Weight-bearing exercise is the best kind of exercise to help strengthen bones because it forces bones to work against gravity, and thus react by becoming stronger. Examples of weight-bearing exercises include resistance training, walking, body weight squats, push-ups, jogging, climbing stairs, and even dancing. Examples of exercises that are not weight-bearing include swimming and bicycling. Although these activities help

FIGURE 2.32

Ligament.

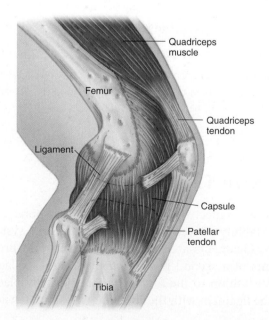

Quadriceps muscle

Femur

Quadriceps tendon

Ligament

Capsule

Patellar tendon

Tibia

build and maintain strong muscles and have excellent cardiovascular and weight control benefits, they are not the best way to exercise your bones (35).

SUMMARY

The skeletal system is the body's framework and is made up of bones and joints in two divisions: axial and appendicular. There are many types of bones, all of which have markings of depressions or processes. Bones are connected (via ligaments) by either synovial or nonsynovial joints, which both provide movement as well as stability. Joints are interconnected, and movement of one will affect the others. Like muscle, bone is living tissue that responds to exercise by becoming stronger. Individuals who exercise regularly generally achieve greater peak bone mass (maximal bone density and strength) than those who do not.

The Muscular System

The nervous system is the control center for movement production, and the skeletal system provides the structural framework for our bodies. However, to complete the cycle of movement production, the body must have a device that the nervous system can command to move the skeletal system. This is the **muscular system Figure 2.33**. Muscles generate internal tension that, under the control of the nervous system, manipulates the bones of our body to produce movements. Muscles are the movers and stabilizers of our bodies.

Muscular system Series of muscles that moves the skeleton.

The Structure of Skeletal Muscle

Skeletal muscle is one of three major muscle types in the body; the others are cardiac and smooth muscle. Skeletal muscle is made up of individual muscle fibers, and the term *muscle* literally refers to multiple bundles of muscle fibers held together by connective tissue **Figure 2.34** (30). Bundles of muscle fibers can be further broken

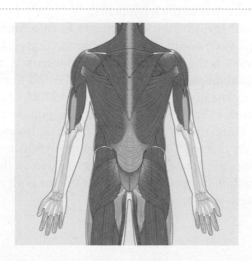

FIGURE 2.33

Muscular system.

Epimysium A layer of connective tissue that is underneath the fascia and surrounds the muscle.

Perimysium The connective tissue that surrounds fascicles.

Endomysium The deepest layer of connective tissue that surrounds individual muscle fibers.

Tendons Connective tissues that attach muscle to bone and provide an anchor for muscles to produce force.

down into layers from the outer surface to the innermost layer. The first bundle is the actual muscle itself wrapped by an outer layer of connective tissue called fascia and an inner layer immediately surrounding the muscle called the **epimysium**. The fascia and epimysium are also connected to bone and help to form the muscle's tendon (8–10,13,15,28–31,38,42). The next bundle of muscle fiber is called a fascicle. Each fascicle is wrapped by connective tissue called **perimysium**. Each fascicle is in turn made up of many individual muscle fibers that are wrapped by connective tissue called **endomysium** (Figure 2.34) (8–10,13,15,28–31,38,42).

Connective tissues within the muscle play a vital role in movement. They allow the forces generated by the muscle to be transmitted from the contractile components of the muscle (discussed next) to the bones, creating motion. Each layer of connective tissue extends the length of the muscle, helping to form the tendon.

Tendons are the structures that attach muscles to bone and provide the anchor from which the muscle can exert force and control the bone and joint (8–10,13,15,28–31,38,42,43). They are very similar to ligaments in that they have poor vascularity (blood supply), which leaves them susceptible to slower repair and adaptation (31,40,43).

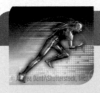

Memory Jogger

As with ligaments, the tendon's poor vascularity will be important to remember when considering the number of days' rest taken and the structure of your daily exercise programming plan when performing high-intensity exercise to ensure you do not develop overuse injuries.

Muscle Fibers and Their Contractile Elements

Muscle fibers are encased by a plasma membrane known as the sarcolemma and contain cell components such as cellular plasma called sarcoplasm (which contains glycogen, fats, minerals, and oxygen-binding myoglobin), nuclei, and mitochondria (which transform energy from food into energy for the cell). Unlike other cells, they also have structures called myofibrils. Myofibrils contain myofilaments that are the actual contractile components of muscle tissue. These myofilaments are known as actin (thin stringlike filaments) and myosin (thick filaments).

Sarcomere The functional unit of muscle that produces muscular contraction and consists of repeating sections of actin and myosin.

The actin (thin) and myosin (thick) filaments form a number of repeating sections within a myofibril. Each one of these particular sections is known as a **sarcomere Figure 2.35**. A sarcomere is the functional unit of the muscle, much like the neuron is for the nervous system. It lies in the space between two Z lines. Each Z line denotes another sarcomere along the myofibril (8–10,13,15,28–31,38,42).

Two protein structures that are also important to muscle contraction are tropomyosin and troponin. Tropomyosin is located on the actin filament and blocks myosin binding sites located on the actin filament, keeping myosin from attaching to actin when the muscle is in a relaxed state. Troponin, also located on the actin filament, plays a role in muscle contraction by providing binding sites for both calcium and tropomyosin when a muscle needs to contract.

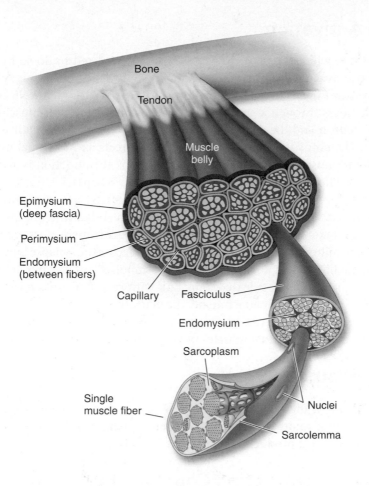

FIGURE 2.34

Structure of the skeletal muscle.

Bone

Tendon

Muscle belly

Epimysium (deep fascia)

Perimysium

Endomysium (between fibers)

Capillary

Fasciculus

Endomysium

Sarcoplasm

Single muscle fiber

Nuclei

Sarcolemma

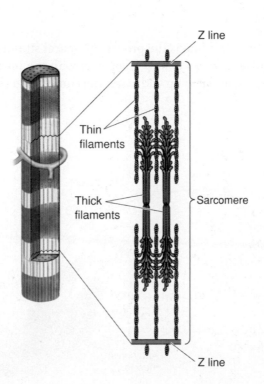

FIGURE 2.35

Sarcomere.

Z line

Thin filaments

Thick filaments

Sarcomere

Z line

Neural Activation

Neural activation The contraction of a muscle generated by neural stimulation.

Motor unit A motor neuron and all of the muscle fibers it innervates.

Neurotransmitters Chemical messengers that cross the neuromuscular junction (synapse) to transmit electrical impulses from the nerve to the muscle.

Skeletal muscles will not contract unless they are stimulated to do so by motor neurons. **Neural activation** is the communication link between the nervous system and the muscular system **Figure 2.36**. Motor neurons originating from the CNS communicate with muscle fibers through a specialized synapse called the neuromuscular junction. One motor neuron and the muscle fibers it connects (innervates) with is known as a **motor unit**. The point at which the motor neuron meets an individual muscle fiber is called the neuromuscular junction (nerve to muscle). This junction is actually a small gap between the nerve and muscle fiber often called a synapse.

Electrical impulses (also known as action potentials) are transported from the central nervous system down the axon of the neuron. When the impulse reaches the end of the axon (axon terminal), chemicals called **neurotransmitters** are released.

Neurotransmitters are chemical messengers that cross the synapse between the neuron and muscle fiber, transporting the electrical impulse from the nerve to the muscle. Once neurotransmitters are released, they link with receptor sites on the muscle fiber specifically designed for their attachment. The neurotransmitter used by the neuromuscular system is acetylcholine (ACh). Once attached, ACh stimulates the muscle fibers to go through a series of steps that initiates muscle contractions (8–10,13,15,28–31,38,42).

Sliding Filament Theory

The sliding filament theory describes how thick and thin filaments within the sarcomere slide past one another, shortening the entire length of the sarcomere and thus shortening muscle and producing force **Table 2.4**; **Figure 2.37**.

Excitation-Contraction Coupling: Putting It All Together

Excitation-contraction coupling is the process of neural stimulation creating a muscle contraction. It involves a series of steps that start with the initiation of a neural message (neural activation) and end up with a muscle contraction (sliding filament theory) **Figure 2.38**.

FIGURE 2.36

Neural activation.

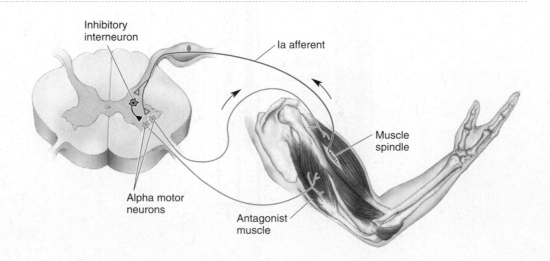

Inhibitory interneuron

Ia afferent

Muscle spindle

Alpha motor neurons

Antagonist muscle

TABLE 2.4	Sliding Filament Theory

Steps in the sliding filament theory are summarized as follows[8,10,13,42]
1. A sarcomere shortens as a result of the Z lines moving closer together.
2. The Z lines converge as the result of myosin heads attaching to the actin filament and asynchronously pulling (power strokes) the actin filament across the myosin, resulting in shortening of the muscle fiber.

Motor Units and the "All or Nothing" Law

Muscles are divided into motor units; a single motor unit consists of one motor neuron (nerve) and the muscle fibers it innervates. As was discussed earlier, if the stimulus is strong enough to trigger an action potential, then it will spread through the whole length of the muscle fiber. More specifically, it will spread through all the muscle fibers supplied by a single nerve. Conversely, if the stimulus is not strong enough, then there will be no action potential and no muscle contraction. Motor units cannot, therefore, vary the amount of force they generate; they either contract maximally or not at all—hence the "all or nothing" law.

As a result of the all or nothing law, the overall strength of a skeletal muscle contraction will depend on the size of the motor unit recruited (i.e., how many muscle fibers are contained within the unit) and the number of motor units that are activated at a given time.

It should also be understood that the size of motor units making up a particular muscle will relate directly to the function of that muscle. For example, muscles that have to control precise movements are made up of many small motor units, e.g., the muscles that control eye movements have as few as 10 to 20 muscle fibers within each motor unit, allowing the fine control that eye movement demands. Conversely, large muscles and muscle groups, such as the gastrocnemius muscle, which are required to generate more powerful, gross movements with far less fine control, have as many as 2,000 to 3,000 muscle fibers in each of their motor units.

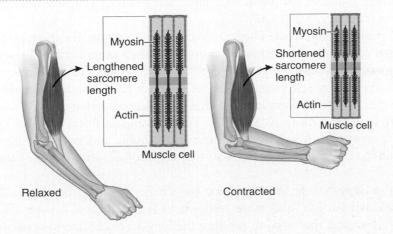

FIGURE 2.37

Sliding filament theory.

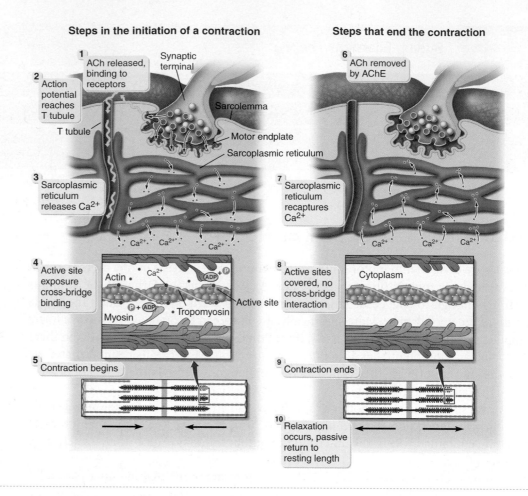

FIGURE 2.38

Excitation-contraction coupling. Ach, acetylcholine; AChE, acetylcholine esterase.

Muscle Fiber Types

Muscle fiber types vary in their chemical and mechanical properties. There are two main categories of muscle fibers, type I and type II fibers Table 2.5 (8–10,13,15,28–31,38,42).

Type I (slow-twitch) muscle fibers contain a large number of capillaries, mitochondria (which transform energy from food into ATP, or cellular energy), and myoglobin, which allows for improved delivery of oxygen. Myoglobin is similar to hemoglobin, the red pigment found in red blood cells, and therefore type I muscle fibers are often referred to as red fibers (8,10,13,42).

Type II (fast-twitch) muscle fibers are subdivided into type IIa and type IIx based again on their chemical and mechanical properties. They generally contain fewer capillaries, mitochondria, and myoglobin. Type II muscle fibers are often referred to as white fibers. Type IIx muscle fibers have a low oxidative capacity (ability to use oxygen) and fatigue quickly. Type IIa muscle fibers have a higher oxidative capacity and fatigue more slowly than type IIx (8,10,13,15,42). Type IIa muscle fibers are also known as intermediate fast-twitch fibers. They can use both aerobic and anaerobic metabolism almost equally to create energy. In this way, they are a combination of type I and type II muscle fibers.

Type I, or slow-twitch, muscle fibers, are smaller in size (diameter), slower to produce maximal tension, and more resistant to fatigue (44–47). Type I fibers are important for muscles that need to produce the long-term contractions necessary for

TABLE 2.5	Muscle Fiber Types
Type	**Characteristic**
Type I (slow-twitch)	More capillaries, mitochondria, and myoglobin
	Increased oxygen delivery
	Smaller in size
	Less force produced
	Slow to fatigue
	Long-term contractions (stabilization)
	Slow twitch
Type II (fast-twitch)	Fewer capillaries, mitochondria, and myoglobin
	Decreased oxygen delivery
	Larger in size
	More force produced
	Quick to fatigue
	Short-term contractions (force and power)
	Fast twitch

stabilization and postural control. An example would include sitting upright, while maintaining ideal posture against gravity, for an extended period of time.

Fast-twitch or type II muscle fibers are larger in size, quick to produce maximal tension, and fatigue more quickly than type I fibers. These fibers are important for muscles producing movements requiring force and power such as performing a sprint.

It is important to note that all muscles have a combination of slow- and fast-twitch fibers that will vary depending on the function of the muscle (8,10,13,15,42). For example, it has been shown that the human anterior tibialis muscle (muscle on the shin) has approximately 73% slow-twitch type I muscle fibers, whereas the lateral head of the gastrocnemius (superficial calf muscle) has approximately 49% slow-twitch type I muscle fibers (48,49).

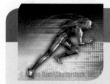

Memory Jogger

When designing a program, it becomes very important for the health and fitness professional to incorporate specific training parameters to fulfill specific muscular requirements (stabilization, strength, and power). This is demonstrated in the OPT™ model and discussed in Chapter 14.

Muscles as Movers

Muscles provide the human body with a variety of functions that allow for the manipulation of forces placed on the body and to produce and slow down movement. These muscle functions categorize the muscle as an agonist, synergist, stabilizer, or antagonist **Table 2.6** (7,28).

Agonist muscles are muscles that act as prime movers, or, in other words, they are the muscles most responsible for a particular movement. For example, the gluteus maximus is an agonist for hip extension.

Synergist muscles assist prime movers during movement. For example, the hamstring complex and the erector spinae are synergistic with the gluteus maximus during hip extension.

Stabilizer muscles support or stabilize the body, whereas the prime movers and the synergists perform the movement patterns. For example, the transversus abdominis, internal oblique, and multifidus (deep muscles in the low back) stabilize the low back, pelvis, and hips (lumbo-pelvic-hip complex) during hip extension.

Antagonist muscles perform the opposite action of the prime mover. For example, the psoas (a deep hip flexor) is antagonistic to the gluteus maximus during hip extension.

TABLE 2.6 Muscles as Movers

Muscle Type	Muscle Function	Exercise	Muscle(s) Used
Agonist	Prime mover	Chest press	Pectoralis major
		Overhead press	Deltoid
		Row	Latissimus dorsi
		Squat	Gluteus maximus, quadriceps
Synergist	Assist prime mover	Chest press	Anterior deltoid, triceps
		Overhead press	Triceps
		Row	Posterior deltoid, biceps
		Squat	Hamstring complex
Stabilizer	Stabilize while prime mover and synergist work	Chest press	Rotator cuff
		Overhead press	Rotator cuff
		Row	Rotator cuff
		Squat	Transversus abdominis
Antagonist	Oppose prime mover	Chest press	Posterior deltoid
		Overhead press	Latissimus dorsi
		Row	Pectoralis major
		Squat	Psoas

Refer to the Appendix D for a more detailed description of all major muscles of the muscular system.

SUMMARY

The muscular system is made up of many individual fibers and attaches to bones by way of tendons. There are different muscle fiber types and arrangements of them that affect how they move. Muscles generate force through neural activation.

The nervous system receives and delivers information throughout the body, by way of neurons. The stimulation of the nervous system activates sarcomeres, which generates tension in the muscles. This tension is transferred through tendons to the bones, and this produces motion.

The Endocrine System

The endocrine system is a system of glands that secrete hormones into the bloodstream to regulate a variety of bodily functions, including the control of mood, growth and development, tissue function, and metabolism **Figure 2.39**. The endocrine system consists of host organs (known as glands), chemical messengers (hormones), and target (receptor) cells. Once a hormone is secreted from a gland, it travels through the bloodstream to target cells designed to receive its message. The target cells have hormone-specifc receptors ensuring that each hormone will communicate only with specific target cells. Along the way, special proteins bind to some hormones, acting as carriers that control the amount of hormone that is available to interact with and affect the target cells (50).

The endocrine system is responsible for regulating multiple bodily functions to stabilize the body's internal environment much like a thermostat regulates the temperature in a room. The term *endocrine* literally means "hormone secreting" (50). Hormones produced by the endocrine system virtually affect all forms of human function including (but not limited to) triggering muscle contraction, stimulating protein and fat synthesis, activating enzyme systems, regulating growth and metabolism, and determining how the body will physically and emotionally respond to stress (50).

Endocrine Glands

The primary endocrine glands are the hypothalamus, pituitary, thyroid, and adrenal glands. The pituitary gland is often referred to as the "master" gland of the endocrine system, because it controls the functions of the other endocrine glands. The pituitary has three different sections or lobes, the anterior, intermediate, and posterior lobes, and each lobe secretes specific types of hormones. The anterior lobe secretes growth hormone, prolactin (to stimulate milk production after giving birth), adrenocorticotropic hormone or ACTH (to stimulate the adrenal glands), thyroid-stimulating hormone or TSH (to stimulate the thyroid gland), follicle-stimulating hormone or FSH (to stimulate the ovaries and testes), and luteinizing hormone or LH (to stimulate the ovaries or testes). The intermediate lobe of the pituitary gland secretes melanocyte-stimulating hormone (to control skin pigmentation), and the posterior lobe secretes antidiuretic

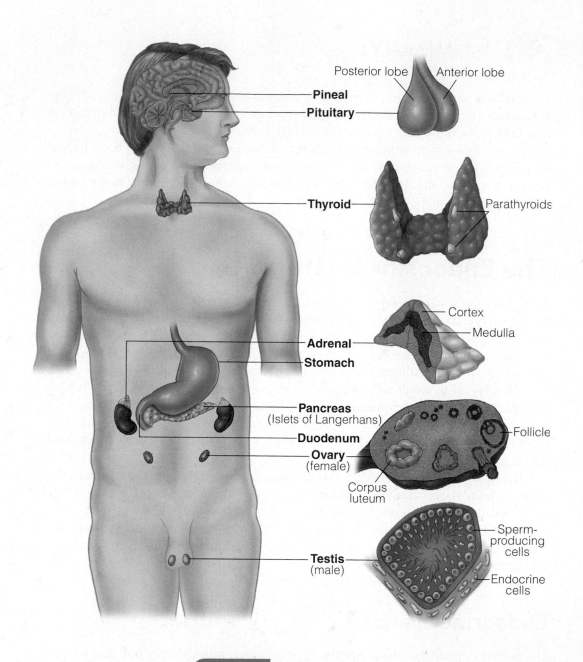

FIGURE 2.39 Endocrine organs.

hormone or ADH (to increase absorption of water into the blood by the kidneys) and oxytocin (to contract the uterus during childbirth and stimulate milk production). The thyroid gland produces hormones that regulate the rate of metabolism and affect the growth and rate of function of many other systems in the body. Adrenal glands secrete hormones such as corticosteroids and catecholamines, including cortisol and adrenaline (epinephrine) in response to stress.

Much of the control of hormonal activity ultimately rests with the hypothalamus and pituitary gland, which are located in the brain. Together they represent an important link between the nervous and endocrine systems (51). As stated earlier, many of the hormones produced in this region directly influence the activities of other glands; thus the pituitary gland is often referred to as the master gland (51). However, for the purposes of this chapter we will focus on those glands and hormones directly involved in exercise activity.

Insulin, Glucagon, and Control of Blood Glucose

Carbohydrate, specifically glucose, is the primary energy source during vigorous exercise. Carbohydrates are the human body's key source of energy, and glucose is the principal fuel for the brain. Any extreme fluctuations in blood glucose levels can be extremely dangerous; too little can inhibit performance, whereas too much can damage the vascular system. Control of blood glucose is regulated by the pancreas, which produces two specific hormones: insulin and glucagon.

Insulin

Insulin helps regulate energy and glucose metabolism in the body. After consuming a meal, glucose enters the blood at the small intestine, causing a rise in blood glucose levels. As the blood is circulated through the pancreas, elevated levels of glucose trigger the release of insulin. The circulating insulin binds with the receptors of its target cells (in this case skeletal muscle or liver cells), and the cell membrane becomes more permeable to glucose. Glucose then diffuses out of the bloodstream and into the cell. The net result is a drop in blood glucose levels. Thus insulin causes cells in the liver, muscle, and fat tissue to take up glucose from the blood, storing it as glycogen in the liver and muscle (50,51).

Glucagon

Glucagon is one of the two hormones secreted by the pancreas that regulate blood glucose levels. Its effect is opposite to that of insulin, as it functions to raise blood glucose levels by triggering the release of glycogen stores from the liver (glycogen is the stored form of glucose). Hours after a meal, or as a result of a combination of normal metabolic processes and physical activity, the body will begin to exhibit lower blood glucose levels. The drop in circulating blood glucose levels triggers the release of glucagon from the pancreas. In contrast to insulin, glucagon has a much more specific effect, stimulating the liver to convert its glycogen stores back into glucose, which is then released into the bloodstream.

The Effects of Exercise

Understanding the effects of exercise is helpful to understanding the interrelationship between insulin and glucagon. As activity levels increase, glucose uptake by the body's cells also increases. This is the result of an increased sensitivity of the cells to insulin; thus, insulin levels will drop during physical activity (52). At the same time glucagon secretion by the pancreas increases, thus helping maintain a steady supply of blood glucose.

Adrenal, Pituitary, Reproductive, and Thyroid Hormones

Catecholamines

The two catecholamines—epinephrine (also known as adrenaline) and norepinephrine—are hormones produced by the adrenal glands, which are situated on top of each kidney. These hormones help prepare the body for activity; more specifically, they are part of the stress response known as the *fight or flight* response. In preparation for activity, the hypothalamus (part of the brain) triggers the adrenal glands to secrete more epinephrine. This will have a number of specific physiological effects that will help sustain exercise activity (51,52):

* increases heart rate and stroke volume
* elevates blood glucose levels
* redistributes blood to working tissues
* opens up the airways

Testosterone and Estrogen

Testosterone is produced in the testes of the male and in small amount in the ovaries and adrenal glands of the female. Males produce up to 10 times more testosterone than females (53), and this is primarily responsible for the development of the male secondary sexual characteristics, such as facial and body hair and greater muscle mass. Estrogen is produced primarily in the ovaries in the female, with small amounts produced in the adrenals in males. Women of reproductive age have significantly higher levels of estrogen than males, which gives rise to female secondary sexual characteristics such as breast development and regulation of the menstrual cycle.

For both males and females, however, testosterone plays a fundamental role in the growth and repair of tissue. Raised levels of testosterone are indicative of an anabolic (tissue-building) training status. Estrogen has many functions, but in particular has an influence on fat deposition around the hips, buttocks, and thighs.

Cortisol

In contrast to testosterone, cortisol is typically referred to as a catabolic hormone (associated with tissue breakdown). Under times of stress, such as exercise, cortisol is secreted by the adrenal glands and serves to maintain energy supply through the breakdown of carbohydrates, fats, and protein. High levels of cortisol brought about through overtraining, excessive stress, poor sleep, and inadequate nutrition can lead to significant breakdown of muscle tissue, along with other potentially harmful side effects (53).

Growth Hormone

The name of this hormone has particular reference to its primary functions. Growth hormone is released from the pituitary gland in the brain and is regulated by the near-by hypothalamus. Growth hormone is stimulated by several factors including estrogen, testosterone, deep sleep, and vigorous exercise. Growth hormone is primarily an anabolic hormone that is responsible for most of the growth and development during childhood up until puberty, when the primary sex hormones take over that control. Growth hormone also increases the development of bone, muscle tissue, and protein synthesis; increases fat burning; and strengthens the immune system.

Thyroid Hormones

The thyroid gland is located at the base of the neck just below the thyroid cartilage, sometimes called the Adam's apple. This gland releases vital hormones that are primarily responsible for human metabolism. The release of thyroid hormones is regulated by the pituitary gland. Thyroid hormones have been shown to be responsible for carbohydrate, protein, and fat metabolism, basal metabolic rate, protein synthesis, sensitivity to epinephrine, heart rate, breathing rate, and body temperature. Low thyroid function has become a well-recognized disorder leading to low metabolism, fatigue, depression, sensitivity to cold, and weight gain.

The Effects of Exercise

Research has indicated that testosterone and growth hormone levels increase after strength training and moderate to vigorous aerobic exercise. A similar pattern also seems to emerge for cortisol (53). The presence of cortisol in the bloodstream is often taken to be indicative of overtraining. This is perhaps a little simplistic as cortisol is a necessary part of maintaining energy levels during normal exercise activity and may even facilitate recovery and repair during the postexercise period (53). Problems may arise, however, as a result of extremely intense or prolonged bouts of endurance training, which have been found to lower testosterone levels while raising cortisol levels. Under these circumstances, catabolism (breakdown) is likely to outstrip anabolism (build up) and give rise to symptoms of overtraining (52,53).

SUMMARY

The endocrine system is responsible for regulating multiple bodily functions to stabilize the body's internal environment. Hormones produced by the endocrine system affect virtually all forms of human function and determine how the body physically and emotionally responds to stress. The endocrine system consists of host organs (known as glands), chemical messengers (or hormones), and target (or receptor) cells. Some of the major endocrine organs include the pituitary, hypothalamus, thyroid, and adrenal glands. Several other organs contain discrete areas of endocrine tissue that also produce hormones, including the pancreas and reproductive organs. Exercise programming has a significant impact on hormone secretion. Health and fitness professionals should become familiar with how pertinent hormones respond to exercise to maximize programming strategies and avoid overtraining.

REFERENCES

1. Cohen H. *Neuroscience for Rehabilitation.* 2nd ed. Philadelphia: Lippincott Williams & Wilkins; 1999.
2. Panjabi MM. The stabilizing system of the spine. Part 1. Function, dysfunction, adaptation, and enhancement. *J Spinal Disord.* 1992; 5:383–389.
3. Liebenson CL. Active muscle relaxation techniques. Part II. Clinical application. *J Manipulative Physiol Ther.* 1990;13(1):2–6.
4. Edgerton VR, Wolf S, Roy RR. Theoretical basis for patterning EMG amplitudes to assess muscle dysfunction. *Med Sci Sports Exerc.* 1996;28(6):744–751.
5. Clark M. Advanced Stabilization Training for performance enhancement. In: Liebenson C, ed. *Rehabilitation of the Spine.* 2nd ed. Baltimore: Williams & Wilkins; 1996: 712–727.
6. Chaitow L. *Muscle Energy Techniques.* New York: Churchill Livingstone; 1997.
7. Clark MA. *Integrated Training for the New Millennium.* Thousand Oaks, CA: National Academy of Sports Medicine; 2001.
8. Milner-Brown A. *Neuromuscular Physiology.* Thousand Oaks, CA: National Academy of Sports Medicine; 2001.
9. Tortora GJ. *Principles of Human Anatomy.* 9th ed. New York: John Wiley & Sons; 2001.
10. Fox SI. *Human Physiology.* 9th ed. New York: McGraw-Hill; 2006.
11. Brooks GA, Fahey TD, White TP, Baldwin, K. *Exercise Physiology: Human Bioenergetics and Its Application.* 4th ed. New York: McGraw-Hill; 2008.
12. Drury DG. Strength and proprioception. *Ortho Phys Ther Clin.* 2000;9(4):549–561.
13. Vander A, Sherman J, Luciano D. *Human Physiology: The Mechanisms of Body Function.* 8th ed. New York: McGraw-Hill; 2001.
14. Biedert RM. Contribution of the three levels of nervous system motor control: Spinal Cord, Lower Brain, Cerebral Cortex. In: Lephart SM, Fu FH, eds. *Proprioception and Neuromuscular Control in Joint Stability.* Champaign, IL: Human Kinetics; 2000:23–30.
15. Enoka RM. *Neuromechanical Basis of Kinesiology.* 4th ed. Champaign, IL: Human Kinetics; 2008.
16. Rose DJ. *A Multi Level Approach to the Study of Motor Control and Learning.* 2nd ed. Upper Saddle River, NJ: Benjamin Cummings; 2005.
17. Barrack RL, Lund PJ, Skinner HB. Knee proprioception revisited. *J Sport Rehab.* 1994;3:18–42.
18. Grigg P. Peripheral neural mechanisms in proprioception. *J Sport Rehab.* 1994;3:2–17.
19. Wilkerson GB, Nitz AJ. Dynamic ankle stability: mechanical and neuromuscular interrelationships. *J Sport Rehab.* 1994;3:43–57.
20. Boyd IA. The histological structure of the receptors in the knee joint of the cat correlated with their physiological response. *J Physiol (Lond).* 1954;124:476–488.
21. Edin B. Quantitative analysis of static strain sensitivity in human mechanoreceptors from hairy skin. *J Neurophysiol.* 1992;67:1105–1113.
22. Edin B, Abbs JH. Finger movement responses of cutaneous mechanoreceptors in the dorsal skin of the human hand. *J Neurophysol.* 1991;65:657–670.
23. Gandevia SC, McClosky DI, Burke D. Kinesthetic signals and muscle contraction. *Trends Neurosci.* 1992;15:62–65.
24. McClosky DJ. Kinesthetic sensibility. *Physiol Rev.* 1978;58:763–820.
25. Lephart SM, Rieman BL, Fu FH. Introduction to the sensorimotor system. In: Lephart SM, Fu FH, eds. *Proprioception and Neuromuscular Control in Joint Stability.* Champaign, IL: Human Kinetics; 2000:xvii–xxiv.
26. Lephart SM, Pincivero D, Giraldo J, Fu F. The role of proprioception in the management and rehabilitation of athletic injuries. *Am J Sports Med.* 1997;25:130–137.
27. Proske U, Schaible HG, Schmidt RF. Joint receptors and kinaesthesia. *Exp Brain Res.* 1988;72:219–224.
28. Hamill J, Knutzen JM. *Biomechanical Basis of Human Movement.* 2nd ed. Baltimore, MD: Lippincott Williams & Wilkins; 2003.
29. Watkins J. *Structure and Function of the Musculoskeletal System.* Champaign, IL: Human Kinetics; 1999.
30. Luttgens K, Hamilton N. *Kinesiology: Scientific Basis of Human Motion.* 11th ed. New York: McGraw-Hill; 2007.
31. Norkin CC, Levangie PK. *Joint Structure and Function: A Comprehensive Analysis.* 3rd ed. Philadelphia: FA Davis Company; 2000.
32. Chaffin DB, Andersson GJ, Martin BJ. *Occupational Biomechanics.* New York: Wiley-Interscience; 1999.
33. Whiting WC, Zernicke RF. *Biomechanics of Musculoskeletal Injury.* Champaign, IL: Human Kinetics; 1998.
34. Bogduk N. *Clinical Anatomy of the Lumbar Spine and Sacrum.* 3rd ed. New York: Churchill Livingstone; 1997.
35. National Institute of Arthritis and Musculoskeletal and Skin Diseases. http://www.niams.nih.gov/Health_Info/bone/Bone_Health/default.asp. Accessed May 5, 2010.
36. National Institute of Neurological Disorders and Stroke. http://www.ninds.nih.gov/disorders/backpain/detail_backpain.htm#102183102. Accessed May 5, 2010.
37. Hertling D, Kessler RM. *Management of Common Musculoskeletal Disorders.* Philadelphia: Lippincott Williams & Wilkins; 1996.
38. Alter MJ. *Science of Flexibility.* 2nd ed. Champaign, IL: Human Kinetics; 1996.
39. Gross J, Fetto J, Rosen E. *Musculoskeletal Examination.* Malden, MA: Blackwell Sciences; 1996.
40. Nordin M, Lorenz T, Campello M. Biomechanics of tendons and ligaments. In: Nordin M, Frankel VH, eds. *Basic Biomechanics of the Musculoskeletal System.* 3rd ed. Philadelphia: Lippincott Williams & Wilkins; 2001:102–126.
41. Solomonow M, Baratta R, Zhou BH, et al. The synergistic action of the anterior cruciate ligament and thigh muscles in maintaining joint stability. *Am J Sports Med.* 1987;15:207–213.
42. McComas AJ. *Skeletal Muscle: Form and Function.* Champaign, IL: Human Kinetics; 1996.
43. Kannus P. Structure of the tendon connective tissue. *Scand J Med Sci Sports.* 2000;10(6):312–320.
44. Al-Amood WS, Buller AJ, Pope R. Long-term stimulation of cat fast twitch skeletal muscle. *Nature.* 1973;244:225–227.
45. Buller AJ, Eccles JC, Eccles RM. Interaction between motorneurones and muscles in respect of the characteristic speeds of their responses. *J Physiol.* 1960;150:417–439.

46. Dubowitz V. Cross-innervated mammalian skeletal muscle: histochemical, physiological and biomechanical observations. *J Physiol*. 1967;193:481–496.

47. Hennig R, Lomo T. Effects of chronic stimulation on the size and speed of long-term denervated and innervated rat fast and slow skeletal muscles. *Acta Physiol Scand*. 1987;130: 115–131.

48. Johnson MA, Polgar J, Weightman D, Appleton D. Data on the distribution of fiber types in thirty-six human muscles. *J Neurol Sci*. 1973;18:111–129.

49. Green HJ, Daub B, Houston ME, Thomson JA, Fraser I, Ranney D. Human vastus lateralis and gastrocnemius muscles. A comparative histochemical analysis. *J Neurol Sci*. 1981;52:200–201.

50. McArdle W, Katch F, Katch V. *Exercise Physiology: Nutrition, Energy and Human Performance*. 7th ed. Philadelphia: Lippincott Williams & Wilkins; 2010.

51. Tortora GJ, Grabowski SR. *Principles of Anatomy and Physiology*. 8th ed. New York: HarperCollins; 1996.

52. Wilmore JH, Costill DL. *Physiology of Sport and Exercise*. Champaign, IL: Human Kinetics; 2004.

53. McArdle W, Katch F, Katch V. *Exercise Physiology: Nutrition, Energy and Human Performance*. 5th ed. Philadelphia: Lippincott Williams & Wilkins; 2001.

The Cardiorespiratory System

After studying this chapter, you will be able to:

✔ Describe the structure and function of the cardiovascular and respiratory systems.

✔ Explain how each of these systems relates to human movement.

✔ Describe how the cardiovascular and respiratory systems work in unison.

✔ Explain the influence that dysfunctional breathing can have on the human movement system.

Introduction to the Cardiorespiratory System

The **cardiorespiratory system** is composed of two closely related systems, the cardiovascular system consisting of the heart, blood vessels, and blood and the respiratory system, which includes the trachea, bronchi, alveoli, and the lungs. These systems work together to provide the body with adequate oxygen and nutrients and to remove waste products such as CO_2 from cells in the body (1–5). This chapter focuses on the structure and function of the cardiovascular and respiratory systems and how each of these systems responds and adapts to exercise.

Cardiorespiratory system A system of the body composed of the cardiovascular and respiratory systems.

Cardiovascular system A system of the body composed of the heart, blood, and blood vessels.

The Cardiovascular System

The **cardiovascular system** is composed of the heart, blood, and blood vessels that transport the blood from the heart to the tissues of the body **Figure 3.1**. A basic understanding of the structure and function of the cardiovascular system is necessary to understand the human movement system.

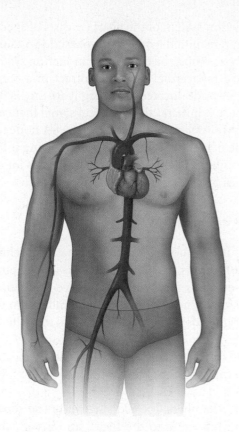

FIGURE 3.1

The cardiovascular system.

The Heart

The **heart** is a muscular pump that rhythmically contracts to push blood throughout the body. It is positioned obliquely in the center of the chest (or thoracic cavity), lying anteriorly (in front) to the spine and posteriorly (behind) to the sternum (4). The left and right lungs lie on either side of the heart (4). The heart is contained in the area of the chest known as the **mediastinum** (6). The adult heart is approximately the size of a typical adult fist and weighs roughly 300 g (approximately 10 ounces) (4,6).

Cardiac muscle is one of three major types of muscle, the others being skeletal and smooth muscle. Cardiac muscle is similar to skeletal muscle in that cardiac muscle cells contain myofibrils and sarcomeres aligned side by side, which give them their striated appearance (1–3,6). Whereas skeletal muscle is a voluntary muscle, cardiac muscle is involuntary muscle, meaning that it cannot typically be consciously controlled.

Heart A hollow muscular organ that pumps a circulation of blood through the body by means of rhythmic contraction.

Mediastinum The space in the chest between the lungs that contains all the internal organs of the chest except the lungs.

Cardiac Muscle Contraction

Cardiac muscle fibers are shorter and more tightly connected than skeletal muscle (1–3). Another unique feature of cardiac muscle is the presence of irregularly spaced dark bands between cardiac cells called intercalated discs. Intercalated discs help hold muscle cells together during contraction and create an electrical connection between the cells that allows the heart to contract as one functional unit. The heart has its own built-in conduction system, unlike skeletal muscle, that sends an electrical signal rapidly throughout all the cardiac cells (1–3). The typical resting heart rate is between 70 and 80 beats per minute (3,4,6).

Sinoatrial (SA) node
A specialized area of cardiac tissue, located in the right atrium of the heart, which initiates the electrical impulses that determine the heart rate; often termed the pacemaker for the heart.

Atrioventricular (AV) node A small mass of specialized cardiac muscle fibers, located in the wall of the right atrium of the heart, that receives heartbeat impulses from the sinoatrial node and directs them to the walls of the ventricles.

Atrium The superior chamber of the heart that receives blood from the veins and forces it into the ventricles.

Ventricle The inferior chamber of the heart that receives blood from its corresponding atrium and, in turn, forces blood into the arteries.

The electrical conduction system of the heart consists of specialized cells that allow an electrical signal to be transmitted from the **sinoatrial (SA) node** through both atria and down into the ventricles. Thus, the electrical conduction system of the heart is what stimulates the mechanical myocardial cells to contract in a regular rhythmic pattern **Figure 3.2** (1–4,6). The SA node, located in the right atrium, is referred to as the pacemaker for the heart because it initiates the electrical signal that causes the heart to beat. The internodal pathways transfer the impulse from the SA node to the **atrioventricular (AV) node**. The AV node delays the impulse before allowing it to move on to the ventricles. The AV bundle conducts the impulse to the ventricles for contraction via the left and right bundle branches of the Purkinje fibers.

Structure of the Heart

The heart is composed of four hollow chambers that are delineated into two interdependent (but separate) pumps on either side. These two pumps are separated by the interatrial septum (separates the atria) and interventricular septum (separates the ventricles) (4–6). Each side of the heart has two chambers: an atrium and a ventricle **Figure 3.3** (1–4,6). The right side of the heart is referred to as the pulmonic side because it receives blood from the body that is low in O_2 and high in CO_2 (deoxygenated) and pumps it to the lungs and then back to the left atria. The left side of the heart is referred to as the systemic side because it pumps blood high in O_2 and low in CO_2 (oxygenated) to the rest of the body.

The **atria** are smaller chambers, located superiorly (on top) on either side of the heart. They gather blood returning to the heart, and act much like a reservoir. The right atrium gathers deoxygenated blood returning to the heart from the entire body, whereas the left atrium gathers oxygenated blood coming to the heart from the lungs.

The **ventricles** are larger chambers located inferiorly (on bottom) on either side of the heart. Unlike the right ventricle, which has thin walls and pumps under low pressure because it only has to pump blood a short distance (to the lungs), the left ventricle

FIGURE 3.2

Conduction system of the heart.

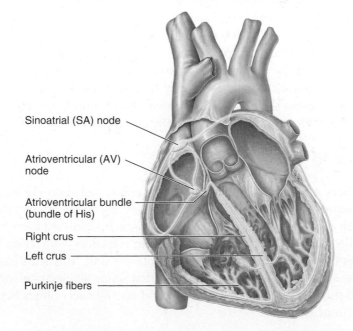

Sinoatrial (SA) node

Atrioventricular (AV) node

Atrioventricular bundle (bundle of His)

Right crus

Left crus

Purkinje fibers

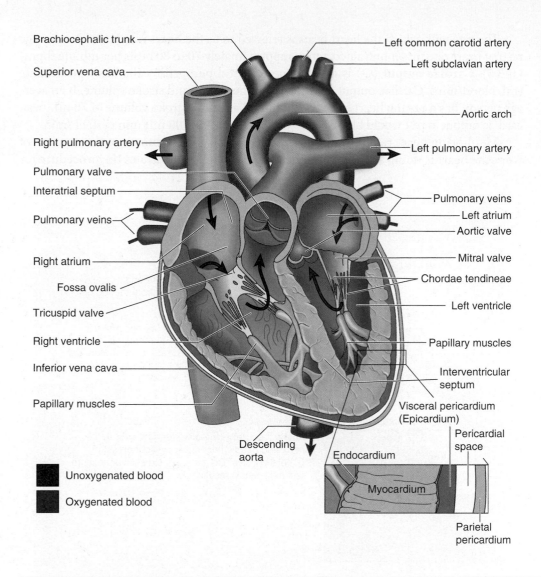

FIGURE 3.3

Atria and ventricles.

Labels (clockwise): Brachiocephalic trunk, Left common carotid artery, Left subclavian artery, Superior vena cava, Aortic arch, Right pulmonary artery, Left pulmonary artery, Pulmonary valve, Pulmonary veins, Interatrial septum, Left atrium, Pulmonary veins, Aortic valve, Mitral valve, Right atrium, Chordae tendineae, Fossa ovalis, Left ventricle, Tricuspid valve, Papillary muscles, Right ventricle, Interventricular septum, Inferior vena cava, Visceral pericardium (Epicardium), Papillary muscles, Pericardial space, Descending aorta, Endocardium, Myocardium, Parietal pericardium

Unoxygenated blood
Oxygenated blood

has thicker walls and pumps under high pressure because it pumps blood out to the rest of the body. The right ventricle receives the deoxygenated blood from the right atrium and then pumps it to the lungs to be saturated with incoming oxygen. The left ventricle receives the oxygenated blood from the left atrium and proceeds to pump it to the entire body. Each chamber of the heart is separated from one another and major veins and arteries via valves to prevent a backflow or spillage of blood back into the chambers. These valves include the atrioventricular valves (tricuspid and mitral valves) and the semilunar valves (pulmonary and aortic valves).

Function of the Heart

The amount of blood pumped out of the heart with each contraction is referred to as **stroke volume (SV)**. The SV is the difference between the ventricular end-diastolic volume (EDV) and the end-systolic volume (ESV). The EDV is the filled volume of the ventricle before contraction, and the ESV is the residual volume of blood remaining in the ventricle after ejection. In a typical heart, the EDV is about 120 mL of blood and the ESV about 50 mL of blood. The difference in these two volumes, 70 mL, represents the SV (1–3,5).

Stroke volume The amount of blood pumped out of the heart with each contraction.

Heart rate (HR) The rate at which the heart pumps.

Cardiac output (Q̇) Heart rate × stroke volume, the overall performance of the heart.

The rate with which the heart beats is referred to as the **heart rate (HR)**. An average resting heart rate for an untrained adult is approximately 70 to 80 beats per minute (bpm) (1–3,5). **Cardiac output (Q̇)** is the volume of blood pumped by the heart per minute (mL blood/min). Cardiac output is a function of heart rate and stroke volume. If an average person has a resting heart rate of 70 bpm and a resting stroke volume of 70 mL/beat, cardiac output at rest would be: 70 bpm × 70 mL/beat = 4,900 mL/min or 4.9 L/min.

Monitoring heart rate during exercise provides a good estimate of the amount of work the heart is doing at any given time (3,7). **Figure 3.4** illustrates the procedure for

FIGURE 3.4

How to manually monitor heart rate.

How To Manually Monitor Heart Rate

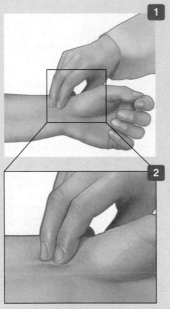

1 Place index and middle fingers around the palm side of the wrist (about one inch from the top of wrist, on the thumb side).

Although some people use the carotid artery in the neck, NASM does not recommend this location for measuring pulse rate. Pressure on this artery reduces blood flow to the brain, which can cause dizziness or an inaccurate measurement.

2 Locate the artery by feeling for a pulse with the index and middle fingers. Apply light pressure to feel the pulse. Do not apply excessive pressure as it may distort results.

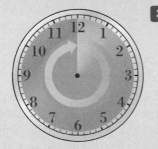

3 When measuring the pulse during rest, count the number of beats in 60 seconds.

There are some factors that may affect resting heart rate, including digestion, mental activity, environmental temperature, biological rhythms, body position, and cardiorespiratory fitness. Because of this, resting heart rate should be measured on waking (or at the very least, after you have had 5 minutes of complete rest).

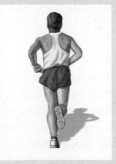

4 When measuring the pulse during exercise, count the number of beats in 6 seconds and add a zero to that number. Adding the zero will provide an estimate of the number of beats in 60 seconds. Or one can simply multiply the number by 10 and that will provide the health and fitness professional with the same number.

Example: Number of beats in 6 seconds = 17. Adding a zero = 170. This gives a pulse rate of 170 bpm or, 17 x 10 = 170

manually monitoring heart rate. Another common procedure used to monitor heart rate is with a heart rate monitor, which is worn on the body and automatically derives the beats per minute.

Blood

Blood is a unique life-sustaining fluid that supplies the body's organs and cells with oxygen and nutrients and helps regulate body temperature, fight infections, and remove waste products (1,2,5). Blood consists of cells suspended in a watery liquid called plasma that also contains nutrients such as glucose, hormones, and clotting agents. There are three kinds of cells in the blood, red blood cells, white blood cells, and platelets. Red blood cells carry oxygen from the lungs throughout the body, white blood cells help fight infection, and platelets help with clotting. Plasma makes up about 55% of the total volume of the blood, and the remaining 45% is made up of red blood cells, white blood cells, and platelets. The average adult has between 4 to 6 L of blood in his or her body (1,2,5). Blood is a vital support mechanism, which provides an internal transportation, regulation, and protection system for the human movement system **Table 3.1**.

Blood Fluid that circulates in the heart, arteries, capillaries, and veins, carries nutrients and oxygen to all parts of the body, and also rids the body of waste products.

Transportation

Blood transports life-sustaining oxygen to all bodily tissues and removes waste products. Blood also transports hormones that act as chemical messengers and nutrients from the gastrointestinal tract to various organs and tissues throughout the body and helps remove heat from internal to external regions of the body (1,2,5).

Regulation

Blood helps regulate body temperature by transferring heat from the internal core out to the periphery of the body as blood circulates throughout the body. As blood travels close to the skin it gives off heat to the environment or can be cooled depending on the environment (1–3,6). Blood is also essential in the regulation of the pH levels (acid balance) in the body as well as maintaining the water content of body cells (6).

TABLE 3.1	Support Mechanisms of Blood	
Mechanism	**Function**	
Transportation	Transports oxygen and nutrients to tissues	
	Transports waste products from tissues	
	Transports hormones to organs and tissues	
	Carries heat throughout the body	
Regulation	Regulates body temperature and acid balance in the body	
Protection	Protects the body from excessive bleeding by clotting	
	Contains specialized immune cells to help fight disease and sickness	

Blood vessels Network of hollow tubes that circulates blood throughout the body.

Arteries Vessels that transport blood away from the heart.

Capillaries The smallest blood vessels, and the site of exchange of chemicals and water between the blood and the tissues.

Protection

Blood provides protection from excessive blood loss through its clotting mechanism, which seals off damaged tissue until a scar forms (1,2,5). It also provides specialized immune cells to fight against foreign toxins within the body, which helps to reduce the risk of disease and illness (1–3,5).

Blood Vessels

Blood vessels form a closed circuit of hollow tubes that allow blood to be transported to and from the heart **Figure 3.5**. There are three major types of blood vessels: **arteries**, which carry the blood away from the heart, the **capillaries**, which are the site of

FIGURE 3.5

Blood vessels.

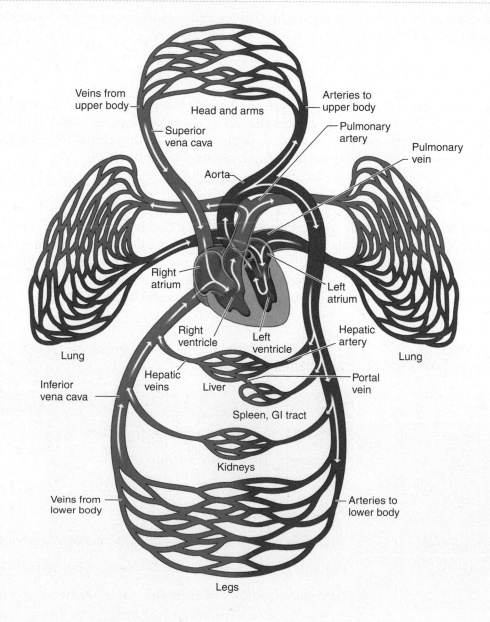

exchange of water and chemicals between the blood and the tissues, and **veins**, which carry blood back to the heart (1,2,4–6).

Arteries

The largest artery in the body is the aorta, which carries blood away from the heart (4,6). The branches of the aorta include medium-sized arteries, including the carotid artery, the subclavian artery, the mesenteric arteries, the renal artery, and the iliac artery (1,2,4–6). These medium-sized arteries further divide into smaller arteries that are called **arterioles** and eventually into microscopic vessels known as capillaries (1,2,4–6). Capillaries are where substances such as oxygen, nutrients, hormones, and waste products are exchanged between tissues (1,2,4–6).

Veins

Vessels that collect blood from the capillaries are called **venules** (1,2,4–6). Venules progressively merge with other venules to form veins. Veins then transport all of the blood from the body back to the heart (1,2,4–6).

SUMMARY

The cardiorespiratory system is composed of the cardiovascular system and the respiratory system. Together, they provide the body with oxygen, nutrients, protective agents, and a means to remove waste products. The cardiovascular system is composed of the heart, blood, and blood vessels. The heart is located in the mediastinum and is made up of involuntary cardiac muscle, which contracts according to a built-in rhythm to regularly pump blood throughout the body. It is divided into four chambers: two atria (which gather blood from the body) and two ventricles (which pump blood out to the body) on each side.

The heart rate and the stroke volume make up the overall performance of the heart. Cardiac output is the combination of how many times the heart beats per minute and how much blood is being pumped out with each beat. Heart rate can be monitored manually or through use of a heart rate monitor.

Blood acts as a medium to deliver and collect essential products to and from the tissues of the body, providing an internal transportation, regulation, and protection system. The blood vessels that transport blood away from the heart are called arteries (which have smaller components called arterioles). The vessels that bring blood back to the heart are called veins (which have smaller components called venules). Capillaries are the smallest blood vessels and connect venules with arterioles.

The Respiratory System

The function of the **respiratory system** (also known as the pulmonary system) is to bring oxygen into the lungs and remove carbon dioxide from the lungs to the outside air. The respiratory system includes airways, lungs, and the respiratory muscles **Figure 3.6**. The primary role of the respiratory system is to ensure proper cellular function (9,10). The respiratory system works intimately with the cardiovascular

Veins Vessels that transport blood from the capillaries toward the heart.

Arterioles Small terminal branches of an artery, which end in capillaries.

Venules The very small veins that connect capillaries to the larger veins.

Respiratory system A system of organs (the lungs and respiratory passageways) that collects oxygen from the external environment and transports it to the bloodstream.

FIGURE 3.6

The respiratory system.

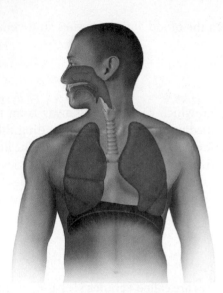

system to accomplish optimal cellular function by transporting oxygen from the environment and transferring it to the bloodstream, and transferring carbon dioxide from the blood to the lungs and eventually transporting it to the environment (10). This entire process is accomplished through the integrated functioning of the respiratory pump to move air in and out of the body and of the respiratory passageways to channel the air (10).

Mechanisms of Breathing

Breathing (or ventilation) is the actual process of moving air in and out of the body and requires optimal functioning of the **respiratory pump** and all its components Table 3.2. Breathing is divided into two phases: **inspiration** (or inhalation) and **expiration** (exhalation). Inspiratory ventilation is active. This means that it requires active contraction of inspiratory muscles to increase the thoracic cavity volume, which decreases the intrapulmonary pressure (or pressure within the thoracic cavity). When the intrapulmonary pressure decreases below that of the atmospheric pressure (or the everyday pressure in the air), air is drawn into the lungs (1–3,9,10). Conversely, expiration is the process of actively or passively relaxing the inspiratory muscles to move air out of the body.

Inspiratory ventilation occurs in two forms: normal resting state (quiet) breathing and heavy (deep, forced) breathing. Normal breathing requires the use of the primary respiratory muscles (i.e., diaphragm, external intercostals), whereas heavy breathing requires the additional use of the secondary respiratory muscles (scalenes, pectoralis minor) (1,2,5,6,9,11).

Expiratory ventilation can be both active and passive. During normal breathing, expiratory ventilation is passive as it results from the relaxation of the contracting inspiratory muscles. During heavy or forced breathing, expiratory ventilation relies on the activity of expiratory muscles to compress the thoracic cavity and force air out (1,2,5,6,9,12).

Breathing also helps regulate blood flow back to the heart. The respiratory pump acts as a mechanism that helps to pump blood back to the heart during inspiration. During inspiration intrathoracic pressure decreases, causing a drop in pressure in the right atrium of the heart, and helps improve blood flow back to the heart.

Respiratory pump
Is composed of skeletal structures (bones) and soft tissues (muscles) that work together to allow proper respiratory mechanics to occur and help pump blood back to the heart during inspiration.

Inspiration The process of actively contracting the inspiratory muscles to move air into the body.

Expiration The process of actively or passively relaxing the inspiratory muscles to move air out of the body.

Respiratory Airways

The purpose of ventilation is to move air in and out of the body. The respiratory passages are divided into two categories, the conducting airways and the respiratory airways.

The conducting airways consist of all the structures that air travels through before entering the respiratory airways Table 3.3. The nasal and oral cavities, mouth, pharynx, larynx, trachea, and bronchioles provide a gathering station for air and oxygen to be directed into the body Figure 3.7. These structures also allow the incoming air to be purified, humidified (or moisture added), and warmed or cooled to match body temperature (1–3,5,7,8,9).

TABLE 3.2	Structures of the Respiratory Pump
	© ilolab/ShutterStock, Inc.
Bones	Sternum
	Ribs
	Vertebrae
Muscles Inspiration	Diaphragm
	External intercostals
	Scalenes
	Sternocleidomastoid
	Pectoralis minor
Expiration	Internal intercostals
	Abdominals

TABLE 3.3	Structures of the Respiratory Passages
	© ilolab/ShutterStock, Inc.
Conducting airways	Nasal cavity
	Oral cavity
	Pharynx
	Larynx
	Trachea
	Right and left pulmonary bronchi
	Bronchioles
Respiratory airways	Alveoli
	Alveolar sacs

Diffusion The process of getting oxygen from the environment to the tissues of the body.

The respiratory airways collect the channeled air coming from the conducting airways (1,2,5,6,8). At the end of the bronchioles sit the alveoli, which are made up of clusters of alveolar sacs (Figure 3.7) (1,2,5,6,8). It is here, in the alveolar sacs, that gases such as oxygen (O_2) and carbon dioxide (CO_2) are transported in and out of the bloodstream through a process known as **diffusion** (1–3,6,8). This is how oxygen gets from the outside environment to the tissues of the body.

FIGURE 3.7

The respiratory passages.

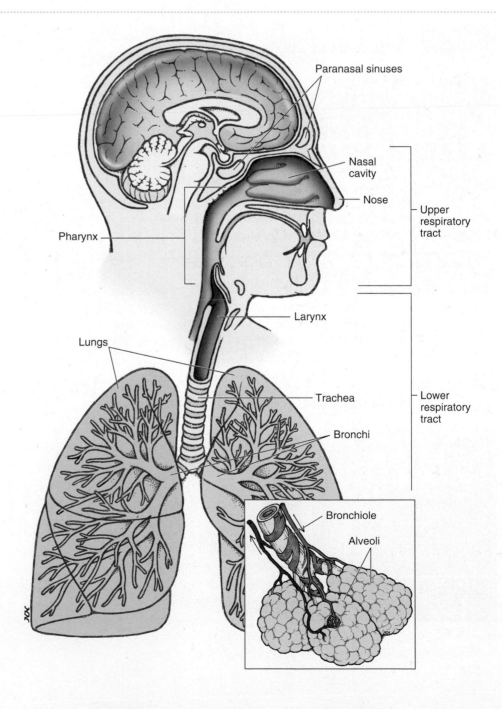

- Paranasal sinuses
- Nasal cavity
- Nose
- Pharynx
- Larynx
- Lungs
- Trachea
- Bronchi
- Bronchiole
- Alveoli

Upper respiratory tract

Lower respiratory tract

SUMMARY

The respiratory system collects oxygen from the environment and transports it to the bloodstream. Breathing is divided into the inspiratory phase (or inhalation) and expiratory phase (or exhalation). Inspiratory ventilation is active, whereas expiratory ventilation can be both active and passive (as during normal breathing, when it results from the relaxation of the contracting inspiratory muscles). There are two groups of respiratory passages. The first is the conducting airways, which consist of all the structures that air travels through before entering the respiratory airways. These structures purify, humidify, and warm or cool air to match body temperature. The second group is the respiratory airways, which collect the channeled air coming from the conducting airways and allow gases such as oxygen and carbon dioxide to be transferred into and out of the bloodstream.

Cardiorespiratory System Function

Together, the cardiovascular and respiratory systems make up the cardiorespiratory system. They form a vital support system to provide the human movement system with many essential elements (such as oxygen), while removing waste products that can cause dysfunction in the body.

An essential element to sustain life is oxygen (3). The respiratory system provides the means to gather oxygen from the environment and transfer it into our bodies. It is inhaled through the nose and mouth, and conducted through the trachea, and then down through the bronchi, where it eventually reaches the lungs and alveolar sacs (1–3,5,6,8). Simultaneously, deoxygenated blood is pumped from the right ventricle to the lungs through the pulmonary arteries. Pulmonary capillaries surround the alveolar sacs, and as oxygen fills the sacs it diffuses across the capillary membranes and into the blood (3). The oxygenated blood then returns to the left atrium through the pulmonary veins, from which it is pumped into the left ventricle and out to the tissues of the body.

As the cells of the body use oxygen they produce carbon dioxide, which needs to be removed from the body (1–3,5,6,8). Carbon dioxide is transported from the tissues back to the heart and eventually to the lungs in the deoxygenated blood. In the alveolar sacs, it diffuses from the pulmonary capillaries into the alveoli and is released through exhalation (1–3,5,6,8). In a simplistic overview, oxygen and carbon dioxide trade places in the tissues of the body, blood, and lungs. As one is coming in, the other is going out.

Oxygen Consumption

The cardiovascular and respiratory systems work together to transport oxygen to the tissues of the body. The capacity to efficiently use oxygen is dependent on the respiratory system's ability to collect oxygen and the cardiovascular system's ability to absorb and transport it to the tissues of the body (14). The use of oxygen by the body is known as oxygen uptake (or oxygen consumption) (1–3,5,6,8,9).

Resting oxygen consumption ($\dot{V}o_2$) is approximately 3.5 mL of oxygen per kilogram of body weight per minute (3.5 mL $\cdot$ kg^{-1} $\cdot$ min^{-1}), typically termed 1 metabolic equivalent or 1 MET (3,5,7,10,14–16). It is calculated as follows:

$$\dot{V}o_2 = \dot{Q} \times a - v\,o_2 \text{ difference}$$

The equation for oxygen consumption is known as the Fick equation. According to the Fick equation, oxygen consumption, $\dot{V}O_2$, is a product of cardiac output, $\dot{Q}$ or (HR $\times$ SV), times the arterial-venous difference (difference in the O_2 content between the blood in the arteries and the blood in the veins), a $-$ v o$_2$. From the Fick equation, it is easy to see how influential the cardiovascular system is on the body's ability to consume oxygen, and that heart rate plays a major factor in determining $\dot{V}O_2$.

Maximal oxygen consumption ($\dot{V}O_{2max}$) may be the best measure of cardiorespiratory fitness (3,5,7,15). $\dot{V}O_{2max}$ is the highest rate of oxygen transport and utilization during maximal exercise (10,14,15). $\dot{V}O_{2max}$ values can range anywhere from 40 to 80 mL $\cdot$ kg^{-1} $\cdot$ min^{-1}, or approximately 11 to 23 METs (7,15). The only way to determine $\dot{V}O_{2max}$ is to directly measure ventilation, oxygen consumption, and carbon dioxide production during a maximal exercise test. However, because the equipment needed to measure $\dot{V}O_{2max}$ is very expensive and not readily available, the use of a submaximal exercise test to estimate or predict $\dot{V}O_{2max}$ is the preferred method (13,15). Some of the tests that can be used to predict $\dot{V}O_{2max}$ include the Rockport Walk Test, the Step Test, and the YMCA bike protocol test (13,15). It is important to note that numerous assumptions are made when predicting versus directly measuring $\dot{V}O_{2max}$, which can lead to overestimates or underestimates of what an individual's true $\dot{V}O_{2max}$ actually is (13,15).

Maximal oxygen consumption ($\dot{V}O_{2max}$) The highest rate of oxygen transport and utilization achieved at maximal physical exertion.

Abnormal Breathing Patterns

Any difficulty or changes to normal breathing patterns can affect the normal response to exercise (16). Common abnormal breathing scenarios associated with stress and anxiety include the following:

- The breathing pattern becomes more shallow, using the secondary respiratory muscles more predominantly than the diaphragm. This shallow, upper-chest breathing pattern becomes habitual, causing overuse to the secondary respiratory muscles such as the scalenes, sternocleidomastoid, levator scapulae, and upper trapezius.
- The respiratory muscles also play a major postural role in the human movement system, all connecting directly to the cervical and cranial portions of the body. Their increased activity and excessive tension may result in headaches, lightheadedness, and dizziness.
- Excessive breathing (short, shallow breaths) can lead to altered carbon dioxide and oxygen blood content and can lead to feelings of anxiety that further initiate an excessive breathing response.
- Inadequate oxygen and retention of metabolic waste within muscles can create fatigued, stiff muscles.
- Inadequate joint motion of the spine and rib cage, as a result of improper breathing, causes joints to become restricted and stiff.

All of these situations can lead to a decreased functional capacity that may result in headaches, feelings of anxiety, fatigue, and poor sleep patterns, as well as poor circulation. As a health and fitness professional, it is not your job to try to diagnose these problems. If a client presents any of these scenarios, refer him or her immediately to a medical professional for assistance.

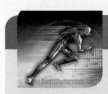

Memory Jogger

Teaching your client to breathe diaphragmatically (through the stomach) can be a way to help avoid these symptoms. Assessing one's breathing pattern ("chest breather") can also help determine potential muscle imbalances.

SUMMARY

The respiratory system gathers oxygen from the environment, and processes it to be delivered to the tissues of the body. As cells use oxygen, they produce carbon dioxide, which is transported back to the heart and lungs in the deoxygenated blood, to be released through exhalation.

The usage of oxygen by the body is known as oxygen consumption. Maximal oxygen consumption, $\dot{V}o_{2max}$, is the highest rate of oxygen transport and utilization achieved at maximal physical exertion. It is generally accepted as the best means of gauging cardiorespiratory fitness. Values can range anywhere from 11 to 23 METs.

Alterations in breathing patterns can directly impact the components of the human movement system and lead to further dysfunction. If the breathing patterns become shallow, the body uses secondary respiratory muscles more than the diaphragm, which can negatively impact posture. This may create excessive muscular tension, resulting in headaches, lightheadedness, and dizziness. Short, shallow breaths can also lead to altered carbon dioxide and oxygen blood content, which causes feelings of anxiety. Inadequate oxygen and retention of metabolic waste within muscles can create stiff muscles and joints. If a client complains of headaches, feelings of anxiety, fatigue, poor sleep patterns, or poor circulation, refer him or her immediately to a medical professional for assistance.

REFERENCES

1. Fox SI. *Human Physiology*. 9th ed. New York: McGraw-Hill; 2006.
2. Vander A, Sherman J, Luciano D. *Human Physiology: The Mechanisms of Body Function*. 9th ed. New York: McGraw-Hill; 2003.
3. Brooks GA, Fahey TD, White TP, Baldwin, KM. *Exercise Physiology: Human Bioenergetics and Its Application*. 3rd ed. New York: McGraw-Hill; 2000.
4. Murray TD, Pulcipher JM. Cardiovascular anatomy. In: American College of Sports Medicine, ed. *ACSM's Resource Manual for Guidelines for Exercise Testing and Prescription*. 4th ed. Baltimore, MD: Lippincott Williams & Wilkins, 2001:65-72.
5. Hicks GH. *Cardiopulmonary Anatomy and Physiology*. Philadelphia: WB Saunders; 2000.
6. Tortora GJ, Nielsen M. *Principles of Human Anatomy*. 11th ed. New York: Wiley; 2008.
7. Swain DP. Cardiorespiratory exercise prescription. In: American College of Sports Medicine, ed. *ACSM's Resource Manual for Guidelines for Exercise Testing and Prescription*. 6th ed. Baltimore, MD: Lippincott Williams & Wilkins; 2006: 448-462.
8. Mahler DA. Respiratory anatomy. In: American College of Sports Medicine, ed. *ACSM's Resource Manual for Guidelines for Exercise Testing and Prescription*. 4th ed. Baltimore, MD: Lippincott Williams & Wilkins; 2001:74-81.
9. Brown DD. Pulmonary responses to exercise and training. In: Garrett WE, Kirkendall DT, eds. *Exercise and Sport Science*. Philadelphia: Lippincott Williams & Wilkins; 2000:117-132.
10. Leech JA, Ghezzo H, Stevens D, Becklake MR. Respiratory pressures and function in young adults. *Am Rev Respir Dis*. 1983;128:17-23.

11. Farkas GA, Decramer M, Rochester DF, De Troyer A. Contractile properties of intercostal muscles and their functional significance. *J Appl Physiol*. 1985;59:528-535.

12. Sharp JT, Goldberg NB, Druz WS, Danon J. Relative contributions of rib cage and abdomen to breathing in normal subjects. *J Appl Physiol*. 1975;39:608-619.

13. Guthrie J. Cardiorespiratory and health-related physical fitness assessments. In: American College of Sports Medicine, ed. *ACSM's Resource Manual for Guidelines for Exercise Testing and Prescription*. 6th ed. Baltimore, MD: Lippincott Williams & Wilkins; 2006:297-331.

14. Franklin BA. Cardiovascular responses to exercise and training. In: Garrett WE, Kirkendall DT, eds. *Exercise and Sport Science*. Philadelphia: Lippincott Williams & Wilkins; 2000: 107-115.

15. *ACSM's Resource Manual for Guidelines for Exercise Testing and Prescription*. 5th ed. Baltimore, MD: Lippincott Williams & Wilkins; 2005.

16. Timmons B. *Behavioral and Psychological Approaches to Breathing Disorders*. New York: Plenum Press; 1994.

© Eky Studio/ShutterStock, Inc.

Exercise Metabolism and Bioenergetics

After studying this chapter, you will be able to:

✔ Describe the primary methods of how the body produces energy for exercise.

✔ Differentiate between aerobic and anaerobic metabolism.

✔ Distinguish which energy pathways predominate for various intensities and durations of exercise.

✔ Understand the interaction of carbohydrate, fat, and protein as fuels for exercise.

✔ State the differences in the energy use during steady state and exhaustive exercise.

✔ Discriminate between the energy requirements of steady state versus intermittent exercise.

✔ Describe basic training-induced adaptations in energy production.

Introduction to Exercise Metabolism and Bioenergetics

Our bodies need a constant supply of energy to function properly to maintain health and internal balance. Exercise places unique and demanding requirements on the body's ability to supply energy and remove metabolic by-products. The food we eat is what provides our cells with the needed energy to survive and function properly. But before food can become a usable form of energy it has to be converted into smaller units called substrates, including carbohydrates, proteins, and fats (1–9). The energy stored in these substrate molecules is then chemically released in cells and stored in

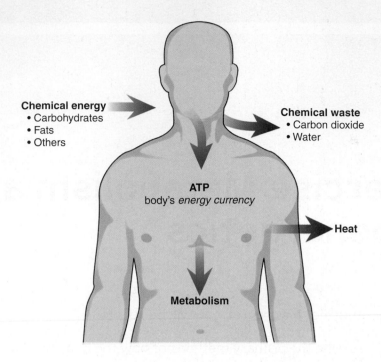

FIGURE 4.1

Basic overview of energy metabolism.

the form of a high-energy compound called adenosine triphosphate (ATP) **Figure 4.1**. The role of energy metabolism during exercise involves understanding how energy is supplied, which energy systems are used during exercise, how quickly energy can be supplied, and how cells generate ATP. This chapter covers basic information on energy metabolism and bioenergetics that will be useful in helping personal trainers plan safe and effective exercise programs for their clients.

Bioenergetics and Metabolism

Bioenergetics The study of energy in the human body.

Metabolism All of the chemical reactions that occur in the body to maintain itself. Metabolism is the process in which nutrients are acquired, transported, used, and disposed of by the body.

Exercise metabolism The examination of bioenergetics as it relates to the unique physiologic changes and demands placed on the body during exercise.

Substrates The material or substance on which an enzyme acts.

Energy metabolism, or **bioenergetics**, is the study of how energy is transformed through various biochemical reactions (6,9). Energy is required to sustain life, support exercise, and help recovery from it. The ultimate source of energy is the sun. Through photosynthesis, energy from the sun produces chemical energy and other compounds that are used to convert carbon dioxide into organic chemicals such as glucose. The word **metabolism** refers to all the chemical reactions that occur in the body to maintain itself (6,9). The main sources of chemical energy for most organisms are carbohydrates, fats, and protein. The energy from the oxidation of carbohydrates, fats, and proteins sustains the biochemical reactions required for life. **Exercise metabolism** refers to the examination of bioenergetics as it relates to the unique physiologic changes and demands placed on the body during exercise (6,9).

Fuel for Energy Metabolism

Dietary food provides energy to sustain life and support physical activity, but not directly; it first has to be broken down by the digestive system into smaller by-products called substrates. Proteins, carbohydrates, and lipids (fats) constitute the main **substrates** used to transfer metabolic energy to be used for all types of cellular activity and life (1–9).

Carbohydrates provide the body with a source of fuel and energy required for all daily activities including exercise (1–9).

Our bodies need a constant supply of energy to function properly, and a lack of carbohydrates in the diet can cause fatigue, poor mental function, and lack of endurance and stamina. The primary end product after the digestion of carbohydrates is the formation of **glucose**. Glucose is absorbed and transported in the blood, where it circulates until it enters cells (with the aid of insulin) and is either used or stored as energy. The storage form of carbohydrates, called **glycogen**, is a string of glucose molecules that can rapidly be broken down into glucose and used for energy during periods of prolonged or intense exercise. Glycogen is stored in the liver and muscle cells.

Another important source of energy is **fat**. The chemical or substrate form in which most fat exists in food as well as in the body is called **triglycerides** (5,6,9). Triglycerides are derived from fats eaten in foods or made in the body from other energy sources such as carbohydrates. When calories are consumed but not immediately needed by cells or tissues they are converted to triglycerides and transported to fat cells where they are stored. One of the benefits of fat as a fuel source is that most people have an inexhaustible supply of fat, which can be broken down into triglycerides and used for energy during prolonged physical activity or exercise.

The third fuel source is **protein**. But protein rarely supplies much energy during exercise and in many descriptions is ignored as a significant fuel for energy metabolism (1–9). When protein becomes a significant source of fuel is in starvation. During a negative energy balance (e.g., low-calorie diet), amino acids are used to assist in energy production. This is called **gluconeogenesis** (1,6,9).

SUMMARY

Our bodies need a constant supply of energy to function properly to maintain health and internal balance. The food we eat is what provides our cells with the needed energy to survive and function properly. But before food can become a usable form of energy it has to be converted into smaller units called substrates, including carbohydrates, proteins, and fats. The energy stored in these substrate molecules is then chemically released in cells and stored in the form of a high-energy compound called ATP.

Bioenergetics is the study of how energy is transformed through various biochemical reactions. The main sources of chemical energy for most organisms are carbohydrates, fats, and protein. Exercise metabolism refers to the examination of bioenergetics as it relates to the unique physiologic changes and demands placed on the body during exercise.

Energy and Work

As stated earlier, one of the primary sources of immediate energy for cellular metabolism is stored in the chemical bonds of a molecule called **adenosine triphosphate (ATP)**. When the chemical bonds that hold ATP together are broken, energy is released for cellular work (such as performing muscle contraction), leaving behind another molecule called **adenosine diphosphate (ADP)** (1–9). One of the functions of energy metabolism is to harness enough free energy to reattach a phosphate group to an ADP and restore ATP levels back to normal to perform more work.

Carbohydrates Organic compounds of carbon, hydrogen, and oxygen, which include starches, cellulose, and sugars, and are an important source of energy. All carbohydrates are eventually broken down in the body to glucose, a simple sugar.

Glucose A simple sugar manufactured by the body from carbohydrates, fat, and to a lesser extent protein, which serves as the body's main source of fuel.

Glycogen The complex carbohydrate molecule used to store carbohydrates in the liver and muscle cells. When carbohydrate energy is needed, glycogen is converted into glucose for use by the muscle cells.

Fat One of the three main classes of foods and a source of energy in the body. Fats help the body use some vitamins and keep the skin healthy. They also serve as energy stores for the body. In food, there are two types of fats, saturated and unsaturated.

Triglycerides The chemical or substrate form in which most fat exists in food as well as in the body.

Protein Amino acids linked by peptide bonds, which consist of carbon, hydrogen, nitrogen, oxygen, and usually sulfur, and that have several essential biologic compounds.

Gluconeogenesis The formation of glucose from noncarbohydrate sources, such as amino acids.

Adenosine triphosphate
Energy storage and
transfer unit within the
cells of the body.

Adenosine diphosphate
A high-energy compound
occurring in all cells
from which adenosine
triphosphate (ATP) is
formed.

Energy and Muscle Contraction

Energy is used to form the myosin-actin cross-bridges that facilitate muscle contraction. At these cross-bridges is an enzyme that separates a phosphate from the ATP, releasing energy. The energy is needed to allow the cross-bridge to ratchet the thin actin filament toward the center of the sarcomere. Once that process is complete, another ATP is needed to release the cross-bridge so that it can flip back and grab the next actin active site and continue the contractile process. Thus, for one cycle of a cross-bridge, two ATPs are needed (6,8,9). When all the ATP is completely depleted, there is no energy to break the connection between cross-bridges and actin active sites, and the muscle goes into rigor.

Energy and Mechanical Work

Any form of exercise can be defined by two factors: intensity and duration. **Figure 4.2** illustrates the relationship of these factors. Lifting weights of very short duration with a high intensity is illustrated at point A. Running 400 meters is a slightly longer duration, still pretty intense activity (point B), whereas distance running is of a long duration and a lower intensity (point C). Identifying where an exercise is located within this relationship helps define the exercise's predominate energy system.

To perform mechanical work, the body needs fuel, which goes through a chemical process to provide energy. As stated earlier, the human body needs energy, which is obtained from the sun through ingestion of food. Moreover, the human body does not technically make energy, but rather transfers energy from the sun through food to the cells to perform their specific cellular and mechanical functions (6,8,9). ATP is a high-energy molecule that stores energy to be used in cellular and mechanical work, including exercise. Only about 40% of the energy released from ATP is actually used for cellular work, like muscle contraction. The remainder is released as heat (6,8,9).

FIGURE 4.2

Energy and mechanical
work.

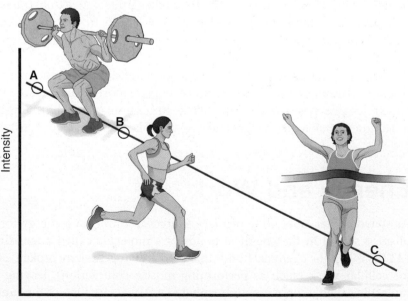

Adenosine Triphosphate

When the enzyme ATPase combines with an ATP molecule, it splits the last phosphate group away, releasing a large amount of free energy, approximately 7.3 kcal per unit of ATP (6,8,9). Once the phosphate group has been split off, what remains is ADP and an inorganic phosphate molecule (Pi).

$$ATP \Leftrightarrow ADP + Pi + energy\ release$$

Before ATP can release additional energy again, it must add back another phosphate group to ADP through a process called phosphorylation. There are three metabolic pathways in which cells can generate ATP:

1. The ATP-PC system
2. The glycolytic system (glycolysis)
3. The oxidative system (oxidative phosphorylation)

ATP-PC System

Once an ATP has been used, it must be replenished before it can provide energy again. By transferring a phosphate (and its accompanying energy) from another high-energy molecule called phosphocreatine (abbreviated as either PC or CP) to an ADP molecule, enough energy can be produced to facilitate one cross-bridge cycle. Together, ATP and PC are called phosphagens, and, therefore, this system is sometimes referred to as the phosphagen system. The process of creating a new ATP molecule from a phosphocreatine molecule (ATP-PC system) is the simplest and fastest of the energy systems **Figure 4.3** and occurs without the presence of oxygen (anaerobic) (1–9). The ATP-PC system provides energy for primarily high-intensity, short-duration bouts of exercise or activity. This can be seen in power and strength forms of training in which heavy loads are used with only a few repetitions, or during short sprinting events. For example, during an all-out sprint, the combination of ATP and PC stores could supply energy to all of the working muscles for only 10 to 15 seconds before complete exhaustion was reached (1–3,6–9). However, this system is activated at the onset of activity, regardless of intensity, because of its ability to produce energy very rapidly in comparison with the other systems (1–3,6–9).

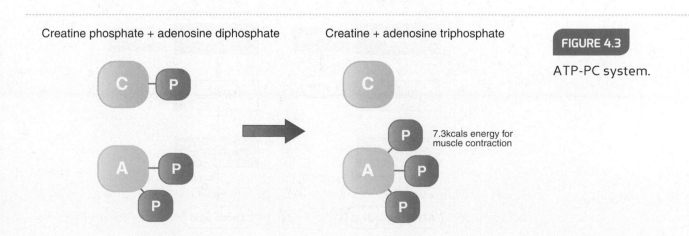

Creatine phosphate + adenosine diphosphate   Creatine + adenosine triphosphate

7.3kcals energy for muscle contraction

FIGURE 4.3

ATP-PC system.

Glycolysis

The other anaerobic means of producing ATP is through the chemical breakdown of glucose, a process referred to as anaerobic glycolysis. Before glucose or glycogen can generate energy, it must be converted to a compound called glucose-6-phosphate (5,6,8,9). It is important to understand at this point that the process of glycolysis does not begin until either glucose or glycogen is broken down into glucose-6-phosphate. And despite the fact that the overall goal of glycolysis is to produce energy, the conversion of glucose to glucose-6-phosphate actually uses up 1 ATP molecule, whereas with glycogen it does not (6,9). The end result of glycolysis in which glucose or glycogen is broken down to either pyruvic acid (aerobic glycolysis) or lactic acid (anaerobic glycolysis) is 2 ATP for each mole or unit of glucose and 3 ATP from each unit of glycogen (6,9) **Figure 4.4**.

Although this system can produce a significantly greater amount of energy than the ATP-PC system, it too is limited to approximately 30 to 50 seconds of duration (1–3,6–9). Most fitness workouts will place a greater stress on this system than the other systems because a typical repetition range of 8 to 12 repetitions falls within this time frame.

The Oxidative System

The most complex of the three energy systems is the process that uses substrates with the aid of oxygen to generate ATP. All three of the oxidative processes involved in the production of ATP involve oxygen and are thus referred to as aerobic processes. The three oxidative or aerobic systems include:

1. Aerobic glycolysis
2. The Krebs cycle
3. The electron transport chain (ETC)

FIGURE 4.4

Glycolysis.

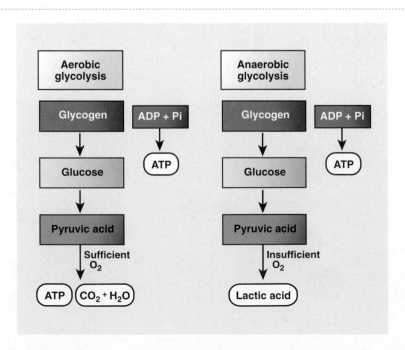

Whether glycolysis is aerobic or anaerobic, the process is the same; the presence of oxygen only determines the fate of the end product, pyruvic acid (without oxygen the end product is lactic acid), but in the presence of oxygen, pyruvic acid is converted into an important molecule in metabolism called acetyl coenzyme A (acetyl CoA) (1–9). Acetyl CoA is an important molecule because it contributes substrates for use in the second process of oxidative production of ATP, called the Krebs cycle. The complete oxidation of acetyl CoA produces two units of ATP and the by-products carbon dioxide and hydrogen **Figure 4.5**. Hydrogen ions released during glycolysis and during the Krebs cycle combine with other enzymes and in the third process of oxidation, ultimately provide energy for the oxidative phosphorylation of ADP to form ATP (electron transport chain). Depending on some details, the complete metabolism of a single glucose molecule produces between 35 and 40 ATP (6,9).

Remember that fat can also be metabolized aerobically. The first step in the oxidation of fat is a process referred to as **β-oxidation** (3–6,8,9). The process of β-oxidation begins with the breakdown of triglycerides into smaller subunits called free fatty acids (FFAs). The purpose of β-oxidation is to convert FFAs into acyl-CoA molecules, which then are available to enter the Krebs cycle and ultimately lead to the production of additional

β-oxidation The breakdown of triglycerides into smaller subunits called free fatty acids (FFAs) to convert FFAs into acyl-CoA molecules, which then are available to enter the Krebs cycle and ultimately lead to the production of additional ATP.

Did You Know?

Lactic Acid and Pain

If the concept of the pain from the acidity of lactic acid seems a little foreign, try running up a few flights of stairs and focus your attention on your thighs. That discomfort is from lactic acid accumulation. Notice also that the pain diminishes pretty quickly as the body metabolizes the lactic acid.

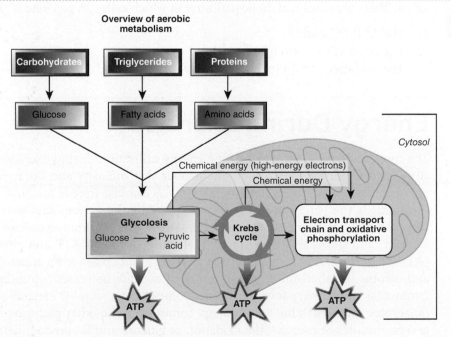

Overview of aerobic metabolism

FIGURE 4.5

The oxidative system.

ATP. Depending on what specific kind of fat is oxidized, say for example palmitic acid, one molecule produces 129 ATP molecules (6,9). Even though fat oxidation produces far more ATP per molecule of fat compared with a molecule of carbohydrate, fat oxidation requires more oxygen to produce ATP; thus carbohydrates are the preferred fuel substrate for the oxidative production of ATP.

The end results of the aerobic metabolism of carbohydrates and fats are water and carbon dioxide, both easily eliminated, especially when compared with lactic acid. The aerobic breakdown of glucose and fat takes much longer than the anaerobic metabolism of glucose and far longer than the ATP-PC cycle. Although speed of ATP production is not its strong point, aerobic metabolism has the capability to produce energy, at least for exercise, for an indefinite period of time. That is because everyone has an ample supply of storage fat.

SUMMARY

One of the primary sources of energy for cellular metabolism is stored in the chemical bonds of a molecule called ATP. When the chemical bonds that hold ATP together are broken, energy is released for cellular work, leaving behind another molecule called ADP. One of the functions of energy metabolism is to harness enough free energy to reattach a phosphate group to ADP and restore ATP levels back to normal.

Energy is used to form the myosin-actin cross-bridges that facilitate muscle contraction. For one cycle of a cross-bridge, two ATPs are needed. When all the ATP is completely depleted, there is no energy to break the connection between cross-bridges and actin active sites, and the muscle goes into rigor. Only about 40% of the energy released from ATP is actually used for cellular work, like muscle contraction. The remainder is released as heat.

Once an ATP has been used, it must be replenished before it can provide energy again. There are three metabolic pathways in which cells can generate ATP:

1. The ATP-PC system
2. The glycolytic system (glycolysis)
3. The oxidative system (oxidative phosphorylation)

Energy During Exercise

The most important factor regulating energy utilization during exercise is the intensity and duration of the exercise. Remember that intensity and duration of exercise are inversely related. In **Figure 4.6**, the x axis is exercise time at maximal capacity and the y axis is the percentage of energy supplied by the various fuel sources. The line labeled *Immediate energy systems* represents a very short-duration execise (for example a sprint) and shows that the primary fuel source is stored ATP and phosphocreatine (ATP-PC system), but a small portion of energy still comes from anaerobic glycolysis and aerobic metabolism. As the duration of exercise increases (up to approximately 2 minutes), the primary source of energy comes from anaerobic metabolism of glucose (anaerobic glycolysis), but some energy comes from the other pathways as well. After several minutes of exercise, the oxidation of glucose and fat predominates as the primary energy source.

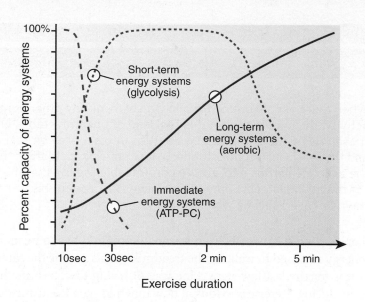

FIGURE 4.6

Energy during exercise.

The amount of energy available from stored ATP and phosphocreatine is small, whereas the amount of energy from stored carbohydrate has a greater capacity, but is still limited. The amount of available fuel for exercise from fats is essentially unlimited. Muscle glycogen also has a limited ability to supply fuel, and when glycogen stores are depleted, exercise intensity begins to slow as the primary energy supply turns from glycogen to fats. After 90 minutes of exercise, the majority of muscle glycogen stores are depleted. Through a combination of training and high carbohydrate intake, it is possible to store significantly greater quantities of glycogen, perhaps up to 50% more, allowing athletes to exercise for longer periods of before fatiguing or reaching a point of exhaustion (1–9).

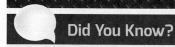

Did You Know?

Glycogen and Endurance

We have all heard that carbohydrate loading (aka glycogen loading, carbohydrate supercompensation, etc.) improves endurance performance. The extra glycogen does not let the runner run faster during the race; it allows the runner to maintain his or her pace for longer, slowing down later.

Metabolism During Steady-State Exercise

The bioenergetics of exercise can be indirectly measured in a laboratory using various modes of exercise (e.g., treadmill, cycle ergometer, rowing ergometer, cross-country ski simulator, swimming flume) while measuring the concentrations of oxygen and carbon dioxide and volume of expired air. Other physiologic functions can be measured as well, including heart rate, blood pressure, and exercise load or work output. Measurements made for the purpose of assessing exercise metabolism are typically made during periods of steady state. Steady-state exercise, as the term suggests, is exercise performed at a constant pace (intensity). For example, steady-state exercise could be described as walking at a brisk pace of 4 mph or 15:00 minutes per mile for a total of 15 minutes or 1 mile.

Did You Know?

Second Wind

When most people go out for a jog, a swim, or any other aerobic activity, the initial few minutes feel kind of uncomfortable, but after these few minutes, the exercise settles into a more comfortable pace and that earlier discomfort fades. Most physiologists think that when the exercise settles into a more comfortable feeling that the body has reached this plateau. Some people have referred to this as reaching their so-called second wind.

When considering steady-state exercise, an assumption has to be made that at the outset, the energy required to walk on the treadmill at this pace is the same for the first few steps as it is for the last few steps. One way of trying to determine how the body supplies energy during exercise is to look at how much oxygen it is using during specific periods of exercise. While standing over the treadmill belt, there is a low energy requirement that rises immediately (in a square wave response) when walking begins, stays constant for the duration of the walk, then declines back to the preexercise requirement immediately on stepping off the treadmill belt. The entire energy requirement of the 15 minutes of exercise can be visualized in **Figure 4.7**.

The oxygen consumption of supine (lying down) rest is less than seated rest, which is less than standing at rest. The simple anticipation of exercise raises the resting oxygen use before stepping on the treadmill, but Figure 4.7 begins with a subject straddling a treadmill belt set at 4 mph (segment A in Figure 4.7). On stepping on the belt, the physical demand on the body increases immediately, but the line showing oxygen consumption does not show the square wave response of the energy requirement. There is a fairly rapid increase in oxygen consumption that, a few minutes later, begins to plateau, and that plateau continues for the duration of the exercise. Once the exercise is complete and our subject steps off the treadmill, the oxygen consumption stays elevated for a short period before starting a rapid decline, then a slower decline before finally returning to baseline. If the caloric requirement exceeds the body's ability to deliver energy aerobically, the body will make up the difference anaerobically, regardless of when this occurs during exercise.

The body prefers aerobic or oxidative metabolism because carbon dioxide and water are more easily eliminated (1,3–6,9). At the start of exercise, however, aerobic metabolic pathways are too slow to meet these initial demands, so the body relies on the

FIGURE 4.7

Metabolism during steady-state exercise.

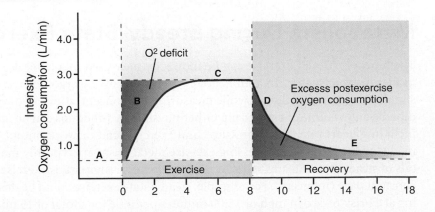

ATP-PC cycle (resulting in a reduction of ATP and PC levels and an increase in ADP and creatine) as well as from anaerobic metabolism of glucose early into the exercise period. The amount of unmet energy demand is the difference between the oxygen consumption curve and the box that represents total energy needs (the shaded area B above the oxygen consumption curve). Gradually, the rate of aerobic ATP production increases, and less and less energy is derived from anaerobic sources. Once the plateau has been reached, the energy demands of the exercise are being met by aerobic production of energy (segment C of Figure 4.7).

When the subject in this example steps off the treadmill, the energy demands fall back to baseline quickly (segment D) and then more slowly (segment E), but the oxygen consumption remains elevated for a short period to keep generating ATP aerobically. This shaded area is often referred to as **excess postexercise oxygen consumption,** or **EPOC** (1–9). ATP above and beyond what is needed (as evidenced by the still elevated oxygen consumption) for recovery is produced to help reestablish baseline levels of ATP and PC and to assist with clearing metabolic end products. Once the ATP and PC levels have been restored and other physiologic processes have returned to normal, oxygen consumption will have returned close to baseline, and immediate recovery will be mostly complete.

Excess postexercise oxygen consumption (EPOC) The state in which the body's metabolism is elevated after exercise.

Metabolism During Intermittent Work

The above example was that of a subject who had an increase in intensity (from rest to a 4-mph walk) followed by recovery. During intermittent exercise, as in many team sports, this same pattern occurs multiple times with every change in work requirement. When an athlete has to increase intensity (e.g., when movement speed transitions from a walk to a jog to a sprint), most of the energy needs come from anaerobic metabolism (1,2,6–9). When intensity is decreased (or the athlete experiences temporary fatigue), there is a continued period of high, but briefly elevated, oxygen consumption in an attempt to recover quickly to be ready for the next bout of higher intensity work (1,2,6–9). If the prior bout of high-intensity work is quite short, meaning it was probably fueled by ATP-PC, the recovery period is correspondingly brief; recovery of the ATP-PC cycle is complete in approximately 90 seconds. If the period of high-intensity work is longer, the recovery period will take longer. During intermittent exercise including sports, the ability to recover quickly is paramount. Moreover, recovery is an aerobic event to set ATP-PC concentrations back toward normal as well as the aerobic elimination of lactic acid. Thus, games really do need to have periods of training that address aerobic energy production despite the fact that games are not constant-pace exercise.

Estimating Fuel Contribution During Exercise

The respiratory quotient (RQ) is the amount of carbon dioxide (CO_2) expired divided by the amount of oxygen (O_2) consumed, measured during rest or at steady state of exercise using a metabolic analyzer (6,9). When $\dot{V}O_2$ and $\dot{V}CO_2$ are measured and the RQ calculated during steady-state exercise, the relative contribution of fats and carbohydrates as fuel sources can be determined. During steady-state exercise, an RQ of 1.0 indicates that carbohydrate is supplying 100% of the fuel, whereas an RQ of 0.7 indicates that fat is supplying 100% of the fuel for metabolism. Any RQ between 0.7 and 1.0 indicates a mixture of carbohydrates and fats are fueling metabolism. Table 4.1 shows just how the mixture of fuel changes depending on the RQ. Notice that this is a nonprotein RQ table as protein's minimal contribution to energy production during exercise is ignored.

TABLE 4.1	RQ and Percentage of Calories from Fats and Carbohydrates	
RQ	**Calories Derived from Carbohydrates (%)**	**Calories Derived from Fats (%)**
0.70	0.0	100.0
0.75	15.6	84.4
0.80	33.4	66.6
0.85	50.7	49.3
0.90	67.5	32.5
0.95	84.0	16.0
1.00	100.0	0.0

The Myth of the Fat-Burning Zone

There is another use of the RQ that some marketing departments of exercise equipment have misinterpreted, and that is the concept of the so-called fat-burning zone. The thought is that people burn more fat at lower-intensity exercise because such easy work does not require getting energy quickly from carbohydrates. Although this might be a logical concept, it is an inaccurate science.

To illustrate the fallacy of the fat-burning zone, it is important to compare two different exercise protocols. For example, an individual partaking in low-intensity fat-burning exercise such as 20 minutes of walking at 3.0 mph may result in an RQ of 0.80. An RQ of 0.80 results in 67% of energy coming from fats and 33% of energy from carbohydrates, respectively. Further, at this pace the individual expends 4.8 calories per minute; 3.2 of which (67%) comes from fat and 1.6 (33%) from carbohydrate. Thus, for the full 20 minutes the individual expends 64 calories from the metabolism of fat and only 32 calories from the metabolism of carbohydrates.

If this same individual doubled the intensity to 6 mph for the same 20 minutes, the added intensity would require more carbohydrate as a fuel source and a subsequent RQ of 0.86. An RQ of 0.86 results in 54% of energy coming from carbohydrates and only 46% of energy from fat. However, this pace resulted in 9.75 calories expended per minute or 5.2 and 4.48 calories per minute from carbohydrates and fats, respectively. Thus, for the full 20 minutes the individual expended 104 calories from carbohydrates and 90 calories from fat. This increase in intensity raised the total caloric expenditure from fats, for the same time investment, above that of the low-intensity walk, to the tune of about a 50% increase. Thus, the marketing statement that decreasing intensity puts one into a fat-burning zone is not entirely accurate. In this example, a slightly higher intensity resulted in a greater contribution from fat despite the increased reliance on carbohydrates as a fuel source.

SUMMARY

Although energy metabolism is very complex and confusing, a basic understanding of how the body uses energy for exercise forms the foundation for all exercise and training advice. A fundamental concept of exercise, training, and fatigue is specificity. Knowing the specific demands of an exercise guides almost all decisions regarding training so that athletes or fitness clients become adept at producing energy using the specific energy pathway for that exercise. Virtually every systemic response to exercise and adaptation to training can be traced back to the predominant source of fuel during any bout of exercise. Knowing this removes the guesswork and allows one to make exercise and training recommendations based on sound science. The body's responses to exercise and adaptations to training are all quite logical when related to energetics, making the adaptations to training outlined in this chapter far easier to understand.

REFERENCES

1. De Feo P, Di Loreto C, Lucidi P, et al. Metabolic response to exercise. *J Endocrinol Invest*. 2003;26:851–854.
2. Gastin PB. Energy system interaction and relative contribution during maximal exercise. *Sports Med*. 2001;31:725–741.
3. Glaister M. Multiple sprint work: physiological responses, mechanisms of fatigue and the influence of aerobic fitness. *Sports Med*. 2005;35:757–777.
4. Grassi B. Oxygen uptake kinetics: old and recent lessons from experiments on isolated muscle in situ. *Eur J Appl Physiol*. 2003;90 (3–4):242–249.
5. Johnson NA, Stannard SR, Thompson MW. Muscle triglyceride and glycogen in endurance exercise: implications for performance. *Sports Med*. 2004;34:151–164.
6. McArdle WD, FI Katch, VL Katch. *Exercise Physiology. Energy, Nutrition, and Human Performance*. 7th ed. Philadelphia: Lippincott Williams & Wilkins; 2010:134–169.
7. McMahon S, Jenkins D. Factors affecting the rate of phosphocreatine resynthesis following intense exercise. *Sports Med*. 2002;32(12):761–784.
8. Wells GD, Selvadurai H, Tein I. Bioenergetic provision of energy for muscular activity. *Paediatr Respir Rev*. 2009;10:83–90.
9. Howley ET, Powers SK. *Exercise Physiology: Theory and Application to Fitness and Performance*. 7th ed. New York: McGraw Hill; 2009:22–46.

Human Movement Science

Stock, Inc.
Relax/ShutterStock, Inc.

After studying this chapter, you will be able to:

✔ Explain the concept of functional multiplanar biomechanics including basic biomechanical terminology.

✔ Describe how muscle actions and outside forces relate to human movement.

✔ Explain the concepts of motor learning and motor control as they relate to exercise training.

Introduction to Human Movement Science

You will recall from chapter two that movement represents the integrated functioning of three main systems within the human body, the nervous system (central and peripheral), the skeletal (articular) system, and the muscular system. These collective components and structures represent the human movement system (HMS). Although separate in structure and function, the HMS relies on a collaborative effort to form interdependent links that form a functional kinetic chain. For example, your arm, shoulder, and spine are interconnected segments that function together to perform movement. If any part of the kinetic chain is injured or not functioning properly, the entire link is compromised, resulting in less than optimal performance. Body segments and their movements must be coordinated to allow for the efficient transfer of energy and power throughout the body, when moving from one body segment to the next **Figure 5.1**.

This chapter focuses on how the HMS works interdependently to learn and produce efficient human movement based on the principles of motor learning and biomechanics.

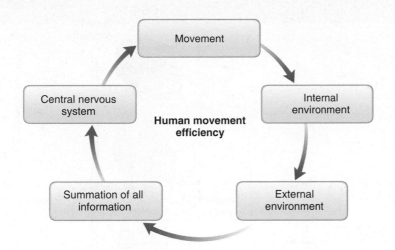

FIGURE 5.1

Human movement efficiency.

Biomechanics

Biomechanics or more appropriately sports biomechanics is the study of applying laws of mechanics and physics to determine how forces affect human movement and to better predict performance in athletic events. This chapter focuses on the motions that the HMS produces and the forces that act on it (1,2). Included within this chapter is a review of basic anatomic terminology, planes of motion, joint motions, muscle actions, force-couples, levers, forces, and the force-velocity relationship.

Biomechanics The science concerned with the internal and external forces acting on the human body and the effects produced by these forces.

Terminology

It is important for personal trainers to understand some of the basic terminology used in the study of biomechanics to be able not only to understand the science of biomechanics better but to apply the principles learned when assessing and prescribing exercise programs to clients.

Anatomic Locations

Anatomic location refers to terms that describe specific locations or landmarks on the body **Figure 5.2**. These include medial, lateral, contralateral, ipsilateral, anterior, posterior, proximal, distal, inferior, and superior.

Superior refers to a position above a reference point. The femur (thigh bone) is superior to the tibia (shin bone). The pectoralis major (chest muscle) is superior to the rectus abdominis (abdominal muscle).

Inferior refers to a position below a reference point. The calcaneus (heel bone) is inferior to the patella (knee bone). The soleus (calf muscle) is inferior to the hamstring complex.

Proximal refers to a position nearest the center of the body or point of reference. The knee is more proximal to the hip than the ankle. The lumbar spine (low back) is more proximal to the sacrum (tailbone) than the sternum (breast bone).

Distal refers to a position away from the center of the body or point of reference. The ankle is more distal to the hip than the knee. The sternum is more distal to the sacrum than the lumbar spine.

Anterior refers to a position on or toward the front of the body. The quadriceps are located on the anterior aspect of the thigh.

Superior Positioned above a point of reference.

Inferior Positioned below a point of reference.

Proximal Positioned nearest the center of the body, or point of reference.

Distal Positioned farthest from the center of the body, or point of reference.

Anterior (or ventral) On the front of the body.

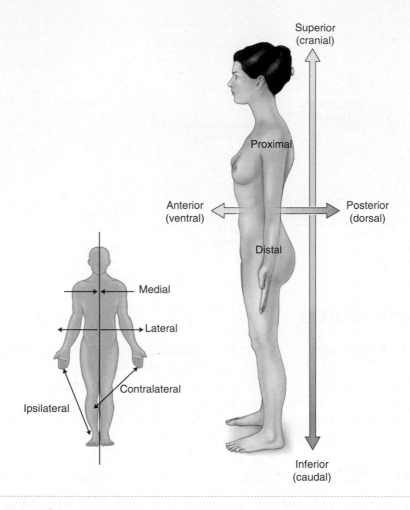

FIGURE 5.2

Anatomic locations.

Posterior refers to a position on or toward the back of the body. The hamstring complex is located on the posterior aspect of the thigh.

Medial refers to a position relatively closer to the midline of the body. The adductors (inner thigh muscles) are on the medial side of the thigh, because they are on the side of the limb closest to the midline of the body. The sternum is more medial than the shoulder.

Lateral refers to a position relatively farther away from the midline or toward the outside of the body. The ears are on the lateral side of the head.

Contralateral refers to a position on the opposite side of the body. The right foot is contralateral to the left hand.

Ipsilateral refers to a position on the same side of the body. The right foot is ipsilateral to the right hand.

Posterior (or dorsal) On the back of the body.

Medial Positioned near the middle of the body.

Lateral Positioned toward the outside of the body.

Contralateral Positioned on the opposite side of the body.

Ipsilateral Positioned on the same side of the body.

Planes of Motion, Axes, and Joint Motions

The universally accepted method of describing human movements is in three dimensions and is based on a system of planes and axes **Figure 5.3**. Three imaginary planes are positioned through the body at right angles so they intersect at the center of mass of the body. They include the sagittal, frontal, and transverse planes. Movement is said to occur more commonly in a specific plane if it is actually along the plane or parallel to it. Although movements can be one-plane dominant, no motion occurs strictly in one plane of motion. Movement in a plane occurs on an axis running perpendicular to that plane, much like the axle that a car wheel revolves around. This is known as *joint*

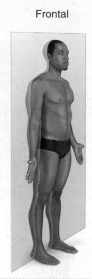 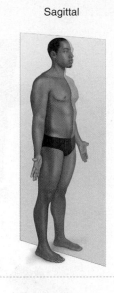 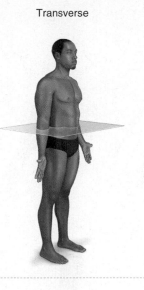

Frontal   Sagittal   Transverse

© Holab/ShutterStock, Inc.

FIGURE 5.3

Planes of motion.

motion. Joint motions are termed for their action in each of the three planes of motion **Table 5.1**. When applying these principles, it is important to keep in mind that anatomic nomenclatures occur according to the body in the **anatomic position**.

The Sagittal Plane

The **sagittal plane** bisects the body into right and left sides. Sagittal plane motion occurs around a coronal axis (1–3). Movements in the sagittal plane include flexion and extension **Figure 5.4**. **Flexion** is a bending movement in which the relative

Anatomic position The position with the body erect with the arms at the sides and the palms forward. The anatomic position is of importance in anatomy because it is the position of reference for anatomic nomenclature. Anatomic terms such as anterior and posterior, medial and lateral, and abduction and adduction apply to the body when it is in the anatomic position.

Sagittal plane An imaginary bisector that divides the body into left and right halves.

Flexion A bending movement in which the relative angle between two adjacent segments decreases.

TABLE 5.1 Examples of Planes, Motions, and Axes

© Holab/ShutterStock, Inc.

Plane	Motion	Axis	Example
Sagittal	Flexion/extension	Coronal	Biceps curl Triceps pushdown Squat Front lunge Calf raise Walking Running Vertical jumping Climbing stairs
Frontal	Adduction/abduction Lateral flexion Eversion/inversion	Anterior-posterior	Side lateral raise Side lunge Side shuffle
Transverse	Internal rotation External rotation Left/right rotation Horizontal adduction Horizontal abduction	Longitudinal	Trunk rotation Throwing Golfing Swinging a bat

FIGURE 5.4

Flexion/Extension movements.
A. Dorsiflexion.
B. Plantar flexion.
C. Knee flexion.
D. Knee extension.
E. Hip flexion: femoral-on-pelvic rotation.
F. Hip flexion: pelvic-on-femoral rotation.
G. Hip extension.
H. Spinal flexion.
I. Spinal extension.
J. Elbow flexion.
K. Elbow extension.
L. Shoulder flexion.
M. Shoulder extension.
N. Cervical flexion.
O. Cervical extension.

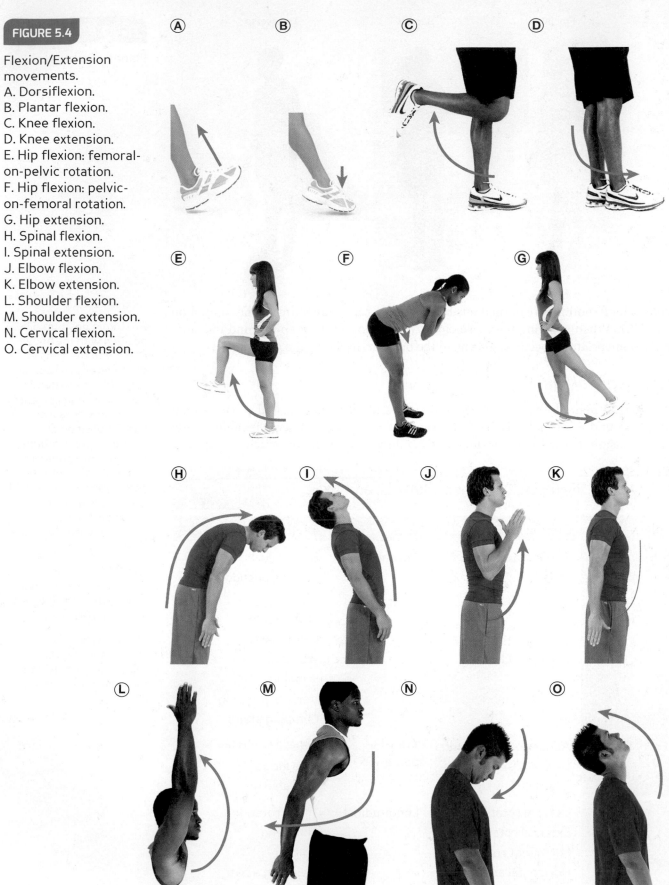

angle between two adjacent segments decreases (2,4). **Extension** is a straightening movement in which the relative angle between two adjacent segments increases (2,5). Note, **hyperextension** is the extension of a joint beyond the normal limit or range of motion and often results in injury. Flexion and extension occur in many joints in the body including the spine, shoulder, elbow, wrist, hip, knee, foot, and hand. At the ankle, flexion is referred to as dorsiflexion and extension is plantar flexion (1,2,5). Examples of predominantly sagittal plane movements include biceps curls, triceps pushdowns, squats, front lunges, calf raises, walking, running, vertical jump, climbing stairs, and shooting a basketball.

Did You Know?

Hip Flexion in the Sagittal Plane

Hip flexion occurs when an individual decreases the angle between the femur (thigh bone) and the pelvis or lumbar spine. This can occur when an individual elevates the knee toward the abdomen (femoral-on-pelvic hip rotation). During this motion the pelvis and spine are fixed while the femur rotates. Another version of hip flexion can occur when an individual bends forward from the trunk (as if touching the toes). In this instance the pelvis and lumbar spine rotate together over a fixed femur (pelvic-on-femoral rotation).

The Frontal Plane

The **frontal plane** bisects the body to create front and back halves. Frontal plane motion occurs around an anterior-posterior axis (1–3). Movements in the frontal plane include abduction and adduction in the limbs (relative to the trunk), lateral flexion of the spine, and eversion and inversion at the foot and ankle complex (1–3,5) **Figure 5.5**. **Abduction** is a movement away from the midline of the body, or similar to extension, it is an increase in the angle between two adjoining segments, but in the frontal plane (1–3,5). **Adduction** is a movement of the segment toward the midline of the body, or like flexion, it is a decrease in the angle between two adjoining segments, but in the frontal plane (1–3,5). Lateral flexion is the bending of the spine (cervical, thoracic, or lumbar) from side to side or simply side-bending (1–3,5). Eversion and inversion follow the same principle, but relate more specifically to the movement of the calcaneus (heel bone) and tarsals (ankle bones) in the frontal plane (1–3,5). Examples of frontal plane movements include side lateral raises, side lunges, and side shuffling.

The Transverse Plane

The **transverse plane** bisects the body to create upper and lower halves. Transverse plane motion occurs around a longitudinal or vertical axis (1–3). Movements in the transverse plane include **internal rotation** and **external rotation** for the limbs, right and left rotation for the head and trunk, **horizontal abduction** and **horizontal adduction** of the limbs, and radioulnar (forearm) pronation and supination **Figure 5.6** (1–3).

The foot, because it is a unique entity, has transverse plane motion termed abduction (toes pointing outward, externally rotated) and adduction (toes pointing inward, internally rotated) (2). Examples of transverse plane movements include cable trunk rotations, dumbbell chest fly, throwing a ball, throwing a Frisbee, golfing, and swinging a bat.

Extension A straightening movement in which the relative angle between two adjacent segments increases.

Hyperextension Extension of a joint beyond the normal limit or range of motion.

Frontal plane An imaginary bisector that divides the body into front and back halves.

Abduction A movement in the frontal plane away from the midline of the body.

Adduction Movement in the frontal plane back toward the midline of the body.

Transverse plane An imaginary bisector that divides the body into top and bottom halves.

Internal rotation Rotation of a joint toward the middle of the body.

External rotation Rotation of a joint away from the middle of the body.

Horizontal abduction Movement of the arm or thigh in the transverse plane from an anterior position to a lateral position.

Horizontal adduction Movement of the arm or thigh in the transverse plane from a lateral position to an anterior position.

© Ilolab/ShutterStock, Inc.

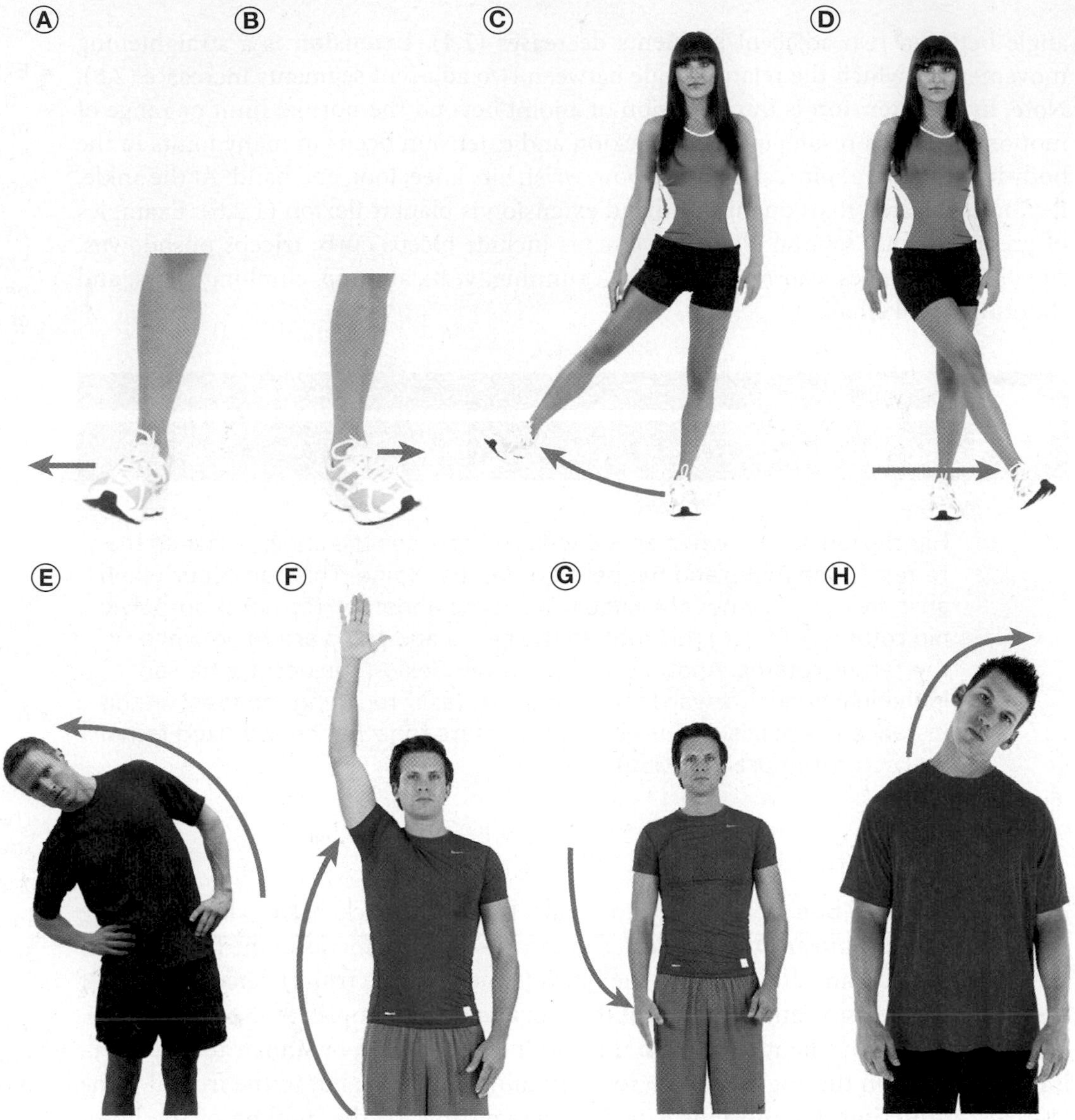

FIGURE 5.5

Adduction
and abduction
movements.
A. Eversion.
B. Inversion.
C. Hip abduction.
D. Hip adduction.
E. Lateral flexion.
F. Shoulder
abduction.
G. Shoulder
adduction.
H. Cervical lateral
flexion.

Scapular Motion

Scapular retraction
Adduction of scapula;
shoulder blades move
toward the midline.

Scapular protraction
Abduction of scapula;
shoulder blades move
away from the midline.

Scapular depression
Downward (inferior)
motion of the scapula.

Scapular elevation
Upward (superior) motion
of the scapula.

Motions of the shoulder blades (or scapulae) are important for the fitness professional to be familiar with to ensure proper movement of the shoulder complex. Scapular movements are primarily retraction (also termed adduction), protraction (also termed abduction), elevation, and depression **Figure 5.7**. **Scapular retraction** occurs when the shoulder blades come closer together. **Scapular protraction** occurs when the shoulder blades move further away from each other. **Scapular depression** occurs when the shoulder blades move downward, whereas **scapular elevation** occurs when the shoulder blades move upward toward the ears.

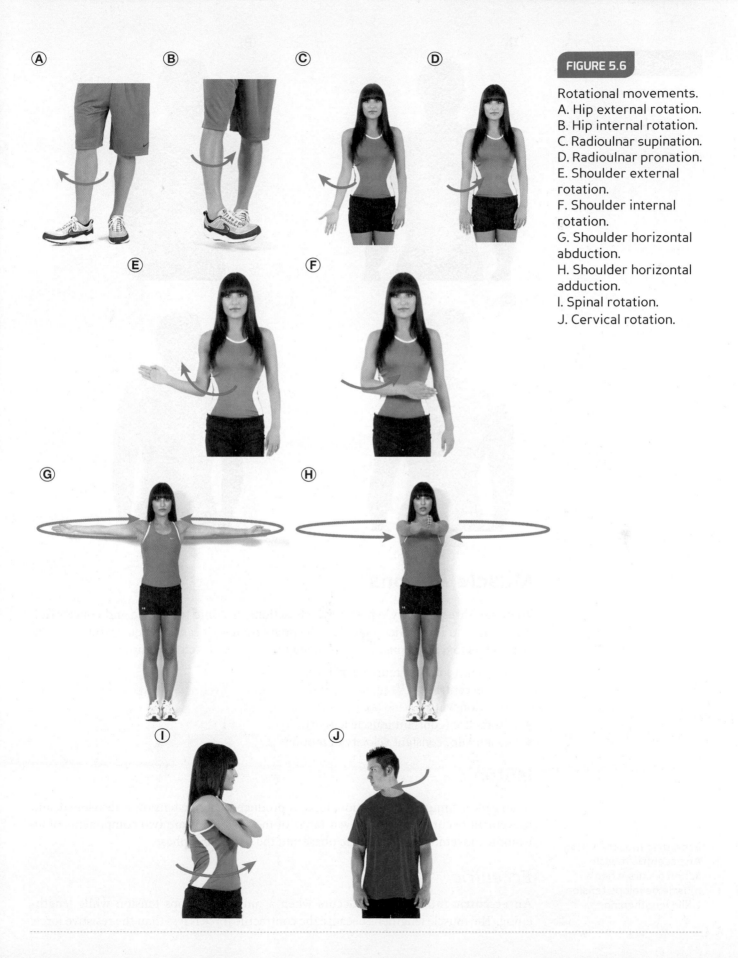

FIGURE 5.6

Rotational movements.
A. Hip external rotation.
B. Hip internal rotation.
C. Radioulnar supination.
D. Radioulnar pronation.
E. Shoulder external rotation.
F. Shoulder internal rotation.
G. Shoulder horizontal abduction.
H. Shoulder horizontal adduction.
I. Spinal rotation.
J. Cervical rotation.

FIGURE 5.7

Scapular movements.
A. Scapular retraction.
B. Scapular protraction.
C. Scapular depression.
D. Scapular elevation.

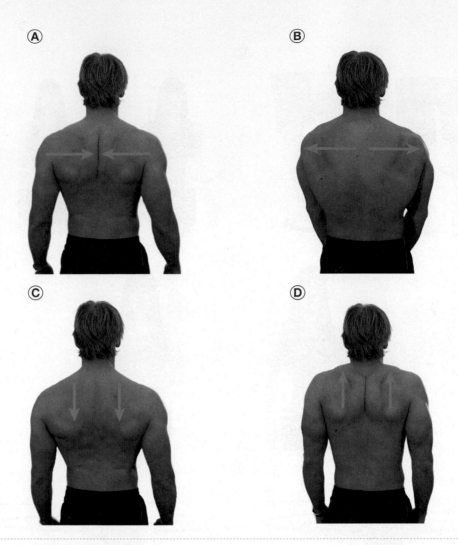

Muscle Actions

There are three primary types of muscle actions: isotonic (eccentric and concentric), isometric, and isokinetic **Table 5.2**. The prefix *iso* means same or equal, and the suffix *tonic* refers to tension, *metric* refers to length, and *kinetic* refers to motion.

- Isotonic (constant muscle tension)
  - » Eccentric
  - » Concentric
- Isometric (constant muscle length)
- Isokinetic (constant velocity of motion)

Isotonic

In an isotonic muscle contraction, force is produced, muscle tension is developed, and movement occurs through a given range of motion. There are two components of an isotonic movement: the eccentric phase and the concentric phase.

Eccentric

Eccentric muscle action
An eccentric muscle action occurs when a muscle develops tension while lengthening.

An **eccentric muscle action** occurs when a muscle develops tension while lengthening. The muscle lengthens because the contractile force is less than the resistive force.

TABLE 5.2	Muscle Action Spectrum

Action	Performance
Isotonic	Force is produced, muscle tension is developed, and movement occurs through a given range of motion
Eccentric	Moving in the same direction as the resistance Decelerates or reduces force
Concentric	Moving in opposite direction of force Accelerates or produces force
Isometric	No visible movement with or against resistance Dynamically stabilizes force
Isokinetic	The speed of movement is fixed, and resistance varies with the force exerted Requires sophisticated training equipment often seen in rehabilitation or exercise physiology laboratories

The overall tension within the muscle is less than the external forces trying to lengthen the muscle. As the muscle lengthens, the actin and myosin cross-bridges are pulled apart and reattach, allowing the muscle to lengthen (2,5). In actuality, the lengthening of the muscle usually refers to its return to a resting length and not actually increasing in its length as if it were being stretched (5).

An eccentric motion is synonymous with deceleration and can be observed in many movements such as landing from a jump, or more commonly seen in a gym as lowering the weight during a resistance exercise. Eccentric muscle action is also known as "a negative" in the health and fitness industry. The term *negative* was derived from the fact that in eccentric movement, work is actually being done on the muscle (because forces move the muscle) rather than the muscle doing the work (or the muscle moving the forces) (2,5). This is related to the fact that eccentric motion moves in the same direction as the resistance is moving (known as direction of resistance) (1,2,5).

In functional activities, such as daily movements and sports, muscles work as much eccentrically as they do concentrically or isometrically (6). Eccentrically, the muscles must decelerate or reduce the forces acting on the body (or force reduction). This is seen in all forms of resistance training exercise. Whether walking on a treadmill or bench pressing, the weight of either the body or the bar must be decelerated and then stabilized to be properly accelerated.

Concentric

A **concentric muscle action** occurs when the contractile force is greater than the resistive force, resulting in shortening of the muscle and visible joint movement. As the muscle shortens, the actin and myosin cross-bridges move together (known as sliding-filament theory), allowing the muscle to shorten (2,5). A concentric muscle action is synonymous with acceleration and can be observed in many movements such as jumping upward, and the "lifting" phase during a resistance training exercise.

Concentric muscle action When a muscle is exerting force greater than the resistive force, resulting in shortening of the muscle.

Isometric

An **isometric muscle action** occurs when the contractile force is equal to the resistive force, leading to no visible change in the muscle length (2,5). An isometric contraction can easily be observed when an individual pauses during a resistance training exercise in between the lifting and lowering phases.

In activities of daily living and sports, isometric actions are used to dynamically stabilize the body. This can be seen in muscles that are isometrically stabilizing a limb from moving in an unwanted direction. For example, the adductors and abductors of the thigh during a squat will dynamically stabilize the leg from moving too much in the frontal and transverse planes (5,6). During a ball crunch, the transversus abdominis and multifidus muscles (deep spine muscles) stabilize the lumbar spine. During a dumbbell bench press, the rotator cuff musculature dynamically stabilizes the shoulder joint.

Isokinetic

During **isokinetic muscle actions**, the muscle shortens at a constant speed over the full range of motion. An isokinetic muscle action requires the use of expensive and sophisticated equipment that measures the amount of force generated by the muscles and adjusts the resistance (load) so that no matter how much muscular tension is produced, movement remains constant. In other words, the harder an individual pushes or pulls, the more resistance they feel. During a full isokinetic contraction, the tension in the muscle is at its maximum throughout the whole range of motion, which is believed to improve strength, endurance, and neuromuscular efficiency. However, the types of movements that are able to be performed on isokinetic machines are rather limited and often only seen in rehabilitation clinics or exercise physiology laboratories.

Example of Muscle Actions

Let's use the example of a biceps curl exercise to illustrate muscle actions. If an individual is performing a biceps curl, the initial movement requires the biceps to shorten to generate force to overcome gravity and the weight of the dumbbell in the individual's hand (or weight stack if using a machine), allowing the elbows to flex and the dumbbells to move up toward the front of the shoulder **Figure 5.8**. This is the concentric phase of the exercise. Once the dumbbells are raised to the front of the shoulder, the individual holds this position. Because the length of the muscle does not change while holding this position, but the biceps muscles are still applying force and under tension, this is considered the isometric portion of the exercise. As the individual lowers the dumbbells down back to the starting position, the biceps muscles must now lengthen (under the control of the nervous system) to decelerate the force of the dumbbells and gravity. This is the eccentric portion of the exercise **Figure 5.9**.

A second example to help illustrate muscle actions is the squat exercise. To initiate the squat from a standing position the individual squats down, flexing at the hips, knees, and ankles **Figure 5.10**. This is an example of an eccentric muscle action. The individual is in the "lowering" phase of a resistance exercise. Moreover, as the individual squats downward, the gluteal muscles and quadriceps mechanically lengthen while simultaneously decelerating the force of their body weight and gravity. The isometric muscle action occurs when the individual pauses at the bottom position and no joint motion is visible. And lastly, the concentric muscle action occurs when the individual returns to the starting position (lifting phase), contracting the gluteal muscles and quadriceps **Figure 5.11**.

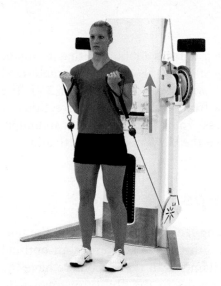

FIGURE 5.8 Biceps curl concentric motion.

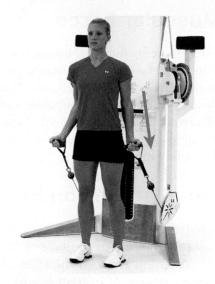

FIGURE 5.9 Biceps curl eccentric motion.

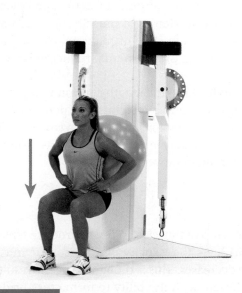

FIGURE 5.10 Squat eccentric motion.

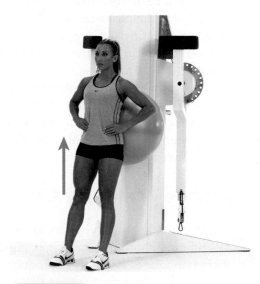

FIGURE 5.11 Squat concentric motion.

Functional Anatomy of Muscles

The traditional perception of muscles is that they work concentrically and predominantly in one plane of motion. However, to more effectively understand motion and design efficient training, reconditioning, and injury prevention programs, it is important to view muscles functioning in all planes of motion and through the entire muscle action spectrum (eccentric, isometric, and concentric). In addition, several muscles work synergistically to produce force, stabilize the body, and reduce force under direct control of the nervous system. Rarely do muscles work in isolation.

The more that functional anatomy is understood, the more specific an exercise prescription can become. A lack of understanding of the synergistic function of the HMS muscles in all three planes of motion commonly leads to a lack of optimal performance and the potential of developing muscle imbalances (see Appendix D for detailed description of HMS muscles).

Muscular Force

Force An influence applied by one object to another, which results in an acceleration or deceleration of the second object.

Force is defined as the interaction between two entities or bodies that result in either the acceleration or deceleration of an object (1,2,7). Forces are characterized by magnitude (how much) and direction (which way they are moving) (1,2,7). The HMS is designed to manipulate variable forces from a multitude of directions to effectively produce movement. As such, the fitness professional must gain an understanding of some of the more pertinent forces that the HMS must deal with and how they affect motion.

Length-Tension Relationships

Length-tension relationship The resting length of a muscle and the tension the muscle can produce at this resting length.

Length-tension relationship refers to the resting length of a muscle and the tension the muscle can produce at this resting length (2,8–13). There is an optimal muscle length at which the actin and myosin filaments in the sarcomere have the greatest degree of overlap **Figure 5.12**. This results in the ability of myosin to make a maximal amount of connections with actin and thus results in the potential for maximal force production of that muscle. Lengthening a muscle beyond this optimal length and then stimulating it reduces the amount of actin and myosin overlap, reducing force production. Similarly, shortening a muscle too much and then stimulating it places the actin and myosin in a state of maximal overlap and allows for no further movement to occur between the filaments, reducing its force output (2,8–13).

It is important for personal trainers to understand the length-tension relationship because if muscle lengths are altered, for example, misaligned joints (i.e., poor posture), then they will not generate the needed force to allow for efficient movement. If one component of the HMS (nervous, skeletal, or muscular) is not functioning as it should, it will have a direct effect on the efficiency of human movement.

Force-Velocity Curve

The force-velocity curve refers to the relationship of muscle's ability to produce tension at differing shortening velocities **Figure 5.13**. As the velocity of a concentric muscle action increases, its ability to produce force decreases. This is thought to be the result of overlapping the actin filament that may interfere with its ability to form cross-bridges with myosin. Conversely, with eccentric muscle action, as the velocity of muscle action

FIGURE 5.12

Length-tension relationship.

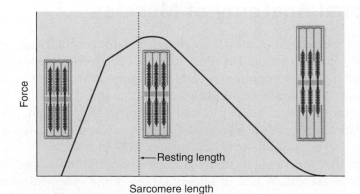

Force

Resting length

Sarcomere length

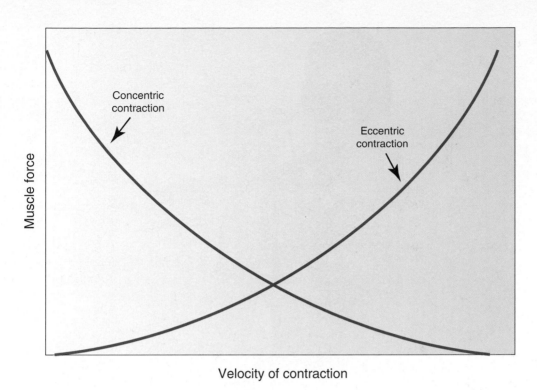

© Holab/ShutterStock, Inc.

FIGURE 5.13

The force-velocity curve.

Concentric contraction

Eccentric contraction

Muscle force

Velocity of contraction

increases, the ability to develop force increases. This is believed to be the result of the use of the elastic component of the connective tissue surrounding and within the muscle (1,5,7,14).

Force-Couple Relationships

Muscles produce a force that is transmitted to bones through their connective tissues (tendons). Because muscles are recruited as groups, many muscles will transmit force onto their respective bones, creating movement at the joints (15–18). This synergistic action of muscles to produce movement around a joint is also known as a **force-couple** (4,5). Muscles in a force-couple provide divergent pulls on the bone or bones they connect with. This is a result of the fact that each muscle has different attachment sites, pulls at a different angle, and creates a different force on that joint. The motion that results from these forces is dependent on the structure of the joint and the collective pull of each muscle involved **Figure 5.14, Table 5.3** (2,5).

In reality, however, every movement produced must involve all muscle actions (eccentric, isometric, concentric) and all functions (agonists, synergists, stabilizers, and antagonists) to ensure proper joint motion as well as to eliminate unwanted or unnecessary motion. Thus, all muscles working in unison to produce the desired movement are said to be working in a force-couple (2). To ensure that the HMS moves properly, it must exhibit proper force-couple relationships, which can only happen if the muscles are at the right length-tension relationships and the joints have proper arthrokinematics (or joint motion). Collectively, proper length-tension relationships, force-couple relationships, and arthrokinematics allow for proper sensorimotor integration and ultimately proper and efficient movement (2).

Force-couple Muscle groups moving together to produce movement around a joint.

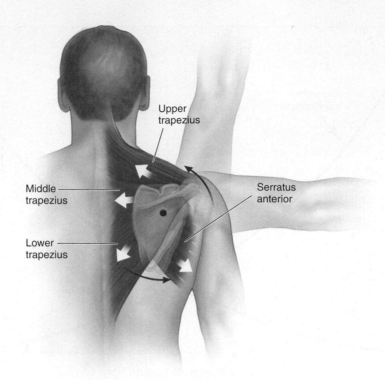

FIGURE 5.14

Force-couple relationship.

TABLE 5.3	Common Force-Couples
Muscles	**Movement Created**
Internal and external obliques	Trunk rotation
Upper trapezius and the lower portion of the serratus anterior	Upward rotation of the scapula
Gluteus maximus, quadriceps, and calf muscles	Produce hip and knee extension during walking, running, stair climbing, etc.
Gastrocnemius, peroneus longus, and tibialis posterior	Performing plantarflexion at the foot and ankle complex
Deltoid and rotator cuff	Performing shoulder abduction

Muscular Leverage and Arthrokinematics

The amount of force that the HMS can produce is not only dependent on motor unit recruitment and muscle size, but also the lever system of the joint. The musculoskeletal system is composed of bones, muscles, tendons, and ligaments, all of which create a series of levers and pulleys that generate force against external objects. Skeletal muscles are attached to bone by tendons, and produce movement by bending the skeleton at movable joints. Joint motion is caused by muscles pulling on bones; muscles cannot actively push. Particular attachments of muscles to bones will determine how much force the muscle is capable of generating. For example the quadriceps muscles can produce more force than muscles of the hand.

Most motion uses the principle of levers. A lever consists of a rigid "bar" that pivots around a stationary fulcrum (pivot point). In the human body, the fulcrum is the joint axis, bones are the levers, muscles create the motion (effort), and resistance can be the weight of a body part, or the weight of an object (such as barbells and dumbbells) (1).

Levers are classified by first, second, and third class, depending on the relations among the fulcrum, the effort, and the resistance **Figure 5.15**. First-class levers have the fulcrum in the middle, like a seesaw. Nodding the head is an example of a first-class lever, with the top of the spinal column as the fulcrum (joint axis). Second-class levers have a resistance in the middle (with the fulcrum and effort on either side), like a load in a wheelbarrow. The body acts as a second-class lever when one engages in a full-body push-up or calf raise. If using the calf raise as an example, the ball of the foot is the fulcrum, the body weight is the resistance, and the effort is applied by the calf musculature. Third-class levers have the effort placed between the resistance and the fulcrum. The effort always travels a shorter distance and must be greater than the resistance. Most limbs of the human body are operated as third-class levers (7). An example of a third-class lever is the human forearm: the fulcrum is the elbow, the effort is applied by the biceps muscle, and the load is in the hand such as a dumbbell when performing a biceps curl.

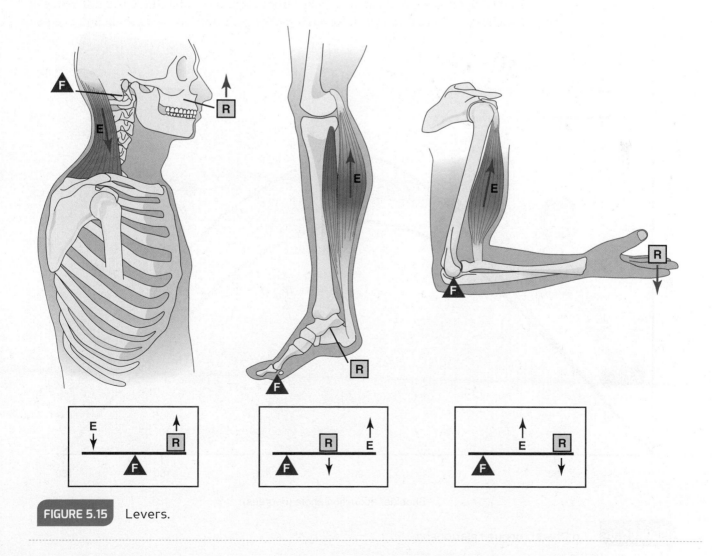

FIGURE 5.15   Levers.

Rotary motion
Movement of the bones around the joints.

Torque A force that produces rotation. Common unit of torque is the newton-meter or Nm.

Applying the principle of the HMS to the concept of levers, bones act as lever arms that move a load from the force applied by the muscles. This movement around an axis can be termed **rotary motion** and implies that the levers (bones) rotate around the axis (joints) (1,2,5). This turning effect of the joint is often referred to as **torque** (1,2,5).

In resistance training, torque is applied so we can move our joints. Because the neuromuscular system is ultimately responsible for manipulating force, the amount of leverage the HMS will have (for any given movement) depends on the leverage of the muscles in relation to the resistance. The difference between the distance that the weight is from the center of the joint and the muscle's attachment and line of pull (direction through which tension is applied through the tendon) is from the joint will determine the efficiency with which the muscles manipulate the movement (1,2,5). As we cannot alter the attachment sites or the line of pull of our muscles through the tendon, the easiest way to alter the amount of torque generated at a joint is to move the resistance. In other words, the closer the weight is to the point of rotation (the joint), the less torque it creates **Figure 5.16**. The farther away the weight is from the point of rotation, the more torque it creates.

For example, when holding a dumbbell straight out to the side at arm's length (shoulder abduction), the weight may be approximately 24 inches from the center of the shoulder joint. The prime mover for shoulder abduction is the deltoid muscle. If its attachment is approximately 2 inches from the joint center, there is a difference of 22 inches (11 times greater). However, if the weight is moved closer to the joint center,

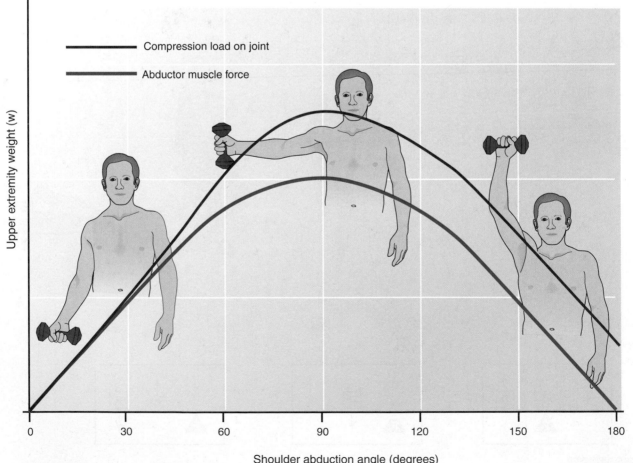

FIGURE 5.16 Load and torque relationship.

to the elbow, the resistance is only approximately 12 inches from the joint center. Now the difference is only 10 inches or 5 times greater. Essentially, the weight was reduced by half. Many people performing side lateral raises with dumbbells (raising dumbbells out to the side) do this inadvertently by bending their elbow and bringing the weight closer to the shoulder joint. Personal trainers can use this principle as a regression to exercises that are too demanding by reducing the torque placed on the HMS, or as a progression to increase the torque and place a greater demand on the HMS.

SUMMARY

The study of biomechanics looks at how internal and external forces affect the way the body moves. To understand the body and communicate about it effectively, a personal trainer must be familiar with the terminology for the various anatomic locations. It is also important to know how the body moves in the sagittal, frontal, and transverse planes as well as the joint motions in each of these planes.

There are three types of muscle movements: eccentrically (to decelerate force), isometrically (to stabilize), or concentrically (to accelerate force). Each muscle should be studied at length to examine its functions as well as how it moves synergistically with others. In addition, an isokinetic muscle action occurs at a constant speed, requiring expensive and sophisticated equipment.

Muscles are influenced by outside forces from a multitude of directions. To compensate they produce corresponding forces in groups to move bones and joints, in force-couple actions. However, the amount of force that can be produced is dependent on leverage (or how far a weight being moved is from the joint). This leverage directly affects rotary motion and torque.

Motor Behavior

Motor behavior is the HMS response to internal and external environmental stimuli. The study of motor behavior examines the manner by which the nervous, skeletal, and muscular systems interact to produce skilled movement using sensory information from internal and external environments.

Motor behavior is the collective study of motor control, motor learning, and motor development (19) **Figure 5.17**. **Motor control** is the study of posture and movements with the involved structures and mechanisms used by the central nervous system to assimilate and integrate sensory information with previous experiences (16,17). Motor control is concerned with what central nervous system structures are involved with motor behavior to produce movement (16). **Motor learning** is the utilization of these processes through practice and experience, leading to a relatively permanent change in one's capacity to produce skilled movements (20). Finally, **motor development** is defined as the change in motor behavior over time throughout the lifespan (21). For the purposes of this text we will confine this section to a brief discussion of motor control and motor learning.

Motor Control

To move in an organized and efficient manner, the HMS must exhibit precise control over its collective segments. This segmental control is an integrated process involving

Motor behavior Motor response to internal and external environmental stimuli.

Motor control How the central nervous system integrates internal and external sensory information with previous experiences to produce a motor response.

Motor learning Integration of motor control processes through practice and experience, leading to a relatively permanent change in the capacity to produce skilled movements.

Motor development The change in motor skill behavior over time throughout the lifespan.

FIGURE 5.17

Motor behavior.

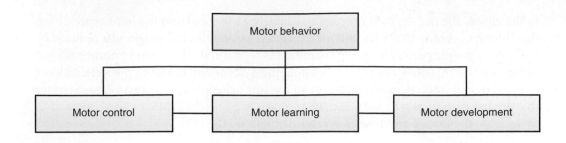

neural, skeletal, and muscular components to produce appropriate motor responses. This process (and the study of these movements) is known as motor control and focuses on the involved structures and mechanisms used by the central nervous system to integrate internal and external sensory information with previous experiences to produce a skilled motor response. Motor control is concerned with the neural structures that are involved with motor behavior and how they produce movement (16,20,22,23).

Muscle Synergies

Muscle synergies
Groups of muscles that are recruited by the central nervous system to provide movement.

One of the most important concepts in motor control is that muscles are recruited by the central nervous system as groups (or **muscle synergies**) (15,16–18). This simplifies movement by allowing muscles and joints to operate as a functional unit (9). Through practice of proper movement patterns (proper exercise technique), these synergies become more fluent and automated Table 5.4.

Proprioception

Proprioception The cumulative sensory input to the central nervous system from all mechanoreceptors that sense position and limb movements.

The mechanoreceptors, discussed in chapter two, collectively feed the nervous system with a form of sensory information known as **proprioception**. Proprioception uses information from the mechanoreceptors (muscle spindle, Golgi tendon organ, and joint receptors) to provide information about body position, movement, and sensation as it pertains to muscle and joint force (17). Proprioception is a vital source of information that the nervous system uses to gather information about the environment to produce the most efficient movement (24). Research has demonstrated that proprioception is altered after injury. This becomes relevant for the personal trainer as 80% of the adult population experiences low-back pain, and an estimated 80,000 to 100,000 anterior cruciate ligament (ACL) injuries occur annually. This means that many of today's health club members may have altered proprioception as a result of past injuries. This provides a rationale for core and balance training to enhance one's proprioceptive capabilities, increasing postural control, and decreasing tissue overload.

Sensorimotor Integration

Sensorimotor integration The cooperation of the nervous and muscular system in gathering and interpreting information and executing movement.

Sensorimotor integration is the ability of the nervous system to gather and interpret sensory information and to select and execute the proper motor response (2,16,24–30). The definition implies that the nervous system ultimately dictates movement. Sensorimotor integration is effective as long as the quality of incoming

TABLE 5.4	Common Muscle Synergies	
Exercise	**Muscle Synergies**	
Squat 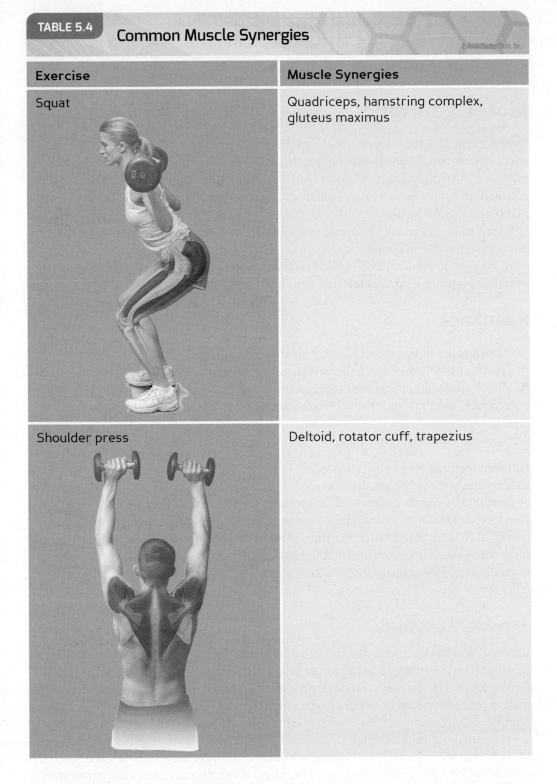	Quadriceps, hamstring complex, gluteus maximus	
Shoulder press	Deltoid, rotator cuff, trapezius	

sensory information is good (2,27–29). Individuals that train using improper form will develop improper sensory information delivered to the central nervous system, leading to movement compensations and potential injury. It is therefore important to create properly designed exercise programs and encourage clients to train with correct technique at all times. For example, if an individual consistently performs a chest press while rounding and elevating the shoulders, it can lead to altered length-tension relationships of muscles (altered muscle length), altered force-couple relationships (improper recruitment pattern of muscles), and altered arthrokinematics (improper joint motion), ultimately leading to shoulder impingement or other forms of shoulder injury.

Motor Learning

Motor learning is the integration of motor control processes, with practice and experience, leading to a relatively permanent change in the capacity to produce skilled movements (2,16,19). The study of motor learning looks at how movements are learned and retained for future use. Examples include riding a bike, throwing a baseball, playing the piano, or even performing a squat. In these examples, proper practice and experience will lead to a permanent change in one's ability to perform the movement efficiently. For a movement to occur repeatedly sensory information and sensorimotor integration must be used to aid the HMS in the development of permanent neural representations of motor patterns, a process referred to as feedback.

Feedback

Feedback The use of sensory information and sensorimotor integration to help the human movement system in motor learning.

Feedback is the utilization of sensory information and sensorimotor integration to aid the HMS in the development of permanent neural representations of motor patterns. Feedback allows for efficient movement, which is achieved through two different forms of feedback, internal (or sensory) feedback and external (or augmented) feedback.

Internal Feedback

Internal feedback The process whereby sensory information is used by the body to reactively monitor movement and the environment.

Internal feedback (or sensory feedback) is the process whereby sensory information is used by the body via length-tension relationships (posture), force-couple relationships, and arthrokinematics to reactively monitor movement and the environment. Internal (sensory) feedback acts as a guide, steering the HMS to the proper force, speed, and amplitude of movement patterns. Thus, it is important to instruct clients to use proper form when exercising to ensure that the incoming sensory feedback is correct information, allowing for optimal sensorimotor integration and ideal structural and functional efficiency.

External Feedback

External feedback Information provided by some external source, such as a health and fitness professional, videotape, mirror, or heart rate monitor, to supplement the internal environment.

External feedback refers to the information provided by an external source, including a personal trainer, videotape, mirror, or heart rate monitor, to help supplement internal feedback (16,31). External feedback provides the client with another source of information that allows him or her to associate whether the achieved movement pattern was "good" or "bad" with what he or she is feeling internally.

Two major forms of external feedback are knowledge of results and knowledge of performance **Figure 5.18** (16,19,20,30,31). *Knowledge of results* is used after the completion of a movement to help inform a client about the outcome of the performance. Effective use and application of knowledge of results involves both the personal trainer and the client's participation. An example of knowledge of results is a personal trainer telling clients that their squats looked "good" followed by asking the clients whether they could "feel" or "see" their good form. By getting clients involved with the knowledge of results, they increase their awareness and augment other forms of sensory feedback, leading to more effective exercise technique. Utilization of knowledge of results

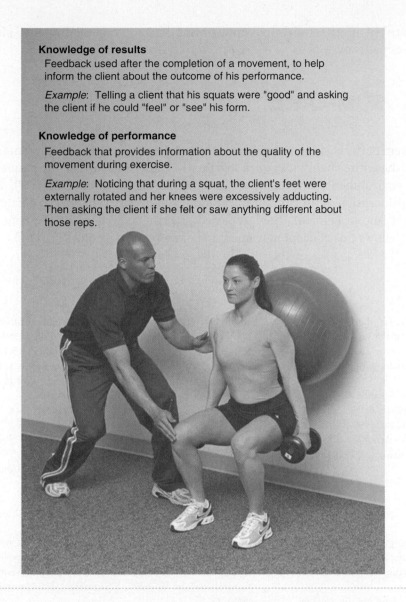

Knowledge of results
Feedback used after the completion of a movement, to help inform the client about the outcome of his performance.

Example: Telling a client that his squats were "good" and asking the client if he could "feel" or "see" his form.

Knowledge of performance
Feedback that provides information about the quality of the movement during exercise.

Example: Noticing that during a squat, the client's feet were externally rotated and her knees were excessively adducting. Then asking the client if she felt or saw anything different about those reps.

FIGURE 5.18

Forms of external feedback.

can be done after each repetition, after a few repetitions, or after the set is completed. As clients become increasingly familiar with the desired technique of a movement (exercise), knowledge of results from the personal trainer can be offered less frequently. Utilization of knowledge of results also improves neuromuscular efficiency as well (31).

Knowledge of performance provides information about the quality of the movement during an exercise. An example would be noticing that during a squat, a client's feet were externally rotated and the knees were excessively adducting, and then asking the client whether he or she felt or looked different during those repetitions. Knowledge of performance gets the client involved in his or her own sensory process. Knowledge of performance should be offered less frequently as the client becomes more proficient (31).

These forms of external feedback allow for the identification of performance errors and help improve effective performance outcomes in the future. They are also an important component of motivation. Furthermore, they provide the client supplemental sensory input to help create an awareness of the desired action (16,19,20,31). It is important that clients not become dependent on external feedback, especially from a personal trainer, as this may detract from their responsiveness to internal sensory input, or internal motivation (16,19,20,31). Excessive use of external feedback can negatively affect sensorimotor integration and motor learning and, ultimately, movement patterns.

SUMMARY

Each system of the HMS (kinetic chain) is interdependent. All of the segments and processes in the entire chain must work together to gather information from internal and external environments to create and learn movements (or motor behavior). The body uses proprioception, sensorimotor integration, and muscle synergies to create efficient movement (motor control). Then, repeated practice, as well as internal and external feedback, allows this efficient movement to be reproduced (motor learning).

REFERENCES

1. Hamill J, Knutzen JM. *Biomechanical Basis of Human Movement.* 2nd ed. Baltimore, MD: Lippincott Williams & Wilkins; 2003.

2. Norkin CC, Levangie PK. *Joint Structure and Function: A Comprehensive Analysis.* 2nd ed. Philadelphia: FA Davis Company; 1992.

3. Kendall FP, McCreary EK, Provance PG. *Muscles: Testing and Function.* 4th ed. Baltimore: Lippincott Williams & Wilkins; 1993.

4. Gambetta V. Everything in balance. *Train Cond.* 1996;1(2):15-21.

5. Luttgens K, Hamilton N. *Kinesiology: Scientific Basis of Human Motion.* 9th ed. Dubuque, IA: Brown & Benchmark Publishers; 1997.

6. Gray GW. *Chain Reaction Festival.* Adrian, MI: Wynn Marketing; 1996.

7. Enoka RM. *Neuromechanical Basis of Kinesiology.* 2nd ed. Champaign, IL: Human Kinetics; 1994.

8. Milner-Brown A. *Neuromuscular Physiology.* Thousand Oaks, CA: National Academy of Sports Medicine; 2001.

9. Fox SI. *Human Physiology.* 5th ed. Dubuque, IA: Wm C Brown Publishers; 1996.

10. Vander A, Sherman J, Luciano D. *Human Physiology: The Mechanisms of Body Function.* 8th ed. New York: McGraw-Hill; 2001.

11. Hamill J, Knutzen JM. *Biomechanical Basis of Human Movement.* Baltimore: Williams & Wilkins; 1995.

12. Watkins J. *Structure and Function of the Musculoskeletal System.* Champaign, IL: Human Kinetics; 1999.

13. Luttgens K, Hamilton N. *Kinesiology: Scientific Basis of Human Motion.* 9th ed. Dubuque, IA: Brown & Benchmark Publishers; 1997.

14. Fleck SJ, Kraemer WJ. *Designing Resistance Training Programs.* 2nd ed. Champaign, IL: Human Kinetics; 1997.

15. Brooks VB. *The Neural Basis of Motor Control.* New York: Oxford University Press; 1986.

16. Rose DJ. *A Multi Level Approach to the Study of Motor Control and Learning.* Needham Heights, MA: Allyn & Bacon; 1997.

17. Newton RA. Neural systems underlying motor control. In: Montgomery PC, Connoly BH, eds. *Clinical Applications for Motor Control.* Thorofare, NJ:SLACK, Inc; 2003. 53-78.

18. Kelso JAS. *Dynamic Patterns. The Self-Organization of Brain and Behavior.* Cambridge, MA: The MIT Press; 1995.

19. Schmidt RA, Lee TD. *Motor Control and Learning: A Behavioral Emphasis.* 3rd ed. Champaign, IL: Human Kinetics; 1999.

20. Schmidt RA, Wrisberg CA. *Motor Learning and Performance.* 2nd ed. Champaign, IL: Human Kinetics; 2000.

21. Gabbard C. *Lifelong Motor Development.* San Francisco: Pearson Benjamin Cummings; 2008.

22. Coker CA. *Motor Learning and Control for Practitioners.* Boston: McGraw-Hill; 2004.

23. Magill RA. *Motor Learning and Control: Concepts and Applications.* Boston: McGraw-Hill; 2007.

24. Ghez C, Krakuer J. Movement. In: Kandel E, Schwartz J, Jessel T, eds. *Principles of Neuroscience.* 4th ed. New York: Elsevier Science; 2000. 654-679.

25. Biedert RM. Contribution of the three levels of nervous system motor control: spinal cord, lower brain, cerebral cortex. In: Lephart SM, Fu FH, eds. *Proprioception and Neuromuscular Control in Joint Stability.* Champaign, IL: Human Kinetics; 2000. 23-29.

26. Boucher JP. Training and exercise science. In: Liebension C, ed. *Rehabilitation of the Spine.* Baltimore: Williams & Wilkins; 1996. 45-56.

27. Janda V, Va Vrova M. Sensory motor stimulation. In: Liebension C, ed. *Rehabilitation of the Spine.* Baltimore: Williams & Wilkins; 1996. 319-328.

28. Gagey PM, Gentez R. Postural disorders of the body axis. In: Liebension C, ed. *Rehabilitation of the Spine.* Baltimore: Williams & Wilkins; 1996. 329-340.

29. Drury DG. Strength and proprioception. *Ortho Phys Ther Clin.* 2000;9(4):549-561.

30. Grigg P. Peripheral neural mechanisms in proprioception. *J Sport Rehab.* 1994;3:2-17.

31. Swinnen SP. Information feedback for motor skill learning: a review. In: Zelaznik HN, ed. *Advances in Motor Learning and Control.* Champaign, IL: Human Kinetics; 1996. 37-60.

Assessments, Training Concepts, and Program Design

CHAPTER 6

Fitness Assessment

After studying this chapter, you will be able to:

✔ Explain the components of and rationale for an integrated fitness assessment.

✔ Understand how to administer a health history questionnaire and then from that be able to stratify a client's overall risk for fitness assessment.

✔ Understand the importance of posture, how it relates to movement observation, and how to assess it.

✔ Understand how to perform a comprehensive health-related fitness assessment, obtain subjective and objective information about clients, and how to use the information collected to help design an exercise program.

Overview of Fitness Assessments

In 2008, the federal government of the United States issued its first-ever physical activity guidelines for Americans. The *2008 Physical Activity Guidelines for Americans* draws attention to the growing problem of physical inactivity among adults, and that little progress has been made to reverse the trend (1). Physical inactivity exposes adults to unnecessary risk for developing a variety of chronic diseases, disabilities, and even musculoskeletal pain, whereas as little as 2.5 hours a week of moderate aerobic physical activity can substantially reduce that risk and lead to significant health benefits. One of the most important goals of the *2008 Physical Activity Guidelines for Americans* is to promote the fact that even in small doses, regular physical activity can help prevent, treat, and in some cases even cure more than 40 of the most common chronic health conditions encountered by primary care physicians, as well as reduce health-care costs and improve the quality and quantity of life for millions of Americans. Unfortunately, only 31% of US adults engage in regular leisure-time physical activity (defined as either three sessions per week of vigorous physical activity lasting

20 minutes or more, or five sessions per week of light-to-moderate physical activity lasting 30 minutes or more) (2).

Clearly, more needs to be done to get American adults to engage in regular bouts of moderate-to-vigorous physical activity and exercise on a regular basis. Another important message to all Americans is that although there are risks associated with physical activity and exercise, primarily musculoskeletal injuries, the benefits of physical activity clearly outweigh the risks. To minimize these risks, *2008 Physical Activity Guidelines for Americans* endorses a "start low and go slow" approach, which is also recommended by NASM.

Moving beyond general public health guidelines for physical activity and exercise, personal trainers need to be able to design safe and effective exercise programs for a wide client population base. Before any fitness professional, including personal trainers, can develop an individualized exercise program for a client, they need to be as absolutely certain as they possibly can that the potential benefits of exercise for an individual client clearly outweigh the potential risks. To achieve this essential objective, personal trainers will need to complete a preparticipation health or medical screening questionnaire with each individual client, stratify each client's overall risk for physical activity and exercise using the results of the screening, and lastly, determine which fitness or health assessments need to be completed before the client starts his or her exercise program.

Designing an individualized, systematic, integrated fitness assessment can only be accomplished by having an understanding of a client's goals, needs, and abilities. This entails knowing what a client wants to gain from a training program, what a client needs from a program to successfully accomplish his or her goal(s), and how capable he or she is (structurally and functionally) of performing the required tasks within an integrated program. The information necessary to create the right program for a specific individual (or group of individuals) comes through a proper fitness assessment. The remainder of this chapter will focus on the components of a fitness assessment for the fitness professional.

Definition

A comprehensive fitness assessment involves a series of measurements that help to determine the current health and fitness level of clients. Once a client's baseline health and fitness level has been determined, personal trainers can recommend the most appropriate exercises for that client. There are a variety of fitness tests and measurements that personal trainers can use to determine an individual's baseline fitness level. The specific tests used in an assessment depend on the health and fitness goals of the individual, the trainer's experience, the type of workout routines being performed, and availability of fitness assessment equipment.

Fitness assessments provide an ongoing way of communicating information between the personal trainer and the client, ensuring that fitness program goals are constantly being monitored and evaluated to make sure client's individual health and wellness goals are achieved. Fitness assessments allow the fitness professional to continually monitor a client's needs, functional capabilities, and physiologic effects of exercise, enabling the client to realize the full benefit of an individualized training program.

It is important that personal trainers understand that a health and fitness assessment is not designed to diagnose medical or health conditions, but instead is designed to serve as a way of observing and documenting a client's individual structural and functional status. Furthermore, the fitness assessment presented by NASM is not intended to replace a medical examination. If a client is identified as high-risk after a preparticipation health screening or exhibits signs or symptoms of underlying health problems or extreme difficulty or pain with any observation or exercise, the personal trainer should refer the client to his or her physician or qualified health-care provider to identify any underlying cause **Table 6.1**.

TABLE 6.1	Guidelines for Health and Fitness Professionals

© ilolab/ShutterStock, Inc.

Do Not	Do
Diagnose medical conditions.	Obtain exercise or health guidelines from a physician, physical therapist, or registered dietician. Follow national consensus guidelines of exercise prescription for medical disorders. Screen clients for exercise limitations. Identify potential risk factors for clients through screening procedures. Refer clients who experience difficulty or pain or exhibit other symptoms to a qualified medical practitioner.
Prescribe treatment.	Design individualized, systematic, progressive exercise programs. Refer clients to a qualified medical practitioner for medical exercise prescription.
Prescribe diets.	Provide clients with general information on healthy eating according to the food pyramid. Refer clients to a qualified dietician or nutritionist for specific diet plans.
Provide treatment of any kind for injury or disease.	Refer clients to a qualified medical practitioner for treatment of injury or disease. Use exercise to help clients improve overall health. Assist clients in following the medical advice of a physician or therapist.
Provide rehabilitation services for clients.	Design exercise programs for clients after they are released from rehabilitation. Provide postrehabilitation services.
Provide counseling services for clients.	Act as a coach for clients. Provide general information. Refer clients to a qualified counselor or therapist.

What Information Does a Fitness Assessment Provide?

A comprehensive fitness assessment provides a variety of subjective and objective information including a preparticipation health screening, resting physiologic measurements (e.g., heart rate, blood pressure, height, weight), and a series of measurements to help determine the fitness level of a client (health-related fitness tests). In addition to documenting resting physiologic measurements and fitness assessment test results, personal trainers should also take the time to discuss with all their new clients such things as past experiences with exercise, current goals, and any exercise likes or dislikes. All of the information collected during a comprehensive fitness assessment helps personal trainers establish safe and effective exercise programs based on the individual needs and goals of clients **Figure 6.1**.

Components of a Fitness Assessment

Subjective Information
  General and medical history:
  Occupation, Lifestyle, Medical and Personal Information

Objective Information
  Physiologic assessments
  Body composition testing
  Cardiorespiratory assessments
  Static and dynamic postural assessments
  Performance assessments

FIGURE 6.1

Components of a fitness assessment.

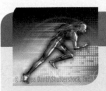

Memory Jogger

Keep in mind that the program you design for your client is only as good as your assessment! The more information you know about your client, the more individualized the program. This ensures the safety and effectiveness of the program, thus creating greater value in the personal trainer.

SUMMARY

A personal trainer's primary responsibility is to provide safe and effective exercise guidance and instruction to help clients successfully attain their personal health and wellness goals. To achieve these goals personal trainers require a comprehensive understanding of each and every client's personal and professional backgrounds, as well as their physical capabilities, health status, goals, and desires. Comprehensive fitness assessments provide a method of systematically gathering subjective and objective information about clients that is used to help ensure that safe and effective exercise programs can be planned and followed. Fitness assessments are *not* designed to diagnose any condition or replace a medical examination, and personal trainers should be knowledgeable enough to know when to refer their clients to qualified health-care providers whenever necessary.

Subjective Information Provided in the Fitness Assessment

Subjective information is gathered from a prospective client to give the health and fitness professional feedback regarding personal history such as occupation, lifestyle, and medical background.

Preparticipation Health Screening

Before allowing a new client to participate in any physical activity, including fitness testing, personal trainers should conduct a preparticipation health screening. A preparticipation health screening includes a medical history questionnaire (such as the PAR-Q discussed next) and a review of their chronic disease risk factors and presence of any signs or symptoms of disease. Once all of the information has been collected, the results should be used to stratify the risk of all new clients according to the following classifications (3):

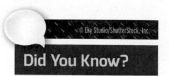

Did You Know?

Cardiovascular disease risk factors include cigarette smoking, dyslipidemia, impaired fasting glucose, obesity, and a sedentary lifestyle.

Low risk	Individuals who do not have any signs or symptoms of cardiovascular, pulmonary, or metabolic disease and have ≤1 cardiovascular disease risk factor.
Moderate risk	Individuals who do not have any signs or symptoms of cardiovascular, pulmonary, or metabolic disease but have ≥2 cardiovascular disease risk factors.
High risk	Individuals who have one or more signs or symptoms of cardiovascular, pulmonary, or metabolic disease.

Once the preparticipation health screening information has been collected and reviewed, and the client's risk stratified, personal trainers are now able to decide whether to proceed with fitness testing or refer the client for further medical evaluation. Additionally, results from the preparticipation health screening provide valuable information to help personal trainers plan safe and effective exercise programs if the client does not require further medical evaluation.

Physical Activity Readiness Questionnaire

Gathering relevant background information from a client helps personal trainers determine whether their client has any medical, health, or physical conditions that could limit or restrict how much or what type of exercise they could do. One of the easiest ways of gathering this information is through the use of a questionnaire **Figure 6.2** (3). The Physical Activity Readiness Questionnaire (PAR-Q) is a questionnaire that has been designed to determine the safety or possible risk of exercising for a client based on the answers to specific health history questions (3,4). The PAR-Q is primarily aimed at identifying individuals who require further medical evaluation before being allowed to exercise because they are at high risk for cardiovascular disease (CVD). When clients answer yes to one or more questions on the PAR-Q, the personal trainers should refer them to a physician for further medical screening before starting an exercise program.

General Health History

A health history is a collection of information that is generally part of a medical physical or medical health history, which discusses relevant facts about the individual's history, including biographic, demographic, occupational, and general lifestyle (physical, mental, emotional, sociocultural, sexual, and sometimes spiritual) data. Two important areas for the personal trainer to focus on are the relevant answers provided about a client's occupation and general lifestyle traits.

Questions		
1. Has your doctor ever said that you have a heart condition and that you should only perform physical activity recommended by a doctor?	☐ Yes	☐ No
2. Do you feel pain in your chest when you perform physical activity?	☐ Yes	☐ No
3. In the past month, have you had chest pain when you are not performing any physical activity?	☐ Yes	☐ No
4. Do you lose your balance because of dizziness or do you ever lose consciousness?	☐ Yes	☐ No
5. Do you have a bone or joint problem that could be made worse by a change in your physical activity?	☐ Yes	☐ No
6. Is your doctor currently prescribing any medication for your blood pressure or for a heart condition?	☐ Yes	☐ No
7. Do you know of *any* other reason why you should not engage in physical activity?	☐ Yes	☐ No

If you have answered "Yes" to one or more of the above questions, consult your physician before engaging in physical activity. Tell your physician which questions you answered "Yes" to. After a medical evaluation, seek advice from your physician on what type of activity is suitable for your current condition.

FIGURE 6.2

Sample Physical Activity Readiness Questionnaire (PAR-Q).

Occupation

Collecting information about a client's occupation helps personal trainers determine common movement patterns, as well as typical energy expenditure levels during the course of an average day. Collecting this kind of information helps personal trainers begin to recognize important clues about the client's musculoskeletal structure and function, potential health and physical limitations, and restrictions that could affect the safety and efficacy of an exercise program. Examples of typical questions are shown in **Figure 6.3**, and each question provides relevant information.

Extended Periods of Sitting

If clients are sitting for long periods throughout the day, their hips are also flexed for prolonged periods of time, which in turn can lead to tight hip flexors (rectus femoris, tensor fascia latae, iliopsoas) and postural imbalances within the human movement system. Moreover, if clients are sitting for prolonged periods of time, especially in front of a computer, there is a tendency for the shoulders and head to fatigue under the constant effect of gravity, which again can lead to postural imbalances including rounding of the shoulders and a forward head. In addition, prolonged periods of sitting are indicative of low energy expenditure throughout the day and potentially poor cardiorespiratory conditioning.

Repetitive Movements

Repetitive movement is a persistent motion that can cause musculoskeletal injury and dysfunction. Repetitive movements can create a pattern overload to muscles and joints, which may lead to tissue trauma and eventually kinetic chain dysfunction, especially in jobs that require a lot of overhead work or awkward positions such as construction or painting (5). Working with the arms overhead for long periods may lead to shoulder

© ilolab/ShutterStock, Inc.

FIGURE 6.3

Sample questions: client occupation.

Questions		
1. What is your current occupation? _____	☐ Yes	☐ No
2. Does your occupation require extended periods of sitting?	☐ Yes	☐ No
3. Does your occupation require extended periods of repetitive movements? (If yes, please explain.) _____	☐ Yes	☐ No
4. Does your occupation require you to wear shoes with a heel (dress shoes)?	☐ Yes	☐ No
5. Does your occupation cause you anxiety (mental stress)?	☐ Yes	☐ No

and neck soreness that may be the result of tightness in the latissimus dorsi and weakness in the rotator cuff. This imbalance does not allow for proper shoulder motion or stabilization during activity.

Dress Shoes

Wearing shoes with a high heel puts the ankle complex in a plantarflexed position for extended periods, which can lead to tightness in the gastrocnemius, soleus, and Achilles tendon, causing postural imbalance, such as decreased dorsiflexion and overpronation at the foot and ankle complex, resulting in flattening of the arch of the foot (6).

Mental Stress

Mental stress or anxiety can cause elevated resting heart rate, blood pressure, and ventilation at rest and exercise. In addition, it can lead to abnormal (or dysfunctional) breathing patterns that may cause postural or musculoskeletal imbalances in the neck, shoulder, chest, and low-back muscles, which collectively can lead to postural distortion and human movement system dysfunction (7,8). For more detailed information, see chapter three (Abnormal Breathing Patterns).

Lifestyle

Lifestyle or personal questions pertain to a client's general lifestyle activities and habits, and might include questions about smoking, drinking, exercise, and sleeping habits as well as recreational activities and hobbies. Examples of typical questions are shown in **Figure 6.4**.

Recreation

Recreation, in the context of assessment, refers to a client's physical activities outside of the work environment, also referred to as leisure time. By finding out what recreational activities a client performs, personal trainers can better design an exercise program to fit the needs of the client. For example, many clients like to golf, ski, play tennis, or perform a variety of other sporting activities in their spare time, and proper exercise

Questions		
1. Do you partake in any recreational activities (golf, tennis, skiing, etc.)? (If yes, please explain.) _____ _____ _____	☐ Yes	☐ No
2. Do you have any hobbies (reading, gardening, working on cars, etc.)? (If yes, please explain.) _____ _____ _____	☐ Yes	☐ No

FIGURE 6.4

Sample questions: client lifestyle.

training must be incorporated to ensure that clients are trained in a manner that optimizes the efficiency of the human movement system, without predisposing it to injury.

Hobbies

Hobbies refer to activities that a client might enjoy participating in on a regular basis, but are not necessarily athletic in nature. Examples include gardening, working on cars, playing cards, reading, watching television, or playing video games. In many instances, many common types of hobbies do not involve any physical activity, and yet still need to be taken into account to create a properly planned integrated exercise training program.

Medical History

Obtaining a client's medical history **Figure 6.5** is vitally important because it provides personal trainers with information about known or suspected chronic diseases, such as coronary heart disease, high blood pressure, or diabetes (3). Furthermore, a medical history provides information about the client's past and current health status, as well as any past or recent injuries, surgeries, or other chronic health conditions.

Past Injuries

All past or recent injuries should be recorded and discussed in sufficient enough detail to be able to make decisions about whether exercise is recommended or a medical referral is necessary. Previous history of musculoskeletal injury is also a strong predictor of future musculoskeletal injury during physical activity (9). The effect of injuries on the functioning of the human movement system is well documented, especially with regard to the following injuries:

1. Ankle sprains: Ankle sprains have been shown to decrease the neural control to the gluteus medius and gluteus maximus muscles. This, in turn, can lead to poor control of the lower extremities during many functional activities, which can eventually lead to injury (10–14).
2. Knee injuries involving ligaments: Knee injury can cause a decrease in the neural control to muscles that stabilize the patella (kneecap) and lead to further injury. Knee injuries that are not the result of contact (noncontact injuries) are often the result of ankle or hip dysfunctions, such as the result of an ankle sprain.

© ilolab/ShutterStock, Inc.

FIGURE 6.5

Sample questions:
client medical history.

Questions

1. Have you ever had any pain or injuries (ankle, knee, hip, back, shoulder, etc.)? (If yes, please explain.) ☐ Yes ☐ No
_____
_____

2. Have you ever had any surgeries? (If yes, please explain.) ☐ Yes ☐ No
_____
_____

3. Has a medical doctor ever diagnosed you with a chronic disease, such as coronary heart disease, coronary artery disease, hypertension (high blood pressure), high cholesterol, or diabetes? (If yes, please explain.) ☐ Yes ☐ No
_____
_____

4. Are you currently taking any medication? (If yes, please list.) ☐ Yes ☐ No
_____
_____

The knee is caught between the ankle and the hip. If the ankle or hip joint begins to function improperly, this results in altered movement and force distribution of the knee. With time, this can lead to further injury (15–31).

3. Low-back injuries: Low-back injuries can cause decreased neural control to stabilizing muscles of the core, resulting in poor stabilization of the spine. This can further lead to dysfunction in the upper and lower extremities (32–39).

4. Shoulder injuries: Shoulder injuries cause altered neural control of the rotator cuff muscles, which can lead to instability of the shoulder joint during functional activities (40–48).

5. Other injuries: Injuries that result from human movement system imbalances include repetitive hamstring strains, groin strains, patellar tendonitis (jumper's knee), plantar fasciitis (pain in the heel and bottom of the foot), posterior tibialis tendonitis (shin splints), biceps tendonitis (shoulder pain), and headaches.

Past Surgeries

Surgical procedures create trauma for the body and may have similar effects on the functioning of the human movement system and safety and efficacy of exercise as those of injuries. Some of the more common surgical procedures personal trainers come across on a frequent basis include:

- Foot and ankle surgery
- Knee surgery
- Back surgery
- Shoulder surgery
- Caesarean section for birth (cutting through the abdominal wall to deliver a baby)
- Appendectomy (cutting through the abdominal wall to remove the appendix)

In each case, surgery will cause pain and inflammation that can alter neural control to the affected muscles and joints if not rehabilitated properly (49,50).

Chronic Conditions

It is estimated that more than 75% of the American adult population does not engage in at least 30 minutes of low-to-moderate physical activity on most days of the week (51). The risk of chronic disease increases dramatically in those individuals who are physically inactive or only meet the minimal standard of physical activity (51,52). Chronic diseases include:

- Cardiovascular disease, coronary heart disease, coronary artery disease, or congestive heart failure
- Hypertension (high blood pressure)
- High cholesterol or other blood lipid disorders
- Stroke or peripheral artery disease
- Lung or breathing problems
- Obesity
- Diabetes mellitus
- Cancer

Medications

A large number of clients seeking fitness and exercise training advice from personal trainers will currently be under the care of a physician or another medical professional and may be taking one or more prescribed medications. It is *not* the role of the personal trainer to administer, prescribe, or educate clients on the usage and effects of any form of legally prescribed medication by a licensed physician or other health-care provider. Personal trainers should always consult with their client's physician or medical professionals regarding the client's health information and which if any medications they may be currently taking.

Table 6.2 briefly outlines some of the primary classes of drugs, and Table 6.3 describes their proposed physiologic effects. These tables are intended to present a basic overview of medications, but are *not* intended to serve as conclusive evidence regarding the medications or their effects. For more complete information regarding medications, contact a medical professional or refer to the *Physician's Desk Reference* (PDR).

TABLE 6.2	Common Medications by Classification
Medication	**Basic Function**
Beta-blockers (β-blockers)	Generally used as antihypertensive (high blood pressure), may also be prescribed for arrhythmias (irregular heart rate)
Calcium-channel blockers	Generally prescribed for hypertension and angina (chest pain)
Nitrates	Generally prescribed for hypertension, congestive heart failure
Diuretics	Generally prescribed for hypertension, congestive heart failure, and peripheral edema
Bronchodilators	Generally prescribed to correct or prevent bronchial smooth muscle constriction in individuals with asthma and other pulmonary diseases
Vasodilators	Used in the treatment of hypertension and congestive heart failure
Antidepressants	Used in the treatment of various psychiatric and emotional disorders

| TABLE 6.3 | Effects of Medication on Heart Rate and Blood Pressure | |

Medication	Heart Rate	Blood Pressure
Beta-blockers (β-blockers)	↓	↓
Calcium-channel blockers	↑	↓
	↔ or ↓	
Nitrates	↑	↔
	↔	↓
Diuretics	↔	↔
		↓
Bronchodilators	↔	↔
Vasodilators	↑	↓
	↔ or ↓	
Antidepressants	↑ or ↔	↔ or ↓

↑, increase; ↔, no effect; ↓, decrease.

SUMMARY

Personal trainers are able to gain insight into their clients' daily physical activity level and health by gathering subjective information about their personal history, including occupation, lifestyle, and medical background. The Physical Activity Readiness Questionnaire (PAR-Q) identifies clients who are at high risk for developing cardiovascular disease, and thus require a medical referral before starting an exercise program. By asking questions that provide important information about the structure and function of a client, it is possible to assess risk factors for chronic disease as well as movement capacities and what kinds of movement patterns are performed throughout the day.

Questions about recreational activities and hobbies reflect what clients do in their leisure time. Proper forms of training for specific activities must be incorporated to increase the efficiency of the human movement system, while avoiding injury. Clients with sedentary hobbies will probably not be at the same level of training as those who participate in recreational sports.

Finding out a client's medical history is crucial to ensuring a safe, effective, and enjoyable exercise experience. Past injuries affect the functioning of the human movement system and are important to ask clients about, as well as surgical procedures that may have similar effects as injuries because they cause pain and inflammation, which can alter neural control to the affected muscles and joints if not rehabilitated properly. It is also important to ask clients about any other chronic health conditions, which are likely to occur in individuals who are habitually sedentary. And finally, many clients who seek out personal training services will be taking one or more prescribed medications, and it is important for personal trainers to know some of the more common medications and their effects on exercise. However, it is important to note that personal trainers do *not* administer, prescribe, or educate on the usage and effects of any type of prescribed medications. Personal trainers should always consult with a client's physician or other medical professionals if they have any questions regarding medications used by one of their clients.

Objective Information Provided in the Fitness Assessment

Objective information collected during a fitness assessment includes resting and exercise physiological measurements (e.g., blood pressure, heart rate), resting anthropometric measurements (e.g., height, weight, body fat percentage, circumference measurements), and specific measures of fitness (e.g., muscular endurance, flexibility, cardiorespiratory fitness). Objective information collected during a fitness assessment can be used to compare beginning baseline measures of fitness with measurements taken weeks, months, or even years later. Moreover, when follow-up data are compared with baseline measurements, ideally improvements of all categories of health-related physical fitness are evident, confirming the effectiveness of the training program. Categories of objective information include:

- Physiological measurements
- Body composition assessments
- Cardiorespiratory assessments
- Static posture assessment
- Movement assessments (dynamic posture)
- Performance assessments

Heart Rate and Blood Pressure Assessment

The assessment of resting heart rate (HR) and blood pressure (BP) is a sensitive indicator of a client's overall cardiorespiratory health as well as fitness status. Through the initial assessment and reassessment of a client's HR and BP, personal trainers are able to gather valuable information that helps in the design, monitoring, and progression of a client's exercise program. For example, resting HR is a *fairly good* indicator of overall cardiorespiratory fitness, whereas exercise HR is a *strong indicator* of how a client's cardiorespiratory system is responding and adapting to exercise.

Pulse

A pulse is created by blood moving or pulsating through arteries each time the heart contracts. Each time the heart contracts or beats, one wave of blood flow or pulsation of blood can be felt by placing one or two fingers on an artery. The artery contracts and relaxes periodically to rhythmically force the blood along its way circulating throughout the body. This coincides with the contraction and relaxation of the heart as it pumps the blood through the arteries and veins. Therefore the pulse rate is also known as the heart rate.

There are seven pulse points, or places where arteries come close enough to the skin to be able to have a pulse felt; the two most common sites used to record a pulse are the radial and carotid arteries.

Heart rate can be recorded on the inside of the wrist (radial pulse; preferred) or on the neck to the side of the windpipe (carotid pulse; use with caution). To gather an accurate recording, it is best to teach clients how to record their resting HR on rising in the morning. Instruct them to test their resting heart rate three mornings in a row and average the three readings.

Radial Pulse

To find the radial pulse, lightly place two fingers along the right side of the arm in line and just above the thumb **Figure 6.6**. Once a pulse is felt, count the pulses for 60 seconds. Record the 60-second pulse rate and average over the course of 3 days. Points to consider:

- The touch should be gentle.
- The test must be taken when the client is calm.
- All three tests must be taken at the same time to ensure accuracy.

Carotid Pulse

To find the carotid pulse, lightly place two fingers on the neck, just to the side of the larynx **Figure 6.7**. Once a pulse is identified, count the pulses for 60 seconds. Record the 60-second pulse rate and average over the course of 3 days. Points to consider:

- The touch should be gentle.
- Excessive pressure can decrease HR and blood pressure, leading to an inaccurate reading, possible dizziness, and fainting (3).
- The test must be taken when the client is calm.
- All three tests should be taken at the same time to ensure accuracy.

Resting HR can vary. As discussed in chapter three the typical resting heart rate is between 70 and 80 beats per minute. However, on average, the resting HR for a male is 70 beats per minute and 75 beats per minute for a female (3).

Personal trainers can use a client's resting HR to calculate the target heart rate (THR) zones in which a client should perform cardiorespiratory exercise **Table 6.4**. The two most common ways to calculate THR are to use a percentage of the client's

FIGURE 6.6

Radial pulse.

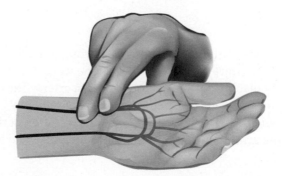

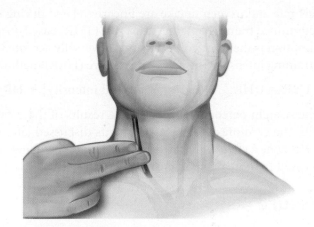

FIGURE 6.7

Carotid pulse.

TABLE 6.4	**Target Heart Rate Training Zones**

© ilolab/ShutterStock, Inc.

Training Zone	Purpose
One	Builds aerobic base and aids in recovery
Two	Increases aerobic and anaerobic endurance
Three	Builds high-end work capacity

estimated maximal heart rate (straight percentage method) or by using a percentage of heart rate reserve (Karvonen method).

STRAIGHT PERCENTAGE METHOD (PEAK MAXIMAL HEART RATE)

A client's estimated maximal heart rate (HR_{max}) is found by subtracting their age from the number 220 (220 − age). Once the client's HR_{max} is determined, multiply the estimated HR_{max} by the appropriate intensity (65–95%) at which the client should work while performing cardiorespiratory exercise to calculate THR.

Zone one	Maximal heart rate × 0.65
	Maximal heart rate × 0.75
Zone two	Maximal heart rate × 0.76
	Maximal heart rate × 0.85
Zone three	Maximal heart rate × 0.86
	Maximal heart rate × 0.95

The results of these calculations should be combined with the cardiorespiratory assessments discussed later in this chapter to establish which HR zone a client will start in. However, exercise intensity levels may need to be lower than 65% (e.g., ~40 to 55%) depending on the client's initial physical condition status (3).

HR RESERVE (HRR) METHOD

Heart rate reserve (HRR), also known as the Karvonen method, is a method of establishing training intensity on the basis of the difference between a client's predicted maximal heart rate and their resting heart rate.

Because heart rate and oxygen uptake are linearly related during dynamic exercise, selecting a predetermined training or target heart rate (THR) based on a given percentage of oxygen consumption is the most common and universally accepted method of establishing exercise training intensity. The heart rate reserve (HRR) method is defined as:

$$\text{THR} = [(\text{HR}_{max} - \text{HR}_{rest}) \times \text{desired intensity}] + \text{HR}_{rest}$$

Similar to the straight percentage method, the results of these calculations should be combined with the cardiorespiratory assessments discussed later in this chapter to establish which HR zone a client will start in. The straight percentage method and HRR method are discussed in more detail in chapter eight.

Blood Pressure

Blood pressure (BP) is the pressure of the circulating blood against the walls of the blood vessels after blood is ejected from the heart. There are two parts to a blood pressure measurement. The first number (sometimes referred to as the top number) is called systolic, and it represents the pressure within the arterial system after the heart contracts. The second number (or bottom number) is called diastolic, and it represents the pressure within the arterial system when the heart is resting and filling with blood. An example of a blood pressure reading is 120/80 (120 over 80). In this example, 120 is the systolic number and 80 is the diastolic number. Blood pressure measurements always consist of both readings. According to the American Heart Association, an acceptable systolic blood pressure measurement for health is ≤120 millimetres (mm) of mercury (Hg) or mm Hg. An acceptable diastolic blood pressure is ≤80 mm Hg.

Blood Pressure Assessment

Blood pressure is measured using an aneroid sphygmomanometer, which consists of an inflatable cuff, a pressure dial, a bulb with a valve, and a stethoscope. To record blood pressure, instruct the client to assume a comfortable seated position and place the appropriate size cuff on the client's arm just above the elbow **Figure 6.8**. Next, rest the arm on a supported chair (or support the arm using your own arm) and place the stethoscope over the brachial artery, using a minimal amount of pressure. Continue by rapidly inflating the cuff to 20 to 30 mm Hg above the point at which the pulse can no longer be felt at the wrist. Next, release the pressure at a rate of

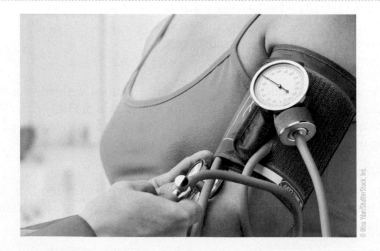

FIGURE 6.8

Proper sphygmomanometer placement.

about 2 mm Hg per second, listening for a pulse. To determine the systolic pressure, listen for the first observation of the pulse. Diastolic pressure is determined when the pulse fades away. For greater reliability, repeat the procedure on the opposite arm (3). It is highly recommended that anyone, including personal trainers, take a professional course in blood pressure assessment before assessing blood pressure with any clients.

Body Composition

Body composition refers to the relative percentage of body weight that is fat versus fat-free tissue, or more commonly reported as "Percent Body Fat." Fat-free mass can be defined as body weight except stored fat, and includes muscles, bones, water, connective and organ tissues, and teeth, whereas fat mass includes both essential fat (crucial for normal body functioning) and nonessential fat (storage fat or adipose tissue). Benefits of body composition assessments include:

- To identify client's health risk for excessively high or low levels of body fat
- To promote client's understanding of body fat
- To monitor changes in body composition
- To help estimate healthy body weight for clients and athletes
- To assist in exercise program design
- To use as a motivational tool (for certain clients)
- To monitor changes in body composition that are associated with chronic diseases
- To assess effectiveness of nutrition and exercise choices

Currently, there is no accepted percent of body fat standard for all ages because most body composition studies use small groups, usually young adults. These studies demonstrate that body fat typically ranges from 10 to 20% for men and 20 to 30% for women (53). Based on these studies, recommendations of 15% for men and 25% for women have been made, discussed in more detail in **Table 6.5** and **Table 6.6** (53).

Body Composition Assessment

There are a variety of methods used to estimate body composition; they vary according to cost, accuracy, and skill needed to perform them.

1. Skinfold measurement: uses a caliper to estimate the amount of subcutaneous fat beneath the skin.

TABLE 6.5	Percent Fat Recommendations for Men and Women
Men	**Women**
Essential body fat: 3–5%	Essential body fat: 8–12%
Athletic: 5–13%	Athletic: 12–22%
Recommended (34 years or less): 8–22%	Recommended (34 years or less): 20–35%
Recommended (35–55 years): 10–25%	Recommended (35–55 years): 23–38%
Recommended (more than 56 years): 10–25%	Recommended (more than 56 years): 25–38%

TABLE 6.6	Percent Fat Recommendations for Active Men and Women			
Men	**Not Recommended**	**Low**	**Mid**	**Upper**
Young adult	<5	5	10	15
Middle adult	<7	7	11	18
Elderly	<9	9	12	18
Women				
Young adult	<16	16	23	28
Middle adult	<20	20	27	33
Elderly	<20	20	27	33

2. Bioelectrical impedance: uses a portable instrument to conduct an electrical current through the body to estimate fat. This form of assessment is based on the hypothesis that tissues that are high in water content conduct electrical currents with less resistance than those with little water (such as adipose tissue).

3. Underwater weighing often referred to as hydrostatic weighing has been the most common technique used in exercise physiology laboratories to determine body composition. The fact that bone, muscle, and connective tissue, collectively known as lean mass, sinks, whereas body fat floats is the main principle behind hydrostatic testing. In essence a person's weight is compared with a person's weight underwater to determine fat percentage. Because bone and muscle are denser than water, a person with a larger percentage of lean body mass will weigh more in the water and ultimately have a lower body fat percentage versus someone with less lean body mass. A person with more body fat will have a lighter body in water and a higher percentage of body fat.

Skinfold Measurements

Most personal trainers do not have an exercise physiology laboratory at their disposal, so the skinfold caliper method will be the method emphasized in this text. Skinfolds (SKF) are an indirect measure of the thickness of subcutaneous adipose tissue. The assumption is that the amount of fat present in the subcutaneous regions of the body is proportional to overall body fatness, and most of the time this is the case. Recommendations for assessing body composition using skinfolds include:

◆ Train with an individual skilled in SKF assessment and frequently compare your results with theirs
◆ Take a minimum of two measurements at each site, and each site must be within 1 to 2 mm to take average at each site
◆ Open jaw of caliper before removing from site
◆ Be meticulous when locating anatomic landmarks
◆ Do not measure SKFs immediately after exercise
◆ Instruct the clients ahead of time regarding test protocol
◆ Avoid performing SKFs on extremely obese clients

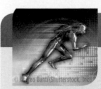

Memory Jogger

Assessing body fat using skinfold calipers can be a sensitive situation, particularly for very overweight individuals. The accuracy of the skinfold measurement in these situations typically decreases; thus, it would be more appropriate to not use this method for assessing body fat. Instead, use bioelectrical impedance (if available), circumference measurements, scale weight, or even how clothes fit to evaluate one's weight loss and body fat reduction progress.

Calculating Body Fat Percentages

The National Academy of Sports Medicine uses the Durnin formula (sometimes known as the Durnin–Womersley formula) to calculate a client's percentage of body fat (54). This formula was chosen for its simple four-site upper body measurement process. The Durnin formula's four sites of skinfold measurement are as follows:

1. Biceps: A vertical fold on the front of the arm over the biceps muscle, halfway between the shoulder and the elbow **Figure 6.9**.
2. Triceps: A vertical fold on the back of the upper arm, with the arm relaxed and held freely at the side. This skin fold should also be taken halfway between the shoulder and the elbow **Figure 6.10**.
3. Subscapular: A 45-degree angle fold of 1 to 2 cm, below the inferior angle of the scapula **Figure 6.11**.
4. Iliac crest: A 45-degree angle fold, taken just above the iliac crest and medial to the axillary line **Figure 6.12**.

All skinfold measurements should be taken on the right side of the body. After the four sites have been measured, add the totals of the four sites, find the appropriate sex and age categories for the body composition on the Durnin–Womersley body fat percentage calculation table **Table 6.7**. For example, a 40-year-old female client with the sum of the skinfolds of 40 has a percent body fat 28.14% (or round down to 28%).

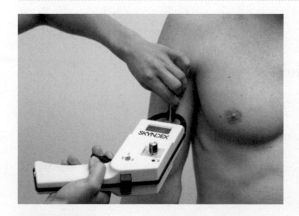

FIGURE 6.9 Biceps measurement.

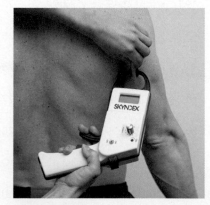

FIGURE 6.10 Triceps measurement.

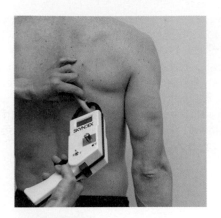

FIGURE 6.11 Subscapular measurement.

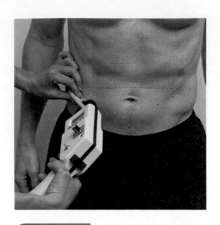

FIGURE 6.12 Iliac crest measurement.

TABLE 6.7 Durnin–Womersley Body Fat Percentage Calculation

© ilolab/ShutterStock, Inc.

Sum of Folds	Men					Women				
	<19	20–29	30–39	40–49	>50	<19	20–29	30–39	40–49	>50
5	−7.23	−7.61	−1.70	−5.28	−6.87	−2.69	−3.97	0.77	3.91	4.84
10	0.41	0.04	5.05	3.30	2.63	5.72	4.88	8.72	11.71	13.10
15	5.00	4.64	9.09	8.47	8.38	10.78	10.22	13.50	16.40	18.07
20	8.32	7.96	12.00	12.22	12.55	14.44	14.08	16.95	19.78	21.67
25	10.92	10.57	14.29	15.16	15.84	17.33	17.13	19.66	22.44	24.49
30	13.07	12.73	16.17	17.60	18.56	19.71	19.64	21.90	24.64	26.83
35	14.91	14.56	17.77	19.68	20.88	21.74	21.79	23.81	26.51	28.82
40	16.51	16.17	19.17	21.49	22.92	23.51	23.67	25.48	28.14	30.56
45	17.93	17.59	20.41	23.11	24.72	25.09	25.34	26.96	29.59	32.10
50	19.21	18.87	21.53	24.56	26.35	26.51	26.84	28.30	30.90	33.49
55	20.37	20.04	22.54	25.88	27.83	27.80	28.21	29.51	32.09	34.75
60	21.44	21.11	23.47	27.09	29.20	28.98	29.46	30.62	33.17	35.91
65	22.42	22.09	24.33	28.22	30.45	30.08	30.62	31.65	34.18	36.99
70	23.34	23.01	25.13	29.26	31.63	31.10	31.70	32.60	35.11	37.98
75	24.20	23.87	25.87	30.23	32.72	32.05	32.71	33.49	35.99	38.91

Sum of Folds	Men					Women				
	<19	20–29	30–39	40–49	>50	<19	20–29	30–39	40–49	>50
80	25.00	24.67	26.57	31.15	33.75	32.94	33.66	34.33	36.81	39.79
85	25.76	25.43	27.23	32.01	34.72	33.78	34.55	35.12	37.58	40.61
90	26.47	26.15	27.85	32.83	35.64	34.58	35.40	35.87	38.31	41.39
95	27.15	26.83	28.44	33.61	36.52	35.34	36.20	36.58	39.00	42.13
100	27.80	27.48	29.00	34.34	37.35	36.06	36.97	37.25	39.66	42.84
105	28.42	28.09	29.54	35.05	38.14	36.74	37.69	37.90	40.29	43.51
110	29.00	28.68	30.05	35.72	38.90	37.40	38.39	38.51	40.89	44.15
115	29.57	29.25	30.54	36.37	39.63	38.03	39.06	39.10	41.47	44.76
120	30.11	29.79	31.01	36.99	40.33	38.63	39.70	39.66	42.02	45.36
125	30.63	30.31	31.46	37.58	41.00	39.21	40.32	40.21	42.55	45.92
130	31.13	30.82	31.89	38.15	41.65	39.77	40.91	40.73	43.06	46.47
135	31.62	31.30	32.31	38.71	42.27	40.31	41.48	41.24	43.56	47.00
140	32.08	31.77	32.71	39.24	42.87	40.83	42.04	41.72	44.03	47.51
145	32.53	32.22	33.11	39.76	43.46	41.34	42.57	42.19	44.49	48.00
150	32.97	32.66	33.48	40.26	44.02	41.82	43.09	42.65	44.94	48.47
155	33.39	33.08	33.85	40.74	44.57	42.29	43.59	43.09	45.37	48.93
160	33.80	33.49	34.20	41.21	45.10	42.75	44.08	43.52	45.79	49.38
165	34.20	33.89	34.55	41.67	45.62	43.20	44.55	43.94	46.20	49.82
170	34.59	34.28	34.88	42.11	46.12	43.63	45.01	44.34	46.59	50.24
175	34.97	34.66	35.21	42.54	46.61	44.05	45.46	44.73	46.97	50.65
180	35.33	35.02	35.53	42.96	47.08	44.46	45.89	45.12	47.35	51.05
185	35.69	35.38	35.83	43.37	47.54	44.86	46.32	45.49	47.71	51.44
190	36.04	35.73	36.13	43.77	48.00	45.25	46.73	45.85	48.07	51.82
195	36.38	36.07	36.43	44.16	48.44	45.63	47.14	46.21	48.41	52.19
200	36.71	36.40	36.71	44.54	48.87	46.00	47.53	46.55	48.75	52.55

Another benefit of assessing body composition is the ability to determine approximately how much of an individual's body weight comes from fat and how much of it is lean body mass. The formula below outlines how to calculate one's fat mass and lean body mass:

1. Body fat % × scale weight = fat mass
2. Scale weight − fat mass = lean body mass

For example, if the above 40-year-old female client weights 130 pounds, her fat mass and lean body mass would be calculated as such:

1. 0.28 (body fat %) × 130 (scale weight) = 36 pounds of body fat
2. 130 (scale weight) − 36 (pounds of body fat) = 94 pounds of lean body mass

Circumference Measurements

A circumference is a measure of the girth of body segments (e.g., arm, thigh, waist, and hip). Circumference methods are affected by both fat and muscle, and therefore do not provide accurate estimates of fatness in the general population.

Some of the uses and benefits of circumference measurements include:

♦ Can be used on obese clients
♦ Good for comparisons and progressions
♦ Good for assessing fat pattern and distribution
♦ Inexpensive
♦ Easy to record
♦ Little technician error
♦ Used for waist circumference
♦ Used for waist-to-hip ratio (WHR)

Circumference measurements can also be another source of feedback used with clients who have the goal of altering body composition. They are designed to assess girth changes in the body. The most important factor to consider when taking circumference measurements is consistency. Remember when taking measurements to make sure the tape measure is taut and level around the area that is being measured.

1. Neck: Across the Adam's apple **Figure 6.13**
2. Chest: Across the nipple line **Figure 6.14**
3. Waist: Measure at the narrowest point of the waist, below the rib cage and just above the top of the hipbones. If there is no apparent narrowing of the waist, measure at the navel **Figure 6.15**.
4. Hips: With feet together, measure circumference at the widest portion of the buttocks **Figure 6.16**.
5. Thighs: Measure 10 inches above the top of the patella for standardization **Figure 6.17**.
6. Calves: At the maximal circumference between the ankle and the knee, measure the calves **Figure 6.18**.
7. Biceps: At the maximal circumference of the biceps, measure with arm extended, palm facing forward **Figure 6.19**.

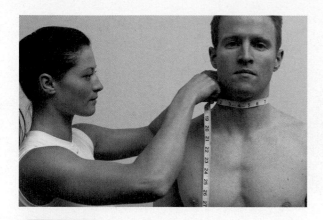

FIGURE 6.13 Neck measurement.

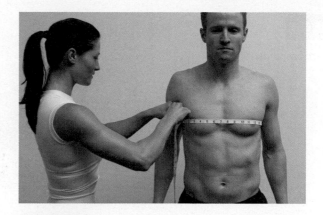

FIGURE 6.14 Chest measurement.

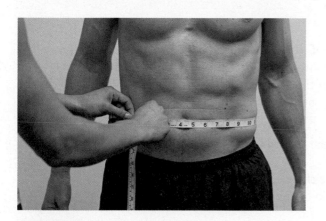

FIGURE 6.15 Waist measurement.

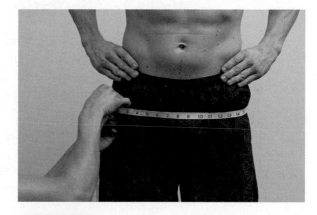

FIGURE 6.16 Hips measurement.

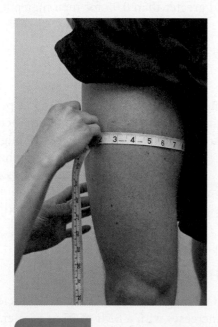

FIGURE 6.17 Thigh measurement.

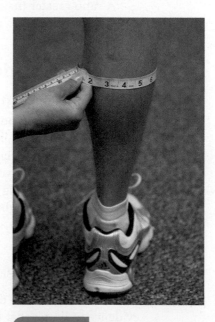

FIGURE 6.18 Calves measurement.

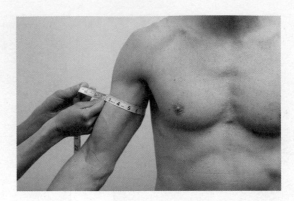

Biceps measurement.

Waist-to-Hip Ratio

The waist-to-hip ratio is one of the most used clinical applications of girth measurements. This assessment is important because there is a correlation between chronic diseases and fat stored in the midsection (3). The waist-to-hip ratio can be computed by dividing the waist measurement by the hip measurement, by doing the following:

1. Measure the smallest part of the client's waist, without instructing the client to draw in the stomach.
2. Measure the largest part of the client's hips.
3. Compute the waist-to-hip ratio by dividing the waist measurement by the hip measurement.
4. For example, if a client's waist measures 30 inches and his or her hips measure 40 inches, divide 30 by 40 for a waist-to-hip ratio of 0.75.

A ratio greater than 0.80 for women and greater than 0.95 for men may put these individuals at risk for a number of diseases.

Body Mass Index (BMI)

Body mass index (BMI) is a rough assessment based on the concept that a person's weight should be proportional to their height. An elevated BMI is linked to increased risk of disease, especially if associated with a large waist circumference. Although this assessment is not designed to assess body fat, BMI is a quick and easy method for determining whether your client's weight is appropriate for their height. BMI is calculated by either dividing the weight in kilograms by the square of the height in meters or dividing body weight in pounds by the square of height in inches and multiplying by 703.

$$BMI = Weight\ (kg)/Height\ (m^2)$$

$$BMI = [Weight\ (lbs)/Height\ (inch^2)] \times 703$$

The lowest risk for disease lies within a BMI range of 22 to 24.9 **Table 6.8**. Scientific evidence indicates that the risk for disease increases with a BMI of 25 or greater. Even though research has proven the risk for premature death and illness increases with a high BMI score, individuals who are underweight are also at risk (55,56).

TABLE 6.8	Body Mass Index Classification	
BMI	**Disease Risk**	**Classification**
<18.5	Increased	Underweight
18.6–21.99	Low	Acceptable
22.0–24.99	Very low	Acceptable
25.0–29.99	Increased	Overweight
30–34.99	High	Obese
35.0–39.99	Very high	Obesity II
≥40	Extremely high	Obesity III

© ilolab/ShutterStock, Inc.

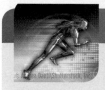

Memory Jogger

Because of its simplicity and measurement consistency, BMI is the most widely used measure to determine overweight and obesity levels. BMI is a useful tool to screen the general population, but its one weakness is that it fails to differentiate fat mass from lean body mass. Using BMI, athletes or bodybuilders with a large amount of muscle mass can mistakenly fall within moderate- to high-risk categories.

SUMMARY

Objective information (such as heart rate, blood pressure, and body composition) provides measurable data that track changes in a client. It can be motivating for a client to assess and reassess body fat, circumference measurements, hip-to-waist ratio, or body mass index. Many clients want to lose body fat, and, as such, it is important to be able to determine a starting body fat percentage. Skinfold calipers are one of the easiest ways to do this in a gym setting. Consistency (in location and administration) is vital when measuring skinfolds. Calculate a client's percentage of body fat by measuring four sites with the calipers, adding the totals of all four sites, and then finding the appropriate sex and age categories on the Durnin–Womersley body fat percentage calculation table.

Circumference measurements and waist-to-hip ratio are other sources of feedback that assess girth changes in the body. Again, consistency in measurements is key. A waist-to-hip ratio greater than 0.80 for women and greater than 0.95 for men may put these individuals at risk for a number of diseases. Finally, the BMI is a good way to determine whether a client's weight is appropriate for his or her height. The chance of having obesity-related health problems potentially increases when a person's BMI exceeds 25.

Cardiorespiratory Assessments

Cardiorespiratory assessments help the personal trainer identify safe and effective starting exercise intensities as well as appropriate modes of cardiorespiratory exercise for clients. The most valid measurement for functional capacity of the cardiopulmonary (heart and lungs) system is Cardiopulmonary Exercise Testing (CPET), also known as maximal oxygen uptake ($\dot{V}o_{2max}$). However, it is not always practical to measure $\dot{V}o_{2max}$ because of equipment requirements, time involved, and willingness of clients to perform at maximal physical capacity. Therefore, submaximal tests are often the preferred method for determining cardiorespiratory functional capacity and fitness.

Submaximal testing allows for the prediction or estimation of $\dot{V}o_{2max}$. These tests are similar to $\dot{V}o_{2max}$ tests, but they differ in that they are terminated at a predetermined heart rate intensity or time frame. There are multiple submaximal tests that have been shown to be valid and reliable predictors of $\dot{V}o_{2max}$, and these tests are often categorized by type (run/walk tests, cycle ergometer tests, and step tests). Any of these tests can be used; however, the space or equipment constraints and specific population (e.g., elderly, youth) to be tested should be considered. Two common submaximal tests for assessing cardiorespiratory efficiency are the YMCA 3-minute step test and the Rockport Walk Test.

YMCA 3-Minute Step Test

This test is designed to estimate an individual's cardiorespiratory fitness level on the basis of a submaximal bout of stair climbing at a set pace for 3 minutes.

Step one: Perform a 3-minute step test on a 12-inch step by having a client perform 96 individual steps per minute (i.e., 24 stepping cycles on and off the step). It is important that the client performs the step test with the correct cadence. A metronome or simply stating out loud, "up, up, down, down" can help keep the client stepping at the correct pace.

Step two: Within 5 seconds of completing the exercise, the client's resting heart rate is measured for a period of 60 seconds and recorded as the recovery pulse.

Step three: Locate the recovery pulse number in one of the following categories:

Men	18–25	26–35	36–45	46–55	56–65	65+
Excellent	50–76	51–76	49–76	56–82	60–77	59–81
Good	79–84	79–85	80–88	87–93	86–94	87–92
Above average	88–93	88–94	92–88	95–101	97–100	94–102
Average	95–100	96–102	100–105	103–111	103–109	104–110
Below average	102–107	104–110	108–113	113–119	111–117	114–118
Poor	111–119	114–121	116–124	121–126	119–128	121–126
Very poor	124–157	126–161	130–163	131–159	131–154	130–151
Women	**18–25**	**26–35**	**36–45**	**46–55**	**56–65**	**65+**
Excellent	52–81	58–80	51–84	63–91	60–92	70–92
Good	85–93	85–92	89–96	95–101	97–103	96–101
Above average	96–102	95–101	100–104	104–110	106–111	104–111

Women	18–25	26–35	36–45	46–55	56–65	65+
Average	104–110	104–110	107–112	113–118	113–118	116–121
Below average	113–120	113–119	115–120	120–124	119–127	123–126
Poor	122–131	122–129	124–132	126–132	129–135	128–133
Very poor	135–169	134–171	137–169	137–171	141–174	135–155

Step four: Determine the appropriate starting program using the appropriate category:

Very poor / Poor	Zone one (65–75% HR_{max})
Below average	Zone one (65–75% HR_{max})
Average / Above average	Zone two (76–85% HR_{max})
Good	Zone two (76–85% HR_{max})
Excellent	Zone three (86–95% HR_{max})

Step five: Determine the client's maximal heart rate by subtracting the client's age from the number 220 (220 – age). Then, take the maximal heart rate and multiply it by the following figures to determine the heart rate ranges for each zone.

Zone one	Maximal heart rate $\times$ 0.65
	Maximal heart rate $\times$ 0.75
Zone two	Maximal heart rate $\times$ 0.76
	Maximal heart rate $\times$ 0.85
Zone three	Maximal heart rate $\times$ 0.86
	Maximal heart rate $\times$ 0.95

Please refer to chapter eight (Cardiorespiratory Fitness Training) for proper use of these zones through specific-stage training programs.

Rockport Walk Test

This test is also designed to estimate a cardiovascular starting point. The starting point is then modified based on ability level. Once determined, refer to the Cardiorespiratory Fitness Training chapter of the text for specific programming strategies.

Step one: First, record the client's weight. Next, have the client walk 1 mile, as fast as he or she can control, on a treadmill. Record the time it takes the client to complete the walk. Immediately record the client's heart rate (beats per minute) at the 1-mile mark. Use the following formula to determine the oxygen consumption ($\dot{V}O_2$) score (57):

$$132.853 - (0.0769 \times Weight) - (0.3877 \times Age) + (6.315 \times Gender) - (3.2649 \times Time)$$
$$- (0.1565 \times Heart\ rate) = \dot{V}O_2\ score$$

Where:

- Weight is in pounds (lbs)
- Gender Male = 1 and Female = 0
- Time is expressed in minutes and 100ths of minutes
- Heart rate is in beats/minute
- Age is in years

Step two: Locate the $\dot{V}O_2$ score in one of the following categories:

Men					
	Heart Rate Zone				
Age	**Poor**	**Fair**	**Average**	**Good**	**Very Good**
20–24	32–37	38–43	44–50	51–56	57–62
25–29	31–35	32–36	43–48	49–53	54–59
30–34	29–34	35–40	41–45	46–51	52–56
35–39	28–32	33–38	39–43	44–48	49–54
40–44	26–31	32–35	36–41	42–46	47–51
45–49	25–29	30–34	35–39	40–43	44–48
50–54	24–27	28–32	33–36	37–41	42–46
55–59	22–26	27–30	31–34	35–39	40–43
60–65	21–24	25–28	29–32	33–36	37–40

Women					
	Heart Rate Zone				
Age	**Poor**	**Fair**	**Average**	**Good**	**Very Good**
20–24	27–31	32–36	37–41	42–46	47–51
25–29	26–30	31–35	36–40	41–44	45–49
30–34	25–29	30–33	34–37	38–42	43–46
35–39	24–27	28–31	32–35	36–40	41–44
40–44	22–25	26–29	30–33	34–37	38–41
45–49	21–23	24–27	28–31	32–35	36–38
50–54	19–22	23–25	26–29	30–32	33–36
55–59	18–20	21–23	24–27	28–30	31–33
60–65	16–18	19–21	22–24	25–27	28–30

Step three: Determine the appropriate starting program using the appropriate category:

Poor	Zone one (65–75% HR_{max})
Fair	Zone one (65–75% HR_{max})
Average	Zone two (76–85% HR_{max})
Good	Zone two (76–85% HR_{max})
Very good	Zone three (86–95% HR_{max})

Step four: Determine the client's maximal heart rate by subtracting the client's age from the number 220 (220 – age). Then, take the maximal heart rate and multiply it by the following figures to determine the heart rate ranges for each zone.

Zone one	Maximal heart rate $\times$ 0.65
	Maximal heart rate $\times$ 0.75
Zone two	Maximal heart rate $\times$ 0.76
	Maximal heart rate $\times$ 0.85
Zone three	Maximal heart rate $\times$ 0.86
	Maximal heart rate $\times$ 0.95

Please refer to chapter eight (Cardiorespiratory Fitness Training) for proper use of these zones through specific-stage training programs.

SUMMARY

There are many ways to determine heart rate zones based on cardiovascular assessments. Once a client's ability level is determined, special programs can be chosen. Two popular cardiorespiratory assessments that can be used to determine one's starting point include the 3-minute step test and the Rockport Walk Test.

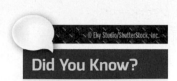
Did You Know?

The Karvonen Formula

The Karvonen formula (HRR) may be used instead of the straight percentage method (220 – age) to determine the appropriate exercise intensity (zones one, two, or three) once establishing the client's baseline cardiorespiratory fitness level.

Posture and Movement Assessments

Importance of Posture

Neuromuscular efficiency is the ability of the nervous system and musculature system to communicate properly producing optimal movement. Proper postural alignment allows optimal neuromuscular efficiency, which helps produce effective and safe movement (58–64). Proper posture ensures that the muscles of the body are optimally aligned at the proper length-tension relationships necessary for efficient functioning of force-couples (58–64). This allows for proper arthrokinematics (joint motion) and effective absorption and distribution of forces throughout the human movement system (kinetic chain), alleviating excess stress on joints (58–64). In other words, proper posture will help keep muscles at their proper length, allowing muscles to properly work together, ensuring proper joint motion, maximizing force production, and reducing the risk of injury.

Proper posture helps the body produce high levels of functional strength. Without it, the body may degenerate or experience poor posture, altered movement patterns, and muscle imbalances. These dysfunctions can lead to common injuries such as ankle sprains, tendonitis, and low-back pain. However, a quick static postural observation can determine any gross deviations in overall posture.

Observing Static Posture

Static posture, or how an individual physically presents himself or herself in stance, could be considered the base from which an individual moves. It is reflected in the alignment of the body. It provides the foundation or the platform from which the extremities function. As with any structure, a weak foundation leads to secondary problems elsewhere in the system.

The use of a static postural assessment has been the basis for identifying muscle imbalances. The static postural assessment may not be able to specifically identify whether a problem is structural in nature or whether it is derived from the development of poor muscular recruitment patterns with resultant muscle imbalances. However, a static postural assessment provides excellent indicators of problem areas that must be further evaluated to clarify the problems at hand. This provides a basis for developing an exercise strategy to target causative factors of faulty movement and neuromuscular inefficiency.

Common Distortion Patterns

How an individual presents himself or herself in static stance is in a sense, a road map of how he or she has been using his or her body with time. What is interesting is that the body has a tendency to compensate in particular patterns or by particular relationships among muscles. These patterns were studied and described by Janda (65) in the early 1970s. Florence and Henry Kendall similarly studied these patterns and took an alternative approach of addressing these postural deviations through the relationship of agonist–antagonist muscle groups. Their work was continued by one of Florence Kendall's students, Shirley Sahrmann (59).

Janda identified three basic compensatory patterns (65). It is not to say that other compensations do not occur. He simply suggested that there was a cascading effect of alterations or deviations in static posture that would more likely than not present themselves in a particular pattern. The three postural distortion patterns to be assessed during a static postural assessment include the pronation distortion syndrome, the lower crossed syndrome, and the upper crossed syndrome.

♦ Pronation distortion syndrome: a postural distortion syndrome characterized by foot pronation (flat feet) and adducted and internally rotated knees (knock knees) **Figure 6.20** and **Table 6.9**.
♦ Lower crossed syndrome: a postural distortion syndrome characterized by an anterior tilt to the pelvis (arched lower back) **Figure 6.21** and **Table 6.10**.
♦ Upper crossed syndrome: a postural distortion syndrome characterized by a forward head and rounded shoulders **Figure 6.22** and **Table 6.11**.

FIGURE 6.20

Pronation distortion syndrome.

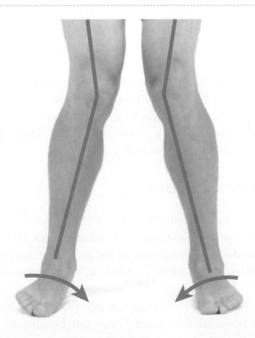

TABLE 6.9	Pronation Distortion Syndrome Summary		
Short Muscles	**Lengthened Muscles**	**Altered Joint Mechanics**	**Possible Injuries**
Gastrocnemius	Anterior tibialis	**Increased:**	Plantar fasciitis
Soleus	Posterior tibialis	Knee adduction	Posterior tibialis tendonitis (shin splints)
Peroneals	Vastus medialis	Knee internal rotation	Patellar tendonitis
Adductors	Gluteus medius/ maximus	Foot pronation	Low-back pain
Iliotibial head	Hip external rotators	Foot external rotation	
Hip flexor complex		**Decreased:**	
Biceps femoris (short head)		Ankle dorsiflexion	
		Ankle inversion	

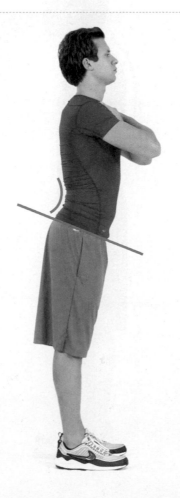

FIGURE 6.21

Lower crossed syndrome.

TABLE 6.10	Lower Crossed Syndrome Summary		
Short Muscles	**Lengthened Muscles**	**Altered Joint Mechanics**	**Possible Injuries**
Gastrocnemius	Anterior tibialis	**Increased:**	Hamstring complex strain
Soleus	Posterior tibialis	Lumbar extension	Anterior knee pain
Hip flexor complex	Gluteus maximus		Low-back pain
Adductors	Gluteus medius	**Decreased:**	
Latissimus dorsi	Transversus abdominis	Hip extension	
Erector spinae	Internal oblique		

© ilolab/ShutterStock, Inc.

FIGURE 6.22

Upper crossed syndrome.

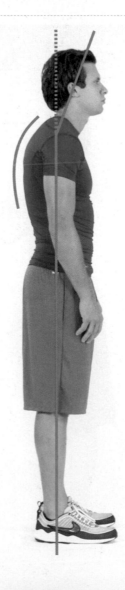

TABLE 6.11

Upper Crossed Syndrome Summary

Short Muscles	Lengthened Muscles	Altered Joint Mechanics	Possible Injuries
Upper trapezius	Deep cervical flexors	**Increased:**	Headaches
Levator scapulae	Serratus anterior	Cervical extension	Biceps tendonitis
Sternocleidomastoid	Rhomboids	Scapular protraction/ elevation	Rotator cuff impingement
Scalenes	Mid-trapezius		Thoracic outlet syndrome
Latissimus dorsi	Lower trapezius	**Decreased:**	
Teres major	Teres minor	Shoulder extension	
Subscapularis	Infraspinatus	Shoulder external rotation	
Pectoralis major/minor			

Static Postural Assessment

There are many elements involved with a detailed static postural assessment. The postural observation discussed here will be a simplified version of an ideal assessment that would be performed by a physician or physical therapist.

In general, one should be checking for neutral alignment, symmetry, balanced muscle tone, and specific postural deformities. It is important that the client be viewed in a weight-bearing position (standing) from multiple vantage points (anterior, posterior, lateral). The fitness professional should look for gross deviations in overall posture.

Kinetic Chain Checkpoints

Postural assessments require observation of the kinetic chain (human movement system). To structure this observation, NASM has devised the use of kinetic chain checkpoints to allow the personal trainer to systematically view the body in an organized fashion. The kinetic chain checkpoints refer to major joint regions of the body including the:

1. Foot and ankle
2. Knee
3. Lumbo-pelvic-hip complex (LPHC)
4. Shoulders
5. Head and cervical spine

Anterior View (Figure 6.23)

- Foot/ankles: Straight and parallel, not flattened or externally rotated
- Knees: In line with toes, not adducted or abducted
- LPHC: Pelvis level with both anterior superior iliac spines in same transverse plane

- ◆ Shoulders: Level, not elevated or rounded
- ◆ Head: Neutral position, not tilted nor rotated

Lateral View (**Figure 6.24**)

- ◆ Foot/ankle: Neutral position, leg vertical at right angle to sole of foot
- ◆ Knees: Neutral position, not flexed nor hyperextended
- ◆ LPHC: Pelvis neutral position, not anteriorly (lumbar extension) or posteriorly (lumbar flexion) rotated
- ◆ Shoulders: Normal kyphotic curve, not excessively rounded
- ◆ Head: Neutral position, not in excessive extension ("jutting" forward)

Posterior View (**Figure 6.25**)

- ◆ Foot/ankle: Heels are straight and parallel, not overly pronated
- ◆ Knees: Neutral position, not adducted or abducted
- ◆ LPHC: Pelvis is level with both posterior superior iliac spines in same transverse plane
- ◆ Shoulders/scapulae: Level, not elevated or protracted (medial borders essentially parallel and approximately 3 to 4 inches apart)
- ◆ Head: Neutral position, neither tilted nor rotated

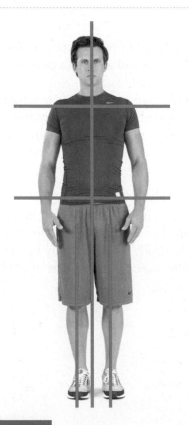

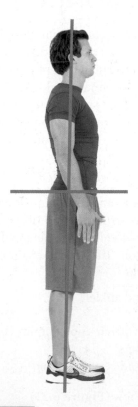

FIGURE 6.23 Kinetic chain checkpoint, anterior view.

FIGURE 6.24 Kinetic chain checkpoint, lateral view.

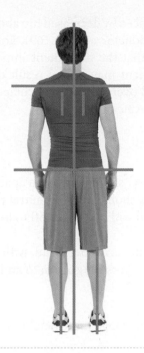

FIGURE 6.25

Kinetic chain checkpoint, posterior view.

Observing Dynamic Posture

Posture is often viewed as being static (or without movement). However, everyday posture is constantly changing to meet the demands placed on the kinetic chain. Thus, once completing a static postural assessment, the dynamic posture assessment should then be performed. The findings from the dynamic postural assessment should further reinforce the observations made during the static postural assessment. In addition, faulty body alignments not revealed during the static postural assessment may be noted during the dynamic postural observations. As such, the dynamic postural assessment (looking at movements) is often the quickest way to gain an overall impression of a client's functional status. Because posture is also a dynamic quality, these observations show postural distortion and potential overactive and underactive muscles in its naturally dynamic setting.

Movement observations should relate to basic functions such as squatting, pushing, pulling, and balancing, in addition to providing crucial information about muscle and joint interplay. The observation process should search for any imbalances in anatomy, physiology, or biomechanics that may decrease a client's results and possibly lead to injury (both in and out of the fitness environment). With the limited time that most fitness professionals have for observation, incorporating a systematic assessment sequence is essential.

Overhead Squat Assessment

Purpose: This is designed to assess dynamic flexibility, core strength, balance, and overall neuromuscular control. There is evidence to support the use of transitional movement assessments such as the overhead squat test (66). These assessments appear to be reliable and valid measures of lower extremity movement patterns when standard protocols are applied. The overhead squat test has been shown to reflect lower extremity movement patterns during jump-landing tasks (67). Knee valgus (knock-knees) during the overhead squat test is influenced by decreased hip abductor and hip external rotation strength (68), increased hip adductor activity (69), and restricted ankle dorsiflexion (69,70). These results suggest that the movement impairments observed during this transitional movement assessment may be the result of alterations in available joint motion, muscle activation, and overall neuromuscular control that some hypothesize point toward people with an elevated injury risk.

Procedure
Position

1. The client stands with the feet shoulders-width apart and pointed straight ahead. The foot and ankle complex should be in a neutral position. It is suggested that the assessment is performed with the shoes off to better view the foot and ankle complex.
2. Have the client raise his or her arms overhead, with elbows fully extended. The upper arms should bisect the torso **Figure 6.26** and **Figure 6.27**.

Movement

1. Instruct the client to squat to roughly the height of a chair seat and return to the starting position.
2. Repeat the movement for 5 repetitions, observing from each position (anterior and lateral).

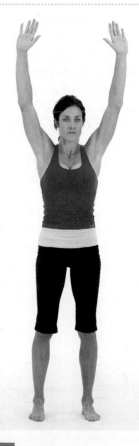

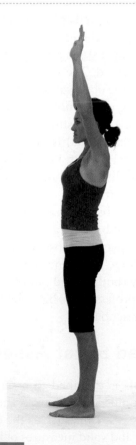

FIGURE 6.26 Overhead squat assessment start, anterior view.

FIGURE 6.27 Overhead squat assessment start, lateral view.

Views

1. View feet, ankles, and knees from the front **Figure 6.28**. The feet should remain straight with the knees tracking in line with the foot (2nd and 3rd toes).
2. View the lumbo-pelvic-hip complex, shoulder, and cervical complex from the side **Figure 6.29**. The tibia should remain in line with the torso while the arms also stay in line with the torso.

Compensations: Anterior View

1. Feet: Do the feet flatten and/or turn out **Figure 6.30** and **Figure 6.31**?
2. Knees: Do the knees move inward (adduct and internally rotate) **Figure 6.32**?

Compensations: Lateral View

3. Lumbo-pelvic-hip complex:

    a. Does the low back arch **Figure 6.33**?
    b. Does the torso lean forward excessively **Figure 6.34**?

4. Shoulder: Do the arms fall forward **Figure 6.35**?

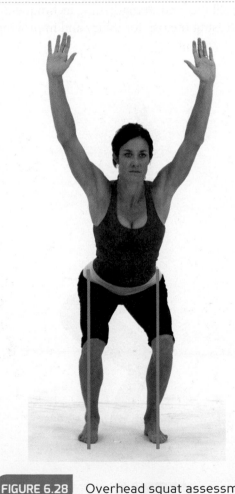
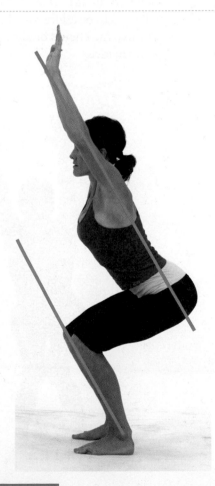

FIGURE 6.28 Overhead squat assessment finish, anterior view.

FIGURE 6.29 Overhead squat assessment finish, lateral view.

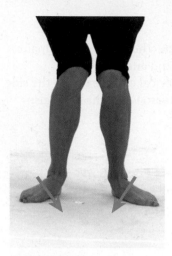

FIGURE 6.30   Feet flatten.

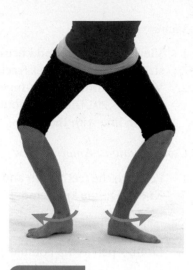

FIGURE 6.31   Feet turn out.

When performing the assessment, record all of your findings **Figure 6.36**. You can then refer to **Table 6.12** to determine potential overactive and underactive muscles that will need to be addressed through corrective flexibility and strengthening techniques to improve the client's quality of movement, decreasing the risk for injury and improving performance.

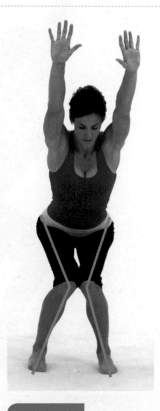

FIGURE 6.32   Knees move inward.

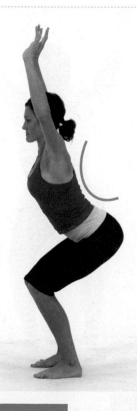

FIGURE 6.33   Low back arches.

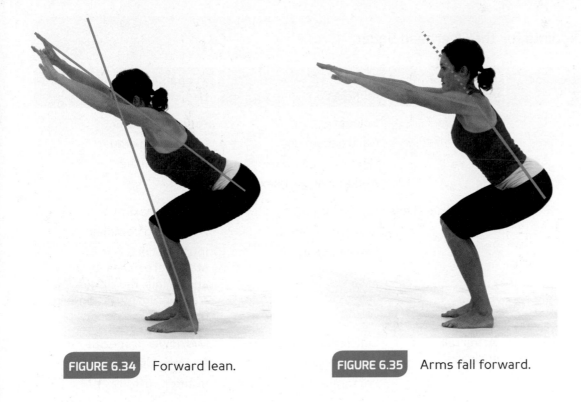

FIGURE 6.34 Forward lean.   **FIGURE 6.35** Arms fall forward.

View	Kinetic chain checkpoints	Movement observation	
Anterior	Feet Knees	• Flatten/Turn out • Moves inward	☐ Yes ☐ Yes
Lateral	Lumbo-pelvic-hip complex Shoulder complex	• Excessive forward lean • Low back arches • Arm falls forward	☐ Yes ☐ Yes ☐ Yes

FIGURE 6.36 Checkpoints for the overhead squat.

Single-Leg Squat Assessment

Purpose: This transitional movement assessment also assesses dynamic flexibility, core strength, balance, and overall neuromuscular control. There is evidence to support the use of the single-leg squat as a transitional movement assessment (66). This assessment appears to be a reliable and valid measure of lower extremity movement patterns when standard application protocols are applied. Knee valgus has been shown to be influenced by decreased hip abductor and hip external rotation strength (68), increased hip adductor activity (66), and restricted ankle dorsiflexion (66,70). These results suggest that the movement impairments observed during the transitional movement assessments may be the result of alterations in available joint motion, muscle activation, and overall neuromuscular control.

TABLE 6.12	Checkpoints for the Overhead Squat			
View	**Checkpoint**	**Compensation**	**Probable Overactive Muscles**	**Probable Underactive Muscles**
Lateral	LPHC	Excessive forward lean	Soleus Gastrocnemius Hip flexor complex Abdominal complex	Anterior tibialis Gluteus maximus Erector spinae
		Low back arches	Hip flexor complex Erector spinae Latissimus dorsi	Gluteus maximus Hamstring complex Intrinsic core stabilizers (transverse abdominis, multifidus, transversospinalis, internal oblique pelvic floor)
	Upper body	Arms fall forward	Latissimus dorsi Teres major Pectoralis major/minor	Mid/lower trapezius Rhomboids Rotator cuff
Anterior	Feet	Turn out	Soleus Lateral gastrocnemius Biceps femoris (short head)	Medial gastrocnemius Medial hamstring complex Gracilis Sartorius Popliteus
	Knees	Move inward	Adductor complex Biceps femoris (short head) TFL Vastus lateralis	Gluteus medius/maximus Vastus medialis oblique (VMO)

Memory Jogger

For some individuals, the single-leg squat assessment may be too difficult to perform (e.g., elderly client). Other options include using outside support for assistance or simply performing a single-leg balance assessment to assess movement compensation and ability to control self in a relatively unstable environment.

Procedure

Position

1. The client should stand with hands on the hips and eyes focused on an object straight ahead.
2. Foot should be pointed straight ahead, and the foot, ankle, and knee and the lumbo-pelvic-hip complex should be in a neutral position **Figure 6.37**.

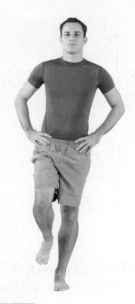 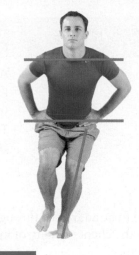

| **FIGURE 6.37** | Single-leg squat start. | **FIGURE 6.38** | Single-leg squat finish. |

Movement

1. Have the client squat to a comfortable level and return to the starting position.
2. Perform up to 5 repetitions before switching sides.

Views

View the knee from the front. The knee should track in line with the foot (2nd and 3rd toes) **Figure 6.38**.

Compensation

1. Knee: Does the knee move inward (adduct and internally rotate) **Figure 6.39**?

Like the overhead squat assessment, record your findings **Figure 6.40**. You can then refer to **Table 6.13** to determine potential overactive and underactive muscles that

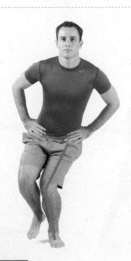

View	Kinetic chain checkpoints	Movement observation	
Anterior	Knees	• Moves inward	☐ Right ☐ Left

| **FIGURE 6.39** | Knee moves inward. | **FIGURE 6.40** | Checkpoints for single-leg squat. |

TABLE 6.13	Checkpoints for the Single-Leg Squat		
Checkpoint	**Compensation**	**Probable Overactive Muscles**	**Probable Underactive Muscles**
Knee	Move inward	Adductor complex Biceps femoris (short head) TFL Vastus lateralis	Gluteus medius/maximus Vastus medialis oblique (VMO)

will need to be addressed through corrective flexibility and strengthening techniques to improve the client's quality of movement, decreasing the risk for injury and improving performance.

Pushing Assessment

Purpose: Like the overhead and single-leg squat assessments, this assessment assesses movement efficiency and potential muscle imbalances during pushing movements.

Procedure

Position

1. Instruct the client to stand with abdomen drawn inward, feet in a split stance and toes pointing forward **Figure 6.41**.

Movement

1. Viewing from the side, instruct the client to press handles forward and return to the starting position.
2. Perform up to 20 repetitions in a controlled fashion. The lumbar and cervical spines should remain neutral while the shoulders stay level **Figure 6.42**.

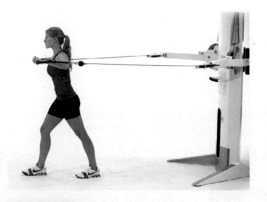

FIGURE 6.41 Pushing assessment start.

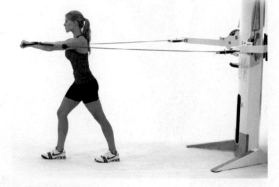

FIGURE 6.42 Pushing assessment finish.

Compensations

1. Low back: Does the low back arch **Figure 6.43**?
2. Shoulders: Do the shoulders elevate **Figure 6.44**?
3. Head: Does the head migrate forward **Figure 6.45**?

Record your findings **Figure 6.46**. You can then refer to **Table 6.14** to determine potential overactive and underactive muscles that will need to be addressed through corrective flexibility and strengthening techniques to improve the client's quality of movement, decreasing the risk for injury and improving performance.

Did You Know?

Pushing Assessment Option

Although it is best to perform this in a standing position to obtain a better representation of the client's functional status, this assessment can also be performed on a machine.

© Sky Studio/ShutterStock, Inc.

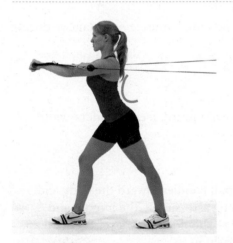

FIGURE 6.43   Low back arches.

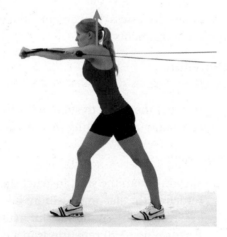

FIGURE 6.44   Shoulders elevate.

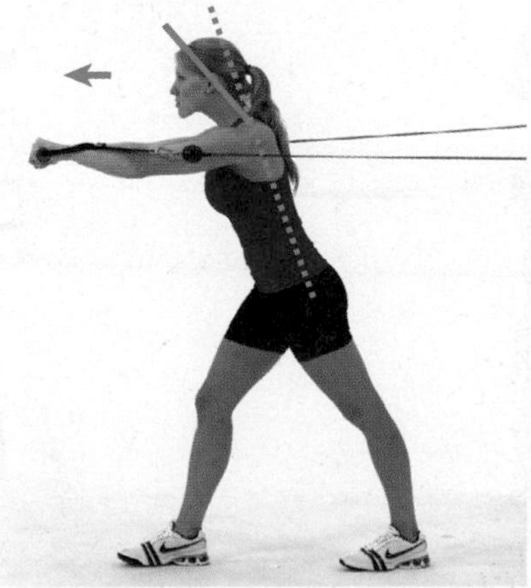

FIGURE 6.45   Head migrates forward.

FIGURE 6.46   Checkpoints for pushing assessment.

Kinetic chain checkpoints	Movement observation	
Lumbo-pelvic-hip complex	• Low back arches	☐ Yes
Shoulder complex	• Shoulders elevate	☐ Yes
Head	• Head migrates forward	☐ Yes

TABLE 6.14	Checkpoints for Pushing Assessment		
Checkpoint	**Compensation**	**Probable Overactive Muscles**	**Probable Underactive Muscles**
LPHC	Low back arches	Hip flexors Erector spinae	Intrinsic core stabilizers
Shoulder complex	Shoulder elevation	Upper trapezius Sternocleidomastoid Levator scapulae	Mid/lower trapezius
Head	Head migrates forward	Upper trapezius Sternocleidomastoid Levator scapulae	Deep cervical flexors

Pulling Assessment

Purpose: To assess movement efficiency and potential muscle imbalances during pulling movements.

Procedure

Position

1. Instruct the client to stand with abdomen drawn inward, feet shoulders-width apart and toes pointing forward **Figure 6.47**.

Movement

1. Viewing from the side, instruct the client to pull handles toward the body and return to the starting position. Like the pushing assessment, the lumbar and cervical spines should remain neutral while the shoulders stay level **Figure 6.48**.
2. Perform up to 20 repetitions in a controlled fashion.

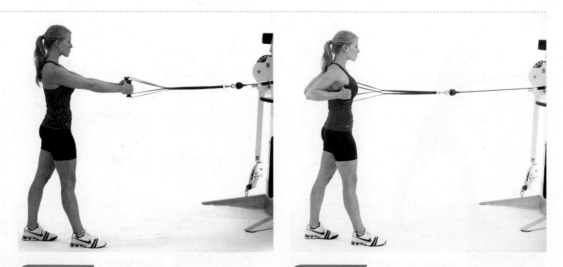

FIGURE 6.47 Pulling assessment start.   **FIGURE 6.48** Pulling assessment finish.

Compensations

1. Low back: Does the low back arch **Figure 6.49**?
2. Shoulders: Do the shoulders elevate **Figure 6.50**?
3. Head: Does the head migrate forward **Figure 6.51**?

Record your findings **Figure 6.52**. You can then refer to **Table 6.15** to determine potential overactive and underactive muscles that will need to be addressed through corrective flexibility and strengthening techniques to improve the client's quality of movement, decreasing the risk for injury and improving performance.

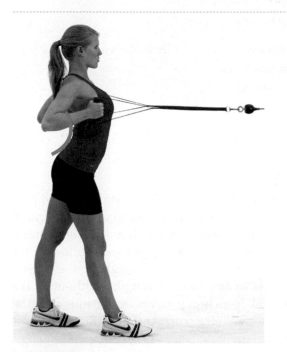

FIGURE 6.49 Low back arches.

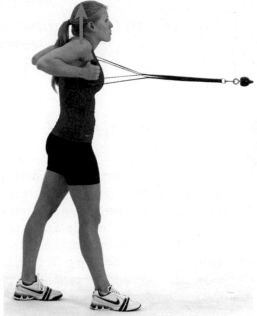

FIGURE 6.50 Shoulders elevate.

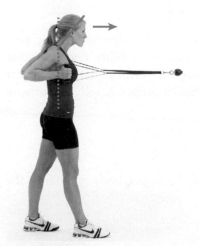

FIGURE 6.51 Head migrates forward.

Kinetic chain checkpoints	Movement observation	
Lumbo-pelvic-hip complex	• Low back arches	☐ Yes
Shoulder complex	• Shoulders elevate	☐ Yes
Head	• Head migrates forward	☐ Yes

FIGURE 6.52 Checkpoints for pulling assessment.

TABLE 6.15	Checkpoints for Pulling Assessment		
Checkpoint	**Compensation**	**Probable Overactive Muscles**	**Probable Underactive Muscles**
LPHC	Low back arches	Hip flexors Erector spinae	Intrinsic core stabilizers
Shoulder complex	Shoulder elevation	Upper trapezius Sternocleidomastoid Levator scapulae	Mid/lower trapezius
Head	Head protrudes forward	Upper trapezius Sternocleidomastoid Levator scapulae	Deep cervical flexors

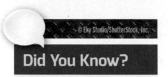

Did You Know?

Pulling Assessment Option

Like the pushing assessment, the pulling assessment can also be performed on a machine.

SUMMARY

Posture is the alignment and function of all parts of the kinetic chain. Its main purpose is to overcome constant forces placed on the body by maintaining structural efficiency. The kinetic chain requires constant postural equilibrium. Proper postural alignment puts the body in a state of optimal neuromuscular efficiency, allowing for proper joint mechanics and effective distribution of force throughout the kinetic chain. It lets the body produce high levels of functional strength. Without it, the body may degenerate or experience postural distortion patterns. A dynamic postural observation examines basic movements and provides crucial information about how muscles and joints interact. It searches for any imbalances in anatomy, physiology, or biomechanics.

Performance Assessments

Performance assessments can be used for clients looking to improve athletic performance. These assessments will measure upper extremity stability and muscular endurance, lower extremity agility, and overall strength. Basic performance assessments include the push-up test, Davies test, shark skill test, bench press strength assessment, and squat strength assessment.

Push-Up Test

Purpose: This test measures muscular endurance of the upper body, primarily the pushing muscles.

Procedure
Position

1. In push-up position (ankles, knees, hips, shoulders, and head in a straight line), the client or athlete lowers the body to touch a partner's closed fist placed under

the chest, and repeats for 60 seconds or exhaustion without compensating (arches low back, extends cervical spine). A variation to this assessment includes performing push-ups from a kneeling position. Additionally, this assessment can be performed with the participant required to touch the chest to the floor (rather than to a partner's fist). Whichever method is performed, be sure to use the same procedure during the reassessment process **Figure 6.53**.

2. Record number of actual touches reported from partner.
3. The client or athlete should be able to perform more push-ups when reassessed.

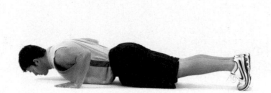
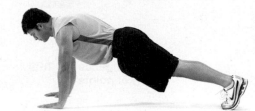

FIGURE 6.53

Push-up test.

Davies Test

Purpose: This assessment measures upper extremity agility and stabilization (71). This assessment may not be suitable for clients or athletes who lack shoulder stability.

Procedure
Position

1. Place two pieces of tape on the floor, 36 inches apart.
2. Have client assume a push-up position, with one hand on each piece of tape **Figure 6.54**.

Movement

1. Instruct client to quickly move his or her right hand to touch the left hand **Figure 6.55**.
2. Perform alternating touching on each side for 15 seconds.
3. Repeat for three trials.
4. Reassess in the future to measure improvement of number of touches.
5. Record the number of lines touched by both hands in **Figure 6.56**.

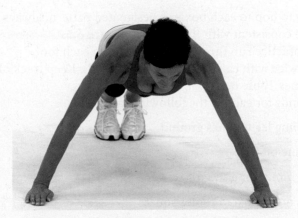

FIGURE 6.54

Davies test start.

FIGURE 6.55

Davies test movement.

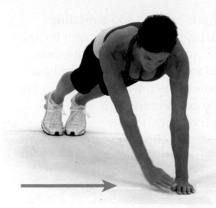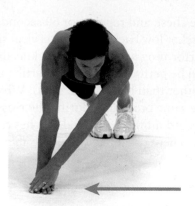

FIGURE 6.56

Checklist for Davies test.

Distance of points	Trial #	Time	Repetitions performed
36 inches	1	15 secs.	☐
36 inches	2	15 secs.	☐
36 inches	3	15 secs.	☐

Shark Skill Test

Purpose: This is designed to assess lower extremity agility and neuromuscular control. (It should be viewed as a progression from the single-leg squat and, as such, may not be suitable for all individuals.)

Procedure

Position

1. Position client in the center box of a grid, with hands on hips and standing on one leg.

Movement:

1. Instruct client to hop to each box in a designated pattern, always returning to the center box. Be consistent with the patterns **Figure 6.57**.
2. Perform one practice run through the boxes with each foot.
3. Perform test twice with each foot (four times total). Keep track of time.
4. Record the times **Table 6.16**.
5. Add 0.10 seconds for each of the following faults:

    i.   Non-hopping leg touches ground

    ii. Hands come off hips

    iii. Foot goes into wrong square

    iv. Foot does not return to center square

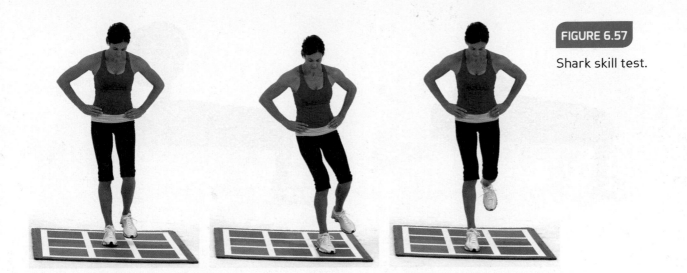

FIGURE 6.57

Shark skill test.

TABLE 6.16   Observation Findings for Shark Skill Test

Trial	Side	Time (seconds)	Deduction Tally	Total Deducted (# of faults × 0.1)	Final Total (time + total deduction)
Practice	Right				
	Left				
One	Right				
	Left				
Two	Right				
	Left				

Upper Extremity Strength Assessment: Bench Press

Purpose: This assessment is designed to estimate the one-rep maximum on overall upper body strength of the pressing musculature. This test can also be used to determine training intensities of the bench press. This is considered an advanced assessment (for strength-specific goals) and, as such, may not be suitable for many clients. Generally speaking, personal trainers should not perform this assessment for clients with general fitness or weight-loss goals.

Position

1. Position client on a bench, lying on his or her back. Feet should be pointed straight ahead. The low back should be in a neutral position **Figure 6.58**.

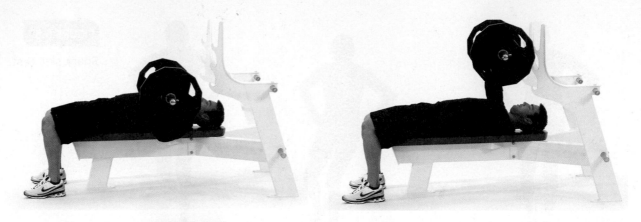

FIGURE 6.58   Bench press strength assessment.

Movement

1. Instruct the client to warm up with a light resistance that can be easily performed for 8 to 10 repetitions.
2. Take a 1-minute rest.
3. Add 10 to 20 pounds (5–10% of initial load) and perform 3 to 5 repetitions.
4. Take a 2-minute rest.
5. Repeat steps 4 and 5 until the client achieves failure between 2 and 10 repetitions (3 to 5 repetitions for greater accuracy).
6. Use the one-rep maximum estimation chart in the appendix to calculate one-repetition max.

Lower Extremity Strength Assessment: Squat

Purpose: This assessment is designed to estimate the one-repetition squat maximum and overall lower body strength. This test can also be used to determine training intensities for the squat exercise. This is considered an advanced assessment (for strength-specific goals) and, as such, may not be suitable for many clients. Generally speaking, personal trainers should not perform this assessment for clients with general fitness or weight-loss goals.

Position

1. Feet should be shoulders-width apart, pointed straight ahead, and with knees in line with the toes. The low back should be in a neutral position **Figure 6.59**.

Movement

1. Instruct the client to warm up with a light resistance that can be easily performed for 8 to 10 repetitions.
2. Take a 1-minute rest.
3. Add 30 to 40 pounds (10–20% of initial load) and perform 3 to 5 repetitions.
4. Take a 2-minute rest.

© ilolab/ShutterStock, Inc.

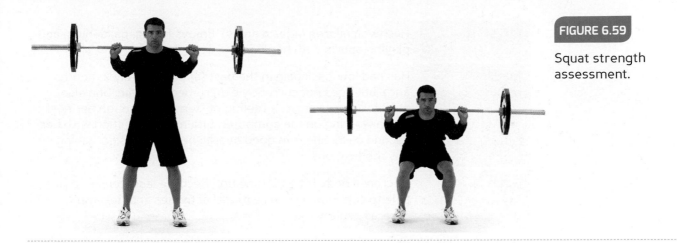

Squat strength assessment.

5. Repeat steps 3 and 4 until the client achieves failure between 2 and 10 repetitions (3 to 5 repetitions for greater accuracy).
6. Use the one-rep maximum estimation chart in the appendix to calculate one-repetition max.

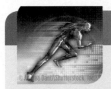

Memory Jogger

Make sure in both the bench press and squat assessments that the individual performs the exercises with minimal movement compensations!

Implementing the Fitness Assessment

Assessment Parameters

The fitness assessment builds the foundation for the entire template. It enables the personal trainer to decide the appropriate selection of flexibility, cardiorespiratory, core, balance, power, and strength training exercises. Listed below are several sample clients, along with the pertinent subjective information that would have been obtained in their first session. From this information, it will also list the appropriate objective assessments that a personal trainer would want to include, ensuring that the program is individualized to these clients' specific goals and needs.

Client 1: Lita

General Information

Age	38
Occupation	Secretary. She spends a lot of time sitting behind a computer and on the phone. Lita is required to wear business attire.

(Continued)

Lifestyle	Has two children (ages 6 and 9). Enjoys hiking, gardening, and playing sports with her kids.
Medical history	Has had low-back pain in the past (approximately 2 months ago), but does not currently experience any pain. She also, at times, experiences a feeling of "tension" through her neck when working on the computer. Lita had a C-section with her second child. She is in good overall health and is not taking any medications.
Goals	Decrease body fat and "tone up." Become less "tense" to be able to continue her recreational activities and be simply "overall healthy."

Recommended Objective Assessments for Lita

- Body fat measurement
- Circumference measurement
- Resting heart rate
- Blood pressure
- Step test or Rockport Walk Test
- Overhead squat assessment
- Single-leg squat or single-leg balance
- Pushing assessment (time permitting)
- Pulling assessment (time permitting)

Client 2: Ron

General Information

Age	72
Occupation	Retired business executive
Lifestyle	Enjoys traveling, long walks with his wife, golf, carpentry, and playing with his seven grandkids.
Medical history	Had triple bypass surgery (10 years ago). Takes medication for high cholesterol. Has lower back and shoulder pain after he plays golf.
Goals	Ron weighs 170 pounds and is not concerned with altering his body composition. He wants to be healthy, increase some overall strength, and decrease his back and shoulder pain to play golf and with his grandkids more easily.

Recommended Objective Assessments for Ron

- Obtain a medical release from Ron's physician
- Resting heart rate
- Blood pressure
- 3-minute step test or Rockport Walk Test
- Overhead squat assessment
- Assisted single-leg squat or single-leg balance

♦   Pushing assessment (time permitting)
♦   Pulling assessment (time permitting)

Client 3: Brian

General Information

Age	24
Occupation	Semiprofessional soccer player
Lifestyle	He travels often, competing in various soccer tournaments. He likes to work out with weights three to four times per week, practices 5 days per week, and plays in an organized game at least two times per week.
Medical history	Had surgery for a torn anterior cruciate ligament in his left knee 3 years ago and has sprained his left ankle two times since his knee surgery. Went through physical therapy for his last ankle sprain 6 months ago and was cleared to work out and play again. For the most part, his knee and ankle have not been giving him any trouble, other than some occasional soreness after games and practice. He has recently gone through a physical to begin playing again, and his physician gave him a clean bill of health.
Goals	He wants to increase his overall performance by enhancing his flexibility, speed, cardiorespiratory efficiency, and leg strength. He also wants to decrease his risk of incurring other injuries. After being out of soccer because of the injury, he increased his body fat percentage and would like to lower it.

Recommended Objective Assessments for Brian

♦   Body fat measurement
♦   3-minute step test or Rockport Walk Test
♦   Overhead squat assessment
♦   Single-leg squat assessment
♦   Davies test
♦   Shark skill test
♦   Lower extremity strength assessment: squat

Filling in the Template

The name should obviously be filled in, to keep proper records of the correct client. The date is necessary to follow a client's progression with time and keep track of what workouts occurred on what dates **Figure 6.60**.

The phase signifies where in the OPT model the client is. This can also act as a reminder about the acute variables significant to this phase. (This will be discussed in detail later in the text.)

FIGURE 6.60

Filled out assessment section of template.

Professional's Name: Brian Sutton

NASM
NATIONAL ACADEMY OF SPORTS MEDICINE

CLIENT'S NAME: JOHN SMITH				DATE: 5/01/13

GOAL: FAT LOSS	PHASE: 1 STABILIZATION ENDURANCE

WARM-UP

Exercise:	Sets	Duration	Coaching Tip

CORE / BALANCE / PLYOMETRIC

Exercise:	Sets	Reps	Tempo	Rest	Coaching Tip

SPEED, AGILITY, QUICKNESS

Exercise:	Sets	Reps	Rest	Coaching Tip

RESISTANCE

Exercise:	Sets	Reps	Tempo	Rest	Coaching Tip

COOL-DOWN

Exercise:	Sets	Duration	Coaching Tip

Coaching Tips:

National Academy of Sports Medicine

REFERENCES

1. US Department of Health and Human Services (USDHHS). Physical Activity Guidelines Advisory Committee Report, 2008. Washington, DC: USDHHS; 2008. http://www.health.gov/paguidelines.

2. National Center for Health Statistics. *Chartbook on Trends in the Health of Americans. Health, United States, 2008.* Hyattsville, MD: Public Health Service; 2008.

3. American College of Sports Medicine. *ACSM's Guidelines for Exercise Testing and Prescription.* 8th ed. Philadelphia: Lippincott Williams & Wilkins; 2010.

4. Thomas S, Reading J, Shephard RJ. Revision of the Physical Activity Readiness Questionnaire (PAR-Q). *Can J Sports Sci.* 1992;17:338-345.

5. Van der Windt DAWM, Thomas E, Pope DP, et al. Occupational risk factors for shoulder pain: a systematic review. *Occup Environ Med.* 2000;57:433-442.

6. MedlinePlus. http://www.nlm.nih.gov/medlineplus/videos/news/high_heels_072010.html. Accessed September 15, 2010.

7. Janda V. Muscles and cervicogenic pain syndromes In: Grant R, ed. *Physical Therapy of the Cervical and Thoracic Spine.* Edinburgh: Churchill Livingstone; 1988:153-166.

8. Leahy PM. Active release techniques: logical soft tissue treatment. In: Hammer WI, ed. *Functional Soft Tissue Examination and Treatment by Manual Methods.* Gaithersburg, MD: Aspen Publishers; 1999:549-559.

9. Kucera KL, Marshall SW, Kirkendall DT, Marchak PM, Garrett WE Jr. Injury history as a risk factor for incident injury in youth soccer. *Br J Sports Med.* 2004;39:462-466.

10. Bullock-Saxton JE. Local sensation changes and altered hip muscle function following severe ankle sprain. *Phys Ther.* 1994;74:17-31.

11. Brown CN, Padua DA, Marshall SW, Guskiewicz KM. Hip kinematics during a stop-jump task in patients with chronic ankle instability. *J Athl Train.* 2011;46(5):461-467.

12. Guskiewicz K, Perrin D. Effect of orthotics on postural sway following inversion ankle sprain. *J Orthop Sports Phys Ther.* 1996;23:326-331.

13. Nitz A, Dobner J, Kersey D. Nerve injury and grades II and III ankle sprains. *Am J Sports Med.* 1985;13:177-182.

14. Wilkerson G, Nitz A. Dynamic ankle stability: mechanical and neuromuscular interrelationships. *J Sport Rehab.* 1994;3:43-57.

15. Barrack R, Lund P, Skinner H. Knee proprioception revisited. *J Sport Rehab.* 1994;3:18-42.

16. Beard D, Kyberd P, O'Connor J, Fergusson C. Reflex hamstring contraction latency in ACL deficiency. *J Orthop Res.* 1994;12:219-228.

17. Boyd I. The histological structure of the receptors in the knee joint of the cat correlated with their physiological response. *J Physiol.* 1954;124:476-488.

18. Corrigan J, Cashman W, Brady M. Proprioception in the cruciate deficient knee. *J Bone Joint Surg Br.* 1992;74B:247-250.

19. DeCarlo M, Klootwyk T, Shelbourne D. ACL surgery and accelerated rehabilitation. *J Sport Rehab.* 1997;6:144-156.

20. Ekholm J, Eklund G, Skoglund S. On the reflex effects from knee joint of the cat. *Acta Physiol Scand.* 1960;50:167-174.

21. Feagin J. The syndrome of the torn ACL. *Orthop Clin North Am.* 1979;10:81-90.

22. Fredericson M, Cookingham CL, Chaudhari AM, Dowdell BC, Oestreicher N, Sahrmann SA. Hip abductor weakness in distance runners with iliotibial band syndrome. *Clin J Sport Med.* 2000;10:169-175.

23. Hewett TE, Lindenfeld TN, Riccobene JV, Noyes FR. The effect of neuromuscular training on the incidence of knee injury in female athletes. A prospective study. *Am J Sports Med.* 1999;27:699-706.

24. Ireland ML, Willson JD, Ballantyne BT, Davis IM. Hip strength in females with and without patellofemoral pain. *J Orthop Sports Phys Ther.* 2003;33:671-676.

25. Irrgang J, Harner C. Recent advances in ACL rehabilitation: clinical factors. *J Sport Rehab.* 1997;6:111-124.

26. Irrgang J, Whitney S, Cox E. Balance and proprioceptive training for rehabilitation of the lower extremity. *J Sport Rehab.* 1994;3:68-83.

27. Johansson H. Role of knee ligaments in proprioception and regulation of muscle stiffness. *J Electromyogr Kinesiol.* 1991;1:158-179.

28. Johansson H, Sjölander P, Sojka P. A sensory role for the cruciate ligaments. *Clin Orthop Relat Res.* 1991;268:161-178.

29. Johansson H, Sjölander P, Sojka P. Receptors in the knee joint ligaments and their role in the biomechanics of the joint. *Crit Rev Biomed Eng.* 1991;18:341-368.

30. Nyland J, Smith S, Beickman K, Armsey T, Caborn D. Frontal plane knee angle affects dynamic postural control strategy during unilateral stance. *Med Sci Sports Exerc.* 2002;34:1150-1157.

31. Powers C. The influence of altered lower-extremity kinematics on patellofemoral joint dysfunction: a theoretical perspective. *J Orthop Sports Phys Ther.* 2003;33:639-646.

32. Bullock-Saxton JE, Janda V, Bullock MI. Reflex activation of gluteal muscles in walking. An approach to restoration of muscle function for patients with low back pain. *Spine.* 1993;18:704-708.

33. Hodges P, Richardson C, Jull G. Evaluation of the relationship between laboratory and clinical tests of transversus abdominis function. *Physiother Res Int.* 1996;1:30-40.

34. Hodges PW, Richardson CA. Inefficient muscular stabilization of the lumbar spine associated with low back pain. A motor control evaluation of transversus abdominis. *Spine.* 1996;21:2640-2650.

35. Hodges PW, Richardson CA. Contraction of the abdominal muscles associated with movement of the lower limb. *Phys Ther.* 1997;77:132-144.

36. Janda V. Muscles and motor control in low back pain: assessment and management. In: Twomey L, ed. *Physical Therapy of the Low Back.* New York, NY: Churchill Livingstone; 1987:253-278.

37. Lewit K. Muscular and articular factors in movement restriction. *Manual Med.* 1985;1:83-85.

38. O'Sullivan P, Twomey L, Allison G, Sinclair J, Miller K, Knox J. Altered patterns of abdominal muscle activation in patients with chronic low back pain. *Aust J Physiother.* 1997;43:91-98.

39. Richardson C, Jull G, Toppenberg R, Comerford M. Techniques for active lumbar stabilization for spinal protection. *Aust J Physiother.* 1992;38:105-112.

40. Broström L-Å, Kronberg M, Nemeth G. Muscle activity during shoulder dislocation. *Acta Orthop Scand.* 1989;60:639-641.

41. Glousman R. Electromyographic analysis and its role in the athletic shoulder. *Clin Orthop Relat Res.* 1993;288:27-34.

42. Glousman R, Jobe F, Tibone J, Moynes D, Antonelli D, Perry J. Dynamic electromyographic analysis of the throwing shoulder with glenohumeral instability. *J Bone Joint Surg Am.* 1988;70A:220-226.

43. Hanson ED, Leigh S, Mynark RG. Acute effects of heavy- and light-load squat exercise on the kinetic measures of vertical jumping. *J Strength Cond Res.* 2007;21:1012-1017.

44. Howell S, Kraft T. The role of the supraspinatus and infraspinatus muscles in glenohumeral kinematics of anterior shoulder instability. *Clin Orthop Relat Res.* 1991;263:128-134.

45. Kedgley A, Mackenzie G, Ferreira L, Johnson J, Faber K. In vitro kinematics of the shoulder following rotator cuff injury. *Clin Biomech (Bristol, Avon).* 2007;22:1068-1073.

46. Kronberg M, Broström L-Å, Nemeth G. Differences in shoulder muscle activity between patients with generalized joint laxity and normal controls. *Clin Orthop Relat Res.* 1991;269:181-192.

47. Yanagawa T, Goodwin C, Shelburne K, Giphart J, Torry M, Pandy M. Contributions of the individual muscles of the shoulder to glenohumeral joint stability during abduction. *J Biomech Eng.* 2008;130:21-24.

48. Yasojima T, Kizuka T, Noguchi H, Shiraki H, Mukai N, Miyanaga Y. Differences in EMG activity in scapular plane abduction under variable arm positions and loading conditions. *Med Sci Sports Exerc.* 2008;40: 716-721.

49. Graven-Nielsen T, Mense S. The peripheral apparatus of muscle pain: evidence from animal and human studies. *Clin J Pain.* 2001;17:2-10.

50. Mense S, Simons D. *Muscle Pain. Understanding Its Nature, Diagnosis, and Treatment.* Philadelphia, PA: Williams & Wilkins; 2001.

51. Lambert E, Bohlmann I, Cowling K. Physical activity for health: understanding the epidemiological evidence for risk benefits. *Int J Sports Med.* 2001;1:1-15.

52. Pate R, Pratt M, Blair S, et al. Physical activity and public health: a recommendation from the Centers for Disease Control and Prevention and the American College of Sports Medicine. *JAMA.* 1995;273:402-407.

53. Going S, Davis R. Body composition. In Roitman JL (Ed.): *ACSM's Resource Manual for Guidelines for Exercise Testing and Prescription.* 4th ed. Philadelphia: Lippincott Williams & Wilkins; 2001:396.

54. Durnin JVGA, Womersley J. Body fat assessed from total body density and its estimation from skinfold thickness measurements on 481 men and women aged 16-72 years. *Br J Nutr.* 1974;32:77-97.

55. Stevens J. The effect of age on the association between body-mass index and mortality. *N Engl J Med.* 1998;338:1-7.

56. American College of Sports Medicine. Position stand; appropriate intervention strategies for weight loss and prevention for weight regain in adults. *Med Sci Sports Exerc.* 2001;33:2145-56.

57. American College of Sports Medicine. *ACSM's Resource Manual for Guidelines for Exercise Testing and Prescription.* 3rd ed. Baltimore: Williams & Wilkins; 1998.

58. Sahrmann SA. *Diagnosis and Treatment of Movement Impairment Syndromes.* St. Louis: Mosby; 2002.

59. Sahrmann SA. Posture and muscle Imbalance. Faulty lumbo-pelvic alignment and associated musculoskeletal pain syndromes. *Orthop Div Rev Can Phys Ther.* 1992;12:13-20.

60. Kendall FP, McCreary EK, Provance PG. *Muscles: Testing and Function.* 4th ed. Baltimore: Williams & Wilkins; 1993.

61. Norkin C, Levangie P. *Joint Structure and Function.* 2nd ed. Philadelphia, PA: FA Davis Company; 1992.

62. Janda V. Muscle strength in relation to muscle length, pain and muscle imbalance. In: Harms–Rindahl K, ed. *Muscle Strength.* Churchill–Livingston, New York, NY, 1993:83-91.

63. Powers CM, Ward SR, Fredericson M, Guillet M, Shellock FG. Patellofemoral kinematics during weight-bearing and non-weight-bearing knee extension in persons with lateral subluxation of the patella: a preliminary study. *J Orthop Sports Phys Ther.* 2003;33:677-685.

64. Newmann D. *Kinesiology of the Musculoskeletal System: Foundations for Physical Rehabilitation.* St. Louis: Mosby; 2002.

65. Janda V. Muscles and motor control in cervicogenic disorders. In: Grant R, ed. *Physical Therapy of the Cervical and Thoracic Spine.* St. Louis, MO: Churchill Livingstone; 2002:182-199.

66. Zeller B, McCrory J, Kibler W, Uhl T. Differences in kinematics and electromyographic activity between men and women during the single-legged squat. *Am J Sports Med.* 2003;31:449-456.

67. Buckley BD, Thigpen CA, Joyce CJ, Bohres SM, Padua DA. Knee and hip kinematics during a double leg squat predict knee and hip kinematics at initial contact of a jump landing task. *J Athl Train.* 2007;42:S81.

68. Ireland ML, Willson JD, Ballantyne BT, Davis IM. Hip strength in females with and without patellofemoral pain. *J Orthop Sports Phys Ther.* 2003;33:671-676.

69. Vesci BJ, Padua DA, Bell DR, Strickland LJ, Guskiewicz KM, Hirth CJ. Influence of hip muscle strength, flexibility of hip and ankle musculature, and hip muscle activation on dynamic knee valgus motion during a double-legged squat. *J Athl Train.* 2007;42:S83.

70. Bell DR, Padua DA. Influence of ankle dorsiflexion range of motion and lower leg muscle activation on knee valgus during a double-legged squat. *J Athl Train.* 2007;42:S84.

71. Goldbeck T, Davies GJ. Test-retest reliability of a closed kinetic chain upper extremity stability test: a clinical field test. *J Sport Rehab.* 2000;9:35-45.

Flexibility Training Concepts

After studying this chapter, you will be able to:

✔ Explain the effects of muscle imbalances on the human movement system (kinetic chain).

✔ Provide a scientific rationale for the use of an integrated flexibility training program.

✔ Differentiate between the various types of flexibility techniques.

✔ Perform and instruct appropriate flexibility techniques for given situations.

Introduction to Flexibility Training

Once all of the assessment data has been collected as described in the Fitness Assessment chapter, the remainder of the programming template can be completed and the focus can be turned to designing the exercise program. The next portion of the Optimum Performance Training™ (OPT™) programming template that needs to be completed is the warm-up section. In designing the warm-up program, the components of flexibility and cardiorespiratory training need should be reviewed. Most clients will require some flexibility training to safely and effectively perform exercise optimally, and that will be the focus of this chapter.

Current Concepts in Flexibility Training

In today's society, nearly everyone is plagued by postural imbalances largely as the result of sedentary lifestyles, advancements in technology, and repetitive movements. Office jobs that require individuals to sit for long hours have led to dramatic increases in work-related injuries, including low-back and neck pain and carpal tunnel syndrome, as well as increased rates of obesity. Flexibility training has become

STRETCH Your Knowledge

Is Lack of Flexibility Associated with Risk of Injury?

Several studies have found an association between altered range of motion (ROM), muscle tightness, or lack of flexibility with increased risk of injury. However, literature reviews have also found studies in which no association was found. More controlled high-quality studies are needed before firm conclusions can be drawn.

- Witvrouw et al. (2003) in a prospective study with 146 male soccer players found that soccer players with increased muscle tightness in the quadriceps and hamstring complex were found to have a statistically greater risk for injury (1).
- Witvrouw et al. (2001) in a prospective study found that decreased flexibility of the hamstring complex and quadriceps significantly contributes to the development of patellar tendonitis in the athletic population (2).
- Cibulka et al. (1998) in a cross-sectional study of 100 patients with unspecified low-back pain demonstrated unilateral hip rotation asymmetry (3).
- Knapik et al. (1991) reported that strength and flexibility imbalances in female collegiate athletes were associated with lower extremity injuries (4).
- Maffey and Emery (2007) found no consistent evidence that adductor tightness increased the risk of groin strains, but also suggested that more research is required before conclusions can be drawn (5).

REFERENCES

1. Witvrouw E, Danneels L, Asselman P, D'Have T, Cambier D. Muscle flexibility as a risk factor for developing muscle injuries in male professional soccer players. A prospective study. *Am J Sports Med.* 2003;31(1):41-46.
2. Witvrouw E, Bellemans J, Lysens R, Danneels L, Cambier D. Intrinsic risk factors for the development of patellar tendinitis in an athletic population. A two-year prospective study. *Am J Sports Med.* 2001;29(2): 190-195.
3. Cibulka MT, Sinacore DR, Cromer GS, Delitto A. Unilateral hip rotation range of motion asymmetry in patients with sacroiliac joint regional pain. *Spine.* 1998;23(9):1009-1015.
4. Knapik JJ, Bauman CL, Jones BH, Harris JM, Vaughan L. Preseason strength and flexibility imbalances associated with athletic injuries in female collegiate athletes. *Am J Sports Med.* 1991;19(1):76-81.
5. Maffey L, Emery C. What are the risk factors for groin strain injury in sport? A systematic review of the literature. *Sports Med.* 2007:37(10):881-894.

increasingly recognized as an important way to help aid in preventing and treating various neuromuscular injuries. Clients without adequate levels of flexibility and joint motion may be at increased risk of injury, and may not be able to achieve their personal fitness goals until these deficits are corrected (1–4). It is important for personal trainers to understand the principles of flexibility training to be able to properly design an integrated training program (1–3).

What Is Flexibility?

Flexibility can be simply described as the ability to move a joint through its complete range of motion. Range of motion (ROM) of a joint is dictated by the normal **extensibility** of all soft tissues surrounding it (1). An important characteristic of soft

Flexibility The normal extensibility of all soft tissues that allows the full range of motion of a joint.

Extensibility Capability to be elongated or stretched.

tissue is that it will only achieve efficient extensibility if optimal control of movement is maintained throughout the entire ROM (5). Optimal control of movement throughout a joint's entire ROM is referred to as **dynamic range of motion**. Dynamic ROM is the combination of flexibility and the nervous system's ability to control this range of motion efficiently. There are various factors that can influence flexibility, including:

◆ Genetics
◆ Connective tissue elasticity
◆ Composition of tendons or skin surrounding the joint
◆ Joint structure
◆ Strength of opposing muscle groups
◆ Body composition
◆ Sex
◆ Age
◆ Activity level
◆ Previous injuries or existing medical issues
◆ Repetitive movements (pattern overload)

Dynamic range of motion The combination of flexibility and the nervous system's ability to control this range of motion efficiently.

Neuromuscular efficiency is the ability of the nervous system to recruit the correct muscles (agonists, antagonists, synergists, and stabilizers) to produce force (concentrically), reduce force (eccentrically), and dynamically stabilize (isometrically) the body's structure in all three planes of motion.

For example, when performing a cable pulldown exercise, the latissimus dorsi (agonist) must be able to concentrically accelerate shoulder extension, adduction, and internal rotation while the middle and lower trapezius and rhomboids (synergists) perform downward rotation of the scapulae. At the same time, the rotator cuff musculature (stabilizers) must dynamically stabilize the glenohumeral (shoulder) joint throughout the motion. If these muscles (force-couples) do not work in tandem efficiently, compensations may ensue, leading to muscle imbalances, altered joint motion, and possible injury.

Neuromuscular efficiency The ability of the neuromuscular system to allow agonists, antagonists, and stabilizers to work synergistically to produce, reduce, and dynamically stabilize the entire kinetic chain in all three planes of motion.

To allow for optimal neuromuscular efficiency, individuals must have proper flexibility in all three planes of motion. This allows for the freedom of movement needed to perform everyday activities effectively, such as bending over to tie shoes or reaching in the top cupboard for dishes **Table 7.1**. To summarize, flexibility requires extensibility, which requires dynamic range of motion, which requires neuromuscular efficiency. This entire chain is achieved by taking an integrated (comprehensive) approach toward flexibility training.

Flexibility training must use a multifaceted approach, which integrates various flexibility techniques to achieve optimal soft tissue extensibility in all planes of motion Table 7.1. To better understand integrated flexibility, a few important concepts must first be reviewed, including the human movement system, muscle imbalances, and neuromuscular efficiency.

Review of the Human Movement System

The human movement system (HMS), also known as the kinetic chain, comprises the muscular, skeletal, and nervous systems. Optimal alignment and function of each component of the HMS is the cornerstone of a sound training program. If one or more segments of the HMS are misaligned and not functioning properly, predictable patterns

TABLE 7.1	Multiplanar Flexibility	
Muscle	Plane of Motion	Movement
Latissimus dorsi	Sagittal	Must have proper extensibility to allow for proper shoulder flexion
	Frontal	Must have proper extensibility to allow for proper shoulder abduction
	Transverse	Must have proper extensibility to allow for proper external humerus rotation
Biceps femoris	Sagittal	Must have proper extensibility to allow for proper hip flexion, knee extension
	Frontal	Must have proper extensibility to allow for proper hip adduction
	Transverse	Must have proper extensibility to allow for proper hip and knee internal rotation
Gastrocnemius	Sagittal	Must have proper extensibility to allow for proper dorsiflexion of ankle
	Frontal	Must have proper extensibility to allow for proper inversion of calcaneus
	Transverse	Must have proper extensibility to allow for proper internal rotation of femur

Postural distortion patters Predictable patterns of muscle imbalances.

of dysfunction develop (5–8). These patterns of dysfunction are referred to as **postural distortion patterns**, which can lead to decreased neuromuscular efficiency and tissue overload **Figure 7.1** (5).

Postural distortion patterns (poor static or dynamic posture) are represented by a lack of structural integrity, resulting from decreased functioning of one (or more) components of the HMS (5–7). A lack of structural integrity can result in altered length-tension relationships (altered muscle lengths), altered force-couple relationships (altered muscle activation), and altered arthrokinematics (altered joint motion). There are several postural distortions that personal trainers must be aware of, all of which are reviewed in the Fitness Assessment chapter (chapter six). Maximal neuromuscular efficiency of the HMS can only exist if all components (muscular, skeletal, and neural) function optimally and interdependently. The ultimate goal of the HMS is to maintain homeostasis (or dynamic postural equilibrium).

FIGURE 7.1

Postural distortion patterns.

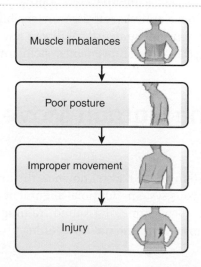

Muscle imbalances → Poor posture → Improper movement → Injury

Poor flexibility can lead to the development of **relative flexibility** (or altered movement patterns), which is the process in which the HMS seeks the path of least resistance, during functional movement patterns (9). A prime example of relative flexibility is seen in people who squat with their feet externally rotated **Figure 7.2**. Because most people have tight calf muscles they lack the proper amount of dorsiflexion at the ankle to perform a squat with proper mechanics. By widening the stance and externally rotating the feet it is possible to decrease the amount of dorsiflexion required at the ankle to perform a squat using good technique. A second example can be seen when people perform an overhead shoulder press with excessive lumbar extension (arched lower back) **Figure 7.3**. Individuals who possess a tight latissimus dorsi will have decreased sagittal-plane shoulder flexion (inability to lift arms directly overhead), and as a result, they compensate for this lack of range of motion at the shoulder in the lumbar spine to allow them to press the load completely above their head.

Relative flexibility The tendency of the body to seek the path of least resistance during functional movement patterns.

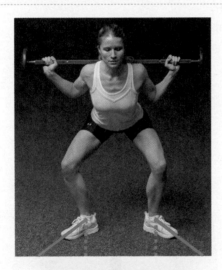

FIGURE 7.2

Squat with externally rotated feet.

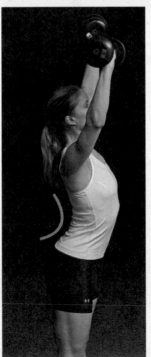

FIGURE 7.3

Overhead shoulder press with lumbar extension.

Muscle Imbalance

Muscle imbalances are alterations in the lengths of muscles surrounding a given joint **Figure 7.4** and **Figure 7.5**, in which some are overactive (forcing compensation to occur) and others may be underactive (allowing for the compensation to occur) (5,7). Examples of such imbalances in the form of movement compensations are discussed in chapter six.

Muscle imbalance can be caused by a variety of mechanisms (1,9). These causes may include:

Muscle imbalance
Alteration of muscle length surrounding a joint.

- ◆ Postural stress
- ◆ Emotional duress
- ◆ Repetitive movement
- ◆ Cumulative trauma
- ◆ Poor training technique
- ◆ Lack of core strength
- ◆ Lack of neuromuscular efficiency

FIGURE 7.4

Muscle balance.

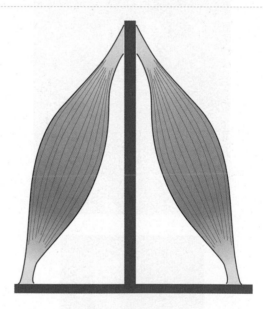

FIGURE 7.5

Muscle imbalance.

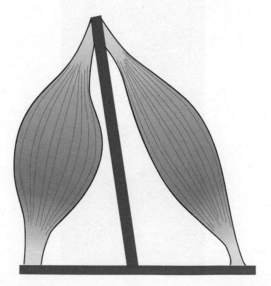

© ilolab/ShutterStock, Inc.

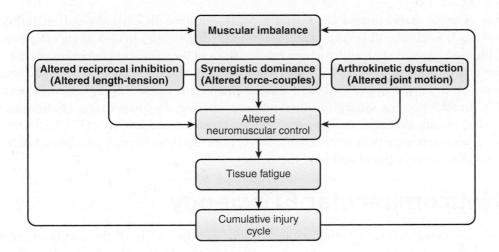

Muscular imbalance.

Muscle imbalances may be caused by or result in altered reciprocal inhibition, synergistic dominance, arthrokinetic dysfunction, and overall decreased neuromuscular control **Figure 7.6**. These concepts are reviewed below.

Altered Reciprocal Inhibition

Reciprocal inhibition is a naturally occurring phenomenon that allows movement to take place. **Reciprocal inhibition** is defined as the simultaneous contraction of one muscle and the relaxation of its antagonist. For example, to perform elbow flexion during a biceps curl, the biceps brachii actively contracts while the triceps brachii (the antagonist muscle) relaxes to allow the movement to occur. However, **altered reciprocal inhibition** is caused by a tight agonist muscle decreasing the neural drive to its functional antagonist (1,5–7,10–16). For example, a tight psoas (hip flexor) would decrease neural drive of the gluteus maximus (hip extensor). Altered reciprocal inhibition alters force-couple relationships, produces synergistic dominance, and leads to the development of faulty movement patterns, poor neuromuscular control, and arthrokinetic (joint) dysfunction.

Synergistic Dominance

Synergistic dominance is a neuromuscular phenomenon that occurs when synergists take over function for a weak or inhibited prime mover (7). For example, if the psoas is tight, it leads to altered reciprocal inhibition of the gluteus maximus, which in turn results in increased force output of the synergists for hip extension (hamstring complex, adductor magnus) to compensate for the weakened gluteus maximus. The result of synergistic dominance is faulty movement patterns, leading to arthrokinetic dysfunction and eventual injury (such as hamstring strains).

Arthrokinetic Dysfunction

The term **arthrokinematics** refers to the motion of the joints. **Arthrokinetic dysfunction** is a biomechanical and neuromuscular dysfunction leading to altered joint motion (5–8). Altered joint motion can be caused by altered length-tension relationships and force-couple relationships, which affect the joint and cause poor movement efficiency.

Reciprocal inhibition The simultaneous contraction of one muscle and the relaxation of its antagonist to allow movement to take place.

Altered reciprocal inhibition The concept of muscle inhibition, caused by a tight agonist, which inhibits its functional antagonist.

Synergistic dominance The neuromuscular phenomenon that occurs when inappropriate muscles take over the function of a weak or inhibited prime mover.

Arthrokinematics The motions of joints in the body.

Arthrokinetic dysfunction Altered forces at the joint that result in abnormal muscular activity and impaired neuromuscular communication at the joint.

For example, performing a squat with excessively externally rotated feet (feet turned outward) forces the tibia (shin bone) and femur (thigh bone) to also rotate externally. This posture alters the length-tension relationships of the muscles at the knees and hips, putting the gluteus maximus in a shortened position and decreasing its ability to generate force. Furthermore, the biceps femoris (hamstring muscle) and piriformis (outer hip muscle) become synergistically dominant, altering the force-couple relationships and ideal joint motion, increasing the stress on the knees and low back (17). With time, the stress associated with arthrokinetic dysfunction can lead to pain, which can further alter muscle recruitment and joint mechanics (5–7).

Neuromuscular Efficiency

As mentioned earlier, neuromuscular efficiency is the ability of the neuromuscular system to properly recruit muscles to produce force (concentrically), reduce force (eccentrically), and dynamically stabilize (isometrically) the entire kinetic chain in all three planes of motion. Because the nervous system is the controlling factor behind this principle, it is important to mention that *mechanoreceptors* (or sensory receptors) located in the muscles and tendons help to determine muscle balance or imbalance. Mechanoreceptors include the muscle spindles and Golgi tendon organs.

Muscle Spindles

As mentioned in chapter two, muscle spindles are the major sensory organ of the muscle and are composed of microscopic fibers that lie parallel to the muscle fiber. Remember that muscle spindles are sensitive to change in muscle length and rate of length change (5,18–25). The function of the muscle spindle is to help prevent muscles from stretching too far or too fast. However, when a muscle on one side of a joint is lengthened (because of a shortened muscle on the opposite side), the spindles of the lengthened muscle are stretched. This information is transmitted to the brain and spinal cord, exciting the muscle spindle and causing the muscle fibers of the lengthened muscle to contract. This often results in micro muscle spasms or a feeling of tightness (1,5,6).

The hamstring complex is a prime example of this response when the pelvis is rotated anteriorly **Figure 7.7**, meaning the anterior superior iliac spines (front of the pelvis) move downward (inferiorly) and the ischium (bottom posterior portion of pelvis, where the hamstrings originate) moves upward (superiorly). If the attachment of the hamstring complex is moved superiorly, it increases the distance between the two attachment sites and lengthens the hamstring complex. In this case, the hamstring

FIGURE 7.7

Effect of the hamstring complex with an anteriorly rotated pelvis.

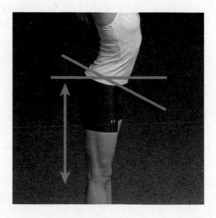

complex does not need to be statically stretched because it is already in a stretched position. When a lengthened muscle is stretched, it increases the excitement of the muscle spindles and further creates a contraction (spasm) response. With this scenario, the shortened hip flexors are helping to create the anterior pelvic rotation that is causing the lengthening of the hamstring complex. Instead, the hip flexors need to be stretched (17). (This will be reviewed later in the chapter.)

Another example includes an individual whose knees adduct and internally rotate (knock-knees) during a squat exercise. The underactive muscle is the gluteus medius (hip abductor and external rotator), and the overactive muscles include the adductors (inner thighs) and tensor fascia latae (a hip flexor and hip internal rotator). Thus, one would not need to stretch the gluteus medius, but instead stretch the adductor complex and tensor fascia latae, which in this case are overactive, pulling the femur into excessive adduction and internal rotation.

Golgi Tendon Organs

As also mentioned in chapter two, Golgi tendon organs are located within the *musculotendinous junction* (or the point where the muscle and the tendon meet) and are sensitive to changes in muscular tension and the rate of tension change (5,18–25). When excited, the Golgi tendon organ causes the muscle to relax, which prevents the muscle from being placed under excessive stress, which could result in injury. Prolonged Golgi tendon organ stimulation provides an inhibitory action to muscle spindles (located within the same muscle). This neuromuscular phenomenon is called **autogenic inhibition** and occurs when the neural impulses sensing tension are greater than the impulses causing muscle contraction (14). The phenomenon is termed *autogenic* because the contracting muscle is being inhibited by its own receptors.

Autogenic inhibition The process by which neural impulses that sense tension are greater than the impulses that cause muscles to contract, providing an inhibitory effect to the muscle spindles.

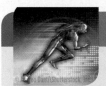

Memory Jogger

Autogenic inhibition is one of the main principles used in flexibility training, particularly with static stretching in which one holds a stretch for a prolonged period. Holding a stretch creates tension in the muscle. This tension stimulates the Golgi tendon organ, which overrides muscle spindle activity in the muscle being stretched, causing relaxation in the overactive muscle and allowing for optimal lengthening of the tissue. In general, stretches should be held long enough for the Golgi tendon organ to override the signal from the muscle spindle (approximately 30 seconds).

SUMMARY

Flexibility training can reduce the risk of muscle imbalances, joint dysfunctions, and overuse injuries. It is important to have proper range of motion in all three planes (sagittal, frontal, transverse), which can be achieved by implementing an integrated approach toward flexibility training. All segments of the kinetic chain must be properly aligned to avoid postural distortion patterns (poor posture) and tissue overload. The adaptive potential of the HMS is decreased by limited flexibility, which forces the body to move in an altered fashion, leading to relative flexibility (faulty movement patterns).

Muscle imbalances result from altered length-tension relationships, force-couple relationships, and arthrokinematics. These imbalances can be caused by poor posture, poor training technique, or previous injury. These muscle imbalances result in altered reciprocal inhibition, synergistic dominance, and arthrokinetic dysfunction, which in turn lead to decreased neuromuscular control and possibly injury.

Scientific Rationale for Flexibility Training

Flexibility training is a key component for all training programs (1,5). It is used for a variety of reasons, including:

- Correcting muscle imbalances
- Increasing joint range of motion
- Decreasing the excessive tension of muscles
- Relieving joint stress
- Improving the extensibility of the musculotendinous junction
- Maintaining the normal functional length of all muscles
- Improving neuromuscular efficiency
- Improving function

Pattern Overload

Pattern overload
Consistently repeating the same pattern of motion, which may place abnormal stresses on the body.

Muscular imbalances are highly prevalent in today's society and are oftentimes caused by **pattern overload**. Pattern overload is consistently repeating the same pattern of motion, such as baseball pitching, long-distance running, and cycling, which with time places abnormal stresses on the body. There are gym members who train with the same routine repetitively. This too may lead to pattern overload and place abnormal stresses on the body.

Pattern overload may not necessarily be directly related to exercise. For example, a loading-dock employee who has a particularly repetitive occupation lifting and loading packages all day is prone to pattern overload. Even sitting for long periods of time while working on a computer is a repetitive stress.

Cumulative Injury Cycle

Poor posture and repetitive movements create dysfunction within the connective tissue of the body (1,5,26–28). This dysfunction is treated by the body as an injury, and as a result, the body will initiate a repair process termed the cumulative injury cycle **Figure 7.8** (5,28).

Any trauma to the tissue of the body creates inflammation. Inflammation, in turn, activates the body's pain receptors and initiates a protective mechanism, increasing muscle tension or causing muscle spasm. Heightened activity of muscle spindles in particular areas of the muscle create a microspasm, and as a result of the spasm, adhesions (or knots) begin to form in the soft tissue **Figure 7.9**. These adhesions form

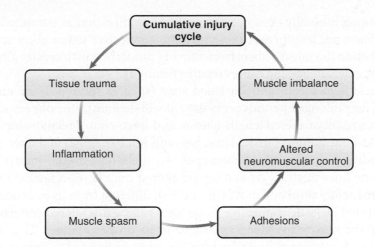

FIGURE 7.8

Cumulative injury cycle.

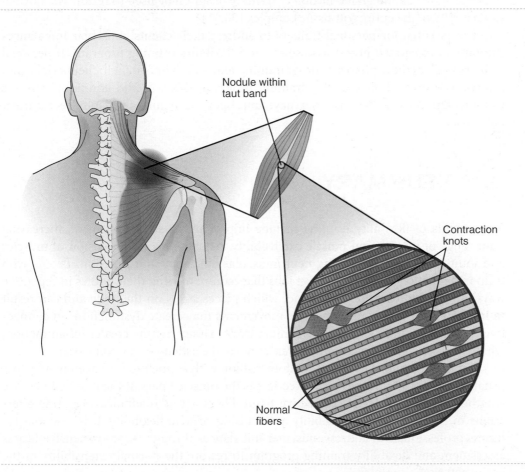

FIGURE 7.9

Myofascial adhesions.

a weak, inelastic matrix (inability to stretch) that decreases normal elasticity of the soft tissue, resulting in altered length-tension relationships (leading to altered reciprocal inhibition), altered force-couple relationships (leading to synergistic dominance), and arthrokinetic dysfunction (leading to altered joint motion) (1,5,28). Left untreated, these adhesions can begin to form permanent structural changes in the soft tissue that is evident by Davis's law.

Davis's law states that soft tissue models along the lines of stress (1,5,29). Soft tissue is remodeled (or rebuilt) with an inelastic collagen matrix that forms in a random

Davis's law States that soft tissue models along the lines of stress.

fashion, meaning it usually does not run in the same direction as the muscle fibers. If the muscle fibers are lengthened, these inelastic connective tissue fibers act as roadblocks, preventing the muscle fibers from moving properly, which creates alterations in normal tissue extensibility and causes relative flexibility (9).

If a muscle is in a constant shortened state (such as the hip flexor musculature when sitting for prolonged periods every day), it will demonstrate poor neuromuscular efficiency (as a result of altered length-tension and force-couple relationships). In turn, this will affect joint motion (ankle, knee, hip, and lumbar spine) and alter movement patterns (leading to synergistic dominance). An inelastic collagen matrix will form along the same lines of stress created by the altered muscle movements. Because the muscle is consistently short and moves in a pattern different from its intended function, the newly formed inelastic connective tissue forms along this altered pattern, reducing the ability of the muscle to extend and move in its proper manner. This is why it is imperative that an integrated flexibility training program be used to restore the normal extensibility of the entire soft tissue complex (30,31).

It is essential for personal trainers to address their clients' muscular imbalances through an integrated fitness assessment and flexibility training program. If personal trainers neglect these phases of programming and simply move their clients right into a resistance or cardiorespiratory training program, this will add additional stresses to joints and muscles because they have improper mechanics and faulty recruitment patterns.

SUMMARY

The benefits of flexibility training include improving muscle imbalances, increasing joint range of motion and muscle extensibility, relieving excessive tension of muscles and joint stress, and improving neuromuscular efficiency and function. People who train in a repetitive fashion (or have jobs that require moving their bodies in repetitive ways) are at risk for pattern overload, which places stress on the body and can result in injury. Poor posture and repetitive movements may create dysfunctions in connective tissue, initiating the cumulative injury cycle. Tissue trauma creates inflammation, which leads to microspasms and decreases normal elasticity of the soft tissue.

Soft tissue rebuilds itself in a random fashion with an inelastic collagen matrix that usually does not run in the same direction as the muscle fibers. If the muscle fibers are lengthened, these inelastic connective tissue fibers act as roadblocks, creating alterations in normal tissue extensibility and causing relative flexibility. It is essential for fitness professionals to address muscular imbalances through a comprehensive fitness assessment and flexibility training program to restore the normal extensibility of the entire soft tissue complex.

The Flexibility Continuum

To better appreciate the benefits and program design considerations, personal trainers need to understand the different types of flexibility training. Flexibility, like any other form of training, should follow a systematic progression known as the flexibility continuum. There are three phases of flexibility training within the OPT model: corrective, active, and functional **Figure 7.10** (1,10,14,32,33). Moreover, it is important to note

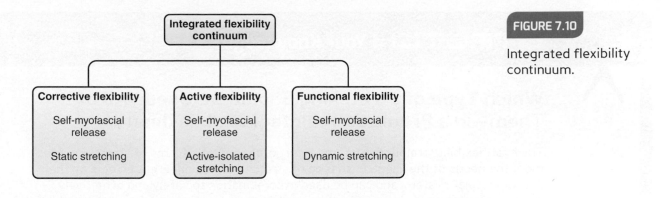

FIGURE 7.10

Integrated flexibility continuum.

that flexibility techniques should only be performed on tissues that have been identified as overactive (tight) during the assessment process.

Corrective Flexibility

Corrective flexibility is designed to increase joint ROM, improve muscle imbalances, and correct altered joint motion. Corrective flexibility includes self-myofascial release (foam roll) techniques and static stretching. Self-myofascial release uses the principle of autogenic inhibition to cause muscle relaxation, whereas static stretching can use either autogenic inhibition or reciprocal inhibition to increase muscle length depending on how the stretch is performed. Corrective flexibility is appropriate at the stabilization level (phase 1) of the OPT model.

Active Flexibility

Active flexibility uses self-myofascial release and active-isolated stretching techniques. Active-isolated stretching is designed to improve the extensibility of soft tissue and increase neuromuscular efficiency by using reciprocal inhibition. Active-isolated stretching allows for agonists and synergist muscles to move a limb through a full range of motion while the functional antagonists are being stretched (14,34,35). For example, a supine straight-leg raise uses the hip flexors and quadriceps to raise the leg and hold it unsupported, while the antagonist hamstring complex is stretched. Active flexibility would be appropriate at the strength level (phases 2, 3, and 4) of the OPT model.

Functional Flexibility

Functional flexibility uses self-myofascial release techniques and dynamic stretching. Dynamic stretching requires integrated, multiplanar soft tissue extensibility, with optimal neuromuscular control, through the full range of motion, or essentially movement without compensations (14). Therefore, if clients are compensating when performing dynamic stretches during training, then they need to be regressed to active or corrective flexibility. This form of flexibility would be appropriate at the power level (phase 5) of the OPT model or before athletic competition. It is important to remember that all functional movements occur in all three planes of motion and that injuries most often occur in the transverse plane. If the appropriate soft tissue is not extensible through the full range of movement, the risk of injury dramatically increases (2,36). Exercises that increase multiplanar soft tissue extensibility and have high levels of neuromuscular demand are preferred.

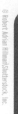

STRETCH Your Knowledge

Which Type of Stretching Should Be Used? All of Them—in a Progressive, Integrated Fashion

The best flexibility training programs incorporate multiple forms of stretching to meet the needs of the client. Each type of stretch creates different effects on the neuromuscular system, and can be used in combination to safely and effectively increase flexibility. The type of exercise will be based on the findings of the evaluation, the goals of the program, and when the stretches will be used (before exercise, after exercise).

Self-Myofascial Release (SMR)

Used to help correct existing muscle imbalances, reduce trigger points (knots within muscle) and inhibit overactive musculature. Can be used before exercise as well as after exercise.

- Hou et al. (1) in a randomized controlled trial of 119 patients found that ischemic compression therapy provides immediate pain relief and trigger point sensitivity suppression.
- Hanten et al. (2) in a randomized trial of 40 adults, found a home program, consisting of ischemic pressure and sustained stretching, was shown to be effective in reducing trigger point sensitivity and pain intensity in individuals with neck and upper back pain.

Static Stretching

Used to correct existing muscle imbalances and lengthen overactive (tight) musculature. Can be used before exercise as well as after exercise. The evidence is strong that static stretching performed daily causes increased flexibility in the stretched muscle.

- Decoster et al. (3), in a systematic review of 28 randomized control trials with 1,338 subjects, found moderately strong evidence that static stretching can increase the flexibility of the hamstring muscles, with varying duration and frequency of stretch.
- Ford et al. (4), in a randomized control trial with 35 subjects with decreased hamstring flexibility, completed static hamstring stretches with durations between 30 and 120 seconds (a control group did no stretching). All four stretching groups increased hamstring flexibility after 5 weeks, and the 30-second hold was just as effective as the 120-second hold.
- Reid and McNair (5), in a randomized controlled trial of 43 males performing 30-second static hamstring stretches for 6 weeks, found a mean gain of 10 degrees in hamstring flexibility compared with the control group.

(Continued)

- Porter et al. (6) in a randomized controlled trial with 94 subjects demonstrated that both sustained (3 minutes, 3 times daily) and intermittent stretching (5 sets of 20-second holds, 2 times daily) for the Achilles' tendon increased flexibility and decreased pain.

Active Stretching

Used to increase the extensibility of soft tissues through reciprocal inhibition. There is moderate evidence that forms of active stretching can increase joint range of motion and muscle flexibility.

- Maddig and Harmer (7) in a randomized controlled trial with 30 recreational athletes found that active-isolated stretching is effective for increasing hamstring range of motion.
- Guroian et al. (8) in a randomized trial found that static stretching and active-isolated stretching were both effective for increased range of motion and flexibility in older adults.

Dynamic Stretching

Dynamic or functional stretching is used to increase flexibility with optimal neuromuscular control. This should be used once clients have demonstrated adequate control over motions to prevent injury.

- Sherry and Best (9) in a prospective randomized comparison study of two rehabilitation programs with 24 athletes demonstrated improved functional outcomes with patients using dynamic functional movements (progressive agility and trunk stabilization) that require stabilization, proprioception, and muscle lengthening to occur simultaneously.

REFERENCES

1. Hou C-R, Tsai L-C, Cheng K-F, Chung K-C, Hong C-Z. Immediate effects of various therapeutic modalities on cervical myofascial pain and trigger-point sensitivity. *Arch Phys Med Rehabil.* 2002;83:1406-1414.
2. Hanten WP, Olson SL, Butts NL, Nowicki AL. Effectiveness of a home program of ischemic pressure followed by sustained stretch for treatment of myofascial trigger points. *Phys Ther.* 2000;80:997-1003.
3. Decoster LC, Cleland J, Altieri C, Russell P. The effects of hamstring stretching on range of motion: a systematic literature review. *J Orthop Sports Phys Ther.* 2005:35(6):377-387.
4. Ford GS, Mazzone MA, Taylor K. The effect of 4 different durations of static hamstring stretching on passive knee-extension range of motion. *J Sport Rehabil.* 2005;14(2):95-107.
5. Reid DA, McNair PJ. Passive force, angle, and stiffness changes after stretching of hamstring muscles. *Med Sci Sports Exerc.* 2004:36(11):1944-1948.
6. Porter D, Barrill E, Oneacre K, May BD. The effects of duration and frequency of Achilles tendon stretching on dorsiflexion and outcome in painful heel syndrome. *Foot Ankle Int.* 2002;23(7):619-624.
7. Maddig TR, Harmer P. Active-isolated stretching is not more effective than static stretching for increased hamstring ROM. *Med Sci Sports Exerc.* 2002;34(5) p S151.
8. Guroian L, Walsh C, Diaz L, Marra A, Wygand J, Otto R. The effects of active isolated stretching on flexibility and function in older adults. *Med Sci Sports Exerc.* 2008;40(5):S373.
9. Sherry MA, Best TM. A comparison of 2 rehabilitation programs in the treatment of acute hamstring strains. *J Orthop Sports Phys Ther.* 2004;34(3):116-125.

SUMMARY

Flexibility training should be progressive, systematic, and based on an assessment. There are three phases of flexibility training: corrective, active, and functional. Corrective flexibility improves muscle imbalances and altered joint motion by using self-myofascial release and static stretching. Active flexibility improves the extensibility of soft tissue and increases neuromuscular efficiency by using self-myofascial release and active-isolated stretching. Functional flexibility improves the extensibility of soft tissue and increases neuromuscular efficiency by using self-myofascial release and dynamic stretches that incorporate multiplanar movements through the full range of motion.

Stretching Techniques

As previously discussed, proper stretching enhances flexibility and can be viewed as a continuum. The flexibility continuum consists of specific forms of stretching. For example, corrective flexibility uses self-myofascial release and static stretching; active flexibility uses self-myofascial release and active-isolated stretching; and functional flexibility uses self-myofascial release and dynamic stretching Table 7.2. Each form of stretching manipulates the receptors of the nervous system, which in turn allows for alteration of muscle extensibility.

TABLE 7.2 Examples of Stretching within the Flexibility Continuum

© Ilolab/ShutterStock, Inc.

Flexibility Type	Type of Stretching	Examples
Corrective flexibility	Self-myofascial release (SMR)	SMR: gastrocnemius/soleus SMR: adductors SMR: latissimus dorsi
	Static stretching	Static gastrocnemius stretch Static adductor stretch Static latissimus dorsi stretch
Active flexibility	Self-myofascial release (SMR)	SMR: adductors SMR: latissimus dorsi SMR: thoracic spine
	Active-isolated stretching	Active standing adductor stretch Active latissimus dorsi ball stretch Active pectoral wall stretch
Functional flexibility	Self-myofascial release (SMR)	SMR: gastrocnemius/soleus SMR: TFL/IT band SMR: latissimus dorsi
	Dynamic stretching	Prisoner squat Multiplanar lunge Tube walking: side to side Medicine ball lift and chop

TFL, tensor fascia latae; IT, iliotibial.

Myofascial Release

Self-myofascial release is a stretching technique that focuses on the neural system and fascial system in the body (or the fibrous tissue that surrounds and separates muscle tissue). By applying gentle force to an adhesion or "knot," the elastic muscle fibers are altered from a bundled position (which causes the adhesion) into a straighter alignment with the direction of the muscle or fascia. The gentle pressure (applied with implements such as a foam roll) will stimulate the Golgi tendon organ and create autogenic inhibition, decreasing muscle spindle excitation and releasing the hypertonicity (tension) of the underlying musculature. In other words, gentle pressure (similar to a massage) breaks up knots within the muscle and helps to release unwanted muscular tension.

It is crucial to note that when a person is using self-myofascial release he or she must find a tender spot (which indicates the presence of muscle hypertonicity) and sustain pressure on that spot for a minimum of 30 seconds. This will increase the Golgi tendon organ activity and decrease muscle spindle activity, thus triggering the autogenic inhibition response. It may take longer, depending on the client's ability to consciously relax. This process will help restore the body back to its optimal level of function by resetting the proprioceptive mechanisms of the soft tissue (37). Self-myofascial release is suggested before stretching because breaking up fascial adhesions (knots) may potentially improve the tissue's ability to lengthen through stretching techniques. In addition, it can be used during the cool-down process.

STRETCHES FOR MYOFASCIAL RELEASE

Gastrocnemius/Soleus (Calves)

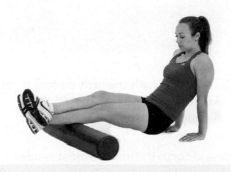

Preparation
1. Place foam roll under mid-calf.
2. Cross left leg over right leg to increase pressure (optional).

Movement
3. Slowly roll calf area to find the most tender spot.
4. Once identified, hold tender spot until the discomfort is reduced (minimum 30 seconds).

Tensor Fascia Latae (TFL)/Iliotibial (IT) Band

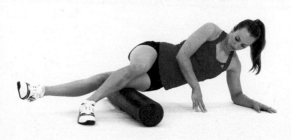

Preparation
1. Lie on one side, the foam roll just in front of the hip. Cross the top leg over lower leg, with foot touching the floor.

Movement
2. Slowly roll from hip joint to lateral knee to find the most tender spot.
3. Once identified, hold tender spot until the discomfort is reduced (minimum 30 seconds).

STRETCHES FOR MYOFASCIAL RELEASE *continued*

Adductors

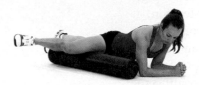

Preparation

1. Lie prone with one thigh flexed and abducted and the foam roll in the groin region, inside the upper thigh.

Movement

2. Slowly roll the inner thigh area to find the most tender spot.
3. Once identified, hold tender spot until the discomfort is reduced (minimum 30 seconds).

Piriformis

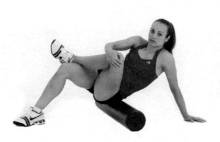

Preparation

1. Sit on top of the foam roll, positioned on the back of the hip. Cross one foot to the opposite knee.

Movement

2. Lean into the hip of the crossed leg. Slowly roll on the posterior hip area to find the most tender spot.
3. Once identified, hold tender spot until the discomfort is reduced (minimum 30 seconds).

Latissimus Dorsi

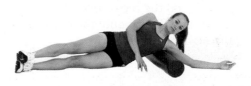

Preparation

1. Lie on the floor on one side with the arm closest to the floor outstretched and thumb facing upward.
2. Place the foam roll under the arm (axillary region).

Movement

3. Slowly move back and forth to find the most tender spot.
4. Once identified, hold tender spot until the discomfort is reduced (minimum 30 seconds).

Static Stretching

Static stretching is the process of passively taking a muscle to the point of tension and holding the stretch for a minimum of 30 seconds (1,2,11). This is the traditional form of stretching that is most often seen in fitness today. It combines low force with longer duration (14,38).

By holding the muscle in a stretched position for a prolonged period, the Golgi tendon organ is stimulated and produces an inhibitory effect on the muscle spindle (autogenic inhibition). This allows the muscle to relax and provides for better elongation of the muscle Table 7.3 (5,39). In addition, contracting the antagonistic musculature while holding the stretch can reciprocally inhibit the muscle being stretched, allowing it to relax and enhancing the stretch. For example, when performing the kneeling hip flexor stretch, an individual can contract the hip extensors (gluteus maximus) to reciprocally inhibit the hip flexors (psoas, rectus femoris), allowing for greater lengthening of these muscles. Another example would be to contract the quadriceps when performing a hamstring stretch.

Static stretching should be used to decrease the muscle spindle activity of a tight muscle before and after activity. Detailed explanations of various static stretching techniques are described below.

> **Static stretching** The process of passively taking a muscle to the point of tension and holding the stretch for a minimum of 30 seconds.

TABLE 7.3	Static Stretching Summary		
Type of Stretch	**Mechanism of Action**	**Acute Variables**	**Examples**
Static stretch	Autogenic inhibition or reciprocal inhibition (depending how stretch is performed)	1–3 sets Hold each stretch 30 seconds	• Gastrocnemius stretch • Kneeling hip flexor stretch • Standing adductor stretch • Pectoral wall stretch

© ilolab/ShutterStock, Inc.

STRETCH Your Knowledge

Does Stretching Decrease Strength?

Recently, researchers have suggested that static stretching, performed immediately before exercise or athletic events, may decrease muscular strength and impair performance. The research in this area is still developing, but there are several studies that have found that static stretching may decrease maximal strength and power for up to 10 minutes (1–5). Naturally, this has caused some controversy for exercise and health professionals. Should patients and clients stop stretching before exercise? Is stretching "bad" for athletic performance?

The best answer is both "yes" and "no." There is mounting scientific evidence that static stretching may decrease strength and power. This appears to be limited to just static stretching, often performed in an acute fashion. However, research has also demonstrated increases in vertical jump, muscular strength, power, and balance ability after a regular (chronic) stretching program (6–11).

(Continued)

In addition, there is no conclusive evidence that patients and clients with known motion limitations and flexibility imbalances have the same reaction to static stretching. Finally, there is little evidence that stretching influences *overall* athletic performance (for example, although quadriceps maximal strength may be decreased, there is no evidence that this prevents a soccer player from kicking the ball with maximal velocity). Therefore, stretching before physical activity may still be beneficial. The current recommendations for the use of stretching before exercise are as follows:

- Acute static stretching, held for more than 30 seconds, may decrease strength and power. Therefore, athletes and others who will be engaging in *maximal effort, explosive* activities (such as high jump, sprinting, or power lifting) may not want to perform static stretching before the event *unless* muscle imbalances are present. If static stretching is used, care should be taken so that only the targeted (tight, overactive) muscles are stretched, and this should be followed by active-isolated or dynamic stretches to increase motorneuron excitability.
- Static stretching may be used to correct muscle imbalances and increase joint range of motion before activity in most patients and clients, as part of a progressive, integrated program.
- Active and dynamic stretching may be used without risking a loss of strength or power. These two forms of stretching may be the most appropriate before physical activity in clients with no identified muscle imbalances.

REFERENCES

1. Fowles JR, Sale DG, MacDougall JD. Reduced strength after passive stretch of the human plantarflexors. *J Appl Physiol.* 2000;89:1179-1188.
2. Knudson D, Noffal G. Time course of stretch-induced isometric strength deficits. *Eur J Appl Physiol.* 2005;94:348-351.
3. Kokkonen J, Nelson AG, Cornwell A. Acute muscle stretching inhibits maximal strength performance. *Res Q Exerc Sport.* 1998;69:411-415.
4. Marek SM, Cramer JT, Fincher AL, et al. Acute effects of static and proprioceptive neuromuscular facilitation stretching on muscle strength and power output. *J Athl Train.* 2005;40:94-103.
5. Power K, Behm D, Cahill F, Carroll M, Young W. An acute bout of static stretching: effects on force and jumping performance. *Med Sci Sports Exerc.* 2004;36:1389-1396.
6. Shrier I. Does stretching improve performance? A systematic and critical review of the literature. *Clin J Sport Med.* 2004;14(5):267-273.
7. Hunter JP, Marshall RN. Effects of power and flexibility training on vertical jump technique. *Med Sci Sports Exerc.* 2002;34(3):478-486.
8. Gajdosik RL, Vander Linden DW, McNair PJ, Williams AK, Riggin TJ. Effects of an eight-week stretching program on the passive-elastic properties and function of the calf muscles of older women. *Clin Biomech (Bristol, Avon).* 2005;20(9):973-983.
9. Kokkonen J, Nelson AG, Eldredge C, Winchester JB. Chronic static stretching improves exercise performance. *Med Sci Sports Exerc.* 2007;39(10):1825-1831.
10. Wilson GJ, Elliott BC, Wood GA. Stretch shorten cycle performance enhancement through flexibility training. *Med Sci Sports Exerc.* 1992;24(1):116-123.
11. LaRoche DP, Lussier MV, Roy SJ. Chronic stretching and voluntary muscle force. *J Strength Cond Res.* 2008;22(2):589-596.
12. Bazett-Jones DM, Gibson MH, McBride JM. Sprint and vertical jump performances are not affected by six weeks of static hamstring stretching. *J Strength Cond Res.* 2008;22(1):25-33.

STATIC STRETCHES

Static Gastrocnemius Stretch

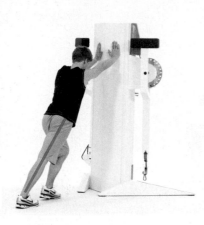

Preparation
1. Stand facing a wall or stable object.
2. Extend one leg back, keeping the knee and foot straight and the back heel on the floor.

Movement
3. Draw navel inward.
4. Keep rear foot flat, with foot pointed straight ahead. Do not allow the rear foot to pronate.
5. Bend arms and lean forward toward the wall. Keep the gluteal muscles and quadriceps tight and the heel on the ground.
6. Hold for 30 seconds.

TECHNIQUE

Make sure the gluteal muscles and quadriceps are activated to keep the knee in full extension. This will enhance the stretch to the gastrocnemius.

Static Standing TFL Stretch

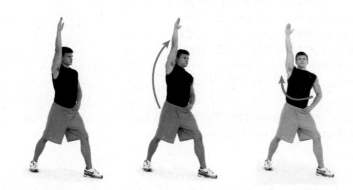

TECHNIQUE

Make sure the gluteal musculature is contracted during the stretch. This will help reciprocally inhibit the TFL, allowing for greater lengthening of the TFL.

Preparation
1. Stand in a staggered stance with the front leg slightly bent and rear leg straight.
2. Externally rotate back leg.

Movement
3. Draw navel inward.
4. Squeeze gluteal muscles while rotating pelvis posteriorly.
5. Slowly move body forward until a mild tension is achieved in the front of the hip being stretched.
6. As a progression, raise the arm (on the same side as the back leg) up and over to the opposite side while maintaining pelvis position.
7. Hold side bend position and slowly rotate posteriorly as illustrated.
8. Hold for 30 seconds.
9. Switch sides and repeat.

STATIC STRETCHES *continued*

Static Kneeling Hip Flexor Stretch

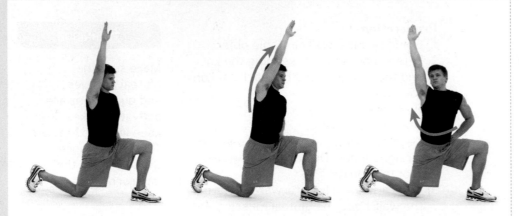

Preparation

1. Kneel with front and back legs bent at a 90-degree angle.
2. Internally rotate back hip to target the psoas musculature or maintain a neutral position to target the rectus femoris.

Movement

3. Draw navel inward.
4. Squeeze gluteal muscles of the side being stretched while rotating pelvis posteriorly.
5. Slowly move body forward until a mild tension is achieved in the front of the hip being stretched.
6. As a progression, raise arm, side bend to opposite side, and rotate posteriorly as illustrated.
7. Hold for 30 seconds.

TECHNIQUE   Placing a foam pad underneath the knee (not illustrated) may improve comfort for the client, especially if stretching on a hard surface.

STATIC STRETCHES *continued*

Static Standing Adductor Stretch

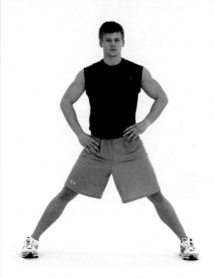 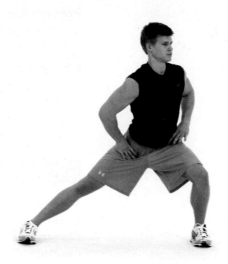

TECHNIQUE

Be sure to take a wider stance than shoulders-width apart to ensure optimal lengthening. This stretch can also be performed from a kneeling position or seated on a stability ball to reduce demand caused by maintaining a static lunge position.

Preparation
1. Stand in a straddled stance with the feet beyond shoulders-width apart. Extend one leg back until the toe of the back leg is in line with the heel of the other foot. Both feet should be pointed straight ahead.

Movement
2. Draw navel inward and posteriorly rotate the pelvis.
3. Slowly move in a sideways motion (side lunge) until a stretch in the straight leg's groin area is felt.
4. Hold for 30 seconds.

Static Latissimus Dorsi Ball Stretch

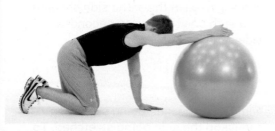

Preparation
1. Kneel in front of a stability ball.
2. Place one arm on ball, with thumb pointed straight up in the air.

Movement
3. Draw navel upward.
4. Posteriorly rotate the pelvis.
5. Slowly reach the arm straight out by rolling the ball forward.
6. Hold for 30 seconds.

TECHNIQUE   If this stretch causes any pinching in the shoulder, perform the stretch with the palm down on the ball. To increase the stretch, slightly adduct the outstretched arm across the body.

STATIC STRETCHES *continued*

Static Pectoral Stretch

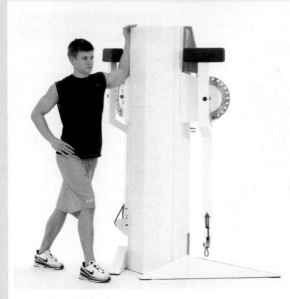

Preparation
1. Stand against an object and form a 90-90-degree angle with your arm.

Movement
2. Draw your navel inward.
3. Slowly lean forward until a slight stretch is felt in the anterior shoulder and chest region.
4. Hold the stretch for 30 seconds.

TECHNIQUE

Make sure the shoulders do not elevate during the stretch. This is an example of relative flexibility and decreases the effectiveness of the stretch.

Static Upper Trapezius/Scalene Stretch

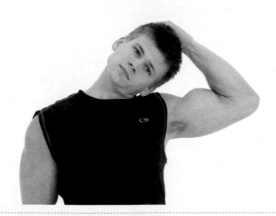

Preparation
1. Stand in optimal posture.

Movement
2. Draw navel inward.
3. Retract and depress the scapula on the side being stretched.
4. Tuck chin and slowly laterally flex the head, pulling one ear toward the same side shoulder.
5. Hold the stretch position for 30 seconds.
6. Switch sides and repeat.

TECHNIQUE

As with the pectoral stretch, keep the shoulder of the side being stretched down and retract it by depressing the scapula on the side being stretched. To help accomplish this, one can place the arm on the side being stretched behind the body.

Active-Isolated Stretching

Active-isolated stretching is the process of using agonists and synergists to dynamically move the joint into a range of motion (14,33). This form of stretching increases motorneuron excitability, creating reciprocal inhibition of the muscle being stretched. The active supine biceps femoris stretch is a good example of active-isolated stretching (1,14). The quadriceps extends the knee. This enhances the stretch of the biceps femoris in two ways. First, it increases the length of the biceps femoris. Second, the contraction of the quadriceps causes reciprocal inhibition (decreased neural drive and muscle spindle excitation) of the hamstring complex, which allows it to elongate.

Active-isolated stretch The process of using agonists and synergists to dynamically move the joint into a range of motion.

Active-isolated stretches are suggested for preactivity warm-up (such as before sports competition or high-intensity exercise), as long as no postural distortion patterns are present. If an individual possesses muscle imbalances, active-isolated stretching should be performed after self-myofascial release and static stretching for muscles determined as tight or overactive during the assessment process. Typically, 5 to 10 repetitions of each stretch are performed and held for 1 to 2 seconds each. Detailed explanations of various active-isolated stretches are given below Table 7.4.

TABLE 7.4	Active-Isolated Stretching Summary		
Type of Stretch	**Mechanism of Action**	**Acute Variables**	**Examples**
Active-isolated stretch	Reciprocal inhibition	1–2 sets Hold each stretch 1–2 seconds for 5–10 repetitions	• Active supine biceps femoris stretch • Active kneeling quadriceps stretch • Active standing adductor stretch • Active pectoral wall stretch

ACTIVE-ISOLATED STRETCHES

Active Gastrocnemius Stretch with Pronation and Supination

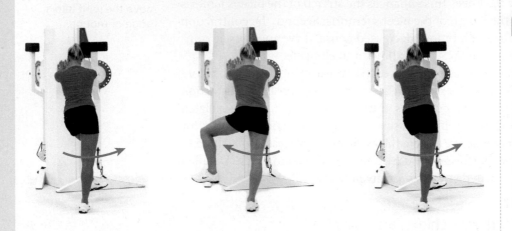

TECHNIQUE

Make sure when performing the stretch that the majority of the motion is coming from internal and external rotation of the hip, which in turn causes rotation at the knee and eversion and inversion on the foot and ankle.

Preparation
1. Stand near a wall or sturdy object.
2. Bring one leg forward for support. Use upper body and lean against object.

Movement
3. Draw navel inward.
4. Keep rear foot on the ground, with opposite hip flexed.
5. Slowly move through hips, creating controlled supination and pronation through the lower extremity.
6. Hold for 1–2 seconds and repeat for 5–10 repetitions.

Active Supine Biceps Femoris Stretch

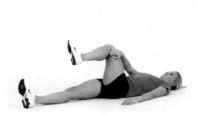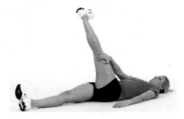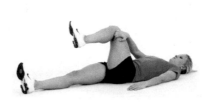

Preparation
1. Lie supine on floor with legs flat.
2. Flex, adduct, and slightly internally rotate the hip of the side being stretched while keeping the knee flexed.
3. Place the opposite hand behind the knee of the leg being stretched.

Movement
4. Draw navel inward.
5. With hand supporting leg, extend the knee.
6. Hold for 1–2 seconds and repeat for 5–10 repetitions.

TECHNIQUE　Adducting and internally rotating the hip places more of an emphasis on the short head of the biceps femoris.

ACTIVE-ISOLATED STRETCHES *continued*

Active Standing TFL Stretch

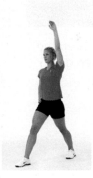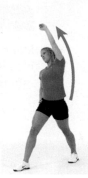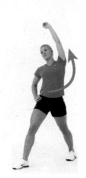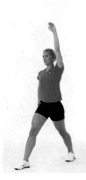

TECHNIQUE

As with the static stretch, make sure the gluteal muscles are contracted when going into the stretch. This will help in enhancing neuromuscular efficiency between the hip flexors and hip extensors.

Preparation
1. Stand in a staggered stance with the front leg slightly bent and rear leg straight.
2. Externally rotate back leg.

Movement
3. Draw navel inward and raise arm overhead.
4. Squeeze gluteal muscles while rotating pelvis posteriorly.
5. Stride forward, in a controlled manner, until a mild tension is achieved in the front of the hip being stretched. Side bend and rotate posteriorly as illustrated.
6. Hold for 1–2 seconds and repeat for 5–10 repetitions.

Active Kneeling Hip Flexor Stretch

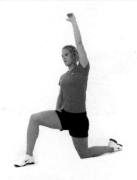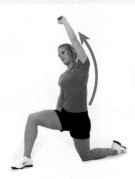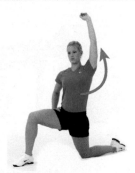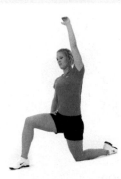

Preparation
1. Kneel with front and back legs bent at a 90-degree angle.
2. Internally rotate back hip to target the psoas musculature or maintain a neutral position to target the rectus femoris.

Movement
3. Draw navel inward and raise arm overhead.
4. Squeeze gluteal muscles of the side being stretched while rotating pelvis posteriorly.
5. Slowly move body forward until a mild tension is achieved in the front of the hip being stretched. Side bend and rotate posteriorly.
6. Hold for 1–2 seconds and repeat for 5–10 repetitions.

TECHNIQUE
Internally rotating the back hip targets the psoas because this muscle concentrically performs hip flexion and external rotation.

© ilolab/ShutterStock, Inc.

ACTIVE-ISOLATED STRETCHES *continued*

© ilolab/ShutterStock, Inc.

Active Standing Adductor Stretch

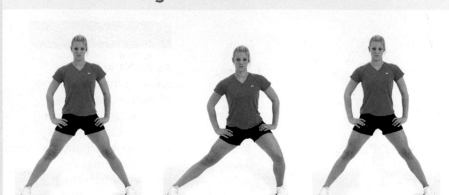

TECHNIQUE

Make sure to keep the hips level when going into the stretch.

Preparation

1. Stand in a straddled stance with the feet more than shoulders-width apart. Extend one leg back until the toe of the back leg is in line with the heel of the other foot. Both feet should be pointed straight ahead.

Movement

2. Draw navel inward and posteriorly rotate the pelvis.
3. Slowly move in a sideways motion (side lunge) until a stretch in the straight leg's groin area is felt.
4. Hold for 1–2 seconds and repeat for 5–10 repetitions.

Active Latissimus Dorsi Ball Stretch

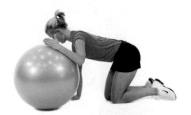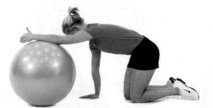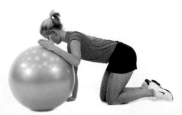

Preparation

1. Kneel in front of stability ball.
2. Place one arm on ball with thumb straight up in the air.

Movement

3. Draw navel upward.
4. Maintaining core control, roll ball out until a comfortable stretch is felt.
5. Hold stretch for 1–2 seconds and repeat for 5–10 repetitions.
6. Switch sides and repeat.

TECHNIQUE Make sure to initiate the stretch by going into a posterior pelvic tilt. This will take the origin and insertion of the latissimus dorsi further apart, enhancing the stretch.

ACTIVE-ISOLATED STRETCHES *continued*

Active Pectoral Stretch

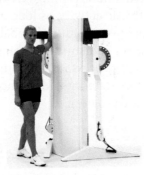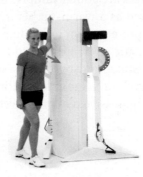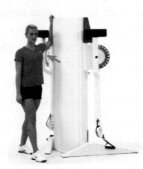

TECHNIQUE

Retract the scapulae when going into the stretch. This will reciprocally inhibit the pectoralis major and minor, enhancing the stretch.

Preparation
1. Stand against an object and form a 90-90-degree angle with the arm as depicted.

Movement
2. Draw navel inward.
3. Slowly lean forward until a slight stretch is felt in the anterior shoulder and chest region.
4. Hold stretch for 1–2 seconds and repeat for 5–10 repetitions.

Active Upper Trapezius/Scalene Stretch

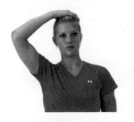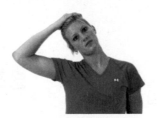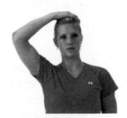

TECHNIQUE

If tingling is felt down the arm and into the finger, decrease the range of motion of the stretch. This will take stress off of the nerve. Also make sure the head stays in a neutral position during the stretch. Do not allow the head to jut forward.

Preparation
1. Stand with optimal posture.

Movement
2. Draw navel inward.
3. Tuck chin and slowly laterally flex the head, pulling one ear toward the same-side shoulder while retracting and depressing the same-side shoulder complex.
4. Hold stretch for 1–2 seconds and repeat for 5–10 repetitions.

Dynamic Stretching

Dynamic stretch The active extension of a muscle, using force production and momentum, to move the joint through the full available range of motion.

Dynamic stretching uses the force production of a muscle and the body's momentum to take a joint through the full available range of motion **Table 7.5**. Dynamic stretching uses the concept of reciprocal inhibition to improve soft tissue extensibility. One can perform one set of 10 repetitions using 3 to 10 dynamic stretches. Hip swings, medicine ball rotations, and walking lunges are good examples of dynamic stretching (1,14). Dynamic stretching is also suggested as a warm-up before athletic activity, as long as no postural distortion patterns are present. If an individual does possess muscle imbalances, self-myofascial release and static stretching should precede dynamic stretching for overactive or tight muscles identified during the assessment process. It is recommended that the client have good levels of tissue extensibility, core stability, and balance capabilities before undertaking an aggressive dynamic stretching program.

TABLE 7.5 Dynamic Stretching Summary

© Ilolab/ShutterStock, Inc.

Type of Stretch	Mechanism of Action	Acute Variables	Examples
Dynamic stretch	Reciprocal inhibition	1–2 sets	• Prisoner squats
		10–15 repetitions	• Multiplanar lunges
		3–10 exercises	• Single-leg squat touchdowns • Tube walking • Medicine ball lift and chop

DYNAMIC STRETCHES

© Ilolab/ShutterStock, Inc.

Prisoner Squat

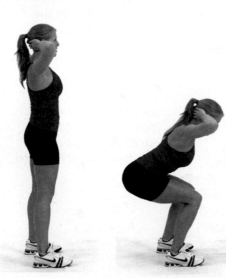

Preparation
1. Stand in proper alignment, with the hands behind the head.

Movement
2. Draw navel inward.
3. Lower to a squat position, under control and without compensation (toes straight ahead, knees in line with the toes).
4. Extend hips, knees, and ankles and repeat.
5. Perform 10 repetitions.

TECHNIQUE

As a progression add a calf raise after extending the hips, knees and ankles.

DYNAMIC STRETCHES *continued*

Multiplanar Lunge with Reach

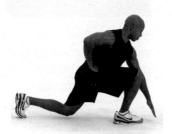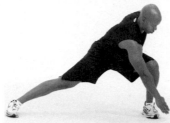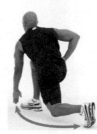

Preparation

1. Stand in proper alignment with hands on hips and feet straight ahead.

Movement

2. Draw navel inward.
3. While maintaining total body alignment, step forward (sagittal plane), and descend into a lunge position while reaching forward as illustrated.
4. Use hip and thigh muscles to push up and back to the start position.
5. Perform 10 repetitions.
6. Repeat on opposite leg.
7. Progress to side lunges with reach (frontal plane), followed by turning lunges with reach (transverse plane).

Single-Leg Squat Touchdown

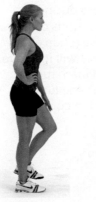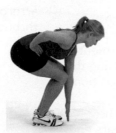

Preparation

1. Stand on one leg in optimal posture, keeping raised leg parallel to the standing leg. Imagine the floating leg is resting on an imaginary phonebook.

Movement

2. Draw navel inward.
3. Squat, in a controlled manner, bending the ankle, knee, and hip while reaching the opposite hand near the standing leg toe.
4. While maintaining drawn-in maneuver and gluteal activity, return to starting position.
5. Perform 10 repetitions.
6. Repeat on opposite side.

TECHNIQUE

Make sure the knee is tracking in line with the second and third toes. Do not allow the knee of the squatting leg to move inside the foot.

DYNAMIC STRETCHES *continued*

Tube Walking: Side-to-Side

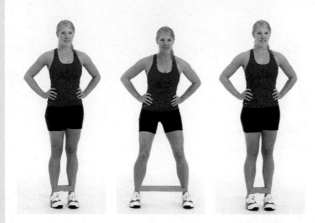

TECHNIQUE

Make sure the toes stay straight ahead and do not turn the feet out when stepping. This exercise is very effective for improving gluteus medius and core activation.

Preparation
1. Stand with feet hip-width apart, knees slightly bent, and feet straight ahead.
2. Place tubing around lower leg.

Movement
3. Draw navel inward.
4. Keep feet straight ahead and take 10 small steps sideways, without allowing knees to cave inward.
5. Repeat in the opposite direction.

Medicine Ball Lift and Chop

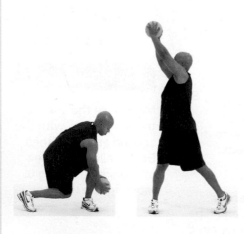

Preparation
1. Stand with feet hip-width apart, knees slightly bent and feet straight ahead.
2. Grasp a medicine ball with both hands and keep elbows fully extended.

Movement
3. Draw belly button inward.
4. Starting from optimal posture, initiate the rotational movement from the trunk outward, lifting the medicine ball from a low position to a high position.
5. Allow the hips to pivot on the back foot as the motion nears end range.
6. Perform 10 repetitions.
7. Repeat on opposite side.

TECHNIQUE

Allow for the hips to rotate during both portions of this exercise (chop and lift). This will improve arthrokinematics through the lumbo-pelvic-hip complex.

SUMMARY

Each type of flexibility training consists of specific stretching techniques. Corrective flexibility uses self-myofascial release and static stretching; active flexibility uses self-myofascial release and active-isolated stretching; and functional flexibility uses self-myofascial release and dynamic stretching. Self-myofascial release applies gentle pressure on muscle hypertonicity for a minimum of 30 seconds. The force applied creates autogenic inhibition, decreasing muscle spindle excitation and releasing the muscle hypertonicity. These techniques are suggested before stretching, as well as for cool-down. Static stretching passively takes a muscle to the point of tension and holds it there for a minimum of 30 seconds. Static stretches can be used before activity to decrease overactivity of tight muscles and to increase range of motion. However, care should be used when static stretching is used before certain activities that involve explosive movements or maximal strength. Static stretches should also be used after activity to reset muscles back to their optimal resting lengths. Active-isolated stretches use agonists and synergists to dynamically move joints into their ranges of motion. These are suggested for preactivity warm-up (5 to 10 repetitions, held for 1–2 seconds each). Dynamic stretches use force production and momentum to take a joint through the full available range of motion. These are suggested for preactivity warm-up as well.

Controversial Stretches

Although stretching and flexibility training have numerous benefits, performing certain types of stretches may cause injury. Flexibility training, like any other physical activity, carries varying degrees of injury risk. Although most stretches (when performed correctly with proper posture and technique) are very safe, there are a few controversial stretches that may be potentially dangerous:

1. Inverted hurdler's stretch **Figure 7.11**: This stretch is believed to place high stress on the inside of the knee (medial collateral ligament) and may cause pain and stress on the kneecap (patella). This stretch should not be performed by anyone with a history of knee or low-back pain, and most health professionals believe this stretch should not be performed by most patients or clients.

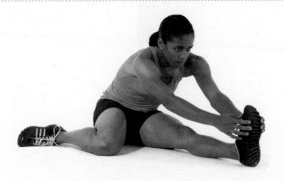

FIGURE 7.11

Inverted hurdler's stretch.

2. Plow **Figure 7.12**: A common posture from yoga. Because of the inverted nature of this stretch (head is lower than the hips), this stretch places high stress on the neck and spine. If this stretch is not done with exact technique, it may place the spine at risk of injury. Patients or clients with a history of neck or back injury should not perform this stretch owing to the high stress it places on these structures. This position should also be avoided by individuals with high blood pressure (hypertension). In addition, many practitioners of yoga will discourage menstruating females from performing inverted stretches (although there is no research to suggest there are negative effects on the body if menstruating females perform these movements).

3. Shoulder stand **Figure 7.13**: Another common posture from yoga, and another inverted stretch. As with the plow, this position places high stress on the neck, shoulders, and spine. It should be avoided in patients with hypertension or any history of neck or spine injury, or if exact technique is not used.

4. Straight-leg toe touch **Figure 7.14**: One of the most common stretches for the hamstring complex. This position may place the vertebrae and the cartilage discs in the low back under high stress. Any client or patient with a history of herniated discs or nerve pain that runs in the back of the leg should avoid this stretch. In addition, clients with poor flexibility may attempt to hyperextend the knees during this stretch, which may place high stress on the ligaments of the knee.

5. Arching quadriceps **Figure 7.15**: This stretch is designed to stretch the quadriceps and hip flexors. This position places very high stress on the kneecap and the

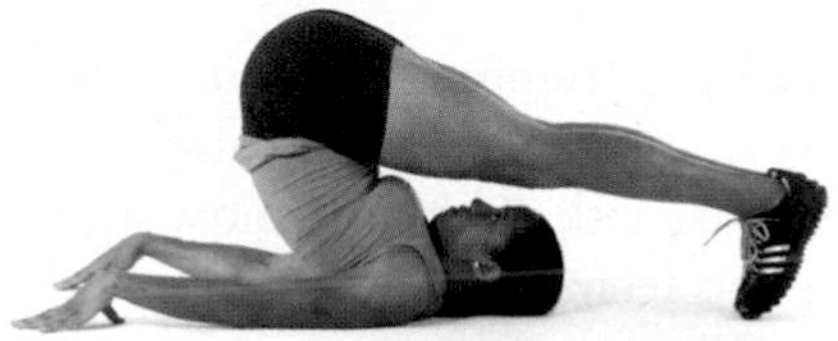

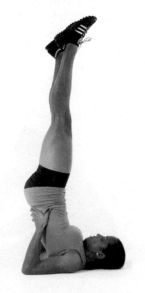

FIGURE 7.12

Plow.

FIGURE 7.13

Shoulder stand.

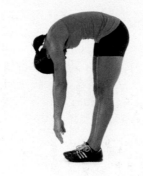

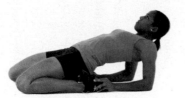

other tissues on the front of the knee joint. Any client or patient with a history of knee injury should avoid this stretch. Owing to the high stress (compression) of the kneecap into the knee during this stretch (which may cause damage to the cartilage), most health-care professionals discourage anyone from performing this exercise.

So, why would anyone perform these stretches if they are dangerous? Some of these positions are required in certain sports or activities (for instance, the inverted hurdler's stretch mimics the position of a hurdler going over a hurdle). Others are traditional positions used in martial arts, gymnastics, or yoga. However, for most clients, there are safer positions that can be used to stretch the targeted muscles. Therefore, all clients should be properly educated about stretching technique and posture, and the safest exercises should be used to meet the goals of the exercise program.

Practical Application of Flexibility Training for Movement Compensations

As previously mentioned, there are some common movement compensations that must be addressed to ensure the safety and effectiveness of a training program. Proper flexibility is the first step to addressing these problems. Table 7.6 provides the common compensations seen during the assessment process, associated overactive and underactive muscles, and corrective strategies for each (flexibility and strengthening exercises). Further chapters in the text will provide proper instruction for the sample strengthening exercises that can be implemented to help strengthen the underactive muscles in each of the compensations.

TABLE 7.6 Compensations, Muscle Imbalances, and Corrective Strategies

View	Check-point	Compensation	Probable Overactive Muscles	Probable Underactive Muscles	Sample SMR (foam roll) and Static Stretch Techniques	Sample Strengthening Exercises
Anterior	Feet	Turn out	Soleus Lateral gastrocnemius Biceps femoris (short head)	Medial gastrocnemius Medial hamstring complex Gracilis Sartorius Popliteus	SMR: Gastrocnemius/soleus SMR: Biceps femoris (short head) Static gastrocnemius stretch Static supine biceps femoris stretch	Single-leg balance reach
	Knees	Move inward	Adductor complex Biceps femoris (short head) Tensor fascia latae Vastus lateralis	Gluteus medius/maximus Vastus medialis oblique (VMO)	SMR: Adductors SMR: TFL/IT band Static supine biceps femoris stretch Static standing TFL stretch	Tube walking: side to side
Lateral	LPHC	Excessive forward lean	Soleus Gastrocnemius Hip flexor complex (TFL, rectus femoris, psoas) Abdominal complex (rectus abdominis, external obliques)	Anterior tibialis Gluteus maximus Erector spinae	SMR: Gastrocnemius/soleus SMR: Quadriceps Static gastrocnemius stretch Static kneeling hip flexor stretch	Quadruped arm/ opposite leg raise Ball wall squats
		Low back arches	Hip flexor complex (TFL, rectus femoris, psoas) Erector spinae Latissimus dorsi	Gluteus maximus Hamstring complex Intrinsic core stabilizers (transverse abdominis, multifidus, transversospinalis, internal oblique, pelvic-floor muscles)	SMR: Quadriceps SMR: Latissimus dorsi Static kneeling hip flexor stretch Static latissimus dorsi ball stretch	Quadruped arm/ opposite leg raise Ball wall squats
	Upper body	Arms fall forward	Latissimus dorsi Teres major Pectoralis major/minor	Mid/lower trapezius Rhomboids Rotator cuff (supraspinatus, infraspinatus, teres minor, subscapularis)	SMR: Thoracic spine SMR: Latissimus dorsi Static latissimus dorsi ball stretch Static pectoral wall stretch	Squat to row
		Shoulders elevate (pushing/pulling assessment)	Upper trapezius Sternocleidomastoid Levator scapulae	Mid/lower trapezius	SMR: Upper trapezius (Thera Cane) Static stretch upper trapezius/ scalene stretch	Ball cobra
		Head protrudes forward (pushing/pulling assessment)	Upper trapezius Sternocleidomastoid Levator scapulae	Deep cervical flexors	SMR: Upper trapezius (Thera Cane) Static stretch upper trapezius/ scalene stretch	Chin tuck (keep head in neutral position during all exercises)

LPHC, lumbo-pelvic-hip complex; TFL, tensor fascia latae; IT, iliotibial.

Filling in the Template

After a fitness assessment, the flexibility portion of the template can now be filled in. On the template, select the form of flexibility your client requires. Go to the warm-up section and input the areas to be addressed **Figure 7.16**. For beginning clients and those requiring correction of postural imbalance, corrective flexibility (self-myofascial release and static stretching) is used before and after training sessions (as well as at home, on off days). Be sure to follow the flexibility guidelines for postural distortion patterns found in this chapter (Table 7.6). Corrective flexibility will be used during the first phase (Stabilization Endurance Training) of the OPT model.

With a proper progression through the flexibility continuum (and as the client's ability dictates), active (self-myofascial release and active-isolated stretching) and functional (self-myofascial release and dynamic stretching) flexibility can be implemented later in the strength and power levels of the OPT model. The use of flexibility techniques can be a great warm-up, but also may be used as a cool-down, especially self-myofascial release and static stretching. On the template, go to the cool-down section and, as for the warm-up, input the form of stretching to be implemented and the areas to be addressed.

Professional's Name: Brian Sutton

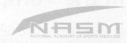

CLIENT'S NAME: JOHN SMITH	DATE: 5/01/13

GOAL: FAT LOSS	PHASE: 1 STABILIZATION ENDURANCE

WARM-UP

Exercise:	Sets	Duration	Coaching Tip
SMR: Calves, IT Band, Adductors	1	30 s.	Hold each tender area for 30 sec
Static Stretch: Calves, Hip Flexors, Adductors	1	30 s.	Hold each stretch for 30 sec

CORE / BALANCE / PLYOMETRIC

Exercise:	Sets	Reps	Tempo	Rest	Coaching Tip

SPEED, AGILITY, QUICKNESS

Exercise:	Sets	Reps	Rest	Coaching Tip

RESISTANCE

Exercise:	Sets	Reps	Tempo	Rest	Coaching Tip

COOL-DOWN

Exercise:	Sets	Duration	Coaching Tip

Coaching Tips:

National Academy of Sports Medicine

FIGURE 7.16 OPT template.

REFERENCES

1. Alter MJ. *Science of Flexibility*. 2nd ed. Champaign, IL: Human Kinetics; 1996.

2. Bandy WD, Irion JM, Briggler M. The effect of time and frequency of static stretching on flexibility of the hamstring muscles. *Phys Ther.* 1997;77(10):1090-1096.

3. Clanton TO, Coupe KJ. Hamstring strains in athletes: diagnosis and treatment. *J Am Acad Orthop Surg.* 1998;6(4):237-248.

4. Condon SA. Soleus muscle electromyographic activity and ankle dorsiflexion range of motion during four stretching procedures. *Phys Ther.* 1987;67:24-30.

5. Chaitow L. *Muscle Energy Techniques*. New York: Churchill Livingstone; 1997.

6. Janda V. Muscle spasm—a proposed procedure for differential diagnosis. *Man Med.* 1999;6136-6139.

7. Liebenson C. Integrating Rehabilitation into chiropractic practice (blending active and passive care). In: Liebenson C, ed. *Rehabilitation of the Spine*. Baltimore: Williams & Wilkins; 1996:13-44.

8. Poterfield J, DeRosa C. *Mechanical Low Back Pain: Perspectives in Functional Anatomy*. Philadelphia: WB Saunders; 1991.

9. Gossman MR, Sahrman SA, Rose SJ. Review of length-associated changes in muscle: experimental evidence and clinical implications. *Phys Ther.* 1982;62:1799-1808.

10. Halbertsma JPK, Van Bulhuis AI, Goeken LNH. Sport stretching: effect on passive muscle stiffness of short hamstrings. *Arch Phys Med Rehabil.* 1996;77(7):688-692.

11. Holcomb WR. Improved stretching with proprioceptive neuromuscular facilitation. *J Natl Strength Cond Assoc.* 2000; 22(1):59-61.

12. Moore MA, Kukulka CG. Depression of Hoffmann reflexes following voluntary contraction and implications for proprioceptive neuromuscular facilitation therapy. *Phys Ther.* 1991;71(4):321-329.

13. Moore MA. Electromyographic investigation of muscle stretching techniques. *Med Sci Sports Exerc.* 1980;12:322-329.

14. Sady SP, Wortman M, Blanke D. Flexibility training: ballistic, static, or proprioceptive neuromuscular facilitation? *Arch Phys Med Rehabil.* 1982;63(6):261-263.

15. Sherrington C. *The Integrative Action of the Nervous System*. New Haven, CT: Yale University Press; 1947.

16. Wang RY. Effect of proprioceptive neuromuscular facilitation on the gait of patients with hemiplegia of long and short duration. *Phys Ther.* 1994;74(12):1108-1115.

17. Bachrach RM. Psoas dysfunction/insufficiency, sacroiliac dysfunction and low back pain. In: Vleeming A, Mooney V, Dorman T, Snijders C, Stoeckart R, eds. *Movement, Stability and Low Back Pain*. London: Churchill Livingstone; 1997: 309-317.

18. Cohen H. *Neuroscience for Rehabilitation*. 2nd ed. Philadelphia: Lippincott Williams & Wilkins; 1999.

19. Liebenson C. Active rehabilitation protocols. In: Liebenson C, ed. *Rehabilitation of the Spine*. Baltimore: Williams & Wilkins; 1996:355-390.

20. Milner-Brown A. *Neuromuscular Physiology*. Thousand Oaks, CA: National Academy of Sports Medicine; 2001.

21. Fox SI. *Human Physiology*. 5th ed. Dubuque, IA: Wm C Brown Publishers; 1996.

22. Vander A, Sherman J, Luciano D. *Human Physiology: The Mechanisms of Body Function*. 8th ed. New York: McGraw-Hill; 2001.

23. Enoka RM. *Neuromechanical Basis of Kinesiology*. 2nd ed. Champaign, IL: Human Kinetics; 1994.

24. McClosky DJ. Kinesthetic sensibility. *Physiol Rev.* 1978;58:763-820.

25. Grigg P. Peripheral neural mechanisms in proprioception. *J Sports Rehab.* 1994;3:2-17.

26. Janda V. Muscles and cervicogenic pain syndromes In: Grant R, ed. *Physical Therapy of the Cervical and Thoracic Spine*. Edinburgh: Churchill Livingstone; 1988:153-166.

27. Lewitt K. *Manipulation in Rehabilitation of the Locomotor System*. London: Butterworth; 1993.

28. Leahy PM. Active release techniques: Logical soft tissue treatment. In: Hammer WI, ed. *Functional Soft Tissue Examination and Treatment by Manual Methods*. Gaithersburg, MD: Aspen Publishers; 1999:549-559.

29. Spencer AM. *Practical Podiatric Orthopedic Procedures*. Cleveland: Ohio College of Podiatric Medicine; 1978.

30. Woo SLY, Buckwalter JA. *Injury and Repair of the Musculoskeletal Soft Tissues*. Park Ridge, IL: American Academy of Orthopedic Surgeons; 1987.

31. Zairns B. Soft tissue injury and repair—biomechanical aspects. *Int J Sports Med.* 1982;3:9-11.

32. Beaulieu JA. Developing a stretching program. *Physician Sports Med.* 1981;9:59-69.

33. Evjenth O, Hamburg J. *Muscle Stretching in Manual Therapy— A Clinical Manual*. Alfta, Sweden: Alfta Rehab; 1984.

34. Tannigawa M. Comparison of the hold-relax procedure and passive mobilization on increasing muscle length. *Phys Ther*. 1972;52:725-735.

35. Voss DE, Ionla MK, Meyers BJ. *Proprioceptive Neuromuscular Facilitation*. 3rd ed. Philadelphia: Harper and Row; 1985.

36. Akeson WH, Woo SLY. The connective tissue response to immobility: biochemical changes in periarticular connective tissue of the immobilized rabbit knee. *Clin Orthop Relat Res*. 1973;93:356-362.

37. Barnes JF. Myofascial release. In: Hammer WI, ed. *Functional Soft Tissue Examination and Treatment by Manual Methods*. 2nd ed. Gaithersburg, MD: Aspen Publishers; 1999:533-547.

38. Sapega A, Quedenfeld T, Moyer R. Biophysical factors in range of motion exercises. *Phys Sports Med*. 1981;9:57-65.

39. Etnyre BR, Abraham LD. Gains in range of ankle dorsiflexion using three popular stretching techniques. *Am J Phys Med*. 1986;65:189-196.

© Eky Studio/ShutterStock, Inc.

© Ilolab/ShutterStock, Inc.

Cardiorespiratory Fitness Training

After studying this chapter, you will be able to:

✔ Define and describe the components associated with cardiorespiratory training.

✔ Describe how various physiologic systems respond and adapt to cardiorespiratory training.

✔ Describe the health-related benefits associated with cardiorespiratory fitness.

✔ Describe current guidelines and recommendations for prescribing safe and effective cardiorespiratory exercise to apparently healthy individuals.

✔ Describe how to design and implement cardiorespiratory training programs to a variety of clients using an individualized approach.

✔ Instruct clients on how to perform safe and effective cardiorespiratory exercise.

OBJECTIVES

Cardiorespiratory Fitness Training

Cardiorespiratory fitness reflects the ability of the circulatory and respiratory systems to supply oxygen-rich blood to skeletal muscles during sustained physical activity. Cardiorespiratory fitness is one of five components to health-related physical fitness; the others include muscular strength, muscular endurance, flexibility, and body composition. Cardiorespiratory fitness is vitally important to health and wellness as well as to the ability to engage in normal activities of daily living (ADLs) without excessive fatigue. Physical activity and exercise training programs should be designed with the intent of improving each of the key components of health-related physical fitness; however, from the standpoint of preventing chronic disease and improving health and quality of life, cardiorespiratory fitness training should always be a top priority when

Cardiorespiratory fitness The ability of the circulatory and respiratory systems to supply oxygen-rich blood to skeletal muscles during sustained physical activity.

201

allocating time and resources during the design and implementation of any exercise training program because of the number of health-related benefits associated with it.

Integrated cardiorespiratory training is a way of planning training programs that systematically progress clients through various stages to achieve optimal levels of physiologic, physical, and performance adaptations by placing stress on the cardiorespiratory system. One of the most common errors made by personal trainers during the planning and implementation of cardiorespiratory exercise programs is the failure to consider *rate of progression*. Rate of progression is critical to helping clients achieve their personal health and fitness goals in the most efficient and effective use of time and energy. In addition, failure to carefully consider and monitor rate of progression of each client on an individual basis can also result in injury if progression is too fast or in poor exercise adherence if the progression is too slow. Thus, applying the principles of the OPT™ model to the design of cardiorespiratory fitness training programs will help ensure that clients maximize their potential to achieve optimal levels of physiologic, physical, and performance adaptation.

Benefits of Cardiorespiratory Fitness

The benefits of regular physical activity and exercise are numerous. Individuals can achieve numerous health-related benefits from modest amounts of moderate-intensity exercise, and even greater benefits from vigorous-intensity exercise, or a combination of both. Engaging in regular, sustained physical activity over the lifespan is one of the most reliable predictors of death and disability. In fact, research has confirmed that an individual's cardiorespiratory fitness level is one of the strongest predictors of morbidity and mortality (1–3). In other words, poor cardiorespiratory fitness is related to a marked increase in risk of premature death from all causes, but particularly from cardiovascular disease. Conversely, an improvement in cardiorespiratory fitness is related to a reduction in premature death from all causes (1–3).

Cardiorespiratory Fitness Training

Exercise training programs should be designed to meet the specific needs and goals of the individual client. Furthermore, the initial exercise prescription should reflect (a) the initial fitness level of the client, (b) fitness assessment results, and (c) whether the client has any significant risk factors or health limitations to exercise. Each exercise training session should also include the following phases:

- Warm-up phase
- Conditioning phase
- Cool-down phase

Warm-Up Phase

A warm-up is generally described as preparing the body for physical activity. It can be either general in nature or more specific to the activity (4,5). A **general warm-up** consists of movements that do not necessarily have any movement specific to the actual activity to be performed. (Examples include warming up by walking on a treadmill or riding a stationary bicycle before weight training.) A **specific warm-up** consists of movements that more closely mimic those of the actual activity, often referred to as dynamic stretches. (Examples include performing body-weight squats and push-ups before weight training.) The proposed benefits of a warm-up are outlined in Table 8.1 (4–7).

Integrated cardiorespiratory training
Cardiorespiratory training programs that systematically progress clients through various stages to achieve optimal levels of physiologic, physical, and performance adaptations by placing stress on the cardiorespiratory system.

General warm-up
Low-intensity exercise consisting of movements that do not necessarily relate to the more intense exercise that is to follow.

Specific warm-up
Low-intensity exercise consisting of movements that mimic those that will be included in the more intense exercise that is to follow.

TABLE 8.1	Benefits and Effects of a Warm-Up	

Benefits	Effects
Increased heart and respiratory rate	Increases cardiorespiratory system's capacity to perform work
	Increases blood flow to active muscle tissue
	Increases the oxygen exchange capacity
Increased tissue temperature	Increases rate of muscle contraction
	Increases efficiency of opposing muscle contraction and relaxation
	Increases metabolic rate
	Increases the soft tissue extensibility
Increased psychological preparation for bouts of exercise	Increases the mental readiness of an individual

The cardiorespiratory portion of a warm-up period typically lasts between 5 and 10 minutes and consists of whole-body, dynamic cardiovascular or muscular movements (well below the anticipated training intensity threshold for conditioning). The purpose of the warm-up period is to increase heart and respiration rates, increase tissue temperature, and psychologically prepare the individual for higher training intensities.

Suggested Warm-Up Activities

NASM recommends that the cardiorespiratory portion of a warm-up last between 5 and 10 minutes and be performed at a low-to-moderate intensity level. However, depending on the client's goals and objectives, these recommendations can be modified by either extending or reducing the time allotted to the warm-up period or by modifying activities based on any known or suspected medical, health, or physical limitations a client may have.

New clients who are sedentary or have medical or health limitations or those with limited previous exercise experience may require up to half or more of their dedicated workout time be directed to warm-up activities, at least initially. Table 8.2 provides examples of suggested warm-ups using flexibility and cardiorespiratory exercise in the stabilization level (Phase 1) of the OPT model. Once a client understands the techniques and activities associated with the warm-up period, including self-myofascial release (foam rolling) and static stretching, they are ready to orient themselves to the cardiorespiratory conditioning segment of their warm-up.

It is vitally important that personal trainers have a comprehensive understanding of safe and effective dynamic and static warm-up activities. Personal trainers should begin each training session with new clients by explaining the benefits to be gained from each new exercise or activity introduced, followed by a demonstration of each new exercise, emphasizing safety and proper technique, and lastly by observing the client perform

TABLE 8.2	Warm-Up for the Stabilization Level Client	
Components	**Examples**	**Time**
Self-myofascial release	Gastrocnemius/soleus Adductors Tensor fascia latae Latissimus dorsi	30 seconds for each muscle
Static stretching	Gastrocnemius/soleus Adductors Tensor fascia latae Latissimus dorsi	30 seconds for each muscle
Cardiorespiratory exercise	Treadmill Stationary bicycle StairClimber Rower Elliptical trainer	5–10 minutes

NOTE: NASM recommends for individuals who possess musculoskeletal imbalances to first perform self-myofascial release to inhibit overactive muscles and then lengthen the overactive muscles through static stretching. This will help decrease movement compensations when performing the cardiorespiratory portion of the warm-up.

each new exercise prescribed to help ensure proper form and technique. Only once a client has demonstrated a complete understanding of the techniques necessary for self-myofascial release (foam rolling), static stretching, and operation of the cardiorespiratory equipment can he or she begin performing the warm-up before the session with the fitness professional. This will then allow for increased training time in which to focus on other aspects of the training program.

Table 8.3 provides a sample warm-up for the client who has progressed to the strength level (Phases 2, 3, and 4) of the OPT model. Strength level clients will use self-myofascial release and active-isolated stretching for muscles determined as tight or overactive during the assessment process before proceeding to the cardiorespiratory portion of the warm-up.

Table 8.4 provides a sample warm-up for the client who has progressed to the power level (Phase 5) of the OPT model. Power level clients will use self-myofascial release and dynamic stretching exercises to complete their warm-up. Keep in mind that dynamic stretches can be performed in a circuit format (performing one exercise after the other), thereby eliminating the need for additional cardiorespiratory warm-up activities.

It should be emphasized that the warm-up period should prepare the body for activity; thus it is important to monitor the intensity at which clients are performing selected warm-up activities to ensure they do not unduly fatigue before the workout portion of their program actually begins. Keeping the activity to a moderate duration and intensity level will help ensure a proper warm-up.

TABLE 8.3	Warm-Up for the Strength Level Client	
Components	**Examples**	**Time/Repetitions**
Self-myofascial release	Gastrocnemius/soleus Adductors Tensor fascia latae Latissimus dorsi	30 seconds for each muscle
Active-isolated stretching	Gastrocnemius/soleus Adductors Tensor fascia latae Latissimus dorsi	1–2 seconds, 5–10 reps for each muscle
Cardiorespiratory exercise	Treadmill Stationary bicycle StairClimber Rower Elliptical trainer	5–10 minutes

TABLE 8.4	Warm-Up for the Power Level Client (Dynamic, Functional Warm-up)	
Components	**Examples**	**Time/Repetitions**
Self-myofascial release	Gastrocnemius/soleus Adductors TFL and Iliotibial band Latissimus dorsi	30 seconds for each muscle
Dynamic stretching	Hip swings: side to side Prisoner squats Lunge with rotation Lateral tube walking Medicine ball lift and chop Single-leg squat touchdown	10 repetitions of each side

Conditioning Phase

Individuals who engage in cardiorespiratory exercise likely do so for a variety of reasons, including burning calories to lose weight, stress reduction, to improve their health, or for a host of other reasons (8–13). An important point that personal trainers should share with their clients is that low-intensity cardiorespiratory exercise will typically result in some improvements in health and well-being, but not necessarily any significant improvements in fitness as compared with higher training intensities (13).

In either scenario, cardiorespiratory exercise has a profound effect on physical and mental health as summarized below (8–16). These benefits accrue as the result of numerous physiologic adaptations to cardiorespiratory training.

Benefits of cardiorespiratory exercise include:

- Stronger and more efficient heart
- Improved ability to pump blood (enhanced cardiac output)
- Reduced risk of heart disease
- Lower resting heart rate
- Lower heart rate at any given level of work
- Improvement of lung ventilation (more efficient breathing)
- Stronger respiratory muscles (e.g., intercostals)
- Thicker articular cartilage and bones with weight-bearing aerobic exercises
- Improved oxygen transport
- Reduced cholesterol levels
- Reduced arterial blood pressure
- Improved blood thinning and reduced risk of clot formation
- Improved fuel supply (improved ability to use fatty acids, sparing muscle glycogen stores)
- Improved ability of muscles to use oxygen
- Improvement in mental alertness
- Reduced tendency for depression and anxiety
- Improved ability to relax and sleep
- Improved tolerance to stress
- Increase in lean body mass
- Increase in metabolic rate
- Reduced risk of obesity or diabetes mellitus

Individuals vary in their response to aerobic training, but if performed properly with due regard for individual abilities, it has a positive effect on many components of health and fitness.

Cool-Down Phase

A cool-down provides the body with a smooth transition from exercise back to a steady state of rest. In essence, a cool-down is the opposite of the warm-up. This portion of a workout is often overlooked and viewed as less important than the other components (6). However, proper use of a cool-down can have a significant impact on a client's overall health. The overarching goal of a cool-down is to reduce heart and breathing rates, gradually cool body temperature, return muscles to their optimal length-tension relationships, prevent venous pooling of blood in the lower extremities, which may cause dizziness or possible fainting, and restore physiologic systems close to baseline. Sufficient time for a cardiorespiratory cool-down period is approximately 5 to 10 minutes (17). The proposed benefits of a cool-down are shown below (6,4,7,17,18).

Benefits of a cool-down include:

- Reduce heart and breathing rates
- Gradually cool body temperature
- Return muscles to their optimal length-tension relationships
- Prevent venous pooling of blood in the lower extremities
- Restore physiologic systems close to baseline

Suggested Cool-Down Activities

During the transition from rest to steady-state cardiorespiratory exercise, the body undergoes numerous and often dramatic physiologic changes, depending on the intensity and duration of the activity. For example, some of the cardiovascular responses to exercise include linear increases in heart rate and systolic blood pressure and an increase in stroke volume (up to 40–60% of maximum), after which it plateaus, and an increase in cardiac output from an average resting value of about 5 L/min to as high as 20 to 40 L/min occurs during intense exercise. In addition, at rest only about 15 to 20% of circulating blood reaches skeletal muscle, but during intense vigorous exercise it increases up to as much as 80 to 85% of cardiac output. During exercise, blood is shunted away from major organs such as the kidneys, liver, stomach, and intestines and is redirected to the skin to promote heat loss. Blood plasma volume also decreases with the onset of exercise, and as exercise continues, increased blood pressure forces water from the vascular compartment to the interstitial space. During prolonged exercise, plasma volume can decrease by as much as 10 to 20%. Thus, with these as well as numerous other physiologic changes with exercise, it is easy to see why the cool-down period is so important. The cool-down period helps gradually restore physiologic responses to exercise close to baseline levels.

Flexibility training should also be included in the cool-down period. Flexibility training, including corrective stretching (self-myofascial release and static stretching), has been shown to be effective at lengthening muscles back to their optimal length-tension relationships, promoting optimal joint range of motion.

Initially, personal trainers should closely monitor new clients during both the warm-up and the cool-down periods to make certain that the activities being performed are appropriate, safe, and effective. It is also important for the client to understand the importance of both the warm-up and the cool-down periods. Table 8.5 provides suggested cool-down activities.

TABLE 8.5 Suggested Cool-Down Activities

© ilolab/ShutterStock, Inc.

Components	Examples	Time
Cardiorespiratory exercise	Treadmill Stationary bicycle StairClimber Rower Elliptical trainer	5–10 minutes
Self-myofascial release	Gastrocnemius/soleus Adductors Tensor fascia latae Latissimus dorsi	30 seconds for each muscle
Static stretching	Gastrocnemius/soleus Adductors Tensor fascia latae Latissimus dorsi	30 seconds for each muscle

1. When used in a warm-up, static stretching should only be used on areas that the assessments have determined are tight or overactive. Each stretch should be held for 20 to 30 seconds at end-range.
2. During the cool-down, static stretching should be used to return muscles to normal resting lengths, focusing on the major muscles used during the workout.

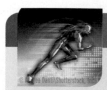

Memory Jogger

Regardless of the goal, always begin an exercise program with movement assessments such as the overhead squat and/or the single-leg squat tests (discussed in chapter six). These assessments help determine the muscles that need to be stretched during a warm-up. If a muscle is overactive or tight, it may be impeding or altering proper movement and as such need to be corrected to enhance movement.

SUMMARY

Cardiorespiratory fitness is one of the most important components of health-related physical fitness. High levels of cardiorespiratory fitness are strongly linked to reduced risk of disease and improved mortality. Cardiorespiratory training should be preceded by a warm-up period and followed by a cool-down period. A warm-up prepares the body for physical activity and can be either general in nature or more specific to the activity. Typically, the cardiorespiratory portion of a warm-up should last 5 to 10 minutes at a low-to-moderate intensity. A cool-down of 5 to 10 minutes provides the body with an essential transition from exercise back to a steady state of rest. Flexibility exercises are also important components of the warm-up and cool-down to reset muscles back to their optimal resting lengths.

General Guidelines for Cardiorespiratory Training

Personal trainers need to understand and appreciate the fact that no two individuals will ever respond and adapt to cardiorespiratory exercise in exactly the same way. In other words, the physiologic and perceptual responses to exercise are highly variable, even among individuals of similar age, fitness, and health. Thus, all exercise training recommendations, including cardiorespiratory exercise, must be individually determined and should always use the FITTE principle **Figure 8.1** (19). FITTE stands for *frequency, intensity, type, time,* and *enjoyment*.

Frequency

Frequency The number of training sessions in a given timeframe.

Frequency refers to the number of training sessions in a given time period, usually expressed as per week. For general health requirements **Table 8.6**, the recommended frequency of activity is preferably every day of the week, for small quantities of time (20). For improved fitness levels, the frequency is 3 to 5 days per week at higher intensities **Table 8.7** (20).

F	Frequency
I	Intensity
T	Time
T	Type
E	Enjoyment

FIGURE 8.1

The FITTE factors.

TABLE 8.6 General Aerobic Activity Recommendations

© ilolab/ShutterStock, Inc.

Frequency	Intensity	Time	Type	Enjoyment
At least 5 days per week	40% to <60% $\dot{V}O_2R$ or 55% to 70% HR_{max}	150 minutes per week	Moderate-intensity aerobic activity (i.e., brisk walking)	Initially, choose endurance activities that require minimal skill or physical fitness to perform.
At least 3 days per week	≥60% $\dot{V}O_2R$ or >70% HR_{max}	75 minutes per week	Vigorous-intensity aerobic activity (i.e., jogging or running)	Initially choose vigorous-intensity endurance activities that require minimal skill to perform.
3–5 days per week	*Combination of Moderate and Vigorous Intensity*: Any combination of moderate and vigorous intensity aerobic (cardiorespiratory fitness) activities.			

$\dot{V}O_2R$ = oxygen uptake reserve; HR_{max} = heart rate max. Source: Adapted from Haskell WL, Lee IM, Pate RR, Powell KE, Blair SN, Franklin BA, Macera CA, Heath GW, Thompson PD, Bauman A. Physical activity and public health updated recommendation for adults from the American College of Sports Medicine and the American Heart Association. *Circulation*. 2007;116;1081–1093.

TABLE 8.7 Relative Intensity

© ilolab/ShutterStock, Inc.

Classification	% $\dot{V}O_2R$ or % HRR	% HR_{max}	RPE (6–20 scale)
Very light	<20	<35	<10
Light	20–39	35–54	10–11
Moderate	40–59	55–69	12–13
Hard	60–84	70–89	14–16
Very hard	≥85	≥90	17–19
Maximal	100	100	20

Intensity

Intensity The level of demand that a given activity places on the body.

Maximal oxygen consumption ($\dot{V}o_2$max) The highest rate of oxygen transport and utilization achieved at maximal physical exertion.

Oxygen uptake reserve ($\dot{V}o_2R$) The difference between resting and maximal or peak oxygen consumption.

Intensity refers to the level of demand that a given activity places on the body. Applied to cardiorespiratory exercise, intensity is established and monitored in numerous ways, including calculating heart rate, power output (watts), or by calculating a percentage of **maximal oxygen consumption ($\dot{V}o_{2max}$)** or **oxygen uptake reserve ($\dot{V}o_2R$)** (19). For general health requirements (shown in Table 8.6), moderate intensity is preferred (19,20). Moderate exercise typically represents an intensity range of less than 60%$\dot{V}o_2R$, which is enough of a demand to increase heart and respiratory rate, but does not cause exhaustion or breathlessness for the average untrained apparently healthy adult (19,20). In other words, the individual should be able to talk comfortably during exercise. Higher intensities greater than 60%$\dot{V}o_2R$ are generally required for improvements in overall fitness and conditioning. However, any combination of the two will also result in improved health.

Methods for Prescribing Exercise Intensity

Peak $\dot{V}O_2$ Method

The traditional gold standard measurement for cardiorespiratory fitness is $\dot{V}o_{2max}$ or the maximal volume of oxygen per kilogram body weight per minute. In other words, $\dot{V}o_{2max}$ is the maximal amount of oxygen that an individual can use during intense exercise. Once $\dot{V}o_{2max}$ is determined, a common method to establish exercise training intensity is to have clients exercise at a percentage of their $\dot{V}o_{2max}$. However, accurately measuring $\dot{V}o_{2max}$ is oftentimes impractical for personal trainers because it requires clients to perform cardiorespiratory exercise at maximal effort and sophisticated equipment to monitor the client's ventilation response (O_2 consumed and CO_2 expired). Thus submaximal tests have become popular for personal trainers to estimate $\dot{V}o_{2max}$.

$\dot{V}O_2$ Reserve Method

$\dot{V}o_2R$ is another method that can be used to establish exercise training intensity, and is now the preferred method according to the most recent position stand by the American College of Sports Medicine. $\dot{V}o_2R$ requires the calculation of $\dot{V}o_{2max}$ and then a simple equation to calculate $\dot{V}o_2R$. The formula is as follows:

$$\text{Target } \dot{V}o_2R = [(\dot{V}o_{2max} - \dot{V}o_{2rest}) \times \text{intensity desired}] + \dot{V}o_{2rest}.$$

In this case, $\dot{V}o_{2max}$ can be estimated using a submaximal test or directly measured, and $\dot{V}o_{2rest}$ is usually always predicted (estimated at 1 MET or 3.5 mL $O_2 \cdot kg^{-1} \cdot min^{-1}$). Consider the following example of a 25-year-old client with a desired training intensity between 70 and 85%. If this 25-year-old client has a $\dot{V}o_{2max}$ of 35 mL $O_2 \cdot kg^{-1} \cdot min^{-1}$ (which is considered average), then the formula would be solved as follows:

$$[(35 - 3.5)] \times .70 + 3.5 = 25.55 \text{ mL } O_2 \cdot kg^{-1} \cdot min^{-1}$$

and

$$[(35 - 3.5)] \times .85 + 3.5 = 30.28 \text{ mL } O_2 \cdot kg^{-1} \cdot min^{-1}$$

NASM has reclassified the relative intensity of exercise in six incremental stages, from "very light" to "maximal effort," with a corresponding oxygen uptake reserve ($\dot{V}o_2R$) or heart rate reserve (HRR) and rating of perceived exertion (RPE) at each progressive level (Table 8.7). The ACSM recommends a relative training intensity of 40 or 50% to 85% of $\dot{V}o_2R$ or HRR, where 50% $\dot{V}o_2R$ or HRR was the threshold intensity for training most adults, and 40% $\dot{V}o_2R$ or HRR was presumably the threshold for training deconditioned individuals. HRR and ratings of perceived exertion will be discussed in more detail in the next sections.

Peak Metabolic Equivalent (MET) Method

One metabolic equivalent or MET is equal to 3.5 mL $O_2 \cdot kg^{-1} \cdot min^{-1}$ or the equivalent of the average resting metabolic rate (RMR) for adults. METs are used to describe the energy cost of physical activity as multiples of resting metabolic rate. MET values are used to relate exercise intensity with energy expenditure. For example, a physical activity with a MET value of 4, such as jogging at a slow pace, would require 4 times the energy that that person consumes at rest (e.g., sitting quietly). There are many resources available for personal trainers that describe common activities and their average MET values.

Peak Maximal Heart Rate (MHR) Method

Calculating maximal heart rate (HR_{max}) is another method for establishing training intensity during cardiorespiratory exercise. Although measuring a client's actual maximal heart rate is impractical for personal trainers because it requires testing clients at maximal capacity, there are many formulas to estimate HR_{max}. Arguably the most commonly used formula for estimating HR_{max} is (220 − age). However, this formula was never intended to be used as an instrument for designing cardiorespiratory fitness programs because maximal heart rate varies significantly among individuals of the same age. Dr. William Haskell (developer of the aforementioned formula) has been quoted as saying, "The formula was never supposed to be an absolute guide to rule people's training" (21). Estimating maximal heart rate from mathematical formulas can produce results that are ±10 to 12 beats per minute off the actual maximal heart rate (22). Accordingly, personal trainers should never use this, or any other formula, as an absolute. However, this equation is very simple to use and can be easily implemented as a general starting point for measuring cardiorespiratory training intensity.

HR Reserve (HRR) Method

Heart rate reserve (HRR), also known as the Karvonen method, is a method of establishing training intensity based on the difference between a client's predicted maximal heart rate and their resting heart rate.

Because heart rate and oxygen uptake are linearly related during dynamic exercise, selecting a predetermined training or target heart rate (THR) based on a given percentage of oxygen consumption is the most common and universally accepted method of establishing exercise training intensity. The heart rate reserve (HRR) method is defined as:

$$THR = [(HR_{max} - HR_{rest}) \times desired\ intensity] + HR_{rest}$$

Consider the following example of a 25-year-old client with a desired training intensity of 85% of his heart rate maximum. If this 25-year-old client has a resting heart rate of 40 bpm (which is considered very good), then the formula would be solved as follows:

$$220 - 25\ (age) = 195\ HR_{max}$$

$$195 - 40\ (resting\ heart\ rate) = 155$$

$$155 \times 85\% = 132$$

$$132 + 40 = 172\ bpm$$

Thus, 172 beats per minute is the client's target heart rate.

Ratings of Perceived Exertion Method

A subjective rating of perceived exertion is a technique used to express or validate how hard a client feels he or she is working during exercise. When using the rating of perceived exertion (RPE) method, a person is subjectively rating the perceived difficulty of exercise. It is based on the physical sensations a person experiences during physical activity, including increased heart rate, increased respiration rate, increased sweating, and muscle fatigue. The client's subjective rating should be reported based on the overall feelings of how hard he or she is working, including an overall sense of fatigue and not just isolated areas of the body, i.e., tired legs during treadmill testing. Although the RPE scale is a subjective measure, if clients report their exertion ratings accurately, RPE does provide a fairly good estimate of the actual heart rate during physical activity. Moderate-intensity activity is equal to "somewhat hard" (12–14) on the 6–20 Borg scale **Figure 8.2.**

Ventilatory threshold (T_{vent}) The point during graded exercise in which ventilation increases disproportionately to oxygen uptake, signifying a switch from predominately aerobic energy production to anaerobic energy production.

Talk Test Method

Up until quite recently, the talk test has been an informal method used to gauge exercise training intensity during exercise. The belief has always been that if clients reach a point at which they are not able to carry on a simple conversation during exercise because they are breathing too hard, then they are probably exercising at too high of an intensity level. A number of studies have now confirmed that there is a correlation between the talk test, $\dot{V}o_2$, **ventilatory threshold (T_{vent})**, and heart rate during both cycle ergometer and treadmill exercise (23,24). Thus, it appears that the talk test can help personal trainers and clients monitor proper exercise intensity without having to rely on measuring heart rate or $\dot{V}o_{2max}$. A summary of methods for prescribing exercise intensity is illustrated in **Table 8.8.**

FIGURE 8.2

Rating of perceived exertion (Borg scale).

6	No exertion at all
7	Extremely light
8	
9	Very light
10	
11	Light
12	
13	Somewhat hard
14	
15	Hard (heavy)
16	
17	Very hard
18	
19	Extremely hard
20	Maximal exertion

TABLE 8.8	Methods for Prescribing Exercise Intensity
Method	**Formula**
Peak $\dot{V}_{O_2}$	Target $\dot{V}_{O_2} = \dot{V}_{O_{2max}} \times$ intensity desired
$\dot{V}_{O_2}$ reserve ($\dot{V}_{O_2}$R)	Target $\dot{V}_{O_2}$R $= [(\dot{V}_{O_{2max}} - \dot{V}_{O_{2rest}}) \times$ intensity desired$] + \dot{V}_{O_{rest}}$
Peak MET $\times$ (% MET)	Target MET $= [(\dot{V}_{O_{2max}}) / 3.5 \text{ mL} \cdot \text{kg}^{-1} \cdot \text{min}^{-}] \times$ % intensity desired
Peak heart rate (HR)	Target HR (THR) $= HR_{max} \times$ % intensity desired
Heart rate reserve (HRR)	Target heart rate (THR) $= [(HR_{max} - HR_{rest}) \times$ % intensity desired$] + HR_{rest}$
Ratings of perceived exertion (RPE)	6- to 20-point scale
Talk test	The ability to speak during activity can identify exercise intensity and ventilatory threshold

Time

Time refers to the length of time engaged in an activity or exercise training session and is typically expressed in minutes. According to the most current public health guidelines on physical activity, the *2008 Physical Activity Guidelines for Americans*, for health benefits, adults should accumulate 2 hours and 30 minutes (150 minutes) of moderate-intensity aerobic activity (i.e., brisk walking) every week or 1 hour and 15 minutes (75 minutes) of vigorous-intensity aerobic activity (i.e., jogging or running) every week or an equivalent mix of moderate- and vigorous-intensity aerobic activity (20).

Time The length of time an individual is engaged in a given activity.

Type

Type refers to the mode or type of activity selected. It should be noted that there are three criteria that must be met for an activity or exercise to be considered "aerobic" exercise. For a mode of exercise to be considered aerobic, it should (a) be rhythmic in nature, (b) use large muscle groups, and (c) be continuous in nature. Some examples of modes of exercise recommended to improve cardiorespiratory fitness include:

Type The type or mode of physical activity that an individual is engaged in.

◆ Running or jogging
◆ Walking
◆ Exercising on cardio equipment
◆ Swimming
◆ Cycling (indoors or outdoors)

Enjoyment

Enjoyment refers to the amount of pleasure derived from engaging in a specific exercise or activity. Unfortunately, this component of the exercise prescription is often overlooked or not considered more seriously. Exercise adherence rates decline significantly when a specific mode of exercise is selected for a client before considering their personality type, previous exercise experiences, and other interests. If the mode of activity or exercise training program in general is not enjoyable to a client, it is highly likely that he or she will not adhere to the training program and thus not achieve their personal

Enjoyment The amount of pleasure derived from performing a physical activity.

health and fitness goals. A client is much more apt to continue with a program that is fun and challenging than one that is dull and boring.

Recommendations

The *2008 Physical Activity Guidelines for Americans* represents the most current and comprehensive set of guidelines published by the US government to date to help Americans aged 6 and older improve their health through appropriate physical activity and exercise. The guidelines, which are based on scientific evidence, recommend adults engage in 150 minutes a week of moderate-intensity activity (i.e., brisk walking) to help improve their overall health and fitness and reduce their risk for developing numerous chronic diseases. The guidelines also recommend that if adults exceed 300 minutes a week of moderate-intensity activity or 150 minutes a week of vigorous-intensity activity, then they will gain even more health benefits.

The guidelines presented in Table 8.6 represent physical activity guidelines for all adults; especially those who are currently sedentary or have little previous experience with exercise. If clients are not able to achieve the suggested minimal guidelines for cardiorespiratory training of 150 minutes per week (or 30 minutes 5 times a week) of moderate-intensity aerobic activity on at least 5 days per week, they can break it up into shorter increments, for example 10 minutes at a time, until 150 minutes per week is met.

SUMMARY

The FITTE guidelines allow for the development of a proper program and quantify its variables. Recommendations are listed below.

- *Frequency:* Refers to the number of training sessions in a given time period, usually expressed as per week. For general health requirements the recommended frequency of activity is preferably every day of the week, for small quantities of time. For improved fitness levels, the frequency is 3 to 5 days per week at higher intensities.
- *Intensity:* Refers to how hard the exercise or activity is or how much work is being done during exercise. For general health requirements, moderate intensity is preferred, of less than 60% $\dot{V}O_{2max}$. Higher intensities of greater than 60% $\dot{V}O_{2max}$ are generally required for improvements in overall fitness and conditioning. There are several methods to identify and monitor training intensity.
- *Time:* Refers to the length of time engaged in an activity or exercise training session and is typically expressed in minutes. Adults should accumulate 2 hours and 30 minutes (150 minutes) of moderate-intensity aerobic activity (i.e., brisk walking) every week or 1 hour and 15 minutes (75 minutes) of vigorous-intensity aerobic activity (i.e., jogging or running) every week or an equivalent mix of moderate- and vigorous-intensity aerobic activity.
- *Type:* Refers to the mode or type of activity selected. It should be noted that there are three criteria that must be met for an activity or exercise to be considered "aerobic" exercise. For a mode of exercise to be considered aerobic, it should (a) be rhythmic in nature, (b) use large muscle groups, and (c) be continuous in nature.
- *Enjoyment:* Refers to the amount of pleasure derived from engaging in a specific exercise or activity. The program and its activities should coincide with the personality, likes, and dislikes of the client.

Cardiorespiratory Training Methods

Cardiorespiratory training, as with any other form of training, falls under *the principle of specificity*. According to the principle of specificity, the body will adapt to the level of stress placed on it and will then require more or varied amounts of stress to produce a higher level of adaptation in the future.

Stage Training

The purpose of stage training is to ensure that cardiorespiratory training programs progress in an organized fashion to ensure continual adaptation and to minimize the risk of **overtraining** and injury. The three different stages of cardiorespiratory training uses three heart rate training zones Table 8.9 that are similar to the three levels of training seen in the OPT model. Each stage helps create a strong cardiorespiratory base to build on in subsequent stages.

Overtraining Excessive frequency, volume, or intensity of training, resulting in fatigue (which is also caused by a lack of proper rest and recovery).

Stage I

Stage I is designed to help improve cardiorespiratory fitness levels in apparently healthy sedentary clients using a target heart rate of 65 to 75% of HR_{max} or approximately 12 to 13 on the rating of perceived exertion scale (zone one). If using the talk test method to monitor training intensity, the client should be able to hold a conversation during the duration of the activity. In stage I, clients should start slowly and gradually work up to 30 to 60 minutes of continuous exercise in zone one Figure 8.3. If the client has never exercised before, he or she might start in zone one for only 5 minutes or reduce the heart rate percentage to the general health activity recommendations discussed in Table 8.6. Clients who can maintain zone one heart rate for at least 30 minutes two to

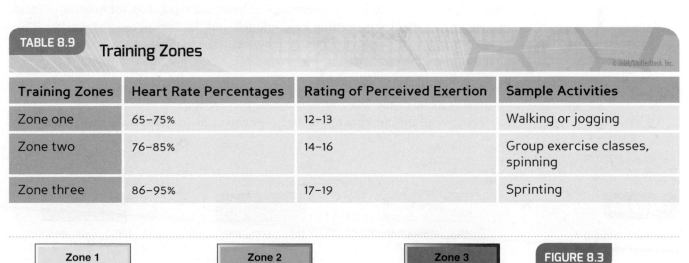

TABLE 8.9	Training Zones		
Training Zones	**Heart Rate Percentages**	**Rating of Perceived Exertion**	**Sample Activities**
Zone one	65–75%	12–13	Walking or jogging
Zone two	76–85%	14–16	Group exercise classes, spinning
Zone three	86–95%	17–19	Sprinting

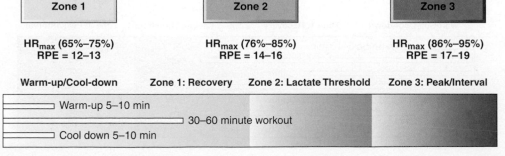

Zone 1	Zone 2	Zone 3	**FIGURE 8.3**
HR_{max} (65%–75%) RPE = 12–13	HR_{max} (76%–85%) RPE = 14–16	HR_{max} (86%–95%) RPE = 17–19	Stage I training parameters.

Warm-up/Cool-down   Zone 1: Recovery   Zone 2: Lactate Threshold   Zone 3: Peak/Interval

Warm-up 5–10 min
30–60 minute workout
Cool down 5–10 min

© Iloiab/ShutterStock, Inc.

three times per week will be ready for stage II. However, a beginning client might take 2 to 3 months to meet this demand. Stage I training also helps a client to better meet the muscular endurance demands of the stabilization level of training in the OPT model.

Stage II

Stage II is designed for clients with low-to-moderate cardiorespiratory fitness levels who are ready to begin training at higher intensity levels **Figure 8.4**. The focus in this stage is on increasing the workload (speed, incline, level) in a way that will help the client alter heart rate in and out of zone one and zone two. Stage II training helps increase the cardiorespiratory capacity needed for the workout styles in the strength level of the OPT model.

Stage II is the introduction to interval training in which intensities are varied throughout the workout. An example of a stage II workout will proceed as follows:

1. Start by warming up in zone one for 5 to 10 minutes.
2. Move into a 1-minute interval in zone two (shown in Figure 8.4). Gradually increase the workload to raise the heart rate up to zone two within that minute. Once the heart rate reaches zone two of maximal heart rate, maintain it for the rest of that minute. It might take 45 seconds to reach that heart rate, which means the client will only be at the top end for 15 seconds before reducing the workload (speed, incline, or level), and returning to zone one.
3. After the 1-minute interval return to zone one for 3 minutes.
4. Repeat this if the client has time and can recover back into the zone one range. The most important part of the interval is to recover back to zone one between the intervals.

During the first workout, questions may need to be asked frequently to determine if adjustments need to be made. For example, did the client get into a zone two heart rate? Was it easy? Could he/she maintain that heart rate, and, if so, for how long? (Also, make sure the client was pushing hard enough and didn't progress the workload too slowly.) Based on the answers to these questions, start to create a more accurate, modified training zone for the client.

1. If the client wasn't able to reach the predicted zone two in 1 minute, then use the heart rate he or she was able to reach as their "85%."
2. Take 9% off this number to get the lower end of the client's readjusted zone.

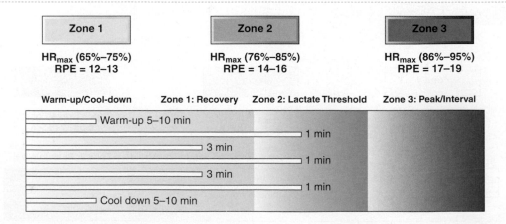

FIGURE 8.4			
Stage II training parameters.	**Zone 1** HR$_{max}$ (65%–75%) RPE = 12–13	**Zone 2** HR$_{max}$ (76%–85%) RPE = 14–16	**Zone 3** HR$_{max}$ (86%–95%) RPE = 17–19

Warm-up/Cool-down   Zone 1: Recovery   Zone 2: Lactate Threshold   Zone 3: Peak/Interval

Warm-up 5–10 min

1 min

3 min

1 min

3 min

1 min

Cool down 5–10 min

3. For example, if 150 beats per minute (bpm) was the predicted 85% of HR_{max}, but the client was only able to work up to 145 bpm during the 1-minute push, 145 bpm should now be considered that client's 85% HR_{max}.
4. Take 9% off 145% (9% of 145 is 13 beats; 145 − 13 = 132). So, 132 bpm is the individual's 76% of HR_{max}.
5. If the client got into the readjusted zone two, and then reaching the zones was fine, work slowly to increase the client's time in this zone.
6. If the client's heart rate goes above the predicted zone and he or she still can recover back to zone one at the end, add a couple of beats per minute to the zone and then work on increasing the time.

In stage II, it is important to alternate days of the week with stage I training. This means alternating sessions every workout. **Figure 8.5** displays an example monthly plan for a 3-days/week schedule. Start with stage I on Monday. Then, move to stage II on Wednesday and go back to stage I on Friday. The next week, start with stage II and so on. Rotate the stages to keep workouts balanced. This will become very important in stage III. The monthly plan is only a general guide and may be changed on the basis of the workout (if any) being performed on that day.

As a general rule, intervals should start out relatively brief as previously demonstrated with a work-to-rest (hard-to-easy) ratio of 1:3 (e.g., 1-minute interval followed by a 3-minute recovery). Once fitness and overall conditioning improves, stage II programs can be progressed using 1:2 and eventually 1:1 work-to-rest ratios. Moreover, the duration of each of these intervals can be gradually increased in regular implements.

Stage III

This stage is for the advanced client who has a moderately high cardiorespiratory fitness level base and will use heart rate zones one, two, and three. The focus in this stage is on further increasing the workload (speed, incline, level) in a way that will help the client alter heart rate in and out of each zone **Figure 8.6**. Stage III training increases the capacity of the energy systems needed at the power level of the OPT model. The workout will proceed as follows:

1. Warm up in zone one for up to 10 minutes.
2. Then, increase the workload every 60 seconds until reaching zone three. This will require a slow climb through zone two for at least 2 minutes.
3. After pushing for another minute in zone three, decrease the workload. This 1-minute break is an important minute to help gauge improvement.
4. Drop the client's workload down to the level he or she was just working in, before starting the zone 3 interval. During this minute, the heart rate will drop.

Week		1						2						3						4					
Day	M	T	W	T	F	S	S	M	T	W	T	F	S	S	M	T	W	T	F	S	S	M	T	W	T	F	S	S
Phase 1																								
Phase 2																								
Phase 3																								
Phase 4																								
Phase 5																								
Cardio	S1		S2		S1			S2		S1		S2			S1		S2		S1			S2		S1		S2		
Flexibility	X		X		X			X		X		X			X		X		X			X		X		X		

S1 = Stage I   S2 = Stage II

FIGURE 8.5

The monthly plan.

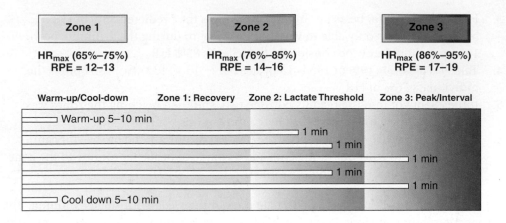

FIGURE 8.6

Stage III training parameters.

5. As improvements are made during several weeks of training, the heart rate will drop more quickly. The faster the heart rate drops, the stronger the heart is getting.

6. If the client is not able to drop to the appropriate heart rate during the 1-minute break, assume that he or she is tired and about to overtrain. The solution is to stay in zone one or two for the rest of the workout. The bottom line is that the client is not rested enough to do that type of exercise on that day (which may be because of a hard workout the day before, not enough sleep, or poor nutrition). Monitoring heart rate is an excellent tool in avoiding overtraining.

7. If the heart rate does drop to a normal rate, then overload the body again and go to the next zone, zone three, for 1 minute.

8. After this minute, go back to zone one for 5–10 minutes and repeat if desired.

It is vital when training at this level to rotate all three stages. There will be a low- (stage I), medium- (stage II), and high-intensity day (stage III) to help minimize the risk of overtraining. The monthly plan **Figure 8.7** is only a general guide and may change based on the workout (if any) that is being performed on that day.

Intervals within zone 3 should start out relatively brief, 30 to 60 seconds. Once fitness and overall conditioning improves, stage III programs can be progressed similarly to stage II workouts, decreasing work-to-rest ratios and increasing the duration of high-intensity intervals. However, the frequency and duration of intervals in zone two and zone three should be client-specific based on their goals, needs, abilities, and tolerance to intense activity.

FIGURE 8.7

The monthly plan.

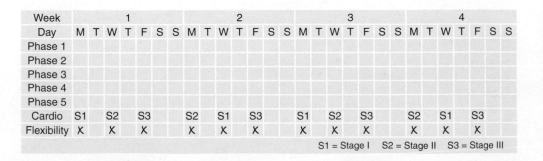

Circuit Training

Another beneficial form of cardiorespiratory training is circuit training. Circuit training allows for comparable fitness results without spending extended periods of time to achieve them. It is a very time-efficient manner in which to train a client and will be thoroughly described as it pertains to cardiorespiratory training.

Circuit-training programs can consist of a series of strength-training exercises that an individual performs, one after the other, with minimal rest. Below are examples of stabilization, strength, and power circuit routines:

Stabilization	Strength	Power
1. Ball dumbbell chest press	1. Dumbbell chest press	1. MB chest pass
2. Ball dumbbell row	2. Machine cable row	2. MB soccer throw
3. Single-leg scaption	3. Seated dumbbell overhead press	3. MB scoop toss
4. Single-leg dumbbell curl	4. Standing barbell curl	4. Squat jump
5. Ball dumbbell triceps extension	5. Machine triceps pushdown	5. Rest
6. Step-up to balance	6. Multiplanar lunges	
7. Rest	7. Rest	

Several research studies have compared the effects of circuit weight training with traditional endurance forms of exercise (such as treadmills, cross-country skiing, jogging, and bicycling), in relation to energy expenditure, strength, and improving physical fitness and found the following results (25–29):

- Circuit training was just as beneficial as traditional forms of cardiorespiratory exercise for improving or contributing to improved fitness levels (25,28,29).
- Circuit training resulted in higher postexercise metabolic rates as well as strength levels (25–27).

It is possible to incorporate traditional exercise training components such as flexibility and cardiorespiratory fitness training into circuit-training routines.

Beginning Client (Stabilization Level)
5–10 minutes	Flexibility (self-myofascial release and static stretching)
5–10 minutes	Stage I cardiorespiratory training
15–20 minutes	Circuit weight training
5–10 minutes	Stage I cardiorespiratory training
5–10 minutes	Flexibility (self-myofascial release and static stretching)

Intermediate Client (Strength Level)
5–10 minutes	Warm-up: flexibility (self-myofascial release and active-isolated stretching)
5–10 minutes	Stage II cardiorespiratory training
15–20 minutes	Circuit weight training
5–10 minutes	Stage II cardiorespiratory training
5–10 minutes	Cool-down: flexibility (self-myofascial release and static stretching)

At the strength level, the warm-up and cool-down may be performed separately by the client, once they have received proper instructions from the fitness professional. This will allow for more time to be spent on the cardiorespiratory and circuit-training components.

Advanced Client (Power Level)

5–10 minutes	Warm-up: flexibility (self-myofascial release and dynamic stretching)
5–10 minutes	Stage III cardiorespiratory training
15–20 minutes	Circuit weight training
5–10 minutes	Stage III cardiorespiratory training
5–10 minutes	Flexibility (self-myofascial release and static stretching)

Similar to the strength level, the warm-up and cool-down may be performed separately by the client as long as he or she has received proper instructions from the fitness professional.

Postural Considerations in Cardiorespiratory Training

As any form of cardiorespiratory training involves movement, it must follow the same kinetic chain technique parameters as flexibility and resistance training exercises. Selecting the appropriate form of cardiorespiratory training is also important for the beginner and should be approached as follows:

Clients Who Possess a Rounded Shoulder and/or Forward Head Posture (Upper Crossed Syndrome)

The fitness professional must watch closely for the following kinetic chain deviations:

- During use of stationary bicycles, treadmills, and elliptical trainers, watch closely for rounding of shoulders forward and a protruding head.
- On steppers and treadmills, watch for the grasping of the handles (with an oversupinated or overpronated hand position), which will cause elevated and protracted shoulders and a forward head. If possible, this equipment should be used without the assistance of the hands to increase the stabilization component, elevating the caloric expenditure and balance requirements.
- In settings in which a television is present, watch for excessive cervical extension (looking upward) or rotation of the head to view the television.

Clients Who Possess an Anteriorly Rotated Pelvis and Arched Lower Back (Lower Crossed Syndrome)

The fitness professional must watch closely for the following kinetic chain deviations:

- Initial use of bicycles or steppers may not be warranted, as the hips are placed in a constant state of flexion, adding to a shortened hip flexor complex. If they are used, emphasize corrective flexibility techniques for the hip flexors before and after use.

◆ Treadmill speed should be kept to a controllable pace to avoid overstriding. The hips may not be able to properly extend and may cause the low back to overextend (arch), placing increased stress on the low back. Corrective flexibility for the hip flexors should be emphasized before and after use.

Clients Whose Feet Turn Out and/or Knees Move In (Pronation Distortion Syndrome)

The fitness professional must watch closely for the following kinetic chain deviations:

◆ Use of the all cardio equipment that involves the lower extremities will require proper flexibility of the ankle joint. Emphasize foam rolling and static stretching for the calves, adductors, biceps femoris (short head), iliotibial (IT) band, and tensor fascia latae (TFL).

◆ Using the treadmill and steppers that require climbing (or aerobics classes) may initially be too extreme for constant repetition, especially if clients are allowed to hold on to the rails and speed up the pace. If these modalities are used, emphasize the flexibility exercises mentioned above and keep the pace at a controllable speed.

SUMMARY

Different cardiorespiratory training programs place different demands on the cardiorespiratory and muscular systems and ultimately affect a client's adaptations and goals. Stage training is a three-stage programming system that uses different heart rate training zones. Zone one consists of a heart rate of approximately 65 to 75% of predicted HR_{max} and is intended for beginners and used as a recovery zone for more advanced clients. Zone two consists of a heart rate of approximately 76 to 85% of predicted HR_{max}, and is intended for individuals who have progressed to the strength level of the OPT model. Zone three is at 86 to 95% of age-predicted HR_{max}, and is intended for short bouts for individuals who have progressed to the power level of the OPT model. These zones can be translated into three stages, which dictate in which zone and for what length of time cardiorespiratory activity should be performed.

Circuit training programs consist of a series of resistance training exercises that an individual performs, one after the other, with minimal rest. Thus, they allow for comparable fitness results in shorter periods of time. It is also a good way to accomplish cardiorespiratory work during weight training.

Because movement is involved, it is vital to monitor all kinetic chain checkpoints with clients who are performing cardiorespiratory activity. For clients who exhibit the upper crossed syndrome, watch for elevated or protracted shoulders and a forward head, particularly on cardio machinery. Individuals with a lower crossed syndrome may hyperextend their low back and minimize hip extension. It may be best to avoid bicycles and steppers for these clients and emphasize hip flexor stretches. Clients who possess the pronation distortion syndrome may need to temporarily limit the use of cardio machinery and stress foam rolling and static stretching techniques for the lower extremities.

Filling in the Template

The information in this chapter allows step 1 of the OPT template to be completed **Figure 8.8**. Here, enter the desired form of cardio that will be used for the warm-up. If a circuit weight training protocol will be used for the workout, the client should still perform some form of cardiorespiratory warm-up after self-myofascial release and static stretching.

FIGURE 8.8

OPT template.

Professional's Name: Brian Sutton

NASM NATIONAL ACADEMY OF SPORTS MEDICINE

CLIENT'S NAME: JOHN SMITH **DATE: 5/01/13**

GOAL: FAT LOSS **PHASE: 1 STABILIZATION ENDURANCE**

WARM-UP

Exercise:	Sets	Duration	Coaching Tip
SMR: Calves, IT Band, Adductors	1	30 s.	Hold each tender area for 30 sec
Static Stretch: Calves, Hip Flexors, Adductors	1	30 s.	Hold each stretch for 30 sec
Treadmill	1	5–10 min	Brisk walk to slow jog

CORE / BALANCE / PLYOMETRIC

Exercise:	Sets	Reps	Tempo	Rest	Coaching Tip

SPEED, AGILITY, QUICKNESS

Exercise:	Sets	Reps	Rest	Coaching Tip

RESISTANCE

Exercise:	Sets	Reps	Tempo	Rest	Coaching Tip

COOL-DOWN

Exercise:	Sets	Duration	Coaching Tip

Coaching Tips:

National Academy of Sports Medicine

REFERENCES

1. Lee DC, Sui X, Ortega FB, et al. Comparisons of leisure-time physical activity and cardiorespiratory fitness as predictors of all-cause mortality in men and women. *Br J Sports Med*. 2010 Apr 23. [Epub ahead of print].

2. Wei M, Kampert JB, Barlow CE, et al. Relationship between low cardiorespiratory fitness and mortality in normal-weight, overweight, and obese men. *JAMA*. 1999;282(16):1547-1553.

3. Blair SN, Kohl HW, Paffenbarger RS Jr, Clark DG, Cooper KH, Gibbons LW. Physical fitness and all-cause mortality: a prospective study of healthy men and women. *JAMA*. 1989;262:2395-2401.

4. Alter MJ. *Science of Flexibility*. 2nd ed. Champaign, IL: Human Kinetics; 1996.

5. Kovaleski JE, Gurchiek LG, Spriggs DH. Musculoskeletal injuries: risks, prevention and care. In: American College of Sports Medicine, ed. *ACSM's Resource Manual for Guidelines for Exercise Testing and Prescription*. 3rd ed. Baltimore: Williams & Wilkins; 1998. 480-487.

6. Brooks GA, Fahey TD, White TP. *Exercise Physiology: Human Bioenergetics and Its Application*. 2nd ed. Mountain View, CA: Mayfield Publishing Company; 1996.

7. Karvonen J. Importance of warm-up and cool-down on exercise performance. *Med Sports Sci*. 1992;35:182-214.

8. Pate RR, Pratt MM, Blair SN, et al. Physical activity and public health: a recommendation from the Centers for Disease Control and Prevention and the American College of Sports Medicine. *JAMA*. 1995;273:402-407.

9. Lambert EV, Bohlmann I, Cowling K. Physical activity for health: understanding the epidemiological evidence for risk benefits. *Int Sport Med J*. 2001;1(5):1-15.

10. Blair SN, Wei M. Sedentary habits, health, and function in older women and men. *Am J Health Promot*. 2000;15(1):1-8.

11. Blair SN, Kohl HW, Barlow CE, Paffenbarger RS Jr, Gibbons LW, Macera CA. Changes in physical fitness and all-cause mortality. A prospective study of healthy and unhealthy men. *JAMA*. 1995;273(14):1093-1098.

12. Blair SN. Physical inactivity and cardiovascular disease risk in women. *Med Sci Sports Exerc*. 1996;28(1):9-10.

13. Smolander J, Blair SN, Kohl HW 3rd. Work ability, physical activity, and cardiorespiratory fitness: 2-year results from Project Active. *J Occup Environ Med*. 2000;42(9):906-910.

14. American College of Sports Medicine. *ACSM's Guidelines for Exercise Testing and Prescription*. 5th ed. Philadelphia: Williams & Wilkins; 1995.

15. Wei M, Schwertner HA, Blair SN. The association between physical activity, physical fitness, and type 2 diabetes mellitus. *Compr Ther*. 2000;26(3):176-182.

16. Andreoli A, Monteleone M, Van Loan M, Promenzio L, Tarantino U, De Lorenzo A. Effects of different sports on bone density and muscle mass in highly trained athletes. *Med Sci Sports Exerc*. 2001;33(4):507-511.

17. Carter R 3rd, Watenpaugh DE, Wasmund WL, Wasmund SL, Smith ML. Muscle pump and central command during recovery from exercise in humans. *J Appl Physiol*. 1999;87(4):1463-1469.

18. Raine NM, Cable NT, George KP, Campbell IG. The influence of recovery posture on post-exercise hypotension in normotensive men. *Med Sci Sports Exerc*. 2001;33(3):404-412.

19. American College of Sports Medicine. *ACSM's Guidelines for Exercise Testing and Prescription*. 8th ed. Philadelphia: Wolters Kluwer Williams & Wilkins; 2010.

20. US Department of Health and Human Services (USDHHS). Physical Activity Guidelines Advisory Committee Report, 2008. Washington, DC: USDHHS; 2008. Available at: http://www.health.gov/paguidelines.

21. Kolata G. 'Maximum' heart rate theory challenged. New York, NY: *New York Times;* April 24, 2001.

22. Visich PS. Graded exercise testing. In: Ehrman JK, Gordon PM, Visich PS, Keteyan SJ, eds. *Clinical Exercise Physiology*. Champaign, IL: Human Kinetics; 2003:79-101.

23. Persinger R, Foster C, Gibson M, Fater DC, Porcari JP. Consistency of the talk test for exercise prescription. *Med Sci Sports Exerc*. 2004;36(9):1632-1636.

24. Foster C, Porcari JP, Anderson J, et al. The talk test as a marker of exercise training intensity. *J Cardiopulm Rehabil Prev*. 2008;28(1):24-30.

25. Kaikkonen H, Yrlama M, Siljander E, Byman P, Laukkanen R. The effect of heart rate controlled low resistance circuit weight training and endurance training on maximal aerobic power in sedentary adults. *Scand J Med Sci Sports*. 2000;10(4):211-215.

26. Jurimae T, Jurimae J, Pihl E. Circulatory response to single circuit weight and walking training sessions of similar energy cost in middle-aged overweight females. *Clin Physiol*. 2000;20(2):143-149.

27. Burleson MA, O'Bryant HS, Stone MH, Collins MA, Triplett-McBride T. Effect of weight training exercise and treadmill exercise on post-exercise oxygen consumption. *Med Sci Sports Exerc*. 1998;30(4):518-522.

28. Gillette CA, Bullough RC, Melby CL. Postexercise energy expenditure in response to acute aerobic or resistive exercise. *Int J Sport Nutr*. 1994;4(4):347-360.

29. Weltman A, Seip RL, Snead D, et al. Exercise training at and above the lactate threshold in previously untrained women. *Int J Sports Med*. 1992;13:257-263.

Core Training Concepts

OBJECTIVES

After studying this chapter, you will be able to:

✔ Understand the importance of the core musculature.

✔ Differentiate between the stabilization system and the movement system.

✔ Discuss the importance of core training.

✔ Design a core training program for clients at any level of training.

✔ Perform, describe, and instruct various core training exercises.

Introduction to Core Training

Core training has become a popular fitness trend in recent years and a common method of training used by personal trainers. The objective of core training is to uniformly strengthen the deep and superficial muscles that stabilize, align, and move the trunk of the body, especially the abdominals and muscles of the back. Historically, physical therapists prescribed core exercises for patients with low-back problems, and more recently core training has become popular among athletes to help improve sports performance. Core training is now commonly incorporated into exercise programs for clients at health clubs to help achieve goals ranging from a flatter midsection to a stronger lower back. A weak core is a fundamental problem inherent to inefficient movement that may lead to predictable patterns of injury (1–6). A properly designed core training program, however, helps an individual gain neuromuscular control, stability, muscular endurance, strength, and power of the core.

This chapter discusses the importance of core training and how to design and incorporate a core component into a client's training program. Successive chapters discuss balance training and plyometric (reactive) training and how these additional training methods can be incorporated into a training program that will enhance overall functional efficiency.

Core Musculature

Personal trainers must have a basic understanding of functional anatomy to understand the principles of core training. The **core** is defined by the structures that make up the lumbo-pelvic-hip complex (LPHC), including the lumbar spine, the pelvic girdle, abdomen, and the hip joint (7–9). The core is where the body's center of gravity (COG) is located and where all movement originates (10–13). A strong and efficient core is necessary for maintaining proper muscle balance throughout the entire human movement system (kinetic chain) **Figure 9.1**.

Optimal lengths (or length-tension relationships), recruitment patterns (or force-couple relationships), and joint motions (or arthrokinematics) in the muscles of the LPHC establish neuromuscular efficiency throughout the entire human movement system. These factors allow for efficient acceleration, deceleration, and stabilization during dynamic movements, as well as the prevention of possible injuries **Figure 9.2** (14,15).

The core musculature has been divided into the local stabilization system, global stabilization system, and the movement system. To maintain core stability, neuromuscular control of the local and global stabilization systems and the movement system is required, ensuring sequential coordinated activation of all systems at the right time with the right amount of force.

> **Core** The structures that make up the lumbo-pelvic-hip complex (LPHC), including the lumbar spine, the pelvic girdle, abdomen, and the hip joint.

Local Stabilization System

The local core stabilizers are muscles that attach directly to the vertebrae. These muscles consist primarily of type I (slow twitch) muscle fibers with a high density of muscle spindles **Table 9.1**. Core stabilizing muscles are primarily responsible for intervertebral and intersegmental stability and work to limit excessive compressive, shear, and rotational forces between spinal segments. Another way to view the function of core stabilizing muscles is that they provide support from vertebra to vertebra. These muscles also aid in proprioception and postural control because of their high density of muscle spindles (16). The primary muscles that make up the local stabilization system include the transverse abdominis, internal obliques, multifidus, pelvic floor musculature, and diaphragm. These muscles contribute to segmental spinal stability by increasing intra-abdominal pressure (pressure within the abdominal cavity) and generating tension in the thoracolumbar fascia (connective tissue of the low back), thus increasing spinal stiffness for improved intersegmental neuromuscular control (17–20).

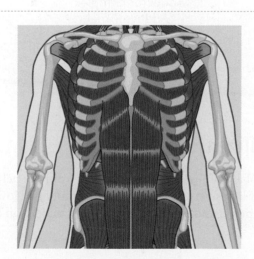

Core musculature.

© ilolab/ShutterStock, Inc.

FIGURE 9.2

Human movement efficiency.

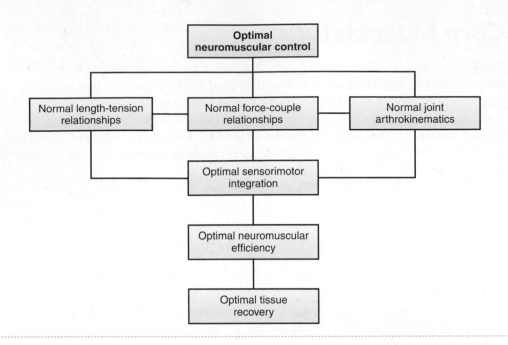

TABLE 9.1 **Muscles of the Core**

© ilolab/ShutterStock, Inc.

Local Stabilization System	Global Stabilization System	Movement System
Transversus abdominis	Quadratus lumborum	Latissimus dorsi
Internal oblique	Psoas major	Hip flexors
Lumbar multifidus	External oblique	Hamstring complex
Pelvic floor muscles	Portions of internal oblique	Quadriceps
Diaphragm	Rectus abdominis	
	Gluteus medius	
	Adductor complex • Adductor magnus • Adductor longus • Adductor brevis • Gracilis • Pectineus	

Global Stabilization System

The muscles of the global stabilization system attach from the pelvis to the spine. These muscles act to transfer loads between the upper extremity and lower extremity, provide stability between the pelvis and spine, and provide stabilization and eccentric control of the core during functional movements (Table 9.1). The primary muscles that make up the global stabilization system include the quadratus lumborum, psoas major, external obliques, portions of the internal oblique, rectus abdominis, gluteus medius, and adductor complex (21).

Movement System

The movement system includes muscles that attach the spine and/or pelvis to the extremities. These muscles are primarily responsible for concentric force production and eccentric deceleration during dynamic activities (Table 9.1). The primary muscles that make up the movement system include the latissimus dorsi, hip flexors, hamstring complex, and quadriceps (22).

Collectively all of the muscles within each system provide dynamic stabilization and neuromuscular control of the entire core (LPHC). These muscles produce force (concentric contractions), reduce force (eccentric actions), and provide dynamic stabilization in all planes of movement during functional activities. In isolation, these muscles do not effectively achieve stabilization of the LPHC; rather it is through their synergistic interdependent functioning that they enhance stability and neuromuscular control.

To better understand how these muscles work to stabilize the LPHC, it helps to view the systems from the inside out (local stabilization system → global stabilization system → movement system). In other words, training the movement system muscles before training the muscles of the global and local stabilization systems would not make sense from both a structural and biomechanical standpoint. Doing so would be analogous to building a house without a foundation. The foundation must be developed first to provide a stable platform for the remaining components of the house to be built on. One must be stable first to move efficiently.

Importance of Properly Training the Stabilization Systems

Some active individuals have developed strength, power, and muscular endurance in the movement system, which enables them to perform functional activities. Few people, however, have properly developed the local stabilization muscles required for intervertebral stabilization (1,23–25). The body's core stabilization system has to be operating with maximal efficiency to effectively use the strength, power, and endurance that has been developed in the prime movers. If the movement system musculature of the core is strong and the local stabilization system is weak, the kinetic chain senses imbalance and forces are not transferred or used properly. This leads to compensation, synergistic dominance, and inefficient movements (1,23–25). Examples include performing a lunge, squat, or overhead press with excessive spinal extension **Figure 9.3**.

A weak core is a fundamental problem that causes inefficient movement and can lead to predictable patterns of injury (1,23–25). This results in lack of stabilization and unwanted motion of the individual vertebrae, thus increasing forces throughout the LPHC that may result in low-back pain (LBP) and injury (26).

FIGURE 9.3

Inefficient core.

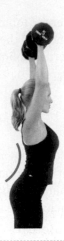

SUMMARY

The core is defined by the structures that make up the LPHC, including the lumbar spine, the pelvic girdle, abdomen, and the hip joint. The core is the origin of all movement and where the center of gravity for the body is located. If the core is unstable during movement, it does not allow optimal stabilization, force reduction, force production, and transference to occur throughout the kinetic chain.

An efficient core is necessary for maintaining proper muscle balance throughout the entire human movement system. Optimal lengths (length-tension relationships), recruitment patterns (force-couple relationships), and joint motions (arthrokinematics) in the muscles of the LPHC establish neuromuscular efficiency throughout the entire human movement system, which allows for efficient acceleration, deceleration, and stabilization during dynamic movements, as well as the prevention of possible injuries.

The core musculature is divided into the local stabilization system, the global stabilization system, and the movement system. The local core stabilizers are muscles that attach directly to the vertebrae. These muscles help provide support from vertebra to vertebra. The global stabilizers are muscles that attach from the pelvis to the spine. These muscles act to transfer loads between the upper extremities and lower extremities and provide stability between the pelvis and spine. The movement system includes muscles that attach the spine and/or pelvis to the extremities. These muscles are primarily responsible for concentric force production and eccentric deceleration during dynamic activities. Collectively, these systems work from the inside out (local stabilization system → global stabilization system → movement system). If the core's movement system musculature is strong and the stabilization systems are weak, the human movement system senses imbalance and forces are not transferred or used properly. This all may result in compensation, synergistic dominance, and inefficient movements.

Scientific Rationale for Core Stabilization Training

Researchers have found that individuals with chronic LBP (~80% of U.S. adults) have decreased activation of certain muscles or muscle groups, including transverse abdominis, internal obliques, pelvic floor muscles, multifidus, diaphragm, and deep erector spinae (1,24,25,27–32). Individuals with chronic LBP also tend to have weaker back extensor muscles (33) and decreased muscular endurance (34,35). Trunk muscle weakness by itself is an independent risk factor for developing LBP (36).

Numerous studies also support the role of core training in the prevention and rehabilitation of LBP. Core stabilization exercises restore the size, activation, and endurance of the multifidus (deep spine muscle) in individuals with LBP (37). In addition, exercise programs that include specific core stabilization training tend to be more effective than manual therapy alone, traditional medical management alone, or other common exercise programs reported to reduce pain and improve function in those with acute and chronic LBP (3,37,38). Clients and athletes with lower extremity pain (5), long-standing adductor (inner thigh) pain (39), hamstring strain (40), iliotibial band syndrome (runner's knee) (41), and LBP (5) have a decreased chance of injury, less recurrence of injury, and improved performance measures after undergoing an active rehabilitation program aimed at improving strength and neuromuscular control of the core (LPHC) muscles.

In addition, a proper application of specific core training programs can reduce pain and help improve function and performance. Specific instructions on the neuromechanical activation of the local stabilization system (**drawing in**) (7,42) and the global movement system (**bracing**) (16) have demonstrated preferential activation of these specifics muscles during the core training continuum. The drawing-in maneuver and bracing will be discussed later in the next section.

Furthermore, traditional low-back hyperextension exercises without proper lumbo-pelvic-hip stabilization have been shown to increase pressure on the discs to

Drawing-in maneuver A maneuver used to recruit the local core stabilizers by drawing the navel in toward the spine.

Bracing Occurs when you have contracted both the abdominal, lower back, and buttock muscles at the same time.

STRETCH Your Knowledge

Low-Back Pain and an Inefficient Core

- Hungerford et al. (1), in a cross-sectional study with 14 men with a clinical diagnosis of back pain, found delayed onset of the transverse abdominis, internal obliques, multifidus, and gluteus maximus during hip flexion on the support leg, suggesting an alteration in the strategy for lumbo-pelvic-hip stability.
- Ebenbichler et al. (2) found that single-leg stance balance in individuals with LBP is less efficient and effective than healthy controls.
- Hodges and Richardson (3) reported that slow speed of contraction of the transverse abdominis during arm and leg movements was well correlated with LBP.
- Hides et al. (4) demonstrated that recovery from acute back pain did not automatically result in restoration of the normal girth of the multifidus.
- Hides et al. (5) demonstrated multifidus atrophy in patients with LBP.

REFERENCES

1. Hungerford B, Gilleard W, Hodges P. Evidence of altered lumbopelvic muscle recruitment in the presence of sacroiliac joint pain. *Spine.* 2003;28(14):1593-1600.
2. Ebenbichler GR, Oddsson LI, Kollmitzer J, Erim Z. Sensory-motor control of the lower back: implications for rehabilitation. *Med Sci Sports Exerc.* 2001;33:1889-1898.
3. Hodges PW, Richardson CA. Delayed postural contraction of transversus abdominis in low back pain associated with movement of the lower limb. *J Spinal Disord.* 1998;11(1):46-56.
4. Hides JA, Richardson CA, Jull GA. Multifidus muscle recovery is not automatic after resolution of acute, first-episode low back pain. *Spine.* 1996;21(23):2763-2769.
5. Hides JA, Stokes MJ, Saide M, Jull GA, Cooper DH. Evidence of lumbar multifidus wasting ipsilateral to symptoms in subjects with acute/subacute low back pain. *Spine.* 1994;19:165-177.

dangerous levels. These unsupported exercises can cause damage to the ligaments supporting the vertebrae, which may lead to a narrowing of openings in the vertebrae that spinal nerves pass through (43–45). Therefore, it is crucial for personal trainers to incorporate a systematic, progressive approach when training the core, ensuring the muscles that stabilize the spine (local stabilization systems) are strengthened before the musculature that moves the spine and extremities (movement system).

Did You Know?

Electromyography (EMG) is a procedure that measures the electrical conducting function of nerves in muscles. An EMG test is able to identify differences in muscle or muscle group activation when performing different movements or exercises.

Drawing-In Maneuver

Research has demonstrated that electromyogram (EMG) activity is increased during pelvic stabilization and transverse abdominis activation when an abdominal drawing-in maneuver is initiated before activity (31,46,47).

Research has found that the transverse abdominis, when properly activated, creates tension in the thoracolumbar fascia, contributing to spinal stiffness, and compresses the sacroiliac joint, increasing stability (48,49). These findings have led other researchers to further understand and demonstrate the important role of the transverse abdominis on spinal stability and LBP.

To perform the drawing-in maneuver, pull in the region just below the navel toward the spine and maintain the cervical spine in a neutral position. Maintaining a neutral spine during core training helps to improve posture, muscle balance, and stabilization. If a forward protruding head is noticed during the drawing-in maneuver, the sternocleidomastoid (large neck muscle) is preferentially recruited, which increases the compressive forces in the cervical spine and can lead to pelvic instability and muscle imbalances as a result of the pelvo-ocular reflex. Because of this reflex it is important to maintain the eyes level during movement (50). If the sternocleidomastoid muscle is hyperactive and extends the upper cervical spine, the pelvis rotates anteriorly to realign the eyes. This can lead to muscle imbalances and decreased pelvic stabilization (51).

Bracing

Bracing is referred to as a co-contraction of global muscles, such as the rectus abdominis, external obliques, and quadratus lumborum. Bracing is also commonly referred to as a "bearing down" or tightening of the global muscles by consciously contracting them. Research has shown that muscular endurance of global and local musculature, when contracted together, create the most benefit for those with LBP compared with traditional LBP training methods (51). Bracing focuses on global trunk stability, not on segmental vertebral stability, meaning that the global muscles, given the proper endurance training, will work to stabilize the spine.

However, both strategies (drawing-in maneuver and bracing) can be implemented in a core training program to help retrain motor control of local and global stabilization systems and movement musculature as well as to help retrain the strength and endurance of these muscles (7,51,52). Activation of the local stabilization system (drawing-in)

(7,52) and the global stabilization system (bracing) (51) has been demonstrated to preferentially activate these specific muscles during core training.

Guidelines for Core Training

A comprehensive core training program should be systematic, progressive, functional, and emphasize the entire muscle action spectrum focusing on force production (concentric), force reduction (eccentric), and dynamic stabilization (isometric) Table 9.2.

TABLE 9.2 Core Training Parameters	
Variables	**Exercise Selection**

• Plane of motion
  • Sagittal
  • Frontal
  • Transverse
	• Progressive
	  • Easy to hard
	  • Simple to complex
	  • Known to unknown
	  • Stable to unstable

• Range of motion
  • Full
  • Partial
  • End-range
	• Systematic
	  • Stabilization
	  • Strength
	  • Power

• Type of resistance
  • Cable
  • Tubing
  • Medicine ball
  • Power ball
  • Dumbbells
  • Kettlebells
	• Activity/Goal-specific
	
	• Integrated
	
	• Proprioceptively challenging
	  • Stability ball
	  • BOSU
	  • Reebok Core Board
	  • Half foam roll
	  • Airex pad
	  • Bodyblade

• Body position
  • Supine
  • Prone
  • Side-lying
  • Kneeling
  • Half-kneeling
  • Standing
  • Staggered-stance
  • Single-leg
  • Standing progression on unstable surface
	• Based in current science

• Speed of motion
  • Stabilization
  • Strength
  • Power	

• Duration	
• Frequency	

• Amount of feedback
  • Fitness Professional's cues
  • Kinesthetic awareness	

A core training program should regularly manipulate plane of motion, range of motion, modalities (tubing, stability ball, medicine ball, BOSU ball, Airex pad, etc.), body position, amount of control, speed of execution, amount of feedback, and specific acute training variables (sets, reps, intensity, tempo, frequency) (Table 9.2).

When designing a core training program, the personal trainer should initially create a proprioceptively enriched (controlled yet unstable training environment), selecting the appropriate exercises to elicit a maximal training response. Core exercises performed in an unstable environment (such as with a stability ball) have been demonstrated to increase activation of the local and global stabilization system when compared with traditional trunk exercises (53,54). As also outlined in Table 9.2, the core exercises must be safe and challenging, and stress multiple planes in a multisensory environment derived from fundamental movement skills specific to the activity.

© Sky Studio/ShutterStock, Inc.

Did You Know?

The use of weight belts for apparently healthy adults engaging in a moderately intense exercise program is not recommended. Weight belts may raise an individual's heart rate and systolic blood pressure and often give individuals a false sense of security and the misconception they can lift heavier loads. Instead, personal trainers need to educate their clients as to appropriate exercise technique and proper activation of the core musculature (the body's natural belt).

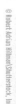

© Robert Adrian Hillman/ShutterStock, Inc.

STRETCH Your Knowledge

Evidence to Support the Use of Core-Stabilization Training

- Cosio-Lima et al. (1) in a randomized controlled trial with 30 subjects demonstrated increased abdominal and back extensor strength and single-leg balance improvements with a 5-week stability ball training program compared with conventional floor exercises.
- Mills and Taunton (2) in a randomized controlled trial with 36 subjects demonstrated that agility and balance were improved after a 10-week specific spinal stabilization training program compared with the control group performing an equivalent volume of traditional, nonspecific abdominal exercises.
- Vera-Garcia et al. (3) in a single-subject design with 8 subjects found that performing abdominal exercises on a labile surface increased activation levels, suggesting increased demand on the motor control system to help stabilize the spine.

(Continued)

- Hahn et al. (4) in a randomized controlled trial with 35 female subjects demonstrated that traditional floor exercises and stability ball exercises significantly increased core strength during a 10-week training period.
- O'Sullivan et al. (5) in a randomized clinical trial demonstrated that pain and function improve initially and at 1- and 3-year follow-up in patients with LBP undergoing specific stabilizing exercises.

REFERENCES

1. Cosio-Lima LM, Reynolds KL, Winter C, et al. Effects of physioball and conventional floor exercises on early phase adaptations in back and abdominal core stability and balance in women. *J Strength Cond Res.* 2003;17(4):721-725.
2. Mills JD, Taunton JE. The effect of spinal stabilization training on spinal mobility, vertical jump, agility and balance. *Med Sci Sports Exerc.* 2003;35(5 Suppl):S323.
3. Vera-Garcia FJ, Grenier SG, McGill SM. Abdominal muscle response during curl-ups on both stable and labile surfaces. *Phys Ther.* 2003;80(6):564-594.
4. Hahn S, Stanforth D, Stanforth PR, Philips A. A 10 week training study comparing resistaball and traditional trunk training. *Med Sci Sports Exerc.* 1998;30(5):199.
5. O'Sullivan PB, Twomey L, Allison GT. Evaluation of specific stabilizing exercises in the treatment of chronic low back pain with radiological diagnosis of spondylosis and spondylolisthesis. *Spine.* 1997;22(24): 2959-2967.

SUMMARY

Clients with chronic LBP activate their core muscles less and have a lower endurance for stabilization. Performing traditional abdominal and low-back exercises without proper spinal and pelvic stabilization may cause abnormal forces throughout the LPHC which may lead to tissue overload and cause damage. However, performing the drawing-in maneuver or bracing can help stabilize the pelvis and spine during core training and other functional movements. In addition, keeping the cervical spine in a neutral position during core training improves posture, muscle balance, and stabilization.

Designing a Core Training Program

The goal of core training is to develop optimal levels of neuromuscular efficiency, stability (intervertebral and lumbopelvic stability—local and global stabilization systems), and functional strength (movement system). Neural adaptations become the focus of the program instead of striving for absolute strength gains. Increasing proprioceptive demand by using a multisensory environment and using multiple modalities (balls, bands, balance equipment) is more important than increasing the external resistance. The quality of movement should be stressed over quantity, and the focus of the program should be on function.

The following is an example of an integrated core training program. The client begins at the highest level at which he or she is able to maintain stability and optimal neuromuscular control (coordinated movement). The client progresses through the program once mastery of the exercises in the previous level has been achieved while demonstrating intervertebral stability and lumbopelvic stability. For example, a client has appropriate intervertebral stability when able to maintain the drawing-in position while performing various exercises. The client has appropriate lumbopelvic stability when able to perform functional movement patterns (squats, lunges, step-ups, single-leg movements, pressing, pushing, etc.) without excessive spinal motion (flexion, extension, lateral flexion, rotation, singly or in combination). It is critical that the core training program is designed to achieve the following functional outcomes. The sequence is critical!

1. Intervertebral stability
2. Lumbopelvic stability
3. Movement efficiency

Levels of Core Training

There are three levels of training within the OPT™ model: stabilization, strength, and power **Figure 9.4**. A proper core training program follows the same systematic progression.

Core-Stabilization Training

In core-stabilization training (Phase 1), exercises involve little motion through the spine and pelvis. These exercises are designed to improve neuromuscular efficiency and intervertebral stability, focusing on drawing-in and then bracing during the exercises (3,55). The client would traditionally spend 4 weeks at this level of core training.
Sample exercises in this level include:

- Marching
- Floor bridge
- Floor prone cobra
- Prone iso-ab

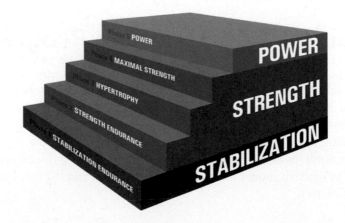

FIGURE 9.4

OPT model.

CORE-STABLIZATION EXERCISES

Marching

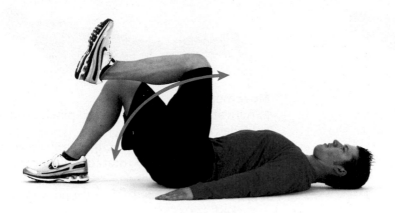

TECHNIQUE

Make sure to keep the abdominals drawn-in throughout the entire movement and the pelvis in a neutral position. Pelvic rotation or abdominal protrusion indicates lack of neuromuscular control of the local core stabilizers.

Preparation
1. Lie supine on floor with knees bent, feet flat, toes pointing straight ahead, and arms by sides.

Movement
2. Lift one foot off the floor only as high as can be controlled. Maintain the drawing-in maneuver.
3. Hold for 1 to 2 seconds.
4. Slowly lower.
5. Repeat on the opposite leg.

Two-Leg Floor Bridge

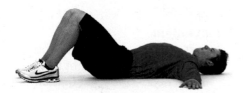 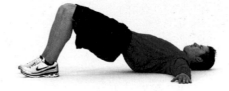

SAFETY

When performing a bridge, do not raise the hips too far up off the floor (hyperextending the low back). This places excessive stress to the lumbar spine. Make sure at the end position, the knees, hips, and shoulders are in alignment and the gluteal muscles are fully contracted.

Preparation
1. Lie supine on the floor with knees bent, feet flat on floor, and toes shoulders-width apart and pointing straight ahead.

Movement
2. Lift pelvis off the floor until the knees, hips, and shoulders are in line.
3. Slowly lower pelvis to the floor.
4. Repeat as instructed.

CORE-STABLIZATION EXERCISES *continued*

Floor Prone Cobra

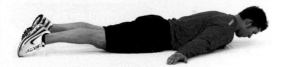 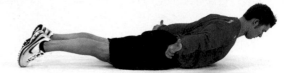

Preparation
1. Lie prone on the floor.

Movement
2. Activate gluteal muscles, and pinch shoulder blades together.
3. Lift chest off the floor with thumbs pointed up and arms externally rotated as illustrated.
4. Hold for 1 to 2 seconds.
5. Slowly return body to the ground, keeping chin tucked.
6. Repeat as instructed.

SAFETY Like the floor bridge, do not come too high off the floor (hyperextending the low back).

Prone Iso-Abs (Plank)

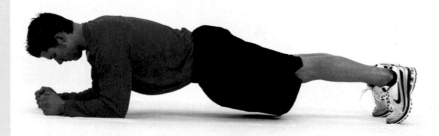

Preparation
1. Lie prone on the floor with feet together and forearms on ground.

Movement
2. Lift entire body off the ground until it forms a straight line from head to toe, resting on forearms and toes.
3. Hold for desired length of time keeping chin tucked and back flat.
4. Repeat as instructed.

TECHNIQUE If this version of the exercise is too difficult for an individual to perform, some regression options include:
• Perform in a standard push-up position.
• Perform in a push-up position with the knees on the floor.
• Perform with the hands on a bench and the feet on the floor.

Core Strength

In core-strength training (Phases 2, 3, and 4), the exercises involve more dynamic eccentric and concentric movements of the spine throughout a full range of motion while clients perform the activation techniques learned in core-stabilization training (drawing-in and bracing). The specificity, speed, and neural demands are also progressed in this level. Clients would traditionally spend 4 weeks at this level of core training. These exercises are designed to improve dynamic stabilization, concentric strength (force production), eccentric strength (force reduction), and neuromuscular efficiency of the entire kinetic chain. Exercises in this level include:

- Ball crunch
- Back extensions
- Reverse crunch
- Cable rotations

CORE-STRENGTH EXERCISES

Ball Crunch

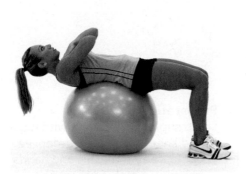 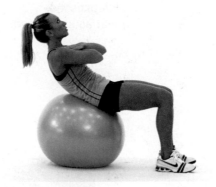

© ilolab/ShutterStock, Inc.

Preparation

1. Lie supine on a stability ball (ball under low back) with knees bent at a 90-degree angle. Place feet flat on floor with toes shoulders-width apart and pointing straight ahead. Allow back to extend over curve of ball. Cross arms across chest or place hands behind ears or head.

Movement

2. Slowly crunch upper body forward, raising shoulder blades off the ball.
3. Slowly lower upper body over the ball, returning to the start position.
4. Repeat as instructed.
5. To progress, perform as a long-lever exercise (arms raised overhead).

CORE-STRENGTH EXERCISES *continued*

© ilolab/ShutterStock, Inc.

Back Extension

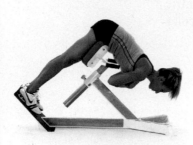 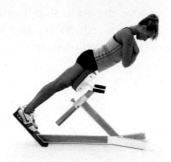

Preparation

1. Lie prone on a back-extension bench with legs straight and toes shoulders-width apart and pointing straight ahead.
2. Place pads on thighs and cross arms over the chest or hands behind ears.

Movement

3. Activate gluteal muscles, tuck chin, and retract shoulder blades.
4. Slowly lower upper body toward the ground to end range.
5. Raise upper body to a neutral position, keeping chin tucked and shoulder blades retracted and depressed.
6. Repeat as instructed.

SAFETY

Make sure that at the end position of the exercise, the ankle, knee, hip, shoulders, and ears are all in alignment. Do not hyperextend the low back.

Reverse Crunch

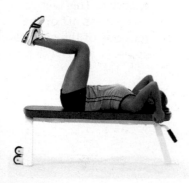 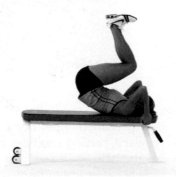

Preparation

1. Lie supine on a bench with hips and knees bent at a 90-degree angle, feet in the air, and hands gripping a stable object for support.

Movement

2. Lift hips off the bench while bringing the knees toward the chest.
3. Slowly lower the hips back to the start position.
4. Repeat as instructed.

TECHNIQUE

Do not swing the legs when performing this exercise. Once you have positioned the lower extremities during the setup, they should not move during the execution of the exercise. Swinging the legs increases momentum, increasing the risk of injury and decreasing the effectiveness of the exercise.

CORE-STRENGTH EXERCISES continued

© ilolab/ShutterStock, Inc.

Cable Rotation

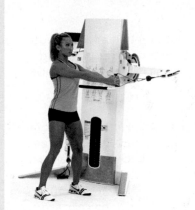 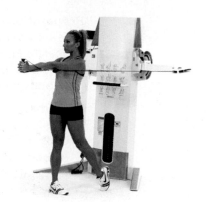

Preparation
1. Stand with feet shoulders-width apart, knees slightly flexed, and toes pointing straight ahead.
2. Hold a cable with both hands directly in front of chest, with arms extended and shoulder blades retracted and depressed.

Movement
3. Rotate body away from the weight stack using abdominals and gluteal muscles. Allow back foot to pivot to achieve triple extension (plantar flexion, knee extension, hip extension).
4. Slowly return to start position.
5. Repeat as instructed.

| TECHNIQUE | To decrease stress to the low back, make sure to pivot the back leg into triple extension: |

- Hip extension
- Knee extension
- Ankle plantarflexion (extension)

This also ensures proper neuromuscular efficiency of the muscles that extend the lower extremities (gluteus maximus, quadriceps, gastrocnemius and soleus).

Core Power

In core-power training (Phase 5), exercises are designed to improve the rate of force production of the core musculature. These forms of exercise prepare an individual to dynamically stabilize and generate force at more functionally applicable speeds. Exercises in this level include:

- Rotation chest pass
- Ball medicine ball (MB) pullover throw
- Front MB oblique throw
- Soccer throw

CORE-POWER EXERCISES

© ilolab/ShutterStock, Inc.

Rotation Chest Pass

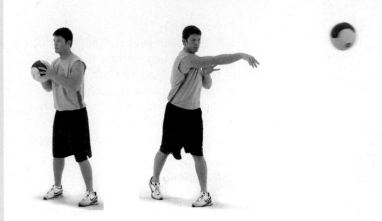

Preparation

1. Stand upright with feet shoulders-width apart and toes pointing straight ahead.
2. Hold a medicine ball (between 5 and 10% of body weight).

Movement

3. Use abdominal muscles and hips to rotate body quickly and explosively 90 degrees. As body turns, pivot back leg and allow it to go into triple extension (hip extension, knee extension, ankle plantarflexion).
4. Throw medicine ball with the rear arm extending and applying force.
5. Catch and repeat as quickly as can be controlled.

SAFETY	It is imperative that individuals demonstrate proper stabilization (core stabilization) and strength (core strength) before performing core-power exercises. Performing these exercises without proper stabilization and strength may lead to movement compensations, muscle imbalances, and eventually injury.

Ball Medicine Ball Pullover Throw

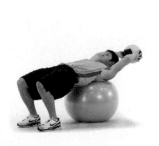 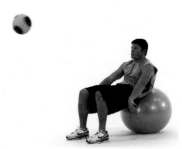

Preparation

1. Lie on a stability ball (ball under low back) with knees bent at a 90-degree angle, feet flat on floor and toes pointing straight ahead.
2. Hold a medicine ball (between 5 and 10% of body weight) overhead with arms extended.

Movement

3. Quickly crunch forward, throwing medicine ball against the wall or to a partner.
4. As the ball releases, allow arms to completely follow through.
5. Catch ball and repeat.

SAFETY	It is important that an individual has proper extensibility of the latissimus dorsi before performing this exercise to decrease stress to the low back and shoulders.

CORE-POWER EXERCISES *continued*

Front Medicine Ball Oblique Throw

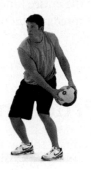 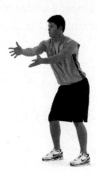

Preparation
1. Stand facing a wall or partner with feet shoulders-width apart, knees slightly bent, and toes pointing straight ahead.
2. Hold a medicine ball (between 5 and 10% of body weight) as illustrated.

Movement
3. Toss the ball against the wall or to a partner with an underhand motion.
4. Use a scooping motion to catch ball.
5. Repeat as quickly as can be controlled.
6. This exercise can be performed continuously to one side or by alternating sides.

SAFETY It is important that with all core-power exercises that you go as fast as you can while maintaining proper exercise technique.

Soccer Throw

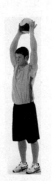 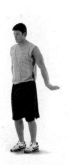

Preparation
1. Stand holding a medicine ball (5 to 10% of body weight) overhead as illustrated.

Movement
2. Quickly throw the medicine ball toward the floor, allowing the arms to follow through.
3. Repeat.

SAFETY It may be easier to perform this exercise using a D-ball (a medicine ball that does not bounce back) or close to a wall for the medicine ball to bounce off of.

SUMMARY

The core musculature helps protect the spine from harmful forces that occur during functional activities. A core-training program is designed to increase stabilization, strength, power, muscle endurance, and neuromuscular control in the LPHC.

Core training programs must be systematic, progressive, activity or goal-specific, integrated, and proprioceptively challenging.

A proper core training program follows the same systematic progression as the OPT model: stabilization, strength, and power. In core-stabilization training (Phase 1), the emphasis is on stabilization of the LPHC. It improves the function of the stabilization system. In core-strength training (Phases 2, 3, and 4), the spine moves dynamically through a full range of motion, with exercises that require greater specificity, speed, and neural demand. These exercises improve neuromuscular efficiency of the entire kinetic chain. Exercises of core-power training (Phase 5) improve the rate of force production in the musculature of the LPHC (movement system).

Implementing a Core Training Program

Implementing a core training program requires that fitness professionals follow the progression of the OPT model (Figure 9.4). For example, if a client is in the stabilization level of training (Phase 1), select core-stabilization exercises. For a different client in the strength level of training (Phases 2, 3, or 4), the fitness professional should select core-strength exercises. For an advanced client in the power level of training (Phase 5), select core-power exercises Table 9.3.

Filling in the Template

To fill in the program template Figure 9.5, go to the section labeled Core/Balance/Plyometric. You will then refer to Table 9.3 for the appropriate type of core exercise (stabilization, strength, or power), the appropriate number of core exercises, and the appropriate acute variables (sets, reps, etc.) specific to the phase of training your client will be working in (Phases 1–5).

TABLE 9.3   Core Training Program Design

© ilolab/ShutterStock, Inc.

Core Systems	OPT Level	Phase(s)	Exercise	Number of Exercises	Sets	Reps	Tempo	Rest
Stabilization	Stabilization	1	Core stabilization	1–4	1–4	12–20	Slow (4/2/1)	0–90 s
Movement	Strength	2, 3, 4	Core strength	0–4[a]	2–3	8–12	Medium	0–60 s
Movement	Power	5	Core power	0–2[b]	2–3	8–12	As fast as can be controlled	0–60 s

[a]For the goal of muscle hypertrophy and maximal strenght, core training may be optional (although recommended).
[b]Because core exercises are typically performed in the dynamic warm-up portion of this program and core-power exercises are included in the resistance training portion of the program, separate core training may not be necessary in this phase of training.

Professional's Name: Brian Sutton

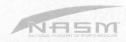

CLIENT'S NAME: JOHN SMITH	DATE: 5/01/13

GOAL: FAT LOSS	PHASE: 1 STABILIZATION ENDURANCE

WARM-UP

Exercise:	Sets	Duration	Coaching Tip
SMR: Calves, IT-Band, Adductors	1	30 s.	Hold each tender area for 30 sec
Static Stretch: Calves, Hip Flexors, Adductors	1	30 s.	Hold each stretch for 30 sec
Treadmill	1	5 – 10 min	Brisk walk to slow jog

CORE / BALANCE / PLYOMETRIC

Exercise:	Sets	Reps	Tempo	Rest	Coaching Tip
Floor Bridge	2	12	Slow	0 s.	
Floor Prone Cobra	2	12	Slow	0 s.	

SPEED, AGILITY, QUICKNESS

Exercise:	Sets	Reps	Rest	Coaching Tip

RESISTANCE

Exercise:	Sets	Reps	Tempo	Rest	Coaching Tip

COOL-DOWN

Exercise:	Sets	Duration	Coaching Tip

Coaching Tips:

National Academy of Sports Medicine

FIGURE 9.5 OPT template.

REFERENCES

1. Hodges PW, Richardson CA. Inefficient muscular stabilization of the lumbar spine associated with low back pain. A motor control evaluation of transversus abdominis. *Spine.* 1996;21: 2640-2650.

2. Nadler SF, Malanga GA, Bartoli LA, Feinberg JH, Prybicien M, Deprince M. Hip muscle imbalance and low back pain in athletes: influence of core strengthening. *Med Sci Sports Exerc.* 2002;34:9-16.

3. O;Sullivan PB, Phyty GD, Twomey LT, Allison GT. Evaluation of specific stabilizing exercise in the treatment of chronic low back pain with radiologic diagnosis of spondylolysis or spondylolisthesis. *Spine.* 1997;22:2959-2967.

4. Hewett TE, Paterno MV, Myer GD. Strategies for enhancing proprioception and neuromuscular control of the knee. *Clin Orthop Relat Res.* 2002 Sep;(402):76-94.

5. Leetun DT, Ireland ML, Willson JD, Ballantyne BT, Davis IM. Core stability measures as risk factors for lower extremity injury in athletes. *Med Sci Sports Exerc.* 2004;36:926-934.

6. Nadler SF, Moley P, Malanga GA, Rubbani M, Prybicien M, Feinberg JH. Functional deficits in athletes with a history of low back pain: a pilot study. *Arch Phys Med Rehabil.* 2002;83: 1753-1758.

7. Arokoski JP, Valta T, Airaksinen O, Kankaanpaa M. Back and abdominal muscle function during stabilization exercises. *Arch Phys Med Rehabil.* 2001;82:1089-1098.

8. Bergmark A. Stability of the lumbar spine. A study in mechanical engineering. *Acta Orthop Scand Suppl.* 1989;230:1-54.

9. Kibler WB, Sciascia A, Dome D. Evaluation of apparent and absolute supraspinatus strength in patients with shoulder injury using the scapular retraction test. *Am J Sports Med.* 2006;34:1643-1647.

10. Gracovetsky S, Farfan H. The optimum spine. *Spine.* 1986; 11:543-573.

11. Gracovetsky S, Farfan H, Heuller C. The abdominal mechanism. *Spine.* 1985;10:317-324.

12. Panjabi MM. The stabilizing system of the spine. Part I: function, dysfunction, adaptation, and enhancement. *J Spinal Disord.* 1992;5:383-389.

13. Panjabi MM, Tech D, White AA. Basic biomechanics of the spine. *Neurosurgery.* 1980;7:76-93.

14. Barr KP, Griggs M, Cadby T. Lumbar stabilization: core concepts and current literature, Part 1. *Am J Phys Med Rehabil.* 2005;84:473-480.

15. Sahrmann S. *Diagnosis and Treatment of Movement Impairment Syndromes.* St. Louis: Mosby; 2002.

16. McGill SM. Low back stability: from formal description to issues for performance and rehabilitation. *Exerc Sport Sci Rev.* 2001;29:26-31.

17. Richardson CA, Jull GA, Hodges PW, Hides JA. *Therapeutic Exercise for Spinal Segment Stabilization in Low Back Pain: Scientific Basis and Clinical Approach.* London: Churchill Livingstone; 1999.

18. Crisco JJ 3rd, Panjabi MM. The intersegmental and multisegmental muscles of the lumbar spine. A biomechanical model comparing lateral stabilizing potential. *Spine.* 1991;16:793-799.

19. Hodges PW. Is there a role for transversus abdominis in lumbo-pelvic stability? *Man Ther.* 1999;4:74-86.

20. O'Sullivan PB, Beales DJ, Beetham JA, et al. Altered motor control strategies in subjects with sacroiliac joint pain during the active straight-leg-raise test. *Spine.* 2002;27:E1-8.

21. Comerford MJ, Mottram SL. Movement and stability dysfunction—contemporary developments. *Man Ther.* 2001;6:15-26.

22. Newmann D. *Kinesiology of the Musculoskeletal System: Foundations for Physical Rehabilitation.* St. Louis: Mosby; 2002.

23. Ferreira PH, Ferreira ML, Hodges PW. Changes in recruitment of the abdominal muscles in people with low back pain: ultrasound measurement of muscle activity. *Spine.* 2004;29:2560-2566.

24. Hodges PW, Richardson CA. Neuromotor dysfunction of the trunk musculature in low back pain patients. In: *Proceedings of the International Congress of the World Confederation of Physical Therapists.* Washington, DC; 1995.

25. Hodges PW, Richardson CA. Contraction of the abdominal muscles associated with movement of the lower limb. *Phys Ther.* 1997;77:132-134.

26. Janda V. Muscle weakness and inhibition (pseudoparesis) in back pain syndromes. In: Grieve GP, ed. *Modern Manual Therapy of the Vertebral Column.* New York: Churchill Livingstone, 1986:197-201.

27. Hodges PW, Richardson CA, Jull G. Evaluation of the relationship between laboratory and clinical tests of transverse abdominus function. *Physiother Res Int.* 1996;1:30-40.

28. O'Sullivan PE, Twomey L, Allison G, Sinclair J, Miller K, Knox J. Altered patterns of abdominal muscle activation in patients with chronic low back pain. *Aus J Physiother.* 1997;43(2):91-98.

29. Richardson CA, Jull G. Muscle control-pain control. What exercises would you prescribe? *Man Med.* 1995;1:2-10.

30. O'Sullivan PB, Twomey L, Allison GT. Altered abdominal muscle recruitment in patients with chronic back pain following a specific exercise intervention. *J Orthop Sports Phys Ther.* 1998;27:114-124.

31. Richardson CA, Snijders CJ, Hides JA, Damen L, Pas MS, Storm J. The relation between the transverse abdominis muscle, sacroiliac joint mechanics and low back pain. *Spine.* 2002;27:399-405.

32. Hodges P, Richardson C, Jull G. Evaluation of the relationship between laboratory and clinical tests of transversus abdominis function. *Physiother Res Int.* 1996;1:30-40.

33. Iwai K, Nakazato K, Irie K, Fujimoto H, Nakajima H. Trunk muscle strength and disability level of low back pain in collegiate wrestlers. *Med Sci Sports Exerc.* 2004;36:1296-1300.

34. McGill SM. *Low Back Stability: Myths and Realities in Low Back Disorders: Evidence Based Prevention and Rehabilitation.* Champaign, IL: Human Kinetics; 2002.

35. Jørgensen K, Nicolaisen T. Trunk extensor endurance: determination and relation to low-back trouble. *Ergonomics.* 1987;30:259-267.

36. Lee J, Hoshino Y, Nakamura K, Kariya Y, Saita K, Ito K. Trunk muscle weakness as a risk factor for low back pain. A 5-year prospective study. *Spine.* 1999;24:54-57.

37. Hides JA, Jull GA, Richardson CA. Long-term effects of specific stabilizing exercises for first-episode low back pain. *Spine.* 2001;26:E243-248.

38. Yílmaz F, Yílmaz A, Merdol F, Parlar D, Sahin F, Kuran B. Efficacy of dynamic lumbar stabilization exercise in lumbar microdiscectomy. *J Rehabil Med.* 2003;35:163-167.

39. Hölmich P, Uhrskou P, Ulnits L, et al. Effectiveness of active physical training as treatment for long-standing adductor-related groin pain in athletes: randomised trial. *Lancet.* 1999;353: 439-443.

40. Sherry MA, Best TM. A comparison of 2 rehabilitation programs in the treatment of acute hamstring strains. *J Orthop Sports Phys Ther.* 2004;34:116-125.

41. Fredericson M, Cookingham CL, Chaudhari AM, Dowdell BC, Oestreicher N, Sahrmann SA. Hip abductor weakness in distance runners with iliotibial band syndrome. *Clin J Sport Med.* 2000;10:169-175.

42. Karst GM, Willett GM. Effects of specific exercise instructions on abdominal muscle activity during trunk curl exercises. *J Orthop Sports Phys Ther.* 2004;34:4-12.

43. Beim G, Giraldo JL, Pincivero DM, Borror MJ, Fu FH. Abdominal strengthening exercises: a comparative EMG study. *J Sports Rehabil.* 1997;6:11-20.

44. Ashmen KJ, Swanik CB, Lephart SM. Strength and flexibility characteristics of athletes with chronic low back pain. *J Sports Rehabil.* 1996;5:275-286.

45. Norris CM. Abdominal muscle training in sports. *Br J Sports Med.* 1993;7(1):19-27.

46. Cresswell AG, Grundstrom H, Thorstensson A. Observations on intra-abdominal pressure and patterns of abdominal intra muscular activity in man. *Acta Physiol Scand.* 1992;144: 409-418.

47. Hides, J, Wilson S, Stanton W, et al. An MRI investigation into the function of the transversus abdominis muscle during "drawing-in" of the abdominal wall. *Spine.* 2006;31(6):175-178.

48. Hodges PW, Richardson CA. Feedforward contraction of transversus abdominis is not influenced by the direction of arm movement. *Exper Brain Res.* 1997;114:362-370.

49. Hodges PW, Richardson CA. Relationship between limb movement speed and associated contraction of the trunk muscles. *Ergonomics.* 1997;40:1220-1230.

50. Lewit K. Muscular and articular factors in movement restriction. *Man Med.* 1985;1:83-85.

51. McGill SM. Low back stability: from formal description to issues for performance and rehabilitation. *Exerc Sport Sci Rev.* 2001;29(1):26-31.

52. Kibler WB, Chandler TJ, Livingston BP, Roetert EP. Shoulder range of motion in elite tennis players. Effect of age and years of tournament play. *Am J Sports Med.* 1996;24(3):279-285.

53. Carter JM, Beam WC, McMahan SG, Barr ML, Brown LE. The effects of stability ball training on spinal stability in sedentary individuals. *J Strength Cond Res.* 2006;20:429-435.

54. Behm D, Leonard A, Young W, Bonsey W, MacKinnon S. Trunk muscle electromyographic activity with unstable and unilateral exercises. *J Strength Cond Res.* 2005;19:193-201.

55. Ng JK, Kippers V, Richardson CA, Parnianpour M. Range of motion and lordosis of the lumbar spine: reliability of measurement and normative values. *Spine.* 2001;26:53-60.

Balance Training Concepts

OBJECTIVES

After studying this chapter, you will be able to:

✔ Define balance and describe its role in performance and injury risk.

✔ Discuss the importance of balance training.

✔ Design a progressive balance training program for clients in any level of training.

✔ Understand and incorporate the principles of selected research outcomes when designing a balance training program.

✔ Perform, describe, and instruct various balance training exercises.

Core Concepts of Balance

Balance When the body is in equilibrium and stationary, meaning no linear or angular movement.

Dynamic balance The ability to move and change directions under various conditions without falling.

A key to all functional movements, whether running down a basketball court, exercising on a stability ball, or walking down stairs, is the ability to maintain balance and postural control. The fundamental definition of **balance** is when the body is in equilibrium and stationary, meaning no linear or angular movement. For example, when a gymnast maintains a handstand without falling over he or she is said to be in balance or balancing. **Dynamic balance** is the ability to move and change directions under various conditions (e.g., running on uneven surfaces) without falling. Dynamic balance is strongly influenced by other neuromuscular skills such as speed, endurance, flexibility, and strength. The integrated performance paradigm **Figure 10.1** shows that adequate force reduction and stabilization are required for optimal force production. The ability to reduce force at the right joint, at the right time, and in the right plane of motion requires optimal levels of dynamic balance and neuromuscular efficiency. Poor balance is associated with injury risk (1–3). Thus it is important for personal trainers to understand that gaining and maintaining proper balance is vital for all of their clients.

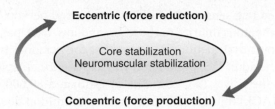

FIGURE 10.1

Integrated performance paradigm.

Balance is dependent on both internal and external factors to maintain the body's center of gravity over its base of support. Balance is often thought of as only a static process, but balance is also a dynamic process involving multiple neurologic pathways. Maintenance of postural equilibrium (or balance) is an integrated process requiring optimal muscular balance (or length-tension relationships and force-couple relationships), joint dynamics (or arthrokinematics), and neuromuscular efficiency using visual, vestibular (inner ear), and proprioceptive inputs.

Scientific Rationale for Balance Training

Research has shown that specific kinetic chain imbalances (such as altered length-tension relationships, force-couple relationships, and arthrokinematics) can lead to altered balance and neuromuscular inefficiency (4–13). Alterations in the kinetic chain before, during, or after exercise can further affect movement quality and bring about flawed movement patterns. Flawed movement patterns alter the firing order of the muscles activated, which disturbs specific functional movement patterns and decreases neuromuscular efficiency (3, 14, 15). Prime movers may be slow to activate, whereas synergists and stabilizers substitute and become overactive (synergistic dominance). The combined effects of flawed movement patterns lead to abnormal joint stress, which affects the structural integrity of the kinetic chain and may lead to pain and joint dysfunction, and further decrease neuromuscular efficiency (6).

Research has shown that joint dysfunction creates muscle inhibition (6, 16, 17). Joint dysfunction leads to joint injury, swelling, and interruption of sensory input from articular, ligamentous, and muscular mechanoreceptors to the central nervous system, which results in a clinically evident disturbance in proprioception **Figure 10.2** (18).

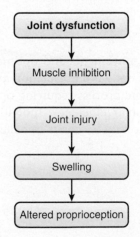

FIGURE 10.2

Effects of joint dysfunction.

It has been demonstrated that sensory feedback to the central nervous system is altered after ankle sprains, ligamentous injuries to the knee, and low-back pain (6, 8, 9, 19–24). The consequences of joint dysfunction are important for personal trainers to understand because 80% of the adult U.S. population will experience an episode of low-back pain at some point in their lives (25, 26), and an estimated 80,000 to 100,000 anterior cruciate ligament (ACL) injuries (27) and another 11 million doctor visits for foot and ankle problems occur annually (28). Therefore, muscle imbalances, joint dysfunctions, pain, and swelling can lead to altered balance. Because the majority of clients with whom personal trainers work may have decreased neuromuscular efficiency, it is imperative to understand balance and how to design a balance routine that caters to the needs of the client.

Importance of Properly Training the Balance Mechanism

Balance training should stress an individual's limit of stability (or balance threshold). An individual's limit of stability is the distance outside of the base of support that he or she can move into without losing control of his or her center of gravity. This threshold must be stressed in a multiplanar, proprioceptively enriched (unstable yet controlled) environment, using functional movement patterns to improve dynamic balance and neuromuscular efficiency. Training functional movements in a proprioceptively enriched environment with appropriate progressions (floor, balance beam, half foam roll, foam pad, balance disc), correct technique, and at varying speeds facilitates maximal sensory input to the central nervous system, resulting in the selection of the proper movement pattern.

Personal trainers are encouraged to implement progressive, systematic training programs to develop consistent, long-term changes in their clients. Traditional training program designs often result in an incomplete training program, which does not challenge the proprioceptive mechanisms of the human movement system. Balance training fills this gap left by traditional training because it focuses on functional movement patterns in a multisensory, unstable environment (29,30). The design and implementation of balance exercises into a training program is critical for developing, improving, and restoring the synergy and synchronicity of muscle firing patterns required for dynamic balance and optimal neuromuscular efficiency (29–32).

SUMMARY

Balance is key to all functional movements and optimal force production, and may help avoid injuries. Balance does not work in isolation and is both static and dynamic. It relies on an integrated, dynamic process requiring optimal muscular relationships, joint dynamics, and neuromuscular efficiency. Individuals with altered neuromuscular control likely have specific kinetic chain imbalances. These affect the quality of movement, create faulty movement patterns, and lead to reduced neuromuscular efficiency. This may contribute to synergistic dominance, which can cause joint dysfunction and pain elsewhere. Joint dysfunction creates muscle inhibition, which alters balance and leads to tissue overload and injury. The majority of fitness clients have decreased neuromuscular efficiency and problems with balance and thus can benefit from balance training programs. Therefore, effective balance ability is necessary for both healthy and injured populations.

Balance training should challenge an individual's ability to stabilize outside the normal base of support. Training in a multisensory environment will increase the demand on the nervous system's ability to activate the right muscles at the right time in the right plane of motion. Training should progress to include unstable environments in which an individual can still safely control movements.

Benefits of Balance Training

Personal trainers must understand the benefits to effectively communicate and efficiently implement a balance training program with their clients. Balance training programs are frequently used to help prevent lower extremity injuries by improving balance ability in many types of individuals including those who are healthy and physically active.

Balance Training Effects on Injury

Research has shown that performing exercises that demand balance can reduce the rate of ankle sprains and other lower extremity injuries (2, 3, 33, 34). Balance exercises are a frequent component of integrated ACL injury prevention programs, which have shown promise in reducing the rate of ACL injuries (35–38). Furthermore, a recent systematic review suggested that integrated injury prevention programs that included balance exercises in addition to plyometric or strength exercises greatly influenced the ability to improve lower extremity biomechanics (39). It is reasonable to believe that these improvements may reduce the risk of lower extremity injuries, such as ACL injuries.

Balance Training Effects on Balance Ability

Several studies have demonstrated success with improving balance ability after healthy, physically active individuals completed a balance training program. On the basis of a recent systematic review (40), balance training programs that are performed for at least 10 minutes a day, 3 times per week for 4 weeks, appear to improve both static and dynamic balance ability.

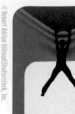

STRETCH Your Knowledge

Effects of Balance Training on Balance Ability and Injury

- Kovacs et al. (1) in a prospective randomized controlled trial with 44 competitive figure skaters found a significant positive effect on postural control when balance training versus traditional training (flexibility and strength training alone) was incorporated into an off-ice training program.
- Emery et al. (2) concluded that a home-based balance training program with wobble boards resulted in improvements in both static and dynamic balance ability in adolescent individuals.
- Gioftsidou et al. (3) performed a unique study comparing the effects of performing a single-leg balance training program either before or after soccer training sessions. The balance training program resulted in improvements in both treatment groups with no changes in the control group. Performing the program after practice appears to be more beneficial than conducting the balance exercises before practice.
- Michell et al. (4) investigated the effect of using exercise sandals during an 8-week balance training program in subjects with stable ankles and functionally unstable ankles. Their results demonstrated that both subject groups were able to improve their postural stability regardless of whether or not the subjects used exercise sandals during the balance training program.
- Emery et al. (5) found that a balance training warm-up and home-based balance program with wobble boards reduced the risk of acute injuries in high school basketball athletes.
- DiStefano et al. (6) implemented an integrated injury prevention program that included static and dynamic balance exercises to 10-year-old soccer athletes and found that the youth athletes were able to improve their dynamic balance ability.
- Soligard et al. (7) demonstrated that an integrated injury prevention program with balance exercises could reduce the risk of all injuries, overuse injuries, and severe injuries in adolescent female soccer athletes.

REFERENCES

1. Kovacs EJ, Birmingham TB, Forwell L, Litchfield RB. Effect of training on postural control in figure skaters: a randomized controlled trial of neuromuscular vs. basic off-ice training programs. *Clin J Sport Med.* 2004; 14(4): 215-224.
2. Emery CA, Cassidy JD, Klassen TP, Rosychuk RJ, Rowe BH. Effectiveness of a home-based balance-training program in reducing sports-related injuries among healthy adolescents: a cluster randomized controlled trial. *Can Med Assoc J.* 2005; 172(6): 749-754.
3. Gioftsidou A, Malliou P, Pafis G, Beneka A, Godolias G, Maganaris CN. The effects of soccer training and timing of balance training on balance ability. *Eur J Appl Physiol.* 2006; 96(6): 659-664. Epub 2006 Jan 17.
4. Michell TB, Ross SE, Blackburn JT, Hirth CJ, Guskiewicz KM. Functional balance training, with or without exercise sandals, for subjects with stable or unstable ankles. *J Athl Train.* 2006; 41(4): 393-398.
5. Emery CA, Rose MS, McAllister JR, Meeuwisse WH. A prevention strategy to reduce the incidence of injury in high school basketball: a cluster randomized controlled trial. *Clin J Sport Med.* 2007; 17(1): 17-24.
6. DiStefano LJ, Padua DA, DiStefano MJ, Marshall SW. Influence of age, sex, technique, and exercise program on movement patterns after an anterior cruciate ligament injury prevention program in youth soccer players. *Am J Sports Med.* 2009; 37(3): 495-505.
7. Soligard T, Myklebust G, Steffen K, et al. Comprehensive warm-up programme to prevent injuries in young female footballers: cluster randomised controlled trial. *BMJ.* 2008; 337: a2469.

SUMMARY

Balance-training programs can effectively reduce injury rates by improving balance ability in many types of individuals, including those who are healthy and physically active.

Designing a Balance Training Program

Balance exercises are a vital component of any integrated training program as they ensure optimal neuromuscular efficiency of the entire human movement system. Balance training exercises must be systematic and progressive. Personal trainers should follow specific program guidelines, proper exercise selection criteria, and detailed program variables Table 10.1. Balance and neuromuscular efficiency are improved through repetitive exposure to a variety of multisensory conditions (31,32).

TABLE 10.1 Balance Training Parameters	
Exercise Selection	**Variables**

• Safe	• Plane of motion
	  • Sagittal
	  • Frontal
	  • Transverse

• Progressive
  • Easy to hard
  • Simple to complex
  • Stable to unstable
  • Static to dynamic
  • Slow to fast
  • Two arms/legs to single-arm/leg
  • Eyes open to eyes closed
  • Known to unknown (cognitive task)
	• Body position
	  • Two-leg/stable
	  • Single-leg/stable
	  • Two-legs/unstable
	  • Single-leg/unstable

• Proprioceptively challenging
  • Floor
  • Balance beam
  • Half foam roll
  • Foam pad[a]
  • Balance disc[a]
  • Wobble board[a]
  • BOSU ball	

[a]These modalities come in many shapes and sizes that will dictate proper progression.

The main goal of balance training is to continually increase the client's awareness of his or her limit of stability (or kinesthetic awareness) by creating *controlled instability*. An example of controlled instability could range from having a 65-year-old client balance on one foot on the floor to having a 25-year-old athlete balance on one foot while standing on a balance disc.

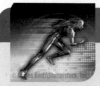

Memory Jogger

There are a number of training modalities on the market today that challenge one's balance, and they all can be very useful tools. However, to ensure the safety and effectiveness of balance training, individuals must start in an environment they can safely control and go through a systematic progression (floor, balance beam, half foam roll, foam pad, and balance disc).

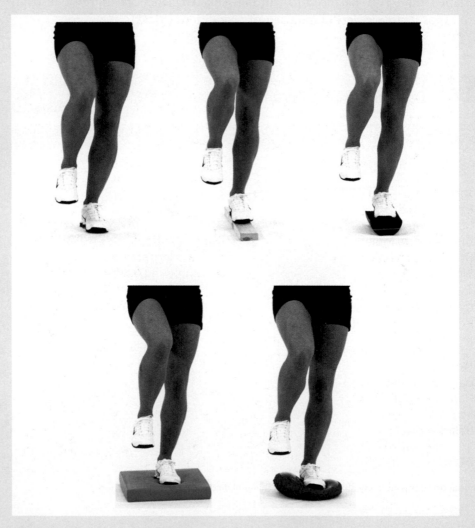

Not following the proper progression can cause movement compensations and improper execution of the exercise, decreasing the effectiveness of the exercise and increasing the risk for injury.

Levels of Balance Training

There are three levels of training within the National Academy of Sports Medicine's OPT™ model—stabilization, strength, and power **Figure 10.3**. A proper balance training program follows the same systematic progression. All three levels can be progressed or regressed by changing the surface, visual condition, and body position or movement that the exercise requires (Table 10.1). Surfaces change in difficulty as an individual moves from stable surfaces (floor) to unstable surfaces (e.g., half foam roll, foam pad, balance disc). Keeping the eyes open during an exercise is easier than having the eyes closed or moving the head around to look at various objects or performing a cognitive task simultaneously. Moving the contralateral limb, trunk, or arms also makes a balance exercise more challenging, whereas standing on two legs versus a single leg simplifies the exercise. Caution should be used to change one variable at a time. Following this strategy of progressions will enable the personal trainer to easily adapt exercises for each individual client, regardless of age or level of fitness.

Balance-Stabilization Exercises

Balance-stabilization exercises involve little joint motion; instead they are designed to improve reflexive (automatic) joint stabilization contractions to increase joint stability. During balance-stabilization training, the body is placed in unstable environments so it learns to react by contracting the right muscles at the right time to maintain balance. Sample exercises in this level include:

- Single-leg balance
- Single-leg balance reach
- Single-leg hip internal and external rotation
- Single-leg lift and chop
- Single-leg throw and catch

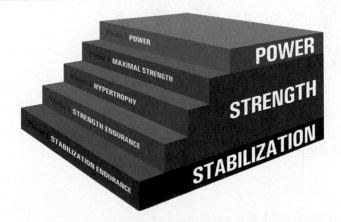

FIGURE 10.3

OPT model.

© ilolab/ShutterStock, Inc.

BALANCE-STABILIZATION EXERCISES

Single-Leg Balance

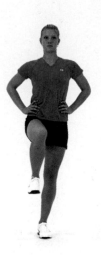

Preparation

1. Stand with feet shoulders-width apart and pointing straight ahead. Hips should be in a neutral position.

Movement

2. Lift one leg directly beside balance leg. Maintain optimal alignment, including level hips and shoulders.
3. Hold for the desired time (typically 5 to 20 seconds).
4. Switch legs and repeat as instructed.

TECHNIQUE

Make sure the gluteal musculature of the balance leg remains contracted while performing this and all balance exercises to help stabilize the lower extremity.

Single-Leg Balance Reach

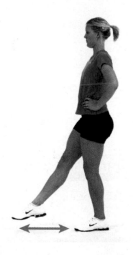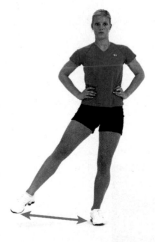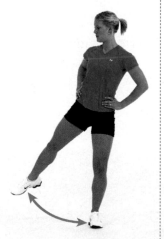

SAFETY

Keep the hips level when performing balance exercises. This will decrease stress to the lumbo-pelvic-hip complex.

Preparation

1. Stand with feet shoulders-width apart and pointing straight ahead. Hips should be level and in a neutral position.

Movement

2. Lift one leg directly beside balance leg.
3. Move lifted leg to the front of the body. Hold for a few seconds.
4. Return to original position and repeat.
5. As a progression, reach the floating leg to the side of the body and then reaching behind the body.

BALANCE-STABILIZATION EXERCISES *continued*

© ilolab/ShutterStock, Inc.

Single-Leg Hip Rotation

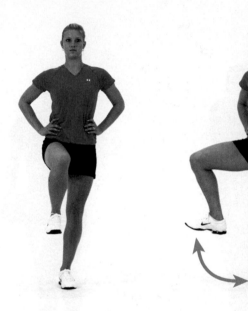

Preparation
1. Stand with feet shoulders-width apart and pointing straight ahead. Hips should be in a neutral position.

Movement
2. Lift one leg while maintaining optimal alignment, including level hips and shoulders.
3. Slowly internally and externally rotate hip of lifted leg, holding each end position for a few seconds.
4. Switch legs and repeat as instructed.

SAFETY Make sure when performing this exercise to rotate through the hip of the balance leg versus the spine. This will decrease stress to the spine and enhance control of the lumbo-pelvic-hip complex.

BALANCE-STABILIZATION EXERCISES *continued*

Single-Leg Lift and Chop

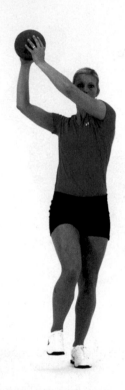
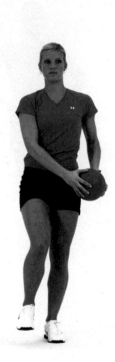

Preparation

1. Stand holding a medicine ball with feet shoulders-width apart and pointing straight ahead. Hips should be in a neutral position.

Movement

2. Lift one leg while maintaining optimal alignment, including level hips and shoulders.
3. Lift medicine ball in a diagonal pattern until medicine ball is overhead as illustrated.
4. Slowly return to original position and repeat.

SAFETY   When performing balance exercises, make sure the knee of the balance leg always stays in line with the toes.

BALANCE-STABILIZATION EXERCISES *continued*

Single-Leg Throw and Catch

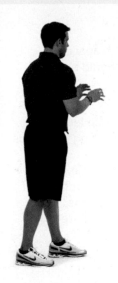 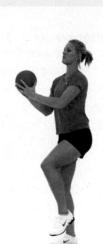 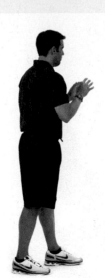 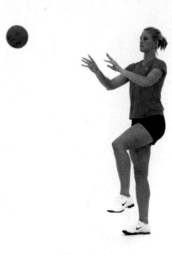

Preparation
1. Stand holding a medicine ball with feet shoulders-width apart and pointing straight ahead. Hips should be in a neutral position.

Movement
2. Lift one leg while maintaining optimal alignment, including level hips and shoulders.
3. Toss the medicine ball to a partner or trainer while maintaining optimal postural alignment as illustrated.
4. Repeat.

SAFETY　There are several methods to increase the demand of this exercise:
- trainer can toss the medicine ball at various heights and across the body
- increase the distance between both individuals
- increase velocity of each throw

Balance-Strength Exercises

Balance-strength exercises involve dynamic eccentric and concentric movement of the balance leg, through a full range of motion. Movements require dynamic control in mid-range of motion, with isometric stabilization at the end-range of motion. The specificity, speed, and neural demand of each exercise are progressed in this level. Strength exercises are designed to improve the neuromuscular efficiency of the entire human movement system. Sample exercises in this level include:

- Single-leg squat
- Single-leg squat touchdown
- Single-leg Romanian deadlift
- Multiplanar step-up to balance
- Multiplanar lunge to balance

BALANCE-STRENGTH EXERCISES

Single-Leg Squat

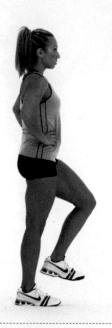

Preparation

1. Stand with feet shoulders-width apart and pointing straight ahead. Hips should be in a neutral position.

Movement

2. Lift one leg directly beside balance leg. Maintain optimal alignment, including level hips and shoulders.
3. Slowly squat as if sitting in a chair, flexing at hips, knees, and ankles. Lower to first point of compensation. Hold for a few seconds.
4. Slowly stand upright and contract gluteal muscles.
5. Repeat as instructed.

SAFETY

As mentioned earlier, make sure the knee always stays in line with the toe and it does not move inside or outside the second and third toe. This will decrease stress to the knee.

Single-Leg Squat Touchdown

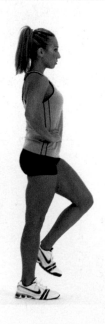

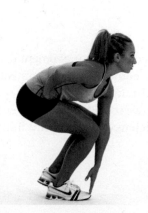

Preparation

1. Stand with feet shoulders-width apart and pointing straight ahead. Hips should be in a neutral position.

Movement

2. Lift one leg directly beside balance leg.
3. Slowly squat as if sitting in a chair, reaching hand opposite of balance leg toward foot.
4. Slowly stand upright using abdominal muscles and gluteal muscles.
5. Repeat as instructed before switching legs.

TECHNIQUE

If individuals cannot touch their foot, have them first work on reaching to their knee, then to the shin, and then to the foot.

BALANCE-STRENGTH EXERCISES *continued*

Single-Leg Romanian Deadlift

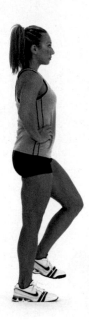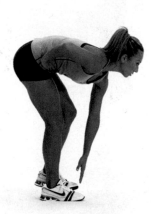

Preparation
1. Stand with feet shoulders-width apart and pointing straight ahead. Hips should be in a neutral position.

Movement
2. Lift one leg directly beside balance leg.
3. Bend from the waist and slowly reach hand down toward the toes of the balance leg. It is important to keep the spine in a neutral position and avoid hunching over.
4. Slowly stand upright using abdominal muscles and gluteal muscles.
5. Repeat as instructed.

TECHNIQUE   One can use the same progression with this exercise as that performed in the single-leg squat touchdown:
1. Reach to the knee
2. Reach to the shin
3. Reach to the foot

BALANCE-STRENGTH EXERCISES *continued*

Multiplanar Step-Up to Balance

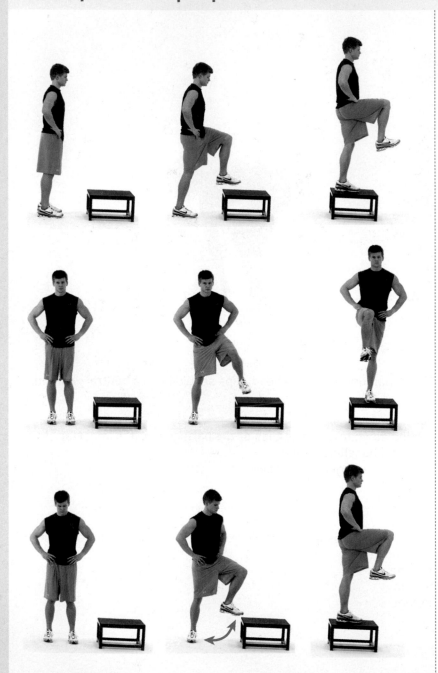

Preparation

1. Stand in front of a box or platform with feet shoulders-width apart and pointing straight ahead. Hips should be in a neutral position.

Movement

2. Step onto box with one leg, keeping toes pointing straight ahead and knee directly over the toes.
3. Push through front heel and stand upright, balancing on one leg.
4. Hold for a few seconds.
5. Return lifted leg to the ground, followed by the opposite leg, keeping toes and knees aligned.
6. Repeat as instructed.
7. As progressions, use the same process and step up from the side (frontal plane) or turn 90 degrees (transverse plane).

TECHNIQUE

Make sure at the end position that the balance leg's hip is in full extension for maximal recruitment of the gluteal musculature.

BALANCE-STRENGTH EXERCISES *continued*

Multiplanar Lunge to Balance

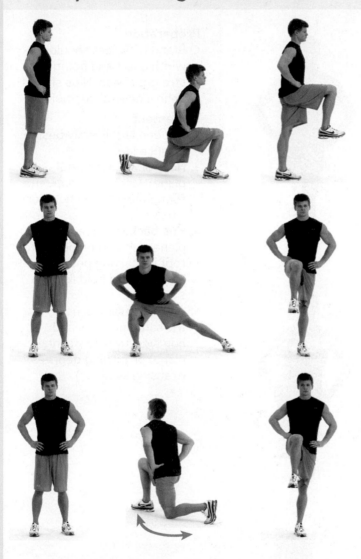

Preparation

1. Stand with feet shoulders-width apart and pointing straight ahead. Hips should be in a neutral position.

Movement

2. Lunge forward with toes pointed straight ahead and knee directly over the toes.
3. Push off of front foot through heel onto back leg and maintain balance on the back leg.
4. Repeat as instructed.
5. As progressions, use the same process and lunge to the side (frontal plane) or turn 90 degrees (transverse plane).

SAFETY

When performing a lunge, make sure the stride length is not too large, particularly if one has tight hip flexors. This can force the spine into excessive extension, increasing stress to the low back.

Balance-Power Exercises

Balance-power exercises are designed to develop proper deceleration ability to move the body from a dynamic state to a controlled stationary position, as well as high levels of eccentric strength, dynamic neuromuscular efficiency, and reactive joint stabilization. Exercises in this level include:

- Multiplanar hop with stabilization
- Mulitplanar single-leg box hop-up with stabilization
- Mulitplanar single-leg box hop-down with stabilization

BALANCE-POWER EXERCISES

Multiplanar Hop with Stabilization (Sagittal, Frontal, and Transverse)

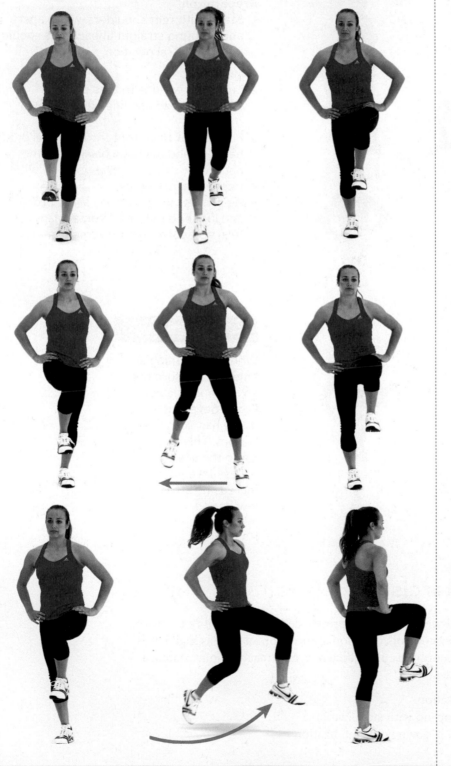

Preparation

1. Stand with feet shoulders-width apart and pointing straight ahead. Hips should be in a neutral position.

Movement

2. Lift one leg directly beside balance leg.
3. Hop forward (sagittal plane), landing on opposite foot. Stabilize and hold for 3 to 5 seconds.
4. Hop backward (sagittal plane), landing on opposite foot in starting position. Stabilize and hold for 3 to 5 seconds.
5. As progressions, use the same process and hop side-to-side (frontal plane) or turning degrees (transverse plane).

SAFETY

For all balance-power exercises, make sure the landing is soft (quiet) to ensure efficient acceptance of forces through the tissues and keep the knee in line with the second and third toes.

BALANCE-POWER EXERCISES *continued*

© ilolab/ShutterStock, Inc.

Multiplanar Single-Leg Box Hop-Up with Stabilization

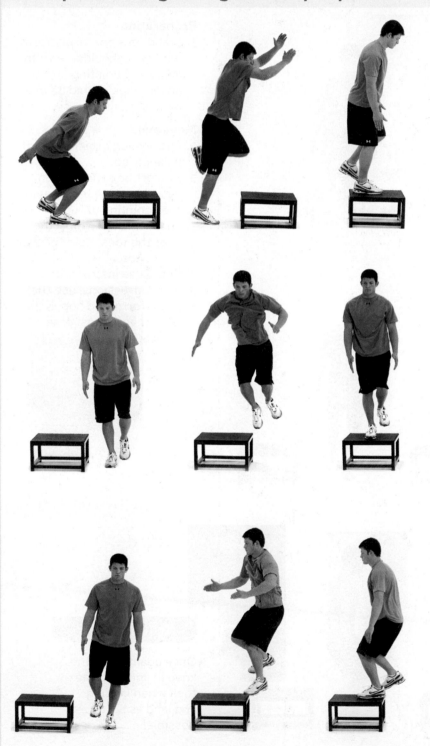

Preparation
1. Stand in front of a box or platform with feet shoulders-width apart and pointing straight ahead. Hips should be in a neutral position.

Movement
2. Lift one leg directly beside balance leg.
3. Hop up and land on top of box on one leg as illustrated. Hold for 3 to 5 seconds.
4. Repeat as instructed.
5. As progressions, use the same format to hop in the frontal and transverse planes.

© ilolab/ShutterStock, Inc.

BALANCE-POWER EXERCISES *continued*

© ilolab/ShutterStock, Inc.

Multiplanar Single-Leg Box Hop-Down with Stabilization

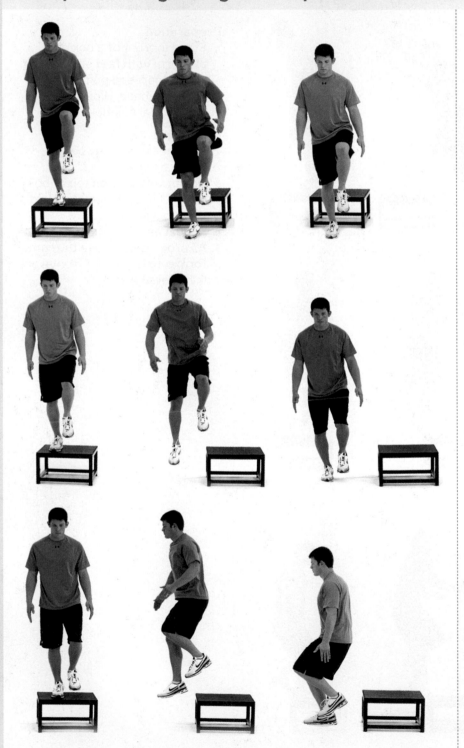

Preparation
1. Stand on a box or platform with feet shoulders-width apart and pointing straight ahead. Hips should be in a neutral position.

Movement
2. Lift one leg directly beside balance leg.
3. Hop off box and land on ground on one leg, keeping toes pointing straight ahead and knee directly over the toes. Hold for 3 to 5 seconds.
4. Repeat as instructed.
5. As progressions, use the same format to hop in the frontal and transverse planes.

TECHNIQUE

Once again, keep the knee in line with the toes when landing and land as softly as possible!

SUMMARY

A well-designed balance training program is designed to ensure optimal neuromuscular efficiency of the entire human movement system. Balance training programs must be systematic and progressive, following specific program guidelines, proper exercise selection criteria, and detailed program variables. A properly designed balance training program follows the same systematic progression as the OPT model—stabilization, strength, and power levels of training. Balance-stabilization exercises do not involve much joint motion. They improve joint stability. During balance-strength exercises, the balancing leg moves dynamically through a full range of motion. These exercises require greater specificity, speed, neural demand, and isometric stabilization at the end-range of motion. They improve neuromuscular efficiency of the entire human movement system. Balance-power exercises improve high levels of eccentric strength, dynamic neuromuscular efficiency, and reactive joint stabilization.

Implementing a Balance Training Program

Implementing a balance training program requires that personal trainers follow the progression of the OPT model. For example, if a client is in the stabilization level of training (Phase 1), select balance-stabilization exercises. For a client in the strength level of training (Phase 2, 3, or 4), the fitness professional should select balance-strength exercises. For an advanced client in the power level of training (Phase 5), select balance-power exercises Table 10.2.

Filling in the Template

To fill in the program template, go to the section labeled Core/Balance/Plyometric of the template Figure 10.4. You will then refer to Table 10.2 for the appropriate type of balance exercise (stabilization, strength, or power), the appropriate number of balance exercises, and the appropriate acute variables specific to the phase of training your client will be working in (Phases 1–5).

TABLE 10.2	Balance Training Program Design						
OPT Level	**Phase(s)**	**Exercise**	**Number of Exercises**	**Sets**	**Reps**	**Tempo**	**Rest**
Stabilization	1	Balance stabilization	1–4	1–3	12–20 6–10 (SL)	Slow	0–90 s
Strength	2, 3, 4	Balance strength	0–4[a]	2–3	8–12	Medium	0–60 s
Power	5	Balance power	0–2[b]	2–3	8–12	Controlled (hold landing position for 3–5 s)	0–60 s

© iíolab/ShutterStock, Inc.

[a] For some goals in this level of training (hypertrophy and maximal strength), balance exercises may not be required. Although recommended, balance training is optional in these phases of training.
[b] Because balance exercises are performed in the dynamic flexibility portion of this program and the goal of the program is power, balance training may not be necessary in this phase of training. Although recommended, balance training is optional.
SL, single leg.

Professional's Name: Brian Sutton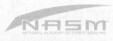

CLIENT'S NAME: JOHN SMITH   **DATE: 5/01/13**

GOAL: FAT LOSS   **PHASE: 1 STABILIZATION ENDURANCE**

WARM-UP

Exercise:	Sets	Duration	Coaching Tip
SMR: Calves, IT-Band, Lats	1	30 s.	Hold each tender area for 30 sec
Static Stretch: Calves, Hip Flexors, Lats	1	30 s.	Hold each stretch for 30 sec
Treadmill	1	5 – 10 min	Brisk walk to slow jog

CORE / BALANCE / PLYOMETRIC

Exercise:	Sets	Reps	Tempo	Rest	Coaching Tip
Floor Bridge	2	12	Slow	0	
Floor Prone Cobra	2	12	Slow	0	
Single-Leg Balance Reach	2	12	Slow	0	

SPEED, AGILITY, QUICKNESS

Exercise:	Sets	Reps	Rest	Coaching Tip

RESISTANCE

Exercise:	Sets	Reps	Tempo	Rest	Coaching Tip

COOL-DOWN

Exercise:	Sets	Duration	Coaching Tip

Coaching Tips:

FIGURE 10.4   OPT template.

REFERENCES

1. McGuine TA, Greene JJ, Best T, Leverson G. Balance as a predictor of ankle injuries in high school basketball players. *Clin J Sport Med.* 2000;10(4):239-244.

2. McGuine TA, Keene JS. The effect of a balance training program on the risk of ankle sprains in high school athletes. *Am J Sports Med.* 2006;34(7):1103-1111. Epub 2006 Feb 13.

3. Olsen OE, Myklebust G, Engebretsen L, Holme I, Bahr R. Exercises to prevent lower limb injuries in youth sports: cluster randomised controlled trial. *BMJ.* 2005;330(7489):449.

4. Edgerton VR, Wolf S, Roy RR. Theoretical basis for patterning EMG amplitudes to assess muscle dysfunction. *Med Sci Sports Exerc.* 1996;28(6):744-751.

5. Janda V. Muscle weakness and inhibition (pseudoparesis) in back pain syndromes. In: Grieve GP, ed. *Modern Manual Therapy of the Vertebral Column.* New York: Churchill Livingstone, 1986:197-201.

6. Lewit K. Muscular and articular factors in movement restriction. *Man Med.* 1985;1:83-85.

7. Janda V, Vavrova M. Sensory Motor Stimulation Video. Brisbane, Australia: Body Control Systems; 1990.

8. Hodges PW, Richardson CA. Neuromotor dysfunction of the trunk musculature in low back pain patients. In: *Proceedings of the International Congress of the World Confederation of Physical Therapists.* Washington, DC; 1995.

9. Hodges PW, Richardson CA. Inefficient muscular stabilization of the lumbar spine associated with low back pain. *Spine.* 1996;21(22):2640-2650.

10. O'Sullivan PE, Twomey L, Allison G, Sinclair J, Miller K, Knox J. Altered patterns of abdominal muscle activation in patients with chronic low back pain. *Aus J Physiother.* 1997;43(2):91-98.

11. Borsa PA, Lephart SM, Kocher MS, Lephart SP. Functional assessment and rehabilitation of shoulder proprioception for glenohumeral instability. *J Sports Rehabil.* 1994;3:84-104.

12. Janda V. *Muscle Function Testing.* London: Butterworth; 1983.

13. Janda V. Muscles, Central nervous system regulation, and back problems. In: Korr IM, ed. *Neurobiologic Mechanisms in Manipulative Therapy.* New York: Plenum Press; 1978:27-41.

14. Liebenson C. Integrating rehabilitation into chiropractic practice (blending active and passive care). In: Liebenson C, ed. *Rehabilitation of the Spine: A Practioner's Manual.* Baltimore: Williams & Wilkins; 1996:165-191.

15. Sahrmann S. Diagnosis and treatment of muscle imbalances and musculoskeletal pain syndrome. Continuing Education Course. St. Louis; 1997.

16. Rowinski MJ. Afferent neurobiology of the joint. In: Gould JA, ed. *Orthopedic and Sports Physical Therapy.* St. Louis: Mosby; 1990:49-63.

17. Warmerdam ALA. Arthrokinetic therapy; manual therapy to improve muscle and joint function. Course manual. Marshfield, WI; 1996.

18. Fahrer H, Rentsch HU, Gerber NJ, Beyler C, Hess CW, Grünig B. Knee effusion and reflex inhibition of the quadriceps. A bar to effective retraining. *J Bone Joint Surg Br.* 1988;70:635-639.

19. Solomonow M, Barratta R, Zhou BH. The synergistic action of the ACL and thigh muscles in maintaining joint stability. *Am J Sports Med.* 1987;15:207-213.

20. Jull G, Richardson CA, Hamilton C, Hodges PW, Ng J. *Towards the Validation of a Clinical Test for the Deep Abdominal Muscles in Back Pain Patients.* Gold Coast, Queensland: Manipulative Physiotherapists Association of Australia; 1995.

21. Ross SE, Guskiewicz KM, Yu B. Single-leg jump-landing stabilization times in subjects with functionally unstable ankles. *J Athl Train.* 2005;40(4):298-304.

22. Ross SE, Guskiewicz KM. Examination of static and dynamic postural stability in individuals with functionally stable and unstable ankles. *Clin J Sport Med.* 2004;14(6):332-338.

23. Wikstrom EA, Tillman MD, Schenker SM, Borsa PA. Jump-landing direction influences dynamic postural stability scores. *J Sci Med Sport.* 2008;11(2):106-111. Epub 2007 Jun 1.

24. Wikstrom EA, Tillman MD, Chmielewski TL, Cauraugh JH, Borsa PA. Dynamic postural stability deficits in subjects with self-reported ankle instability. *Med Sci Sports Exerc.* 2007;39(3):397-402.

25. Walker BF, Muller R, Grant WD. Low back pain in Australian adults: prevalence and associated disability. *J Man Physiol Ther.* 2004;27(4):238-244.

26. Cassidy JD, Carroll LJ, Cote P. The Saskatchewan Health and Back Pain Survey. The prevalence of low back pain and related disability in Saskatchewan adults. *Spine.* 1998;23(17):1860-1866.

27. Griffin LY, Agel J, Albohm MJ, et al. Noncontact anterior cruciate ligament injuries: risk factors and prevention strategies. *J Am Acad Orthop Surg.* 2000;8(3):141-150.

28. Centers for Disease Control and Prevention. Ambulatory care visits to physician offices, hospital outpatient departments, and emergency departments: United States, 2001–2002. *Vital Health Stat. 13* 2006;13(159). Available at http://www.cdc.gov/nchs/data/series/sr_13/sr13_159.pdf. Accessed Feb 8, 2006.

29. Tippet S, Voight M. *Functional Progressions for Sports Rehabilitation.* Champaign, IL: Human Kinetics; 1995.

30. Voight M, Cook G. Clinical application of closed kinetic chain exercise. *J Sport Rehabil.* 1996;5(1):25-44.

31. Lephart SM. Re-establishing proprioception, kinesthesia, joint position sense, and neuromuscular control in rehabilitation. In: Prentice WE, ed. *Rehabilitation Techniques in Sports.* 2nd ed. St. Louis: Mosby; 1993:118-137.

32. Guskiewicz KM, Perrin DM. Research and clinical applications of assessing balance. *J Sport Rehabil.* 1996;5:45-63.

33. Wedderkopp N, Kaltoft M, Holm R, Froberg K. Comparison of two intervention programmes in young female players in European handball—with and without ankle disc. *Scand J Med Sci Sports.* 2003;13(6):371-375.

34. Cumps E, Verhagen E, Meeusen R. Efficacy of a sports specific balance training programme on the incidence of ankle sprains in basketball. *J Sports Sci Med.* 2007;6:212-219.

35. Soligard T, Myklebust G, Steffen K, et al. Comprehensive warm-up programme to prevent injuries in young female footballers: cluster randomised controlled trial. *BMJ.* 2008;337:a2469. doi: 10.1136/bmj.a2469 (Published 9 December 2008).

36. Hewett TE, Lindenfeld TN, Riccobene JV, Noyes FR. The effect of neuromuscular training on the incidence of knee injury in female athletes: a prospective study. *Am J Sports Med.* 1999;27:699-706.

37. Gilchrist J, Mandelbaum BR, Melancon H, et al. A randomized controlled trial to prevent noncontact anterior cruciate ligament injury in female collegiate soccer players. *Am J Sports Med.* 2008;36(8):1476-1483.

38. Mandelbaum BR, Silvers HJ, Watanabe DS, et al. Effectiveness of a neuromuscular and proprioceptive training program in preventing anterior cruciate ligament injuries in female athletes: 2-year follow-up. *Am J Sports Med.* 2005;33;1003-1010.

39. Padua DA, DiStefano LJ. Sagittal plane knee biomechanics and vertical ground reaction forces are modified following ACL injury prevention programs: a systematic review. *Sports Health.* 2009;1(2):165-173.

40. DiStefano LJ, Padua DA, Clark MA. Evidence supporting balance training in healthy individuals: a systematic literature review. *J Strength Cond Res.* 2009;23(9):2718-2731.

Plyometric (Reactive) Training Concepts

OBJECTIVES

After studying this chapter, you will be able to:

✔ Define plyometric (reactive) training and describe its uses.

✔ Discuss the importance of plyometric training.

✔ Design a plyometric training program for clients at various levels of fitness.

✔ Perform and instruct various plyometric training exercises.

Principles of Plyometric Training

Plyometric training, also known as jump or reactive training, is a form of exercise that uses explosive movements such as bounding, hopping, and jumping to develop muscular power. Plyometric training is a form of training in which the individual reacts to the ground surface in such a way that they develop larger than normal ground forces that can then be used to project the body with a greater velocity or speed of movement. The term *reactive training* refers to the reaction stimulus clients encounter during plyometric training, which is the ground surface in this case. Therefore, reactive and plyometric training are used interchangeably throughout this chapter.

It is important for personal trainers to understand that individual clients must possess adequate core strength, joint stability, and range of motion, and have the ability to balance efficiently *before* performing any plyometric exercises. Plyometric training is generally not an appropriate form of training for individuals with selected chronic diseases or other health or functional limitations. This purpose of this chapter is to review the importance of plyometric training and the methods involved in designing and implementing a plyometric training routine into a client's existing exercise program.

What Is Plyometric Training?

Enhanced performance during functional activities emphasizes the ability of muscles to exert maximal force output in a minimal amount of time (also known as **rate of force production**). Success in everyday activities and sport depends on the speed at which muscular force is generated. Speed of movement and reactive neuromuscular control are a function of muscular development and neural control; the first is a function of training and the other of learning. The key then is muscular overload and rapid movements during the execution of the training exercises.

Plyometric (reactive) training involves exercises that generate quick, powerful movements involving explosive concentric muscle contraction preceded by an eccentric muscle action (1). In other words, there is a "cocking" or loading phase described as an eccentric muscle action that dampens or slows the downward movement of the body (deceleration) followed immediately by an explosive concentric muscle contraction (1). These types of explosive muscular contractions can be seen in practical instances such as rebounding in basketball. Watch good basketball players as they prepare to jump up for a loose ball, and you will see them prepare by lowering their body slightly by flexing at the ankles, knees, and hips. They may even drop their arms to assist in takeoff. At a fairly shallow point, players will reverse this downward motion and rapidly project themselves from the ground extending their ankles, knees, hips, and arms upward. The overall height that they will achieve is determined by their vertical velocity or how fast they leave the ground. This is the essence of a plyometric exercise and uses a characteristic of muscle known as the stretch-shortening cycle of the **integrated performance paradigm Figure 11.1,** The integrated performance paradigm states that to move with precision, forces must be loaded (eccentrically), stabilized (isometrically), and then unloaded or accelerated (concentrically).

Three Phases of Plyometric Exercise

There are three distinct phases involved in plyometric training, including the eccentric or loading phase, the amortization phase or transition phase, and the concentric or unloading phase (2).

The Eccentric Phase

The first stage of a plyometric movement can be classified as the eccentric phase, but has also been called the deceleration, loading, yielding, counter movement, or cocking phase (3). This phase increases muscle spindle activity by prestretching the muscle before activation (4). Potential energy is stored in the elastic components of the muscle during this loading phase much like stretching a rubber band.

Rate of force production Ability of muscles to exert maximal force output in a minimal amount of time.

Plyometric (reactive) training Exercises that generate quick, powerful movements involving an explosive concentric muscle contraction preceded by an eccentric muscle action.

Integrated performance paradigm To move with efficiency, forces must be dampened (eccentrically), stabilized (isometrically), and then accelerated (concentrically).

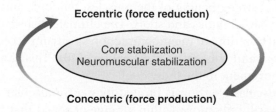

FIGURE 11.1

Integrated performance paradigm.

The Amortization Phase

This phase involves dynamic stabilization and is the time between the end of the eccentric muscle action (the loading or deceleration phase) and the initiation of the concentric contraction (the unloading or force production phase) (5). The amortization phase, sometimes referred to as the transition phase, is also referred to as the electromechanical delay between the eccentric and concentric contraction during which the muscle must switch from overcoming force to imparting force in the intended direction (6). A prolonged amortization phase results in less than optimal neuromuscular efficiency from a loss of elastic potential energy (7). A rapid switch from an eccentric loading phase to a concentric contraction leads to a more powerful response (5,6).

The Concentric Phase

The concentric phase (or unloading phase) occurs immediately after the amortization phase and involves a concentric contraction (5,6,8), resulting in enhanced muscular performance after the eccentric phase of muscle contraction. This is synonymous with releasing a rubber band after it was stretched.

Importance of Plyometric Training

Plyometric exercises enhance the excitability, sensitivity, and reactivity of the neuromuscular system and increase the rate of force production (power), motor unit recruitment, firing frequency (rate coding), and motor unit synchronization. These training exercises are a progression that can be incorporated once a client has achieved an overall strength base, proper core strength, and balance stabilization capabilities. Adequate isometric stabilization strength (developed through core, balance, and resistance-stabilization exercises) decreases the time between the eccentric muscle action and concentric contraction, resulting in shorter ground contact times, which result in decreased tissue overload and potential injury when performing plyometric training. Plyometric exercises also use the stimulation of the body's proprioceptive mechanism and elastic properties to generate maximal force output in the minimal amount of time.

All movement patterns that occur during functional activities involve a series of repetitive stretch-shortening cycles (eccentric and concentric contractions). Stretch-shortening cycles require the neuromuscular system to react quickly and efficiently after an eccentric muscle action to produce a concentric contraction and impart the necessary force (or acceleration) in the appropriate direction. The purpose of this activity is to produce the necessary force to change the direction of an object's center of mass efficiently (9). Therefore, functional movements such as "cutting or change-of-direction" require training exercises that emphasize plyometric training to prepare each client for the functional demands of a specific activity.

Plyometric training provides the ability to train specific movement patterns in a biomechanically correct manner at a more functionally appropriate speed. This provides better functional strengthening of the muscles, tendons, and ligaments to meet the demands of everyday activities and sport. The ultimate goal of plyometric training is to decrease the reaction time of the muscle action spectrum (eccentric deceleration, isometric stabilization, and concentric acceleration) (10). This is also what results in increased speed of movement in the individual.

The speed of muscular exertion is limited by neuromuscular coordination. This means that the body will only move within a range of speed that the nervous system has been programmed to allow (9). Plyometric training improves neuromuscular efficiency and improves the range of speed set by the central nervous system. Optimal reactive performance of any activity depends on the speed at which muscular forces can be generated.

This is another component of program design that is often overlooked in traditional training programs. Plyometric training is often perceived by many to be too dangerous, and as potentially increasing the risk of injury. However, plyometric training has a systematic progression sequence that allows a client to begin with less demanding exercises and progress to more demanding exercises as he or she adapts. This is no different than any other form of training. If too-advanced exercises are assigned to a client, he or she will not have the ability to perform them correctly and will compensate. This leads to synergistic dominance (synergists compensating for weak prime movers) and faulty movement patterns. When placed within the proper programming scheme with proper progression, plyometric training can be a vital component to achieving optimal performance of any activity at any level of ability.

For example, a 60-year-old woman and a 25-year-old male professional athlete may not both need to train for maximal strength. However, they both need stabilization, strength, and endurance as well as the ability to produce force quickly to perform daily

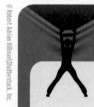

STRETCH Your Knowledge

Evidence to Support the Use of Plyometric Training for Injury Prevention and Performance Enhancement

- Chimera et al. (2004) in a pretest and posttest with control group design using 20 healthy Division I female athletes found that a 6-week plyometric training program improved hip abductor and adductor coactivation ratios to help control varus (bowlegged) and valgus (knock-knees) moments at the knee during landing (1).
- Wilkerson et al. (2004) in a quasi-experimental design with 19 female basketball players demonstrated that a 6-week plyometric training program improved hamstring to quadriceps ratio, which has been shown to enhance dynamic knee stability during the eccentric deceleration phase of landing (2). This is one of the factors contributing to the high incidence of anterior cruciate ligament (ACL) injuries in female athletes.
- Luebbers et al. (2003) in a randomized controlled trial with 19 subjects demonstrated that 4-and 7-week plyometric training programs enhanced anaerobic power and vertical jump height (3).
- Hewett et al. (1996) in a prospective study demonstrated decreased peak landing forces, enhanced muscle-balance ratio between the quadriceps and hamstrings, and decreased rate of anterior cruciate ligament injuries in female soccer, basketball, and volleyball players who incorporated plyometric training into their program (4).

REFERENCES

1. Chimera NJ, Swanik KA, Swanik CB, Straub SJ. Effects of plyometric training on muscle-activation strategies and performance in female athletes. *J Athl Train.* 2004;39(1):24-31.
2. Wilkerson GB, Colston MA, Short NI, Neal KL, Hoewischer PE, Pixley JJ. Neuromuscular changes in female collegiate athletes resulting from a plyometric jump training program. *J Athl Train.* 2004;39(1):17-23.
3. Luebbers PE, Potteiger JA, Hulver MW, Thyfault JP, Carper MJ, Lockwood RH. Effects of plyometric training and recovery on vertical jump performance and anaerobic power. *J Strength Cond Res.* 2003;17(4):704-709.
4. Hewett TE, Stroupe AL, Nance TA, Noyes FR. Plyometric training in female athletes. Decreased impact forces and increased hamstring torques. *Am J Sports Med.* 1996;24(6):765-773.

activities efficiently. Therefore, the ability to react and produce sufficient force to avoid a fall or an opponent is paramount. The specificity of training concept dictates that both clients are trained in a more velocity-specific environment (11). The speed of the repetition or movement is at a faster tempo, similar to movements seen in daily life or sport-related activities.

SUMMARY

The ability to react and generate force quickly is crucial to overall function and safety during movement. Plyometric (reactive) training involves exercises that generate quick, powerful movements involving an explosive concentric muscle contraction preceded by an eccentric muscle action. Plyometric training can enhance one's ability to dynamically stabilize, reduce, and produce forces at speeds that are functionally applicable to the tasks at hand.

The nervous system recruits muscles only at speeds at which it has been trained to do so. If it is not trained to recruit muscles quickly, when met with a demand for fast reaction, the nervous system will not be able to respond appropriately. The ultimate goal of plyometric training is to decrease the reaction time of muscle action (or increase the rate of force production). It is important to note, however, that plyometric training should only be incorporated into an individual's exercise program once the individual has obtained a proper base of total body strength, flexibility, core strength, and balance capabilities. This reiterates the importance of using a progressive and systematic approach when designing the plyometric component of your client's training regimen.

Designing a Plyometric Training Program

Plyometric Training Design Parameters

A plyometric training program is a vital component of any integrated training program. The program must be systematic and progressive. A client must exhibit proper levels of total body strength, core strength, and balance before progressing into plyometric training. Health and fitness professionals must follow specific program guidelines, proper exercise selection criteria, and detailed program variables **Figure 11.2**. Moreover, plyometric training should only be performed by individuals wearing supportive shoes, and on a proper training surface such as a grass field, basketball court, or tartan track.

Levels of Plyometric Training

There are three levels of training within NASM's OPT™ model: (1) *stabilization*, (2) *strength*, and (3) *power* **Figure 11.3**.

Plyometric Stabilization Exercises

In plyometric-stabilization training, exercises involve little joint motion. They are designed to establish optimal landing mechanics, postural alignment, and reactive

Exercise Selection
- Safe
- Done with supportive shoes
- Performed on a proper training surface
  - Grass field
  - Basketball court
  - Tartan track surface
  - Rubber track surface
- Performed with proper supervision
- Progressive
  - Easy to hard
  - Simple to complex
  - Known to unknown
  - Stable to unstable
  - Body weight to loaded
  - Activity-specific

Variables
- Plane of motion
  - Sagittal
  - Frontal
  - Transverse
- Range of motion
  - Full
  - Partial
- Type of resistance
  - Medicine ball
  - Power ball
- Type of implements
  - Tape
  - Cones
  - Boxes
- Muscle action
  - Eccentric
  - Isometric
  - Concentric
- Speed of motion
- Duration
- Frequency
- Amplitude of movement

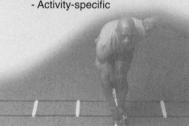

FIGURE 11.2

Program design parameters for reactive training.

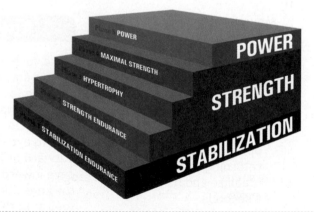

FIGURE 11.3

OPT model.

neuromuscular efficiency (coordination during dynamic movement). When an individual lands during these exercises, he or she should hold the landing position (or stabilize) for 3 to 5 seconds. During this time individuals should make any adjustments necessary to correct faulty postures before repeating the exercise. Exercises in this level include the following:

- Squat jump with stabilization
- Box jump-up with stabilization
- Box jump-down with stabilization
- Multiplanar jump with stabilization

PLYOMETRIC-STABILIZATION EXERCISES

Squat Jump with Stabilization

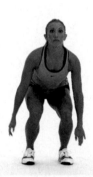
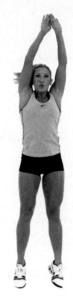
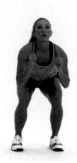

Preparation

1. Stand with feet shoulders-width apart and pointed straight ahead. Hips should be in a neutral position, and knees should be aligned over mid-foot with arms held at sides.

Movement

2. Squat slightly as if sitting in a chair.
3. Jump up, extending arms overhead.
4. Land softly, with the ankles, knees, and hips slightly flexed, maintaining optimal alignment and returning arms to sides. Stabilize and hold for 3 to 5 seconds.
5. Repeat as instructed.

TECHNIQUE

Make sure the knees always stay in line with the toes, both before jumping and on landing. Do not allow feet to excessively turn outward or knees to cave inward. Also keep the knees behind the toes at both takeoff and landing, which can be observed from the side view.

PLYOMETRIC-STABILIZATION EXERCISES *continued*

Box Jump-Up with Stabilization

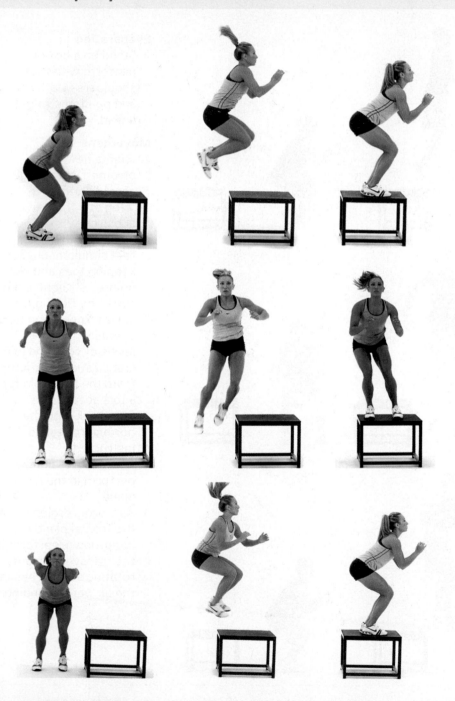

Preparation

1. Stand in front of a box or platform with feet shoulders-width apart and toes and knees pointed straight ahead.

Movement

2. Squat slightly as if sitting in a chair.
3. Using arms, jump up and land on top of box, keeping toes pointed straight ahead and knees directly over the toes. Hold for 3 to 5 seconds.
4. Land softly with the ankles, knees, and hips flexed. Note: hips and knees will be flexed to a deeper level than the prior exercise. Do not let the client "stick" the landing with the legs straight.
5. Step off box and repeat as instructed.
6. As a progression, perform this drill by jumping laterally in the frontal plane to the top of the box.
7. As a progression from the frontal plane box jump-up, perform in the transverse plane, rotating 90 degrees in the air before landing.

SAFETY   Adjust the height of the box to be consistent with the physical capabilities of the individual performing the exercise.

PLYOMETRIC-STABILIZATION EXERCISES *continued*

Box Jump-Down with Stabilization

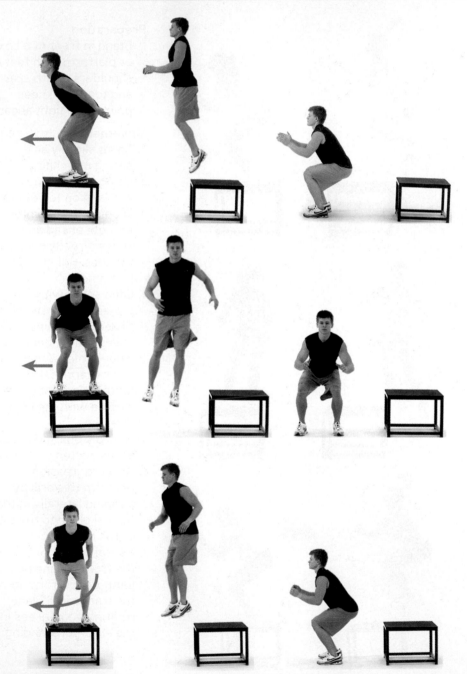

Preparation
1. Stand on a box or platform with feet shoulders-width apart and pointed straight ahead.

Movement
2. Clients new to plyometric training should attempt to "step off" the box and drop to the floor landing with both feet simultaneously, keeping toes and knees pointed straight. Land softly, by flexing the ankles, knees, and hips. Clients with higher levels of core and joint stabilization may jump from the box. Hold for 3 to 5 seconds.
3. Step back onto the box and repeat as instructed.
4. As a progression, perform in the frontal plane.
5. As a progression from the frontal plane box jump-down, perform in the transverse plane, rotating 90 degrees in the air before landing.

TECHNIQUE Attempt to make sure the client steps off and drops from the prescribed height when initially attempting this exercise. Jumping from the box presents different variables and levels of load or intensity of the exercise and can used as a progression. Make sure the individual lands softly and quietly on the ground to ensure proper force transmission through the tissues of the body. Do not let the client "stick" the landing with the legs straight.

PLYOMETRIC-STABILIZATION EXERCISES *continued*

Multiplanar Jump with Stabilization

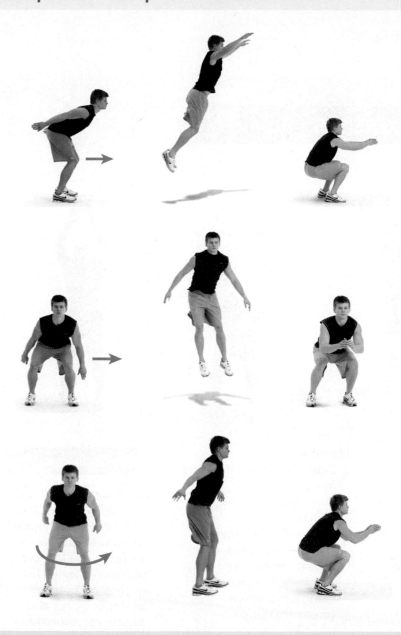

Preparation

1. Stand with feet shoulders-width apart and pointed straight ahead.

Movement

2. Squat slightly as if sitting in a chair.
3. Jump forward (long jump) as far as can be controlled.
4. Land softly, maintaining flexion in the knees and hips, but do not collapse to the ground. Maintain optimal postural alignment and hold for 3 to 5 seconds.
5. Return to the start and repeat as instructed.
6. As a progression, perform in the frontal plane by jumping laterally to the side.
7. As a progression from the lateral jump, perform a transverse plane jump, rotating 90 degrees before landing.

Plyometric Strength Exercises

In plyometric-strength training, exercises involve more dynamic eccentric and concentric movement through a full range of motion. The specificity, speed, and neural demand may also be progressed at this level. These exercises are intended to improve dynamic joint stabilization, eccentric strength, rate of force production, and neuromuscular efficiency of the entire human movement system. These exercises are performed in a repetitive fashion (spending a relatively short amount of time on the ground before repeating the drill). Some exercises in this level include the following:

- Squat jump
- Tuck jump
- Butt kick
- Power step-up

PLYOMETRIC-STRENGTH EXERCISES

Squat Jump

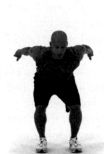 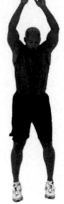 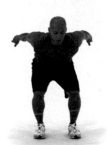 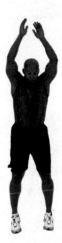

Preparation
1. Stand with feet shoulders-width apart and pointed straight ahead.

Movement
2. Squat slightly as if sitting in a chair.
3. Jump up, extending arms overhead.
4. Land softly, maintaining optimal alignment and repeat for the desired number of repetitions using a repetitive (medium) tempo.

TECHNIQUE

Make sure to land with the ankles, knees, and hips flexed and pointed straight ahead, which becomes the takeoff position as well. This will ensure optimal joint mechanics and muscle recruitment. Perform the exercise with a repetitive (medium) tempo.

PLYOMETRIC-STRENGTH EXERCISES *continued*

Tuck Jump

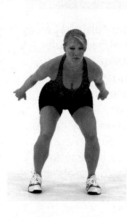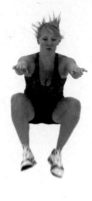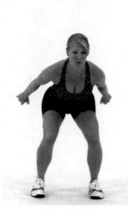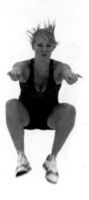

Preparation

1. Stand with feet shoulders-width apart and pointed straight ahead.

Movement

2. Squat slightly as if sitting in a chair.

3. Jump up, bringing both knees toward the chest. Attempt to have the thighs parallel with the ground.

4. Land softly, maintaining optimal alignment on landing keeping the feet, knees, and hips pointed straight ahead.

5. Attempt to keep the jumps in a small area so that the body is not moving excessively forward, backward, or laterally. Consider these jumps as if you were jumping on a particular spot. Repeat for the desired number of repetitions.

| SAFETY | Now that the exercises are becoming more dynamic, proper alignment and landing mechanics will be even more important to maximize force production and prevent injury. |

PLYOMETRIC-STRENGTH EXERCISES *continued*

Butt Kick

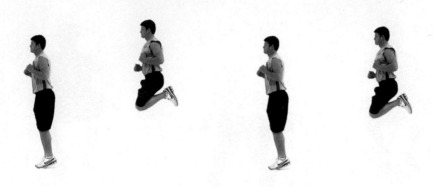

Preparation

1. Stand with feet shoulders-width apart and pointed straight ahead.

Movement

2. Squat slightly as if sitting in a chair.
3. Jump up, bringing heels to gluteal muscles and avoiding arching of the lower back.
4. Land softly, maintaining optimal alignment, and repeat for the desired number of repetitions using a repetitive (medium) tempo.

SAFETY

It is important that an individual has ample amounts of flexibility of the quadriceps to ensure proper execution. Tight quadriceps may cause an individual to arch the lower back when bringing the heels toward the gluteal muscles.

Power Step-Up

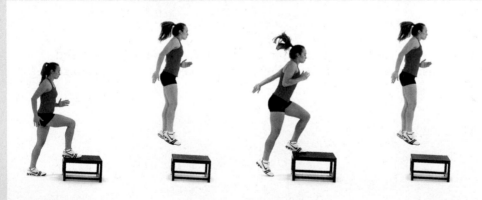

Preparation

1. Stand in front of a box or platform with feet in a staggered stance, pointed straight ahead, with one foot on top of the box.

Movement

2. Forcefully push off of leg on top of box, pushing the ankles, knees, and hips into full extension.
3. Switch legs in the air, landing with the opposite foot on top of the box.
4. Repeat as instructed.

TECHNIQUE

Make sure the knees always stay in line with the toes throughout the jumping phases of takeoff and landing.

Plyometric Power Exercises

In plyometric-power training, exercises involve the entire muscle action spectrum and contraction-velocity spectrum used during integrated, functional movements. These exercises are designed to further improve the rate of force production, eccentric strength, reactive strength, reactive joint stabilization, dynamic neuromuscular efficiency, and optimal force production (9,10). These exercises are performed as fast and as explosively as possible. Some exercises in this level include the following:

- Ice skaters (also known as skater jumps)
- Single-leg power step-up
- Proprioceptive plyometrics

PLYOMETRIC-POWER EXERCISES

Ice Skaters

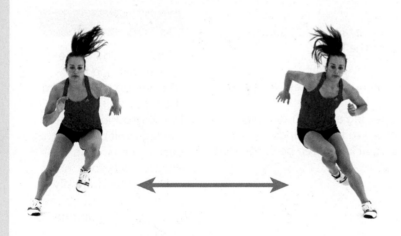

TECHNIQUE

One can start by hopping side-to-side from one foot to the other as fast as possible and then progress by adding a reach with the opposite hand to make it more integrated (skating action).

Preparation
1. Stand with feet shoulders-width apart and pointed straight ahead.

Movement
2. Quickly push from side to side, landing on the opposite foot while maintaining optimal alignment during the side-to-side hopping movement.
3. Repeat as quickly as can be controlled for the prescribed repetitions or time interval.

© ilolab/ShutterStock, Inc.

PLYOMETRIC-POWER EXERCISES *continued*

© ilolab/ShutterStock, Inc.

Single-Leg Power Step-Up

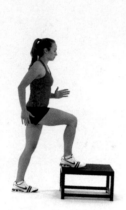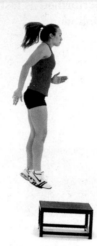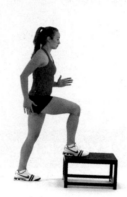

Preparation
1. Stand in front of a box or platform with feet in a staggered stance, pointed straight ahead, with one foot on top of the box.

Movement
2. Forcefully push off of leg on top of box, extending the ankles, knees, and hips and achieving maximal vertical height.
3. Land on same leg, keeping weight on the upper leg and maintaining optimal alignment. The opposite foot will return to the ground.
4. Repeat as instructed, jumping as high and as quickly as can be controlled.

TECHNIQUE

Client must be made aware that one foot will land on the box and the other will continue to the ground so that the legs will be offset during the landing phase. Therefore, he or she must be mentally prepared to absorb the landing in this unique position.

PLYOMETRIC-POWER EXERCISES *continued*

Proprioceptive Plyometrics

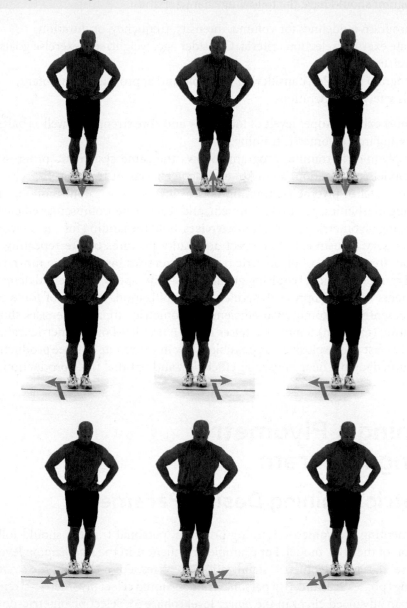

Preparation

1. Stand with feet shoulders-width apart and pointed straight ahead.

Movement

2. Jump (two legs) or hop (one leg) front-to-back, side-to-side, or in a diagonal pattern over lines, cones, hurdles, or other implements.
3. Land softly, maintaining optimal alignment with short ground contact times.
4. Repeat as instructed, as quickly as can be controlled.

TECHNIQUE

If cones or hurdles are not available, you can also place tape on the floor in the form of an X and perform the exercise by jumping in different quadrants.

SUMMARY

A plyometric training program is designed to enhance neuromuscular efficiency, increase rate of force production, and improve functional eccentric strength. To do so, a training program should have the following characteristics:

- Specific program guidelines for volume, intensity, frequency, or duration.
- Appropriate exercise selection criteria. Consider age, weight, sex, exercise goals, fitness level, etc.
- Proper program variables, considering available and appropriate equipment, along with safety considerations.

A client must exhibit proper levels of total body and core strength as well as balance before progressing into plyometric training.

A proper plyometric training program follows the same systematic progression as the OPT model: stabilization, strength, and power levels of training. Exercises in the *stabilization* level of plyometric training do not involve much joint motion. They improve landing mechanics, postural alignment, and reactive neuromuscular efficiency. When performing plyometric-stabilization exercises, hold the landing for 3 to 5 seconds and make necessary adjustments to correct any faulty postures before repeating the exercise. In the *strength* level of plyometric training, exercises involve more movement through a full range of motion, requiring greater specificity, speed, and neural demand. These movements further improve dynamic joint stabilization, the rate of force production, and eccentric neuromuscular efficiency. Plyometric-strength exercises should utilize a repeating (medium) tempo. Exercises in the *power* level of plyometric training are performed as fast and explosively as possible. They improve rate of force production, reactive strength, dynamic neuromuscular efficiency, and optimal force production.

Designing a Plyometric Training Program

Plyometric Training Design Parameter

When implementing a plyometric training program, personal trainers should follow the progression of the OPT model. For example, if a client is in the *stabilization* level of training (phase 1), select plyometric-stabilization exercises. For a client in the *strength* level of training (phases 2, 3, and 4), a personal trainer should select plyometric-strength exercises. For an advanced client in the *power* level (phase 5), select plyometric-power exercises. Exercises from the prior levels of training may be included at the fitness professional's discretion to fit the needs and goals of the client.

Filling in the Template

To fill in the program template **Figure 11.4**, go to the section labeled Core, Balance, Plyometric. You will then refer to **Table 11.1** for the appropriate type of plyometric exercise (stabilization, strength, or power), the appropriate number of plyometric exercises, and the appropriate acute variables specific to the phase of training your client will be working in (phases 1–5).

TABLE 11.1	Plyometric Training Program Design						
OPT Level	Phase(s)	Exercise	Number of Exercises	Sets	Reps	Tempo	Rest
Stabilization	1	Plyometric-stabilization exercises	0–2[a]	1–3	5–8	Controlled (hold stabilization position for 3–5 seconds)	0–90 s
Strength	2, 3, 4	Plyometric-strength exercises	0–4[b]	2–3	8–10	Medium (repeating)	0–60 s
Power	5	Plyometric-power exercises	0–2[c]	2–3	8–12	As fast as possible	0–60 s

[a]Reactive exercises may not be appropriate for an individual in this phase of training if he or she does not possess the appropriate amount of total body strength, core strength, and balance capabilities.
[b]Because of the goal of certain phases in this level (hypertrophy and maximal strength), plyometric training may not be necessary.
[c]Because one is performing plyometric-power exercises in the resistance training portion of this phase of training, separate plyometric exercises may not be necessary.

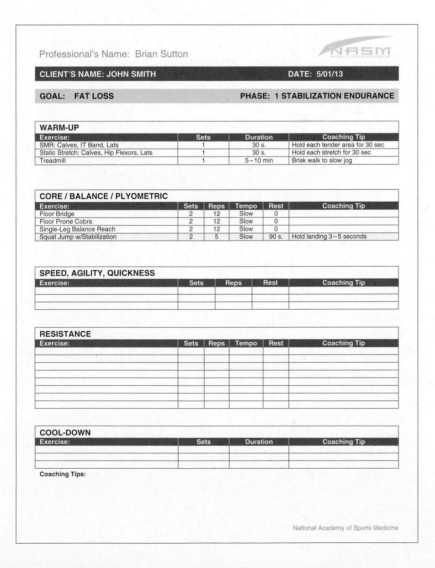

FIGURE 11.4

OPT template.

REFERENCES

1. Chu DA. Jumping into Plyometrics. 2nd ed. Champaign, IL: Human Kinetics; 1998.

2. Chmielewski TL, Myer GD, Kauffman D, Tillman SM. Plyometric exercise in the rehabilitation of athletes: physiological responses and clinical application. *J Orthop Sports Phys Ther.* 2006;36:308-319.

3. Lundin PE. A review of plyometric training. *Natl Strength Conditioning Assoc J.* 1985;73:65-70.

4. Kubo K, Kanehisa H, Kawakami Y, Fukunaga T. Influence of static stretching on viscoelastic properties of human tendon structures in vivo. *J Appl Physiol.* 2001;90:520-527.

5. Wilk KE, Voight ML, Keirns MA, Gambetta V, Andrews JR, Dillman CJ. Stretch-shortening drills for the upper extremities: theory and clinical application. *J Orthop Sports Phys Ther.* 1993;17:225-239.

6. Voight ML, Wieder DL. Comparative reflex response times of vastus medialis obliquus and vastus lateralis in normal subjects and subjects with extensor mechanism dysfunction. An electromyographic study. *Am J Sports Med.* 1991;19:131-137.

7. Wilson GJ, Wood GA, Elliott BC. Optimal stiffness of series elastic component in a stretch-shorten cycle activity. *J Appl Physiol.* 1991;70:825-833.

8. Ishikawa M, Niemelä E, Komi PV. Interaction between fascicle and tendinous tissues in short-contact stretch-shortening cycle exercise with varying eccentric intensities. *J Appl Physiol.* 2005;99:217-223.

9. Voight M, Draovitch P. Plyometrics. In: Albert M, eds. *Eccentric Muscle Training in Sports and Orthopedics.* New York: Churchill Livingstone; 1991:45-73.

10. Voight M, Brady D. Plyometrics. In: Devies GL, ed. *A Compendium of Isokinetics in Clinical Usage.* 4th ed. Onalaska WI: S&S Publishers, 1992. 226-240.

11. Allman FL. *Sports Medicine.* New York: Academic Press; 1974.

© Eky Studio/ShutterStock, Inc.

© ilolab/ShutterStock, Inc.

Speed, Agility, and Quickness Training

OBJECTIVES

After studying this chapter, you will be able to:

✔ Define and describe speed, agility, and quickness training and its purpose.

✔ Discuss the importance of speed, agility, and quickness training for a variety of populations.

✔ Design a speed, agility, and quickness training program for clients at any level of training.

✔ Perform, describe, and instruct various speed, agility, and quickness training exercises.

Concepts in Speed, Agility, and Quickness Training

The programming component of speed, agility, and quickness (SAQ) training is similar to plyometric (reactive) training in which the individual reacts to the ground surface in such a way that they develop larger than normal ground forces that can then be used to project the body with a greater velocity or speed of movement. The term *speed* as it is used throughout this text simply refers to the speed or velocity of distance covered divided by time (i.e., straight ahead speed). *Agility* refers to short bursts of movement that involve a change of movement direction, cadence, or speed. *Quickness* refers to the ability to react to a stimulus and appropriately change the motion of the body.

SAQ training allows clients to enhance their ability to accelerate, decelerate, and dynamically stabilize their entire body during higher-velocity acceleration and deceleration movements in all planes of motion (such as running, cutting, and changing direction). In addition, SAQ training may further help the nervous system to respond or react more efficiently to demands placed on it and enhance muscular recruitment and coordination when performed with correct mechanics (1).

Speed

Speed The ability to move the body in one intended direction as fast as possible.

Stride rate The number of strides taken in a given amount of time (or distance).

Stride length The distance covered with each stride.

Speed is the ability to move the body in one intended direction as fast as possible. It is the product of stride rate and stride length (2,3). **Stride rate** is the number of strides taken in a given amount of time (or distance). It may be improved with proper core strength, plyometric training, and technique. **Stride length** is the distance covered in one stride, during running. Although certain aspects of speed are dependent on genetic factors, it is a skill that can be learned through an integrated training program as seen in the OPT™ model (4). Magnitude of movement speed is relative and population specific. Movement speed should be addressed with a variety of populations, including both apparently healthy individuals and those with a chronic health condition or functional limitation because of its implications for power and force production, particularly of the lower limbs.

Proper Sprint Mechanics

Frontside mechanics Proper alignment of the lead leg and pelvis during sprinting, which includes ankle dorsiflexion, knee flexion, hip flexion, and neutral pelvis.

Backside mechanics Proper alignment of the rear leg and pelvis during sprinting, which includes ankle plantarflexion, knee extension, hip extension, and neutral pelvis.

Proper running mechanics allows the client to maximize force generation through biomechanical efficiency, allowing maximal movement velocity to be achieved in the shortest time possible. Two important aspects of sprint technique are frontside and backside mechanics. **Frontside mechanics** involves triple flexion of the ankle, knee, and hip in appropriate synchrony. Improved frontside mechanics is associated with better stability, less braking forces, and increased forward driving forces. **Backside mechanics** involves triple extension of the ankle, knee, and hip in appropriate synchrony. Improved backside mechanics are associated with a stronger push phase, including hip-knee extension, gluteal contraction, and backside arm drive. Frontside and backside mechanics work in synchrony to apply force to the ground, recover from a stride cycle, and propel the body forward effectively. When executing either frontside or backside mechanics drills, it is essential that the pelvis stay neutral to facilitate proper range of motion and force production **Table 12.1**.

Agility

Agility The ability to accelerate, decelerate, stabilize, and change direction quickly while maintaining proper posture.

Agility is the ability to start (or accelerate), stop (or decelerate and stabilize), and change direction quickly, while maintaining proper posture (5). Agility requires high levels of neuromuscular efficiency to be able to maintain one's center of gravity over their base of support while changing directions at various speeds. Agility training can enhance eccentric neuromuscular coordination, dynamic flexibility, dynamic postural control, functional core strength, and proprioception. Proper agility training can also help prevent injury by enhancing the body's ability to effectively control eccentric forces in all planes of motion as well as by improving the structural integrity of the connective tissue. Proper technique for agility drills should follow the guidelines in Table 12.1.

TABLE 12.1	Kinetic Chain Checkpoints During Running Movements
Body Position	**Comments**
Foot/ankle complex	The foot and ankle should be pointing straight ahead in a dorsiflexed position when it hits the ground.
	Excessive flattening or external rotation of the foot will create abnormal stress throughout the rest of the kinetic chain and decrease overall performance.
Knee complex	The knees must remain straight ahead.
	If the athlete demonstrates excessive adduction and internal rotation of the femur during the stance phase, it decreases force production and leads to overuse injuries.
Lumbo-pelvic-hip complex (LPHC)	The body should have a slight lean during acceleration.
	During maximal velocity, the LPHC should be fairly neutral, without excessive extension or flexion, unless to reach for an object.
Head	The head should remain in line with the LPHC, and the LPHC should be in line with the legs.
	The head and neck should not compensate and move into extension, unless necessary to track an object (such as a ball), as this can affect the position of the LPHC (pelvo-ocular reflex).

Quickness

Quickness (or reaction time) is the ability to react and change body position with maximal rate of force production, in all planes of motion and from all body positions, during functional activities. Quickness involves the ability to assess visual, auditory, or kinesthetic stimuli and to provide the appropriate physical response as fast as possible (such as hitting a baseball or swerving to avoid a car accident). Proper technique for quickness drills should follow the guidelines in Table 12.1.

Quickness The ability to react and change body position with maximal rate of force production, in all planes of motion and from all body positions, during functional activities.

Speed, Agility, and Quickness for Nonathletic Populations

Although speed, agility, and quickness training is a widely used and accepted way to improve sports performance in athletes, components of an SAQ program can also significantly improve the physical health profile of apparently healthy sedentary adults and those with medical or health limitations. The increased neuromuscular, biomechanical, and physiological demand for such training can aid in weight loss, coordination, movement proficiency, and injury prevention when applied safely and effectively as seen in the OPT model. In addition, individuals from a variety of populations find SAQ training fun and invigorating, increasing exercise compliance, adherence, and effectiveness.

Unlike the more common steady-state, moderate-intensity modalities (such as treadmill walking) often prescribed for nonathletic populations, SAQ drills require greater integration of a variety of the body's biologic systems. An individual must accelerate, decelerate, and change direction, all in response to a variety of both predictable and unpredictable stimuli at a relatively high rate of speed. Thus, SAQ training provides a unique challenge to the biologic systems of nonathletic individuals, facilitating constant responses and adaptation. Such rapid adaptation to SAQ training is critical in the development, maintenance, and improvement of neuromuscular, physiologic, and biomechanical proficiency from childhood through the senior years. Because of the elevated intensity of biologic demand with SAQ protocols, it is essential that personal trainers perform extensive client evaluations examining exercise experience, movement quality, health history, and injury profile before beginning an SAQ training program. Moreover, SAQ training should always follow a comprehensive warm-up protocol.

SAQ Training Programs for Youth

Children are constantly growing, developing, and maturing until early adulthood. From birth, children are programmed to develop progressively higher neuromuscular capabilities in line with their physical and mental maturation. Much of this development is innate at the very early stages, for example, crawling progresses to standing, standing progresses to walking, and walking progresses to running. Once a child has developed basic ambulation, the rate and magnitude at which he or she progresses beyond that point often depend on an external interaction with the environment (6). To continue developing effectively, the environment must challenge children's biologic systems; in other words, they must learn through external measures how to adapt and apply appropriate movement patterns.

SAQ training for youth is an effective way of providing a variety of exposures to various physiologic, neuromuscular, and biomechanical demands, resulting in the further development of physical ability. The majority of youth today spend little if any time performing generalized, unstructured physical activity (play-time) that would facilitate the development of SAQ skills (7). SAQ programs for youth have been found to decrease the likelihood of athletic injury (6–10), increase the likelihood of exercise participation later in life (11,12), and improve physical fitness (13,14).

Example SAQ Drills for Youth Populations

Red Light, Green Light

1. Participants line up shoulder-to-shoulder along the base of a designated field (minimum, 20 yards long).
2. One participant is chosen as the "stop light" and begins at the opposite end of the field.
3. The stop light turns his or her back to the other participants and calls "green light."
4. On calling green light, the participants all move as quickly as possible toward the stop light.
5. Still with his or her back to the group, the stop light yells "red light!" and then immediately turns around.
6. On hearing red light, the participants are to stop movement and remain motionless.
7. If the stop light sees anyone move, he or she calls them to start over at the base of the field.
8. This is repeated at arbitrary intervals until a participant is able to reach and touch the stop light.
9. This participant then becomes the stop light.

Follow the Snake

1. The instructor or trainer lays 5–10 jump ropes (or one long rope) on the ground in a random *S* type pattern.
2. Participants line up on one side of the ropes and keeping a foot on each side of the rope, they follow the pattern of the rope first forward to the end, then backward to the beginning.
3. Participants can be timed to create a competition.

SAQ Training for Weight Loss

Interval training in which participants exhibit short, repeated bouts of high-intensity activity has been found to be highly effective in improving a variety of health-related factors. High-intensity, short-duration programs have been found to match or surpass results for functional capacity, muscular power, fat and weight loss, and other metabolic adaptations when compared with moderate-intensity, long-duration exercise protocols (15–20). The high-intensity, short bouts of SAQ drills make them a valid choice for interval training modalities with appropriate nonathletic populations. Although athletes use these drills to improve their sport-specific abilities, weight-loss clients benefit from the increased exercise intensity and variety of movements offered. The exercise variety provides further benefit by making a program fun and engaging for the participant, increasing adherence (21). When designing SAQ programs for weight loss, the primary focus of the program is to keep the heart rate appropriately elevated to increase fat oxidation and caloric expenditure. This can be done by creating a small circuit of SAQ exercises. However, it is critical that a thorough evaluation be administered before beginning an SAQ protocol with a weight-loss client and exercise intensities remain appropriate based on the client's abilities and fitness level.

SAQ Circuits for Weight-Loss Populations

Circuit 1

A. Jump Rope: 30 seconds (using various foot patterns)
B. Rest 20 seconds
C. Cone Shuffles: 30 seconds

    a. Place 8 cones in a line about 30 inches apart.
    b. Participant lines up facing the line of cones.
    c. The participant lowers his or her center of gravity and side-shuffles in and out of the cones without hitting them.
    d. Participant first performs this facing forward and then facing backward,
    e. This is repeated for the duration of the station.
    f. Other foot patterns such as forward, backward, and stepping over the cones can be used as well.

D. Rest 20 seconds
E. Any 3 Ladder Drills: 30 seconds (see Agility Ladder Drills)

Circuit 2

A. 5-10-5 Drill: 30 seconds (see 5-10-5 Drill)
B. Rest 20 seconds
C. Modified Box Drill: 30 seconds (see Modified Box Drill)
D. Rest 20 seconds
E. Partner Mirror Drill: 30 seconds

    a. Place two cones 10 yards apart.
    b. Two participants stand in between the cones facing one another.
    c. One partner is designated the "leader," the other is designated the "mirror."
    d. Staying in between the cones, the leader moves in a variety of patterns, shuffling, jumping, dropping to the ground, turning around, etc.
    e. The mirror is to mimic the motion of the leader without falling behind.
    f. The leader and the mirror switch each time the drill is done.

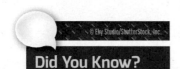

Did You Know?

High-intensity interval training can burn more subcutaneous fat than long-duration, low-to-moderate–intensity endurance training (20).

SAQ Training for Seniors

A primary function of SAQ training in seniors is to prevent age-related decreases in bone density, coordinative ability, and muscular power. This aids in the prevention of injury and an increase in the quality of life (22,23). Although some loss of physiologic, neuromuscular, and biomechanical capacity is an inevitability of the aging process, recent research has determined that these losses can be minimized by appropriate exercise interventions. Osteopenia, or loss of bone density, is often related to the aging processes, particularly in women. This increases the likelihood for fractures and other acute and chronic skeletal disorders such as osteoporosis. Research has determined that properly administered programs requiring an elevated degree of load on the skeletal system such as those found in SAQ protocols are safe and effective in slowing and potentially reversing osteopenia in older adults (24,25).

Movement confidence and proficiency are essential in senior populations to aid in the prevention of falls and maintain activities of daily life. The coordinative abilities required for safe, effective movement often dissipate with age as a result of under-use (26). To maintain and improve these abilities, it is essential that older populations practice coordinative skills on a regular basis. SAQ-based programs have been found to increase coordinative ability and movement confidence, eliciting a decreased likelihood of falling or other movement-related injury (27,28).

Sarcopenia, or age-related loss of skeletal muscle mass, can be detrimental to maintaining functional capacity in older adults. Resistance training as well as SAQ-based interventions has been found to help slow and reverse this process. Of particular relevance to slowing and reversing sarcopenia are interventions requiring increased speed of movement and rate of force production similar to those found in SAQ protocols (29–31).

When designing an SAQ program for seniors, the personal trainer must take specialized care in ensuring safety for the participants. Drills should focus around activities the individuals will need for daily life such as standing up from a chair, walking up stairs, navigating ground obstacles, etc.

Did You Know?

A 10% loss of bone density at the hip can result in a 2.5 times greater risk for hip fracture (32).

SAQ Drills for Seniors

Varied Size Cone/Hurdle Step-Overs

1. In a line 10–15 yards long, place various size cones, hurdles, and other objects about 24 inches apart.
2. Participants line up facing sideways to the line of objects and step over each, moving down the line and then back to the start.
3. Participants can be timed.

Stand-Up to Figure 8

1. The participant begins seated in a chair.
2. Two cones are placed directly in front of the chair, the first 10–15 feet away; the second is 20–25 feet away, directly behind it.
3. On the instructor's command, the participant stands up from the chair as quickly as possible.
4. Then, as quickly as possible, he or she moves to the left of the first cone, then to the right of the second cone while turning around to come back to the chair to complete a "figure 8" around the cones.
5. Participant then repeats the figure 8 in the opposite direction and finishes by sitting in the chair.
6. Participant is timed.

SUMMARY

Similar to plyometric training, speed, agility, and quickness training emphasizes prescribing modalities to improve one's ability to quickly and efficiently create a relatively high rate of movement in the appropriate direction and orientation dependent on a variety of stimuli. The physiologic, neuromuscular, and biomechanical demands presented by an SAQ training program can benefit athletic as well as nonathletic clientele. These benefits are seen in the development, improvement, and maintenance of physical fitness and functional ability throughout the course of life.

SAQ Drills and Programming Strategies

SAQ exercises should be integrated carefully into a client's overall training program. It should be emphasized that the programming guidelines presented in Table 12.2 are only meant to be suggestions and should be gauged on the total volume of training for all components (core, balance, plyometric, and resistance) in a workout. As the demands for movement speed and reactivity increase, so does the risk of injury. The safety and success of an SAQ program is dependent on the client's core, balance, and reactive capabilities. The better a personal trainer can match drills appropriate to the client's capabilities, the more safe and effective the program will be. All exercises should be performed with precise technique and kinetic chain control to minimize risk of injury.

TABLE 12.2 SAQ Program Design					
OPT Level	Phase(s)	SAQ Exercise	Sets	Reps	Rest
Stabilization	1	4–6 drills with limited horizontal inertia and unpredictability such as Cone Shuffles and Agility Ladder Drills	1–2	2–3 each	0–90 s
Strength	2, 3, 4	6–8 drills allowing greater horizontal inertia but limited unpredictability such as the 5-10-5, T-Drill, Box Drill, Stand Up to Figure 8, etc.	3–4	3–5 of each	0–60 s
Power	5	6–10 drills allowing maximal horizontal inertia and unpredictability such as Modified Box Drill, Partner Mirror Drill, and timed drills.	3–5	3–5 of each	0–90 s

SAQ SPEED LADDER DRILLS

One-Ins

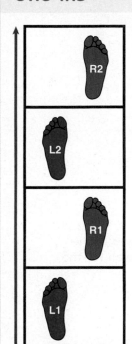

Two-Ins

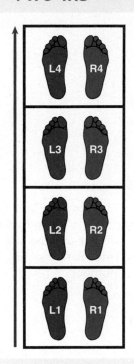

Side Shuffle

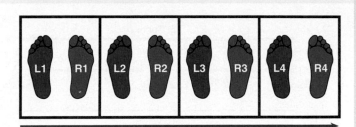

In-In-Out-Out

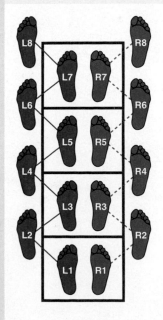

In-In-Out (Zigzag)

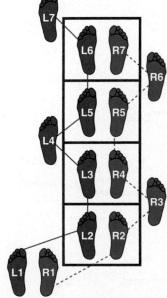
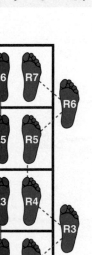

Ali Shuffle

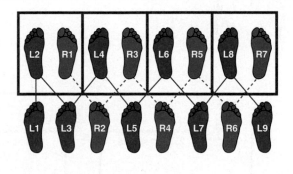

SAQ CONE DRILLS

5-10-5 Drill

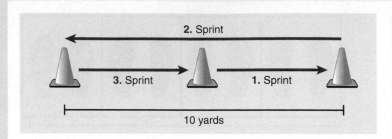

2. Sprint

3. Sprint   1. Sprint

10 yards

Modified Box Drill

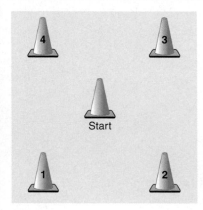

4   3

Start

1   2

For this drill, the client begins at the middle cone. The trainer then calls out a cone number and the client moves to the appropriate cone and returns to the middle to wait for the trainer to call another number.

T-Drill

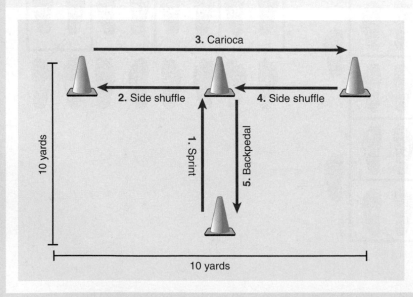

3. Carioca

2. Side shuffle   4. Side shuffle

10 yards

1. Sprint

5. Backpedal

10 yards

SAQ CONE DRILLS *continued*

Box Drill

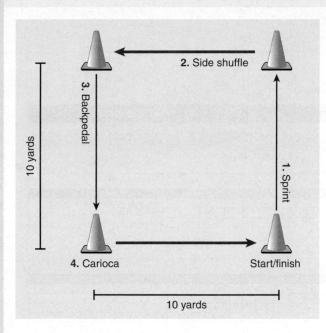

L.E.F.T. Drill

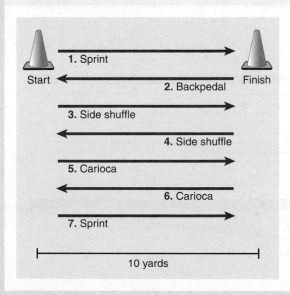

Filling in the Template

As mentioned previously, SAQ training can be used by athletic and nonathletic populations and does not need to be reserved for athletes who solely have performance enhancement goals. Performance enhancement is relative to the needs of the individual. **Figure 12.1** shows how a workout template would look and where speed, agility, and

FIGURE 12.1

Filled-out SAQ section of the template.

Professional's Name: Brian Sutton

NASM

CLIENT'S NAME: JOHN SMITH		DATE: 5/01/13

GOAL: FAT LOSS	PHASE: 1 STABILIZATION ENDURANCE

WARM-UP

Exercise:	Sets	Duration	Coaching Tip
SMR: Calves, IT Band, Adductors	1	30 s.	Hold each tender area for 30 sec
Static Stretch: Calves, Hip Flexors, Adductors	1	30 s.	Hold each stretch for 30 sec
Treadmill	1	5 – 10 min	Brisk walk to slow jog

CORE / BALANCE / PLYOMETRIC

Exercise:	Sets	Reps	Tempo	Rest	Coaching Tip
Floor Bridge	2	12	Slow	0	
Floor Prone Cobra	2	12	Slow	0	
Single-Leg Balance Reach	2	12	Slow	0	
Squat Jump w/Stabilization	2	5	Slow	90 s.	Hold landing 3 – 5 seconds

SPEED, AGILITY, QUICKNESS

Exercise:	Sets	Reps	Rest	Coaching Tip
Cone Shuffles	1	2	60 s.	
1-ins, 2-ins, In-In-Out-Out, Ali Shuffle	1	2	60 s.	

RESISTANCE

Exercise:	Sets	Reps	Tempo	Rest	Coaching Tip

COOL-DOWN

Exercise:	Sets	Duration	Coaching Tip

Coaching Tips:

National Academy of Sports Medicine

quickness exercises would be performed when implemented into an integrated OPT workout. If speed, agility, and quickness training are to be used in the program, you will refer to Table 12.2 for the appropriate type of exercises, the appropriate number of exercises, and the appropriate acute variables specific to the phase of training your client will be working in (phases 1–5).

However, owing to its uniqueness and versatility, SAQ training can also be used as its own workout separate from an integrated training program. In this instance, the volume of the program will typically be higher depending on the capabilities, goals, and conditioning level of the client.

SUMMARY

Programming guidelines must be gauged on the total volume of training for all components in a workout. A client's core, balance, and reactive capabilities will determine the success and safety of the program. Precise technique and kinetic chain control are required to minimize risk of injury. Various speed ladders, cone drills, and other drills requiring the attributes of speed, agility, and quickness may be used in the programming.

REFERENCES

1. Brown LE, Ferrigno VA, Santana JC. *Training for Speed, Agility, and Quickness.* Champaign, IL: Human Kinetics; 2000.
2. Luhtanen P, Komi PV. Mechanical factors influencing running speed. In: Asmussen E, Jorgensen K, eds. *Biomechanics: VI-B.* Baltimore, MD: University Park Press, 1978:23-29.
3. Mero A, Komi PV, Gregor RJ. Biomechanics of sprint running. *Sports Med.* 1992;13(6):376-392.
4. Salonikidis K, Zafeiridis A. The effects of plyometric, tennis-drills, and combined training on reaction, lateral and linear speed, power, and strength in novice tennis players. *J Strength Cond. Res* 2008;22(1):182-191.
5. Parsons LS, Jones MT. Development of speed, quickness and agility for tennis athletes. *Strength Cond J.* 1998;20:14-19.
6. Drabik J. *Children and Sports Training.* Island Pond, VT: Stadion Publishing; 1996.
7. Sokolove M. *Warrior Girls.* New York, NY: Simon & Schuster; 2008.
8. Etty Griffin LY. Neuromuscular training and injury prevention in sports. *Clin Orthop Relat Res.* 2003;409:53-60.
9. Olsen OE, Myklebust G, Engebretsen L, Holme I, Bahr R. Exercises to prevent lower limb injuries in youth sports: cluster randomised control group. *BMJ.* 2005;330:449.
10. Ortega FB, Ruiz JR, Castillo MJ, Sjöström M. Physical fitness in childhood and adolescence: a powerful marker of health. *Int J Obes (Lond).* 2008;32:1-11.
11. Wrotniak BH, Epstein LH, Dorn JM, Jones KE, Kondilis VA. The relationship between motor proficiency and physical activity in children. *Pediatrics.* 2006;118(6):e1758-1765.
12. Janz K, Dawson J, Mahoney L. Increases in physical fitness during childhood improve cardiovascular health during adolescence: the Muscatine Study. *Int J Sports Med.* 2002;23 (Suppl 1):15-21.
13. Balciunas M, Stonkus S, Abrantes C, Sampaio J. Long term effects of different training modalities on power, speed, skill, and anaerobic capacity in young male basketball players. *J Sports Sci Med.* 2006;5:163-170.
14. Ruiz JR, Rizzo NS, Hurtig-Wennlöf A, Ortega FB, Wärnberg J, Sjöström M. Relations of total physical activity and intensity to fitness and fatness in children: the European Youth Heart Study. *Am J Clin Nutr.* 2006;84(2):299-303.
15. Gibala MJ, Little JP, van Essen M, et al. Short-term sprint interval versus traditional endurance training: similar initial adaptations in human skeletal muscle and exercise performance. *J Physiol.* 2006;575:901-911.
16. Iaia FM, Hellsten Y, Nielsen JJ, Fernström M, Sahlin K, Bangsbo J. Four weeks of speed endurance training reduces energy expenditure during exercise and maintains muscle oxidative capacity despite a reduction in training volume. *J Appl Physiol.* 2009;106:73-80.
17. Schmidt D, Biwer C, Kalscheuer L. Effects of long versus short bout exercise on fitness and weight loss in overweight females. *J Am Coll Nutr.* 2001;20(5):494-501.
18. Talanian JL, Galloway SD, Heigenhauser GJ, Bonen A, Spriet LL. Two weeks of high intensity aerobic interval training increases the capacity for fat oxidation during exercise in women. *J Appl Physiol.* 2007;102:1439-1447.

19. Tjønna AE, Lee SJ, Rognmo Ø, et al. Aerobic interval training versus continuous moderate exercise as a treatment for the metabolic syndrome: a pilot study. *Circulation*. 2008;118:346-354.

20. Trembley A, Simaneau J, Bouchard C. Impact of exercise intensity on body fatness and skeletal muscle metabolism. *Metabolism*. 1994;43(7):814-818.

21. Jakicic JM, Wing RR, Butler BA, Robertson RJ. Prescribing exercise in multiple short bouts versus one continuous bout: effects on adherence, cardiorespiratory fitness, and weight loss in overweight women. *Int J Obes Relat Metab Disord*. 1995;19(12):893-901.

22. Liu-Ambrose TY, Khan KM, Eng JJ, Lord SR, Lentle B, McKay HA. Both resistance and agility training reduce back pain and improve health-related quality of life in older women with low bone mass. *Osteoporos Int*. 2005;16(11):1321-1329.

23. Bean J, Kiely D, Herman S, et al. The relationship between leg power and physiological performance in mobility-limited people. *J Am Geriatr Soc*. 2002;50(3):461-467.

24. Heinonen A, Kannus P, Sievänen H, et al. Randomised controlled trial of effect of high-impact exercise on select risk factors for osteoporotic fractures. *Lancet*. 1996;348(9038):1343-1347.

25. Iwamoto J, Takeda T, Ichimura S. Effect of exercise training and detraining on bone mineral density in postmenopausal women with osteoporosis. *J Orthop Sci*. 2001;6(2):128-132.

26. Laroche DP, Knight CA, Dickie JL, Lussier M, Roy SJ. Explosive force and fractionated reaction time in elderly low-and high-active women. *Med Sci Sports Exerc*. 2007;39(9):1659-1665.

27. Liu-Ambrose T, Khan KM, Eng JJ, Janssen PA, Lord SR, McKay HA. Resistance and agility training reduce fall risk in women aged 75 to 85 with low bone mass: A 6-month randomized, controlled trial. *J Am Geriatr Soc*. 2004;52(5):657-665.

28. Sundstrup E, Jakobsen MD, Andersen JL, et al. Muscle function and postural balance in lifelong trained male footballers compared with sedentary men and youngsters. *Scand J Med Sci Sports*. 2010;20(Suppl 1):90-97.

29. Newton RU, Hakkinen K, Hakkinen A, McCormick M, Volek J, Kraemer WJ. Mixed-methods resistance training increases power and strength of young and older men. *Med Sci Sports Exerc*. 2002;34(8):1367-1375.

30. Porter MM. Power training for older adults. *Appl Physiol Nutr Metab*. 2006;31:87-94.

31. Bean JF, Herman S, Kiely DK, et al. Increased velocity exercise specific to task (InVEST) training: a pilot study exploring effects on leg power, balance, and mobility in community-dwelling older women. *J Am Geriatr Soc*. 2004;52:799-804.

32. Klotzbuecher CM, Ross PD, Landsman PB, Abbott TA 3rd, Berger M. Patients with prior fractures have an increased risk of future fractures: A summary of the literature and statistical synthesis. *J Bone Miner Res*. 2000;15:721-739.

Resistance Training Concepts

After studying this chapter, you will be able to:

☑ Describe the stages of the general adaptation syndrome.

☑ Define and describe the principle of adaptation and specificity.

☑ Define stability, muscular endurance, muscular hypertrophy, strength, and power.

☑ List and define the various stages of strength and training systems.

Introduction to Resistance Training

The final step in completing the OPT™ template is planning the resistance training component of an exercise program. The resistance training section of the OPT template requires filling in the appropriate exercises for each body part (chest, back, shoulders, legs, etc.), the sets, repetitions, tempo (speed of repetition), and rest interval (amount of rest between each exercise) based on assessment outcomes and goals for each client. Personal trainers need to understand the science and principles of resistance training to be effective at designing individually tailored safe and appropriate resistance training workouts. This chapter explores some of the most important concepts involved in designing and implementing resistance training programs for a variety of clients. The focus of this chapter includes principles of adaptation, progressive strength adaptations derived from resistance training, training systems used to acquire strength, and specific resistance training exercise progressions.

Principle of Adaptation

One of the many unique qualities of the human body is its ability to adapt or adjust its functional capacity to meet the desired needs **Figure 13.1** (1–6). The ability of the human body to respond and adapt to an exercise stimulus is perhaps one of the

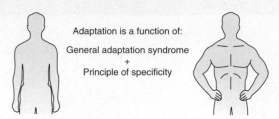

FIGURE 13.1

Resistance training
principle of adaptation.

most important concepts of training and conditioning. Some form of adaptation is the primary goal of most exercise training programs. Whether the goal is cosmetic in nature or health- or performance-related, resistance training has been shown to produce a variety of desirable effects Table 13.1.

General Adaptation Syndrome

The optimal state for the human movement system to be in is one of physiologic balance or homeostasis. The **general adaptation syndrome** (GAS) is a term used to describe how the body responds and adapts to stress. In this case the stress being placed on the body is the weight being lifted during resistance training. This general pattern of adaptation was first described by Hans Selye, a Canadian physician, who stated that exercise, including resistance training, can be considered a good form of stress called "eustress" that over time allows the human movement system to adapt and thus be able to maintain homeostatic states under a variety of conditions. For adaptation to occur, the body must be confronted with a stressor or some form of stress that creates the need for a response Table 13.2 (6). Selye outlined three stages of response to stress (6):

**General adaptation
syndrome** a term used
to describe how the body
responds and adapts to
stress.

◆   Alarm reaction
◆   Resistance development
◆   Exhaustion

TABLE 13.1	Adaptive Benefits of Resistance Training	

© ilolab/ShutterStock, Inc.

Physiologic	Physical	Performance
Improved cardiovascular efficiency	Increased tissue (muscle, tendons, ligaments) tensile strength	Increased neuromuscular control (coordination)
Beneficial endocrine (hormone) and serum lipid (cholesterol) adaptations	Increased cross-sectional area of muscle fibers	Increased endurance
Increased bone density	Decreased body fat	Increased strength
Increased metabolic efficiency (metabolism)		Increased power

TABLE 13.2	The General Adaptation Syndrome
Stage	**Reaction**
Alarm reaction	Initial reaction to stressor such as increased oxygen and blood supply to the necessary areas of the body
Resistance development	Increased functional capacity to adapt to stressor such as increasing motor unit recruitment
Exhaustion	A prolonged intolerable stressor produces fatigue and leads to a breakdown in the system or injury

Alarm Reaction Stage

The **alarm reaction** is the initial reaction to a stressor. The alarm reaction activates a number of physiological and psychological protective processes within the body. During the initial sessions of resistance training programs, the body is forced to try and adapt to increased amounts of force on bones, joints, muscles, connective tissues, and the nervous system. During the alarm stage of resistance training, numerous physiologic responses occur, including an increase in oxygen and blood supply as well as neural recruitment to the working muscles. Initially, an individual's body may be very inefficient at responding to the demands placed on it during resistance training. But gradually over time and by applying the principle of progressive overload, the body increases its ability to meet the demands being placed on it (6).

Consider the typical response to either unaccustomed exercise or a sudden increase in a training program. The new work is performed, and during the next 2 to 3 days, the muscles may exhibit classic **delayed-onset muscle soreness** or DOMS (7). During this period of DOMS, any attempt at replicating or advancing the soreness-inducing exercise will be limited by the factors contributing to the soreness. This could be considered an "alarm reaction." Most experts agree minimizing DOMS involves starting a progressive training program at a low intensity and introducing overload gradually (7).

Resistance Development Stage

During the **resistance development** stage, the body increases its functional capacity to adapt to the stressor. After repeated training sessions, the human movement system will increase its capability to efficiently recruit muscle fibers and distribute oxygen and blood to the proper areas in the body. Once adaptation has occurred, the body will require increased stress or overload to produce a new response and a higher level of fitness (6).

Personal trainers often understand this adaptation response, but use it improperly by *only* manipulating the amount of weight the client uses when, in fact, this is but one of many ways to increase stress on the body. Chapter fourteen will discuss the importance of manipulating the many acute variables (sets, reps, intensity, rest periods, exercise selection, etc.) for optimal adaptation while avoiding breakdown or exhaustion.

In the example of unaccustomed exercise, once the DOMS subsides, further work will be met with less and less soreness so that performance may gradually advance. This would be "resistance development." Performance will continue to improve until some new performance plateau is reached and will be maintained if training is maintained.

Alarm reaction The alarm reaction is the initial reaction to a stressor.

Delayed-onset muscle soreness Pain or discomfort often felt 24 to 72 hours after intense exercise or unaccustomed physical activity.

Resistance development The body increases its functional capacity to adapt to the stressor.

Exhaustion Stage

Exhaustion Prolonged stress or stress that is intolerable and will produce exhaustion or distress to the system.

Prolonged stress or intolerable amounts of stress can lead to **exhaustion** or distress. When a stressor is too much for any one of the physiologic systems to handle, it causes a breakdown or injury such as (6):

♦ Stress fractures
♦ Muscle strains
♦ Joint pain
♦ Emotional fatigue

In turn, many of these types of injuries can lead to the initiation of the cumulative injury cycle.

Avoiding the pitfalls of the exhaustion stage is one of the main reasons for using the OPT model (a systematic, progressive training program) that is based on science and proven application. Resistance training, as well as other forms of training, must be cycled through different stages that increase stress placed on the human movement system, but also allow for sufficient rest and recuperation periods. The term used to describe this approach, in which a training program is divided into smaller, progressive stages, is **periodization**. Additional information on periodization of training (OPT model) is detailed in chapter 14.

Periodization Division of a training program into smaller, progressive stages.

In the above example, if the resistance is continually increased with the intention of stressing specific muscles or muscle groups to produce an increase in size or strength, it can lead to injury of the muscle, joint, or connective tissue, especially if the resistance is added too quickly or inadequate rest and recovery periods are not planned for. Training-related injuries occur more often to connective tissue (such as ligaments and tendons) than muscles because connective tissues lack blood supply (8). Different tissues in the body (muscle fibers versus connective tissue) each have their own adaptive potential to stresses. Thus, training programs should provide a variety of intensities and stresses to optimize the adaptation of each tissue to ensure the best possible results. Adaptation can be more specifically applied to certain aspects of the human movement system depending on the training technique(s) used, which is the basis of the principle of specificity.

© Sky Studio/ShutterStock, Inc.

Did You Know?

Overtraining syndrome commonly occurs in athletes or fitness enthusiasts who are training beyond the body's ability to recover. When an individual is performing excessive amounts of exercise without proper rest and recovery, there may be some harmful side effects. Some of these side effects may include decreased performance, fatigue, altered hormonal states, poor sleeping patterns, reproductive disorders, decreased immunity, loss of appetite, and mood disturbances (9).

The Principle of Specificity: The SAID Principle

The **principle of specificity**, often referred as the SAID (**specific adaptation to imposed demands**) principle, states that the body will specifically adapt to the type of demand placed on it. For example, if someone repeatedly lifts heavy weights, that person will produce higher levels of maximal strength. Conversely, if a person repeatedly lifts lighter weights for many repetitions, that person will develop higher levels of muscular endurance.

According to the principle of specificity, training programs should reflect the desired outcome(s). When applying the SAID principle to any training program, it is important to remember that the body is made up of many types of tissues, and these tissues may respond differently to the same stimulus. To make the principle of specificity a safe and effective tool, it must be used appropriately.

Remember that type I muscle fibers function differently than type II muscle fibers. Type I or slow-twitch muscle fibers are smaller in diameter, slower to produce maximal tension, and more resistant to fatigue. Type I fibers are important for muscles that need to produce long-term contractions necessary for stabilization, endurance, and postural control. Type II or fast-twitch muscle fibers are larger in size, quick to produce maximal tension, and fatigue more quickly than type I fibers. These fibers are important for muscles producing movements requiring force and power such as performing a sprint. To train with higher intensities, proper postural stabilization is required. Therefore, tissues need to be trained differently to prepare them for higher levels of training. This is the specific purpose behind periodization and the OPT model **Figure 13.2**.

The degree of adaptation that occurs during training is directly related to the mechanical, neuromuscular, and metabolic specificity of the training program (3,5). To effectively achieve program goals for clients, personal trainers need to consistently evaluate the need to manipulate the exercise routine to meet actual training goals. Remember, the body can only adapt if it has a reason to adapt.

Principle of specificity or **specific adaptation to imposed demands (SAID principle)** Principle that states the body will adapt to the specific demands that are placed on it.

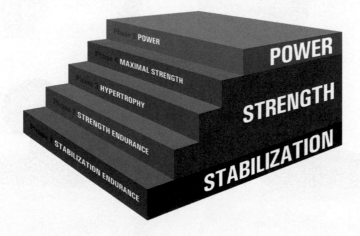

FIGURE 13.2

The OPT model.

Mechanical specificity
Refers to the weight and movements placed on the body.

Neuromuscular specificity Refers to the speed of contraction and exercise selection.

Metabolic specificity Refers to the energy demand placed on the body.

♦ **Mechanical specificity** refers to the weight and movements placed on the body (3,5). To develop muscular endurance of the legs requires light weights and high repetitions when performing leg-related exercises. To develop maximal strength in the chest, heavy weights must be used during chest-related exercises.

♦ **Neuromuscular specificity** refers to the speed of contraction and exercise selection (10–12). To develop higher levels of stability while pushing, chest exercises will need to be performed with controlled, unstable exercises, at slower speeds **Figure 13.3**. To develop higher levels of strength, exercises should be performed in more stable environments with heavier loads to place more of an emphasis on the prime movers **Figure 13.4**. To develop higher levels of power, low-weight, high-velocity contractions must be performed in a plyometric manner **Figure 13.5**.

♦ **Metabolic specificity** refers to the energy demand placed on the body. To develop endurance, training will require prolonged bouts of exercise, with minimal rest periods between sets. Endurance training primarily uses aerobic pathways to supply energy for the body. To develop maximal strength or power, training will require longer rest periods, so the intensity of each bout of exercise remains high. Energy will be supplied primarily via the anaerobic pathways (13,14).

FIGURE 13.3

Training for stability.

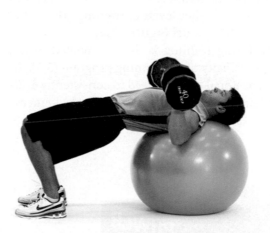
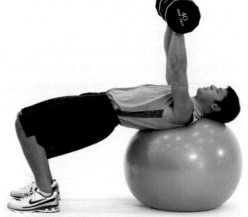

FIGURE 13.4

Training for strength.

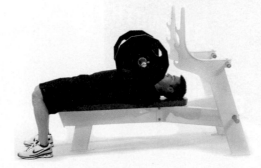
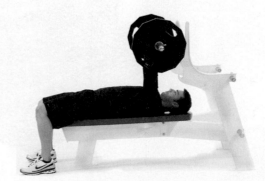

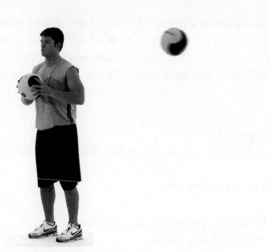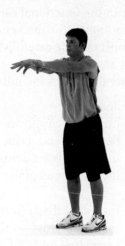

FIGURE 13.5

Training for power.

It is important for personal trainers to remember that a client's training program should be designed to meet the specific demands of their daily life and health and wellness goals. The following example applies the concept of specificity to a client whose goal is body fat reduction (15–18).

1. Mechanically, the body burns more calories when movements are performed while standing (versus a seated or lying position) and using moderate weights. An example would be performing standing cable rows versus seated machine rows.
2. From a neuromuscular standpoint, the body burns more calories when more muscles are being used for longer periods in controlled, unstable environments. An example would be performing a single-leg dumbbell shoulder press versus a seated machine shoulder press.
3. Metabolically, the body burns more calories when rest periods are short to minimize full recuperation. An example would be to have your clients perform resistance training exercises in a circuit fashion with no rests between sets.

Applying the principles of specificity to a training program for weight loss, the client should perform the majority of exercises while standing and using moderate weights. The client should also recruit and use as many muscles as possible during each exercise and carefully monitor rest periods for greater caloric expenditure.

SUMMARY

A well-designed, integrated training program produces optimal levels of:

- Flexibility
- Endurance
- Neuromuscular control
- Alterations in body composition
- Strength
- Power

To achieve optimal training results, the body must adapt to specifically imposed demands and stresses. The ability to adapt to stress is known as the general adaptation syndrome. There are three stages of response to stress: (1a) alarm reaction (or initial activation of protective processes within the body), (b) resistance development (or an increase in the functional capacity to adapt to a stressor), and (c) exhaustion (or stress that is too much for the system and causes an injury). To avoid injury, adaptive programs must include carefully and methodically planned (periodization) cycles through different stages, which allows for sufficient rest and recuperation. Adaptive programs have several benefits, including:

- Physiologic
  - » Improved cardiovascular efficiency
  - » Beneficial endocrine (hormone) and serum lipid (cholesterol) adaptations
  - » Increased bone density
  - » Increased metabolic efficiency (metabolism)
- Physical
  - » Increased tissue (muscles, tendons, ligaments) tensile strength
  - » Increased cross-sectional area of muscle fibers
  - » Decreased body fat
- Performance
  - » Increased neuromuscular control (coordination)
  - » Increased endurance
  - » Increased strength
  - » Increased power

The type of training adaptation and the goals of the client should determine (or dictate) the design of the training program. There are different types of strength and different systems of strength training that can be used to create a more individualized and systematic program for clients. In addition, different tissues in the body each respond to different stresses as seen in the principle of specificity or specific adaptation to imposed demands (or SAID principle). Training programs should provide a variety of intensities and stresses to optimize the adaptation of each tissue to ensure the best possible results. The degree of adaptation that occurs during training is directly related to the mechanical, neuromuscular, and metabolic specificity of the training program.

Progressive Adaptations from Resistance Training

The concept of adaptation makes it clear that some type of change will occur based on the stresses placed on the body. Resistance training programs are designed to produce changes that result in various adaptations. Whether the goal is to increase muscle endurance, strength, hypertrophy, or power or to reduce body fat and improve overall health, the use of resistance training is an important component of any fitness program. This will help ensure optimal health and longevity for the client. As clients develop greater strength and endurance, they can train for longer periods before reaching the exhaustion stage (general adaptation syndrome), which leads to greater degrees of change and adaptation realized over time. The main adaptations that occur from resistance training include stabilization, muscular endurance, hypertrophy, strength, and power.

Stabilization

Stabilization is the human movement system's ability to provide optimal dynamic joint support to maintain correct posture during all movements. In other words, stabilization is getting the right muscles to fire, with the right amount of force, in the proper plane of motion, and at the right time. This requires high levels of muscular endurance for optimal recruitment of prime movers to increase concentric force production and reduce eccentric force. Repeatedly training with controlled, unstable exercises increases the body's ability to stabilize and balance itself (19–21). Conversely, if training is not performed with controlled unstable exercises, clients will not gain the same level of stability and may even worsen (21–23). Research shows that improper stabilization can negatively affect a muscle's force production (24). Stability is an important training adaptation because it increases the ability of the kinetic chain to stabilize the lumbo-pelvic-hip complex and joints during movement to allow the arms and legs to work more efficiently.

Muscular Endurance

Muscular endurance is the ability to produce and maintain force production for prolonged periods of time. Improving muscular endurance is an integral component of all fitness programs. Developing muscular endurance helps to increase core and joint stabilization, which is the foundation on which hypertrophy, strength, and power are built. Training for muscular endurance of the core focuses on the recruitment of muscles responsible for postural stability, namely, type I muscle fibers.

> **Muscular endurance** The ability to produce and maintain force production for prolonged periods of time.

Research has shown that resistance training protocols using high repetitions are the most effective way to improve muscular endurance (25–27). In addition, a periodization training program can enhance local muscular endurance as well (26,28,29), and after an initial training effect in previously untrained individuals, multiple sets of periodized training may prove superior to single-set training for improving muscle endurance (26). Campos et al. (25) found that higher repetitions (2 sets of 20–28 repetitions with 1-minute rest periods beginning at 2 days/week) increased local muscle endurance and hypertrophy in untrained men after an 8-week training program, whereas Marx et al. (26) found that after the initial 12 weeks of training, multiple sets of up to 15 repetitions, 4 times a week for 6 months, resulted in a threefold decrease in body fat and an increase in local muscle endurance, as well as a significant increase in lean body mass.

Muscular Hypertrophy

Muscular hypertrophy is the enlargement of skeletal muscle fibers in response to being recruited to develop increased levels of tension, as seen in resistance training (30). Muscle hypertrophy is characterized by an increase in the cross-sectional area of individual muscle fibers resulting from an increase in myofibril proteins (myofilaments). Although the visible signs of hypertrophy may not be apparent for many weeks (4 to 8 weeks) in an untrained client, the process begins in the early stages of training, regardless of the intensity of training used (31–33).

> **Muscular hypertrophy** Enlargement of skeletal muscle fibers in response to overcoming force from high volumes of tension.

Resistance training protocols that use low to intermediate repetition ranges with progressive overload lead to muscular hypertrophy. Structured progressive resistance training programs using multiple sets help to increase muscular hypertrophy in both younger and older men and women alike (25,28,34–37). Kraemer et al. (4) demonstrated that 24 weeks of training 3 days per week with 3 sets of 8–12 repetitions per exercise improved muscle hypertrophy and body composition. Thus, progressive resistance training programs using moderate to low repetition protocols with progressively higher loads will result in increased hypertrophy in older adults and men and women.

Strength

Strength is the ability of the neuromuscular system to produce internal tension (in the muscles and connective tissues that pull on the bones) to overcome an external force. Whether the external force demands the neuromuscular system to produce stability, endurance, maximal strength, or power, internal tension within the muscles is what leads to force production. The degree of internal tension produced is the result of *strength adaptations*. The specific form of strength or internal tension produced from training is based on the type and intensity of training used by the client (principle of specificity).

Resistance training programs have traditionally focused on developing maximal strength in individual muscles, emphasizing one plane of motion (typically the sagittal plane) (3). Because all muscles function eccentrically, isometrically, and concentrically in all three planes of motion (sagittal, frontal, and transverse) at different speeds, training programs should be designed using a progressive approach that emphasizes the appropriate exercise selection, all muscle actions, and repetition tempos. This is discussed in greater detail in chapter 15.

Because muscle operates under the control of the central nervous system, strength needs to be thought of not as a function of muscle, but as a result of activating the neuromuscular system. Strength gains can occur rapidly in beginning clients and can increase with a structured, progressive resistance training program. One factor in increased strength is an increase in the number of motor units recruited, especially early in a training program (38–40). Using heavier loads increases the neural demand and recruitment of more muscle fibers until a recruitment plateau is reached, after which further increases in strength are a result of fiber hypertrophy (41–44).

Strength cannot be thought of in isolation. Strength is built on the foundation of stabilization requiring muscles, tendons, and ligaments to be prepared for the load that will be required to increase strength beyond the initial stages of training. Whereas stabilization training is designed with the characteristics of type I slow-twitch muscle fibers in mind (slow-contracting, low tension output, and resistant to fatigue), strength training is designed to match the characteristics of type II muscle fibers (quick-contracting, high tension output, prone to fatigue). Thus acute variables (sets, reps, intensities, etc.) are manipulated to take advantage of the specific characteristics of each fiber type. The majority of strength increases will occur during the first 12 weeks of resistance training from increased neural recruitment and muscle hypertrophy (26,29,34,45–48). Intermediate and advanced lifters will find it necessary to carry out a more demanding program in terms of training volume and intensity by following a sound periodized schedule.

Power

Power is the ability of the neuromuscular system to produce the greatest possible force in the shortest possible time. This is represented by the simple equation of force multiplied by velocity (49). Power adaptations build on stabilization and strength adaptations and then apply them at more realistic speeds and forces seen in everyday life and sporting activities. The focus of power-resistance training is getting the neuromuscular system to generate force as quickly as possible (rate of force production).

An increase in either force or velocity will produce an increase in power. Training for power can be achieved by increasing the weight (force), as seen in the strength adaptations, or increasing the speed with which weight is moved (velocity) (42,50–57). Power training allows for increased rate of force production by increasing the number of motor units activated, the synchronization between them, and the speed at which they are activated (42,58,59). The general adaptation syndrome and principle of specificity both dictate that to maximize training for this type of adaptation, both heavy and light loads must be moved as fast as possible (in a controlled fashion). Thus, using both training methods in a superset fashion can create the necessary adaptations to enhance the body's ability to recruit a large number of motor units and increase the rate (speed) of activation (50–57). Early isokinetic work underscored the importance of speed of exercise, showing that training performed at high speeds led to better performance at the training speed and all movement speeds below the training speed.

SUMMARY

Resistance training programs produce physiologic changes that result in a variety of strength adaptations. Strength is the ability of the neuromuscular system to produce internal tension to overcome an external force. Traditionally, resistance training programs focused on developing maximal strength in individual muscles, whereas contemporary training programs emphasize appropriate exercise selection, all muscle actions, multiple planes of motion, and repetition tempos. Training adaptations can be divided into stabilization, muscular endurance, hypertrophy, strength, and power.

Stabilization adaptations should be the starting point for clients new to resistance training. Stabilization adaptations are best achieved using high repetitions with low to moderate volume and low to moderate intensity in a postural position that challenges the stability of the body.

Muscular endurance is the ability to produce and maintain force production for prolonged periods of time. Research has shown that resistance training protocols using high repetitions are the most effective way to improve muscular endurance.

Muscular hypertrophy is the enlargement of skeletal muscle fibers in response to increased volumes of tension resulting from resistance training. Resistance training protocols that use low to intermediate repetition ranges with progressive overload lead to muscular hypertrophy.

Strength is the ability of the neuromuscular system to produce internal tension (in the muscles and connective tissues that pull on the bones) to overcome an external force. The specific form of strength produced is based on the type and intensity of training used by the client (principle of specificity). Generally, strength adaptations should use low to moderate repetition routines with moderate to high volume and moderate to high intensity. Heavier weights and higher volumes of training are used to improve the function of motor units, while placing stress on the muscles to increase size or strength.

Power is the ability of the neuromuscular system to produce the greatest possible force in the shortest possible time. An increase in either force (weight) or velocity (speed with which weight is moved) will produce an increase in power. To maximize training for this adaptation, both heavy and light loads must be moved as fast and as controlled as possible.

Resistance Training Systems

Originally, power lifters, Olympic lifters, and bodybuilders designed most resistance training programs. Many of these styles of resistance training programs remain popular today because of good marketing or "gym science," not because they have been proven to be scientifically superior to other forms of training programs that bring about increases in stabilization, strength, and power. Research has shown that following a systematic, integrated training program and manipulating key training variables achieve optimal gains in strength, neuromuscular efficiency, hypertrophy, and performance (4,27,28).

There are numerous training systems that can be used to structure resistance training programs for a variety of effects. Several of the most common training systems currently used in the fitness industry are presented in this chapter Table 13.3.

The Single-Set System

As the name suggests, the single-set system uses 1 set per exercise. It is usually recommended that single-set workouts be performed two times per week to promote sufficient development and maintenance of muscle mass (60). Although multiple-set training is promoted as being more beneficial for strength and hypertrophy gains in advanced clients, the single-set system has been shown to be just as beneficial for beginning-level clients (61–65).

Personal trainers are encouraged to explore the benefits and options of single-set workouts to further customize individual program design options. Single-set training systems are often negatively perceived for not providing enough stimuli for adaptation. However, when reviewing the physiology of how the human movement system operates, this notion may not be true (65). In fact, most beginning clients could follow a single-set program to allow for proper adaptive responses of the connective tissue and nervous system before engaging in more rigorous training systems. By encouraging clients to avoid lifting more than they can handle, synergistic dominance (synergists overcompensating for weak prime movers) and injury can be avoided.

TABLE 13.3	Resistance Training Systems
Type	**Definition**
Single-set	Performing one set of each exercise
Multiple-set	Performing a multiple number of sets for each exercise
Pyramid	Increasing (or decreasing) weight with each set
Superset	Performing two exercises in rapid succession with minimal rest
Drop-sets	Performing a set to failure, then removing a small percentage of the load and continuing with the set
Circuit training	Performing a series of exercises, one after the other, with minimal rest
Peripheral heart action	A variation of circuit training that uses different exercises (upper and lower body) for each set through the circuit
Split-routine	A routine that trains different body parts on separate days
Vertical loading	Performing exercises on the OPT template one after the other, in a vertical manner down the template
Horizontal loading	Performing all sets of an exercise (or body part) before moving on to the next exercise (or body part)

The Multiple-Set System

The multiple-set system, on the other hand, consists of performing multiple numbers of sets for each exercise. The resistance (load), sets, and repetitions performed are selected according to the goals and needs of the client (66). Multiple-set training can be appropriate for both novice and advanced clients, but has been shown to be superior to single-set training for more advanced clients (29,66,67). The increased volume (sets, reps, and intensity) is necessary for further improvement, but must be administered appropriately to avoid overtraining (5).

The Pyramid System

The pyramid system involves a progressive or regressive step approach that either increases weight with each set or decreases weight with each set **Figure 13.6**. In the *light-to-heavy system*, the individual typically performs 10 to 12 repetitions with a light load and increases the resistance for each following set, until the individual can perform 1 to 2 repetitions, usually in 4 to 6 sets. This system can easily be used for workouts that involve only 2 to 4 sets or higher repetition schemes (12 to 20 repetitions). The *heavy-to-light system* works in the opposite direction, in which the individual begins with a heavy load (after a sufficient warm-up) for 1 to 2 repetitions, then decreases the load and increases the repetitions for 4 to 6 sets.

The Superset System

The superset system uses two exercises performed in rapid succession of one another. There are multiple variations of the superset system.

The first variation includes performing two exercises for the same muscle group back to back. For example, an individual may perform the bench press exercise immediately followed by push-ups to fatigue the chest musculature. Completing two exercises in this manner will improve muscular endurance and hypertrophy because the volume of work performed is relatively high. This style of supersets can use two, three (a tri-set), or more exercises (a giant set) for the target muscle group. The greater the number of exercises used, the greater the degree of fatigue experienced and demands on muscular endurance.

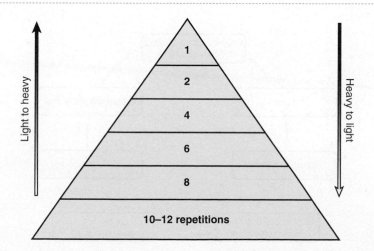

FIGURE 13.6

The pyramid system.

The second variation consists of performing two exercises back to back that involve antagonist muscle groups (e.g., chest and back or quadriceps and hamstring complex). Performing supersets in this manner allows a significant load to be placed on the target muscle during each set. This is possible because while the agonist is working, the antagonist is recovering, and vice versa.

Supersetting typically involves sets of 8 to 12 repetitions with no rest between sets or exercises; however, any number of repetitions can be used. The superset system is popular among bodybuilders and may be beneficial for muscular hypertrophy and muscular endurance.

Drop-Sets

A drop-set is a resistance training system that is popular among bodybuilders. It is a technique that allows a client to continue a set past the point at which it would usually terminate. Drop-sets involve performing a set to failure, then removing a small percentage of the load (5–20%) and continuing with the set, completing a small number of repetitions (usually 2–4). This procedure can be repeated several times (typically 2 to 3 drops per set). A set to failure followed by three successive load decrements performed with no rest would be referred to as a triple drop. Drop-sets are considered an advanced form of resistance training suitable for experienced lifters.

The Circuit-Training System

The circuit-training system consists of a series of exercises that an individual performs one after the other, with minimal rest between each exercise **Figure 13.7**. The typical acute variables for a circuit-training program include low to moderate number of sets (1–3), with moderate to high repetitions (8–20) and short rest periods (15–60 seconds) between exercises; however, these variables can be manipulated to enhance the desired effect (68,69). Circuit training is a great training system for individuals with limited time and for those who want to alter body composition (68,69).

The Peripheral Heart Action System

The peripheral heart action system is another variation of circuit training that alternates upper body and lower body exercises throughout the circuit. This system of training distributes blood flow between the upper and lower extremities potentially improving

FIGURE 13.7

Example circuit.

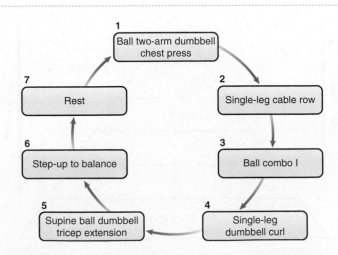

circulation. The number of exercises per sequence varies with the program's goal. The individual performs 8 to 20 repetitions per exercise, depending on the desired adaptation and phase of training they are using in the OPT model. This system is very beneficial for incorporating an integrated, multidimensional program and for altering body composition (38,70). An example for each of the three main adaptations is shown in **Table 13.4**.

The Split-Routine System

A split-routine system involves breaking the body up into parts to be trained on separate days. Many bodybuilders and mass-dominant and strength athletes (football, shot put, etc.) use the split-routine system. Bodybuilders typically perform numerous exercises on the same day for the same body part to bring about optimal muscular hypertrophy. By breaking up the body into parts that can be trained on different days, more work can be performed for the allotted time per workout. Examples of several different split-routines are shown in **Table 13.5**. Any variation of these outlined routines can be used, but the important issue with some of these routines is recovery time. When training each body part more than once a week, volume and intensity should be accounted for.

TABLE 13.4　Peripheral Heart Action System: Sample Workout

Set 1: Stabilization	Set 2: Strength	Set 3: Power
1. Ball dumbbell chest press	1. Bench press	1. Medicine ball chest pass
2. Ball squat	2. Barbell squat	2. Squat jump
3. Single-leg cable row	3. Seated row	3. Soccer throw
4. Step-up to balance	4. Romanian deadlift	4. Power step-up
5. Single-leg dumbbell shoulder press	5. Seated dumbbell shoulder press	5. Front medicine ball oblique throw

TABLE 13.5　Split-Routine System: Sample Workouts

Routine	Day(s) Performed	Body Parts Trained
2-Day	Monday	Chest, shoulders, triceps
	Thursday	Back, biceps, legs
3-Day	Monday	Chest, shoulders, triceps
	Wednesday	Legs
	Friday	Back, biceps
4-Day	Monday and Thursday	Chest, shoulders, triceps
	Tuesday and Friday	Back, biceps, legs

(Continued)

5-Day	Monday	Chest
	Tuesday	Legs
	Wednesday	Back
	Thursday	Shoulders
	Friday	Arms
6-Day	Monday and Friday	Chest, shoulders, triceps
	Tuesday and Saturday	Legs
	Wednesday and Sunday	Back, biceps

Vertical Loading and Horizontal Loading

Vertical loading
Alternating body parts trained from set to set, starting from the upper extremity and moving to the lower extremity.

Vertical loading is a resistance training system used by NASM and follows the OPT model. It progresses a workout vertically down the template by alternating body parts trained from set to set **Table 13.6**. When looking at the OPT template, it can be seen that the resistance training section involves the following exercises:

1. Total body exercise
2. Chest
3. Back
4. Shoulders
5. Biceps
6. Triceps
7. Legs

In a vertically loaded workout, the client would perform the first exercise (total body) for the required repetitions and then move to the chest exercise for the next set of repetitions. After the chest exercise, the client would move on to the back exercise and so forth, until all exercises have been completed. Once completed, the client would then start back at the first exercise (total body) and run through the exercises again for the desired amount of sets. This can also be done in a circuit style, by minimizing the rest periods between exercises.

This vertical loading system of training can be very beneficial for allowing maximal recovery to each body part while minimizing the amount of time wasted on rest. For example, if it takes 1 minute to perform each exercise, by the time the client returns to the chest exercise, 7 to 10 minutes could have passed, which should be sufficient time to allow for full adenosine triphosphate (ATP)/phosphocreatine (PC) recovery. Even though 7 to 10 minutes have passed, the client has been constantly moving and has performed one set of every exercise in his or her workout.

Horizontal loading
Performing all sets of an exercise or body part before moving on to the next exercise or body part.

Horizontal loading refers to performing all sets of an exercise or body part before moving on to the next exercise or body part **Table 13.7**. For example, if performing three sets of a chest exercise and three sets of a back exercise, the client would perform all three sets of the chest exercise before moving on to the back exercise. The progression of exercises is therefore said to be horizontal across the template. This is the method most commonly used in health club environments and is appropriate for maximal strength and power training when longer rest periods are required between sets (71–74).

The drawback to the horizontal loading system is the amount of time typically spent resting, which can often be more time than the actual workout itself. Horizontal loading can be a metabolic progression if rest periods are monitored and limited to 30 to 90 seconds between sets. If the same muscle groups are forced to work with minimal recovery it can lead to faster development of metabolic and hypertrophy-related adaptations in the muscle (14,75,76).

TABLE 13.6	**Vertical Loading**				© ilolab/ShutterStock, Inc.
Exercise	**Sets**	**Reps**	**Tempo**	**Rest**	**Coaching Tips**
Total Body					Complete exercises for each body part before beginning next set
Chest					
Back					
Shoulders					
Biceps					
Triceps					
Legs					

TABLE 13.7	**Horizontal Loading**				© ilolab/ShutterStock, Inc.
RESISTANCE					
Exercise	**Sets**	**Reps**	**Tempo**	**Rest**	**Coaching Tip**
Total Body					Complete all sets before moving to next exercise
Chest					
Back					
Shoulders					
Biceps					
Triceps					
Legs					

SUMMARY

The OPT method follows a progressive, systematic approach that enables personal trainers to make consistent gains with all clients by manipulating key variables to achieve various goals. There are numerous training systems that can be used to structure a resistance training program for a variety of effects.

The single-set system consists of performing one set of each exercise, usually of 8 to 12 repetitions. This system has been shown to be beneficial for strength and hypertrophy gains in beginning clients. The multiple-set system of training consists of performing a multiple number of sets for each exercise, with resistance, sets, and repetitions adjusted according to the goals and needs of the client. This system is superior to single-set training for more advanced clients.

The pyramid system involves a progressive or regressive step approach that either increases weight with each set or decreases weight with each set. The superset system uses two exercises performed in rapid succession of one another. This system is popular among bodybuilders for muscular hypertrophy and muscular endurance.

The circuit-training system programs consist of a series of exercises that an individual performs one immediately after the other, with minimal rest. This is a good system for clients with limited time and those who want to alter body composition. The peripheral heart action system is another variation of circuit training that alternates upper body and lower body exercises (of varied numbers) throughout the circuit. A split-routine system involves breaking the body up into parts to be trained on separate days so that more work can be performed for the allotted time per workout. When training each body part more than once a week, recovery period, volume, and intensity should be accounted for.

Vertical loading and horizontal loading progress a workout vertically or horizontally down the template. In a vertically loaded workout, the client would perform each exercise until all exercises have been completed and then run through the exercises again for the desired amount of sets. This can also be done in a circuit style, by minimizing the rest periods between exercises to allow maximal recovery to each body part and minimize the amount of time wasted on rest. In a horizontally loaded workout, the client would perform all sets of an exercise or body part before moving on to the next exercise or body part.

RESISTANCE TRAINING EXERCISES

Total Body Exercise Descriptions

Total Body–Stabilization Exercises

Ball Squat, Curl to Press

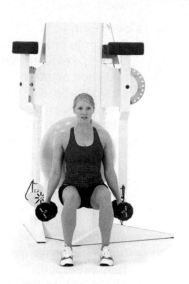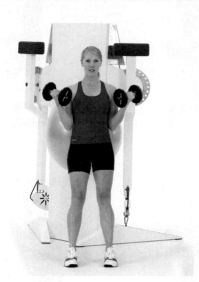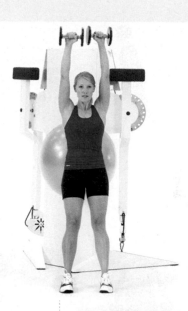

Preparation

1. Begin with both feet shoulders-width apart pointing straight ahead and knees over the second and third toes. Position the ball in the low-back region as shown.

Movement

2. Lower into a squat position, keeping lower extremities in proper alignment.
3. Stand to a fully upright position while contracting the gluteal muscles and quadriceps.
4. Once stabilized, curl and press the dumbbells overhead until both arms are fully extended.
5. Slowly return to the start position and repeat.
6. Regression
   a. Decrease range of motion
7. Progression
   a. Alternating-arm
   b. One-arm
   c. Single-leg

TECHNIQUE

When performing any form of a ball squat, try to use the ball to *guide* one through the squatting motion (sitting into a chair) versus relying on the ball for support (leaning back on the ball).

RESISTANCE TRAINING EXERCISES *continued*

Multiplanar Step-Up Balance, Curl, to Overhead Press

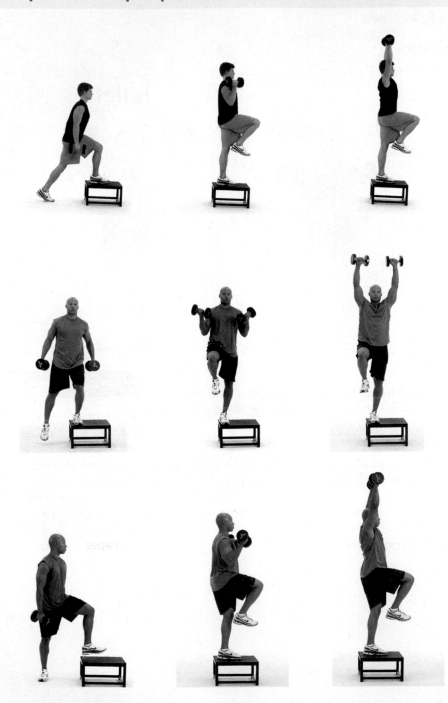

Preparation
1. Stand in front of a box with feet shoulders-width apart.

Movement
2. Step onto box with one leg, keeping foot and knee pointed straight ahead.
3. Push through heel and stand up straight, balancing on one leg.
4. Flex the other leg at the hip and knee.
5. Once balance has been established, curl and press the dumbbells overhead until both arms are fully extended.
6. Slowly return the dumbbells to the starting position.
7. Return opposite leg to the ground and step off the box.
8. Repeat on other leg.
9. Regression
   a. Omit balance
10. Progression
    a. Frontal plane
    b. Transverse plane

TECHNIQUE When pressing overhead, make sure the low back does not arch. This may indicate tightness of the latissimus dorsi and weakness of the intrinsic core stabilizers.

RESISTANCE TRAINING EXERCISES *continued*

Total Body–Strength Exercises

Lunge to Two-Arm Dumbbell Press

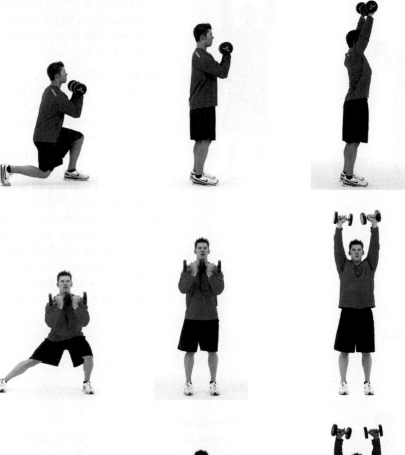

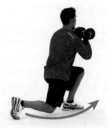

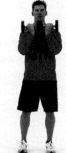

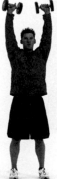

Preparation

1. Begin with both feet shoulders-width apart.
2. Hold two dumbbells in hands at chest level (palms facing body).

Movement

3. Lunge forward, come to a stabilized position with front foot pointing straight ahead and knee directly over second and third toes.
4. Both knees should be bent at a 90-degree angle, front foot should be flat on the ground, and back foot should have the heel lifted off the ground.
5. From this position, drive off of front foot and back into a standing position.
6. Press the dumbbells overhead until arms are fully extended.
7. Lower weight and repeat.

TECHNIQUE

When performing any squatting or lunging motion, make sure the foot stays straight and the knees stay in line with the toes. This ensures proper joint mechanics (arthrokinematics) and optimal force generation (via proper length-tension relationships and force-couple relationships), increasing the benefit of the exercise and decreasing its risk.

RESISTANCE TRAINING EXERCISES *continued*

Squat, Curl, to Two-Arm Press

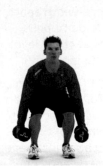
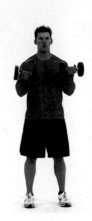
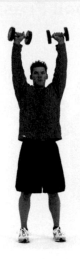

Preparation
1. Begin with both feet shoulders-width apart and pointing straight ahead, and knees over the second and third toes.

Movement
2. Perform a squat as low as can be safely controlled, keeping lower extremities in proper alignment.
3. Before any compensation occurs, activate gluteal muscles and stand to a fully upright position.
4. Once stabilized, curl and press the dumbbells overhead until both arms are fully extended, with palms facing away.
5. Slowly return the dumbbells to the start position and repeat.

Total Body–Power Exercises

Two-Arm Push Press

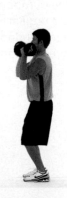
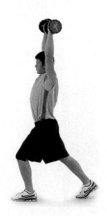

Preparation
1. Stand with feet shoulders-width apart.
2. Hold two dumbbells in hands at shoulder level.

Movement
3. Quickly drive dumbbells up, as if doing a shoulder press.
4. At the same time, drive the legs into a stagger stance position. Back leg should be in triple extension (plantar flexion, knee extension, hip extension) with the front leg bent slightly.
5. Maintain optimal alignment on the return to the starting position and repeat.

SAFETY One must establish proper stability (stabilization level training) and prime mover strength (strength level training) before progressing to the power exercises.

RESISTANCE TRAINING EXERCISES *continued*

Barbell Clean

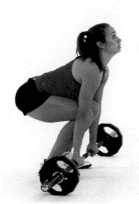
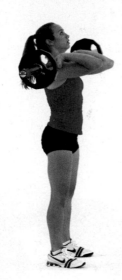

Preparation

1. Squat down next to bar, keeping feet flat on floor.
2. Arms grasp the bar fully extended slightly wider than shoulders-width apart.
3. Position shoulders over or slightly ahead of the bar, and the pelvis should be in a neutral position.

Movement

4. Initiate the first pull by extending knees and hips, lifting bar straight up (keeping the bar close to the shins) with elbows extended.
5. Continue to move bar upward by explosively extending hips, knees, and ankles (plantarflexion) in a jumping motion.
6. At maximal plantarflexion, elevate shoulders and flex and pull with the arms.
7. Pull bar as high as possible before rotating elbows under the bar.
8. Hyperextend wrists as the elbows move under the bar.
9. Point elbows forward.
10. Rack the bar across the front of the shoulders, keeping torso erect.
11. Flex hips and knees to absorb the weight of the bar.

SAFETY

This is a simplified description and illustration of performing the barbell clean. The barbell clean is an advanced power exercise and requires proper instruction before attempting.

RESISTANCE TRAINING EXERCISES *continued*

Chest Exercise Descriptions

Chest–Stabilization Exercises

Ball Dumbbell Chest Press

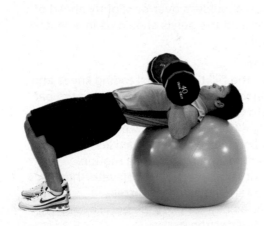 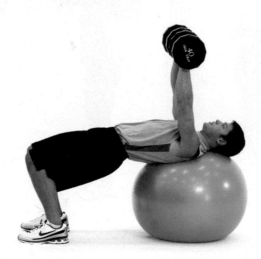

Preparation
1. Lie on stability ball as shown.
2. Maintain a bridge position by contracting gluteal muscles and keeping shoulders, hips, and knees at the same level.
3. Feet should be shoulders-width apart with toes pointing straight ahead.
4. Hold one dumbbell in each hand, at chest level.

Movement
5. Press both dumbbells straight up and then together, by extending elbows and contracting chest.
6. Hold.
7. Slowly return dumbbells toward body by flexing elbows.
8. Regression
   a. Dumbbell chest press progression on bench
9. Progressions
   a. Alternating-arm
   b. Single-arm

SAFETY To ensure proper alignment, the ears, shoulders, hips, and knees should all be in line with one another.

© ilolab/ShutterStock, Inc.

RESISTANCE TRAINING EXERCISES *continued*

© ilolab/ShutterStock, Inc.

Push-Up

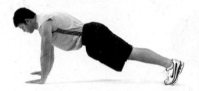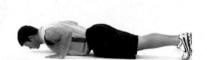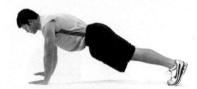

Preparation
1. Begin in a push-up position as shown.
2. Draw in navel and contract gluteal muscles.

Movement
3. Keeping pelvis in a neutral position, slowly lower body toward ground, by flexing elbows and retracting and depressing shoulder blades.

4. Push back up to starting position, by extending elbows and contracting chest. Do not allow head to jut forward.
5. Regressions
   a. On knees   b. Hands on bench, feet on floor
   c. Hands on wall, feet on floor
6. Progressions
   a. Lower extremities on ball   b. Hands on medicine balls   c. Hands on stability ball

| SAFETY | A common compensation that occurs when performing a push-up is the low back arching (stomach falls toward the ground). This is an indicator that the individual possesses weak intrinsic core stabilizers, and the exercise must be regressed. |

Chest–Strength Exercises

Flat Dumbbell Chest Press

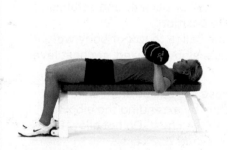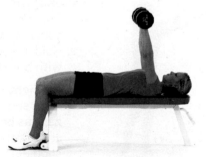

TECHNIQUE

When performing chest presses, the range of motion at the shoulder joint (how far the elbows go down) will be determined by the load one is lifting (control) and tissue extensibility. The key is to only go as far as one can control without compensating.

Preparation
1. Lie on flat bench with knees bent and feet flat on the floor.
2. Hold one dumbbell in each hand, at chest level.

Movement
3. Press both dumbbells straight up and then together, by extending elbows and contracting chest.
4. Hold.
5. Slowly return dumbbells toward body by flexing elbows and allowing shoulders to retract and depress.

RESISTANCE TRAINING EXERCISES *continued*

© ilolab/ShutterStock, Inc.

Barbell Bench Press

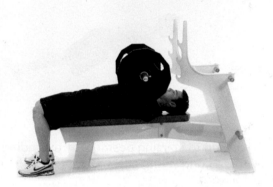
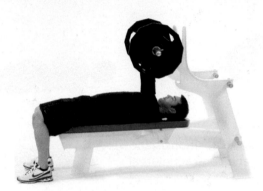

Preparation
1. Lie on flat bench, feet flat on floor and toes pointing straight ahead.
2. Hold a barbell and grasp the bar with hands slightly wider than shoulders-width apart.

Movement
3. Slowly lower the bar toward the chest by flexing elbows. Avoid letting the back arch or the head jut off the bench.
4. Press the bar back up, extending arms and contracting chest, until elbows are fully extended.

Chest–Power Exercises

Two-Arm Medicine Ball Chest Pass

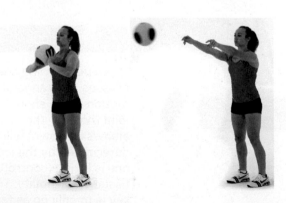

Preparation
1. Stand facing a wall or partner and establish a squared stance position.
2. Hold a medicine ball (5 to 10% of body weight) with both hands, elbows flexed, at chest level

Movement
3. Push and release the ball straight ahead as hard as possible, by extending the elbows and contracting the chest. Do not allow the shoulders to elevate.
4. Catch and repeat as quickly as possible..

TECHNIQUE   If it is not an option to be able to perform power exercises with a medicine ball (facility-dependent, equipment), this exercise can also be done using tubing or cable. Just make sure to adjust the weight or resistance accordingly so one can still perform the movement quickly and under control without compensation.

RESISTANCE TRAINING EXERCISES *continued*

Rotation Chest Pass

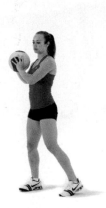 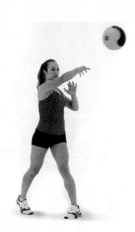

Preparation

1. Stand, with body turned at a 90-degree angle from a wall or partner.
2. Hold a medicine ball (5 to 10% of body weight) with both hands, elbows flexed, at chest level.

Movement

3. Use abdominal muscles, hips, and gluteal muscles to rotate body quickly and explosively toward the wall.
4. As body turns, pivot back leg and allow it to go into triple extension (plantarflexion, knee extension, hip extension).
5. With the upper body, push the medicine ball using the back arm to extend and apply force as shown.
6. Catch and repeat as quickly as possible, under control.

RESISTANCE TRAINING EXERCISES *continued*

Back Exercise Descriptions

Back–Stabilization Exercises

Standing Cable Row

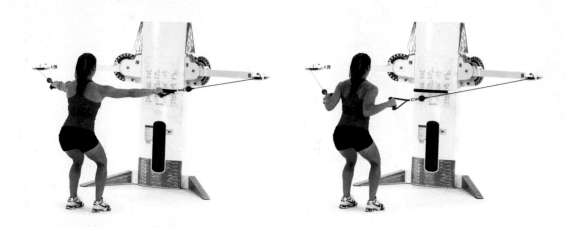

Preparation
1. Stand facing a cable machine with feet pointing straight ahead.
2. Hold cables, with arms extended at chest level.

Movement
3. With knees slightly flexed, row cable by flexing elbows, retracting and depressing the shoulder blades.
4. Do not allow the head to jut forward or shoulders to elevate.
5. Hold.
6. Slowly return arms to original position, by extending the elbows.
7. Regression
   a. Seated
8. Progressions
   a. Two-legs, alternating-arm
   b. Two-legs, one-arm
   c. Single-leg, two-arms
   d. Single-leg, alternating-arm
   e. Single-leg, one-arm

| TECHNIQUE | When performing rows, initiate the movement by retracting and depressing the shoulder blades (scapulae). Do not allow the shoulders to elevate. |

RESISTANCE TRAINING EXERCISES *continued*

Ball Dumbbell Row

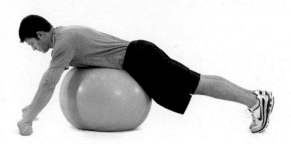 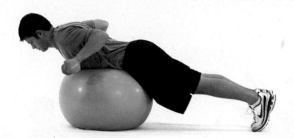

Preparation
1. Begin in a prone position, with stability ball under abdomen.
2. Keep feet pointed down, legs completely straight.
3. Hold dumbbells in each hand and extend arms in front of body.

Movement
4. Contract gluteal muscles and quadriceps.
5. Row the dumbbells by flexing elbows and retracting and depressing shoulder blades.
6. Hold.
7. Return dumbbells slowly to ground, by extending elbows.
8. Regression
    a. Kneeling over ball
9. Progression
    a. Alternating-arm
    b. One-arm

TECHNIQUE   Performing exercises in a prone position can be uncomfortable. When working with overweight individuals, it may be more appropriate to perform these exercises in a seated or standing position.

RESISTANCE TRAINING EXERCISES *continued*

Back–Strength Exercises

Seated Cable Row

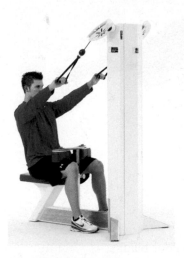 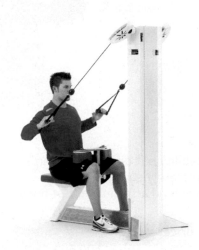

Preparation
1. Sit facing a cable machine, with feet shoulders-width apart and pointing straight ahead.
2. Hold cables, with arms extended.

Movement
3. Row cable by flexing elbows and pulling the handles toward the trunk.
4. Bring thumbs toward the armpits, keeping the shoulder blades retracted and depressed.
5. Do not allow the head to jut forward.
6. Hold.
7. Slowly return arms to original position by extending the elbows.

| TECHNIQUE | To increase the effectiveness of the exercise and decrease the risk of injury, keep the torso stationary throughout the execution of the exercise; flexing and extending the torso while performing the row creates momentum, which decreases the effectiveness of the exercise and places stress on the low back. |

RESISTANCE TRAINING EXERCISES *continued*

Seated Lat Pulldown

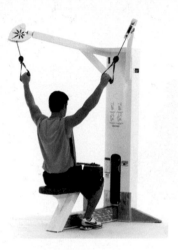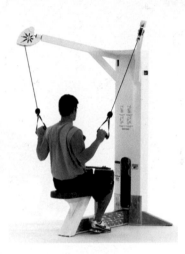

Preparation
1. Sit upright with feet on the floor pointing straight ahead.

Movement
2. Pull handles toward the body, by flexing elbows and depressing the shoulder blades. Do not arch back, allow head to jut forward, or elevate the shoulders.
3. Hold at end range.
4. Slowly return weight to original position, by extending elbows.

SAFETY — Performing lat pulldowns with a bar behind the neck is not advised as this places stress to the shoulder joints and cervical spine. If performing the lat pulldown exercise with a bar (instead of cables as illustrated), the bar should pass in front of the face approximately to shoulder height.

RESISTANCE TRAINING EXERCISES *continued*

Back–Power Exercises

Medicine Ball Pullover Throw

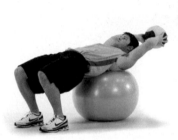
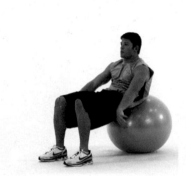

Preparation

1. Place stability ball under low back, bend knees at a 90-degree angle, and keep feet flat and toes pointing straight ahead.
2. Hold a medicine ball (5 to 10% of body weight) overhead with both hands, with arms extended.

Movement

3. Using abdominals, quickly crunch forward.
4. Throw the medicine ball straight ahead keeping elbows fairly straight.
5. As the ball releases, continue pulling the arms through all the way to the sides of the body.
6. Keep chin tucked throughout the exercise.
7. Repeat as quickly as possible, under control.

SAFETY To decrease stress to the shoulder and low back, it will be important that one has optimal extensibility through the latissimus dorsi musculature before performing these back-power exercises.

Soccer Throw

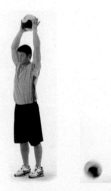
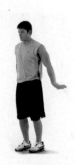

Preparation

1. Stand holding a medicine ball (5 to 10% of body weight) overhead as illustrated.

Movement

2. Quickly throw the medicine ball toward the floor, allowing the arms to follow through.
3. Repeat.

RESISTANCE TRAINING EXERCISES *continued*

Shoulder Exercise Descriptions

Shoulder–Stabilization Exercises

Single-Leg Dumbbell Scaption

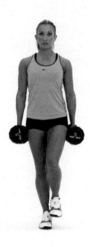
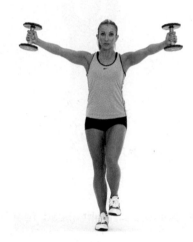

Preparation
1. Hold dumbbells at side, with palms facing side of body.
2. Raise one foot off the floor as illustrated.

Movement
3. Raise both arms, thumbs up, at a 45-degree angle in front of the body, until hands reach approximately eye level.
4. Keep shoulder blades retracted and depressed throughout the exercise. Do not allow the back to arch.
5. Hold.
6. Slowly return arms back to sides of body and repeat.
7. Regression
   a. Two-legs
   b. Seated
8. Progression
   a. Single-leg, alternating-arm
   b. Single-leg, single-arm
   c. Proprioceptive modalities

TECHNIQUE   Performing shoulder exercises in the scapular plane decreases the risk of the supraspinatus muscle becoming impinged between the head of the humerus and the coracoacromial arch of the scapula.

RESISTANCE TRAINING EXERCISES continued

© ilolab/ShutterStock, Inc.

Seated Stability Ball Military Press

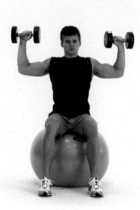 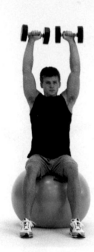

Preparation
1. Sit on a stability ball, keeping the toes pointed straight ahead, feet hips-width apart.
2. Hold dumbbells at shoulder level.

Movement
3. Press the dumbbells overhead until both arms are fully extended, with palms facing away.
4. Hold.
5. Slowly return dumbbells to the start position and repeat.
6. Regression
   a. Seated on a bench
7. Progression
   a. Alternating-arm
   b. One-arm
   c. Standing

| SAFETY | Performing exercises on a stability ball can be uncomfortable for some people. It may be required for the health and fitness professional to hold the ball while the individual performs the exercise to provide some additional support (both mentally and physically). |

RESISTANCE TRAINING EXERCISES *continued*

Shoulder–Strength Exercises

Seated Dumbbell Shoulder Press

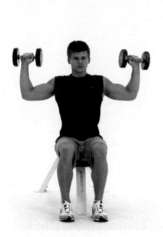 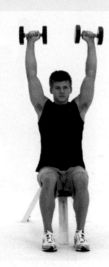

Preparation
1. Sit on a bench, feet flat on floor, and toes pointing straight ahead.
2. Hold dumbbells in each hand as illustrated.

Movement
3. Press arms directly overhead by extending elbows. Do not allow head to jut forward or back to arch.
4. Slowly return to starting position and repeat.

SAFETY   When performing overhead presses, make sure the cervical spine stays neutral (head drawn back). Do not allow the head to migrate forward as this places excessive stress on the posterior neck muscles and cervical spine.

RESISTANCE TRAINING EXERCISES *continued*

Seated Shoulder Press Machine

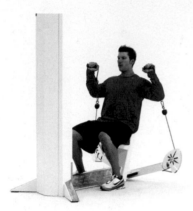 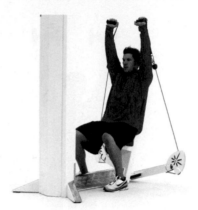

Preparation

1. Sit at machine with feet straight ahead.
2. Make any adjustments necessary to fit body.
3. Select desired weight.
4. Keep the chin tucked.

Movement

5. Press weight overhead until arms are fully extended.
6. Hold.
7. Slowly return weight to original position by flexing elbows and allowing shoulder blades to retract and depress.

Shoulder–Power Exercises

Front Medicine Ball Oblique Throw

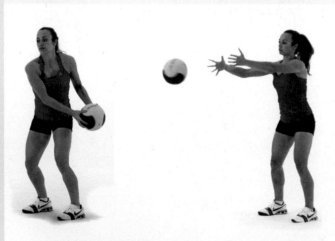

Preparation

1. Stand facing a wall or partner with feet shoulders-width apart, knees slightly bent, and toes pointing straight ahead.
2. Hold a medicine ball (between 5 and 10% of body weight) as illustrated.

Movement

3. Toss the ball against the wall or to a partner with an underhand motion.
4. Use a scooping motion to catch ball.
5. Repeat as quickly as can be controlled.
6. This exercise can be performed continuously to one side or by alternating sides.

TECHNIQUE   If a partner is unavailable, you can perform the exercise by tossing the medicine ball against a wall.

RESISTANCE TRAINING EXERCISES *continued*

Overhead Medicine Ball Throw

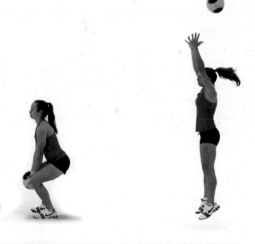

Preparation
1. Stand with back to wall in a semi-squat position holding a medicine ball as shown.

Movement
2. Jump off the ground explosively, extending arms overhead.
3. Throw the medicine ball off the wall.
4. Release the ball before arms pass ears. Do not allow the back to go into hyperextension.
5. Land in a controlled and stable manner, avoiding all compensations.

Biceps Exercise Descriptions

Biceps–Stabilization Exercises

Single-Leg Dumbbell Curl

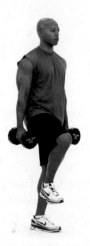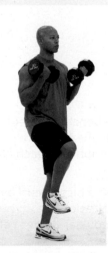

Preparation
1. Stand on one foot and allow arms to extend and hang to the sides of the body with a dumbbell in each hand.

Movement
2. Perform a biceps curl by performing elbow flexion and supination.
3. Slowly return dumbbells to their original position.
4. Regression
   a. Two-leg
5. Progression
   a. Alternating-arm
   b. Single-arm
   c. Proprioceptive modalities

TECHNIQUE Keeping the scapulae retracted during the exercise ensures proper scapular stability, placing more of an emphasis on the biceps musculature.

© ilolab/ShutterStock, Inc.

RESISTANCE TRAINING EXERCISES *continued*

© ilolab/ShutterStock, Inc.

Single-Leg Barbell Curl

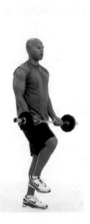
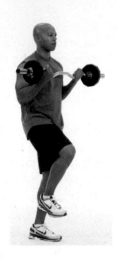

Preparation
1. Stand on one foot while holding a barbell in both hands as shown.

Movement
2. Perform a barbell curl by flexing both elbows, keeping the shoulder blades retracted.
3. Curl bar up to chest level.
4. Slowly lower the bar back to original position by extending the elbows.
5. Regression
   a. Two-leg
6. Progression
   a. Proprioceptive modalities

SAFETY   To decrease stress on the elbow, do not grip too close or too wide on the bar. To determine grip width, extend your elbows so your hands fall naturally to your sides, palms facing forward. Where your hands fall at your sides is the position where they should be when they grip the bar.

Biceps–Strength Exercises

Seated Two-Arm Dumbbell Biceps Curl

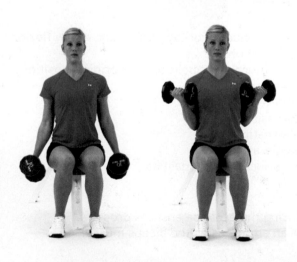

Preparation
1. Sit on a bench with feet flat on the floor, pointing straight ahead.
2. Hold dumbbell in each hand with arms at sides.

Movement
3. Perform a biceps curl by performing elbow flexion and supination.
4. Keep shoulder blades retracted throughout the exercise.
5. Slowly return dumbbells to their original position.

RESISTANCE TRAINING EXERCISES *continued*

Biceps Curl Machine

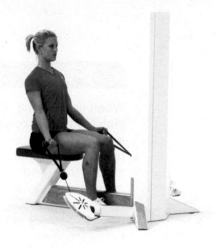 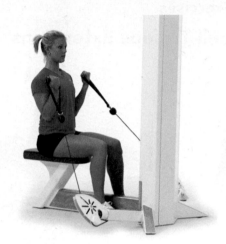

Preparation

1. Sit at machine.
2. Make any adjustments necessary to fit body.
3. Select desired weight.

Movement

4. Perform a curl by flexing elbows, while keeping shoulder blades retracted. Do not allow head to jut forward.
5. Curl until end range.
6. Slowly return weight to original position by extending elbows.

TECHNIQUE	When performing biceps curls it is important to keep an upright posture. Do not allow your torso to excessively flex or extend to cheat the movement.

RESISTANCE TRAINING EXERCISES *continued*

Triceps Exercise Descriptions

Triceps–Stabilization Exercises

Supine Ball Dumbbell Triceps Extensions

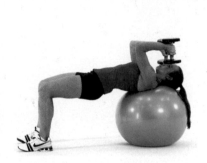 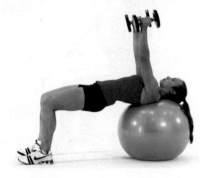

SAFETY

When performing stability ball exercises in a supine position, make sure position is such that head comfortably rests on the ball. This will decrease stress to the cervical spine.

Preparation
1. Lie on a stability ball, with ball between shoulder blades.
2. Maintain a bridge position by contracting gluteal muscles and keeping shoulders, hips, and knees level.
3. Feet should be shoulders-width apart with toes pointing straight ahead.

Movement
4. Extend elbows until arms are straight.
5. Return dumbbells slowly to the start position by flexing elbows.
6. Regression
   a. On bench
7. Progressions
   a. Alternating-arms
   b. One-arm

Prone Ball Dumbbell Triceps Extensions

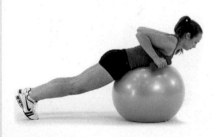 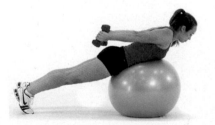

TECHNIQUE

To ensure optimal alignment, make sure the ankles, knees, hips, elbows, shoulders, and ears are all in alignment and maintained throughout the exercise.

Preparation
1. Lie in a prone position, with stability ball under abdomen.
2. Keep feet pointed down, legs completely straight, and navel drawn in.
3. Hold dumbbells in each hand with elbows bent and shoulder blades retracted and depressed.

Movement
4. Maintain a retracted scapular position, and extend elbows so that they are parallel to the side of the body.
5. Hold.
6. Slowly return dumbbells to original position by flexing elbows.

7. Regression
   a. Standing with cable
8. Progression
   a. Alternating-arms
   b. Single-arm

RESISTANCE TRAINING EXERCISES *continued*

Triceps–Strength Exercises

Cable Pushdown

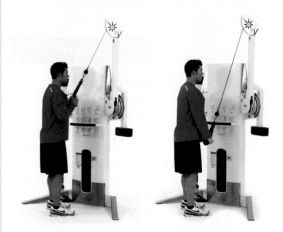

Preparation
1. Stand with feet shoulders-width apart, pointed straight ahead, and knees slightly flexed.
2. Grasp a cable, with elbows flexed.
3. Keep shoulder blades retracted and depressed.

Movement
4. Contract triceps by pushing hands toward the ground until arms are fully extended.
5. Hold.
6. Slowly return to the starting position.
7. Repeat.

TECHNIQUE	Using a rope when performing cable pushdowns will allow the elbows to track through their natural path of motion versus having the hands closely fixed on a bar. This may help decrease the risk of compensation when performing the exercise.

Supine Bench Barbell Triceps Extension

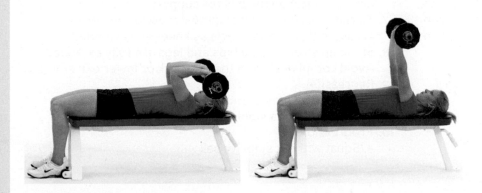

SAFETY

As with barbell curls, keeping the hands too close on the bar can increase stress on the elbow. Having your hands closer to shoulders-width apart can help to decrease stress to the elbow and compensation.

Preparation
1. Lie on flat bench.
2. Feet should be flat with toes pointing straight ahead.
3. Hold barbell in both hands with elbows flexed as illustrated.

Movement
4. Extend elbows until arms are straight.
5. Hold.
6. Slowly lower barbell toward forehead by flexing the elbows.
7. Repeat.

© iliolab/ShutterStock, Inc.

RESISTANCE TRAINING EXERCISES *continued*

© iliolab/ShutterStock, Inc.

Leg Exercise Descriptions

Leg–Stabilization Exercises

Ball Squat

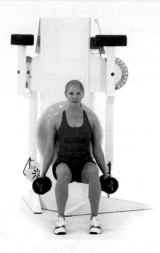 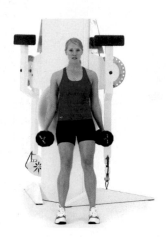

Preparation

1. Stand with feet shoulders-width apart, toes pointing forward, and knees over second and third toes. Hold dumbbells to the side of the body.
2. Rest back against a stability ball, which is placed on a wall.
3. Ideally, keep feet under the knees. For individuals who lack ankle dorsiflexion (tight calves), place the feet slightly in front of the knees.

Movement

4. Slowly begin to squat down, bending knees and flexing hips, keeping feet straight (as if sitting into a chair). Keep the knees in line with the toes and abdominals activated.
5. Allow the pelvis to sit back under the ball while maintaining a neutral spine.
6. Keep the chest up and put pressure through the heels. Do not rely solely on the ball for support.
7. To rise back up, contract gluteal muscles and place pressure through the heels as knees are extended.
8. Stand up straight until hips and legs are fully extended. Avoid compensation in the low back or lower extremities.
9. Regression
   a. Decrease range of motion
   b. Holding on to a stable support
10. Progression
    a. Squat without stability ball

RESISTANCE TRAINING EXERCISES *continued*

Multiplanar Step-Up to Balance

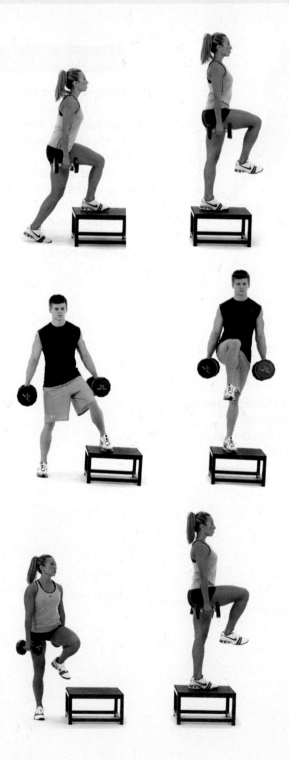

Preparation
1. Stand in front of box, with feet pointed straight ahead. Hold dumbbells to the side.

Movement
2. Step onto box with one leg, keeping foot pointed straight ahead and knee lined up over mid-foot.
3. Push through heel and stand up straight, balancing on one leg.
4. Flex the other leg at the hip and knee and dorsiflex the foot.
5. Return "floating" leg to the ground and step off the box, maintaining optimal alignment.
6. Repeat on other leg.
7. Regression
   a. Omit balance
   b. Decrease step height
8. Progression
   a. Frontal plane step-up
   b. Transverse plane step-up

TECHNIQUE

Lunges are excellent lower-extremity strengthening exercises; however, many individuals lack the flexibility and stabilization requirements to execute the exercise properly. Step-ups are a great way to regress the lunge until one develops proper flexibility and stabilization capabilities to perform the lunge correctly.

RESISTANCE TRAINING EXERCISES *continued*

Leg–Strength Exercises

Leg Press (Hip Sled)

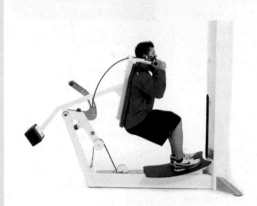 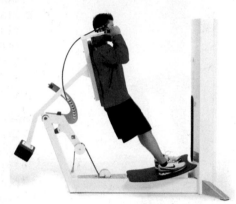

TECHNIQUE

Make sure the feet are positioned on the platform hips-to shoulders-width apart, toes are pointed straight, and the knees track in line with the toes. This will decrease stress to the knees, hips, and low back.

Preparation
1. Stand in machine.
2. Make any adjustments necessary to fit body.
3. Place feet shoulders-width apart, with toes pointing forward and knees directly over second and third toes.

Movement
4. Slowly perform a squat to a depth that can be safely controlled. Keep optimal alignment of the lower extremities throughout the movement.
5. Before any compensation occurs, activate gluteal muscles and apply pressure through heels extending hips and knees back to the starting position.

RESISTANCE TRAINING EXERCISES *continued*

Barbell Squat

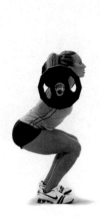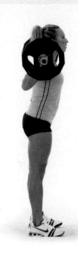

Preparation
1. Stand with feet shoulders-width apart, toes pointing straight ahead, and knees over second and third toes.
2. Rest barbell on shoulders, behind neck, with hands grasping the bar wider than shoulders-width apart.

Movement
3. Slowly begin to squat down, bending knees and flexing hips, keeping feet straight. Do not allow the knees to move inward.
4. Keep the chest up and put pressure through the heels.
5. Squat to a depth that can be safely controlled while maintaining ideal posture.
6. To rise back up, contract gluteal muscles and place pressure through the heels as knees and hips are extended.
7. Stand up straight until hips and legs are fully extended. Avoid compensation in the low back or lower extremities.

SAFETY

How far down should you squat? Only as far as can be controlled without compensating. As one develops more flexibility and stabilization strength, the range of motion can be increased, assuming no compensations occur.

RESISTANCE TRAINING EXERCISES *continued*

Leg–Power Exercises

Squat Jump

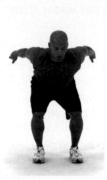
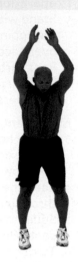

Preparation
1. Stand with feet shoulders-width apart and pointing straight ahead.

Movement
2. Squat down slightly.
3. Jump up into the air while extending arms overhead.
4. Bring arms back to sides during landing.
5. Land softly on the mid-foot in a controlled manner with feet and knees pointing straight ahead. Repeat as quickly as can be controlled.

Tuck Jump

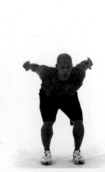
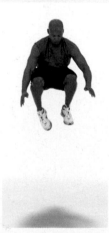

Preparation
1. Stand with feet shoulders-width apart and pointing straight ahead.

Movement
2. Jump up off the ground and, while in the air, bring knees up to chest.
3. Land softly on the midpoint of the feet, in a controlled manner, with feet straight and knees over mid-foot.
4. Repeat, as quickly as can be controlled.

TECHNIQUE   When performing power exercises, make sure you land behind the ball of the foot (not on the ball of the foot or on the heel). This will ensure proper force distribution through the foot and lower extremity, improving force production capabilities.

Filling in the Template

The information contained in this chapter provides personal trainers with the essentials to effectively design safe and effective resistance training programs for the needs of a variety of clients. The information provided in this chapter combined with the information contained in chapter 15 allows the personal trainer to properly complete the resistance training portion of the OPT program template. The template should be completed according to the example in **Figure 13.8**.

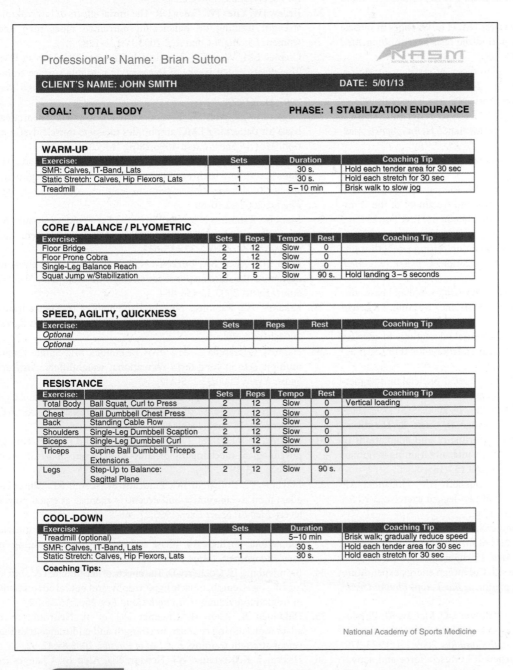

Professional's Name: Brian Sutton

NASM
NATIONAL ACADEMY OF SPORTS MEDICINE

CLIENT'S NAME: JOHN SMITH   **DATE: 5/01/13**

GOAL: TOTAL BODY   **PHASE: 1 STABILIZATION ENDURANCE**

WARM-UP

Exercise:	Sets	Duration	Coaching Tip
SMR: Calves, IT-Band, Lats	1	30 s.	Hold each tender area for 30 sec
Static Stretch: Calves, Hip Flexors, Lats	1	30 s.	Hold each stretch for 30 sec
Treadmill	1	5–10 min	Brisk walk to slow jog

CORE / BALANCE / PLYOMETRIC

Exercise:	Sets	Reps	Tempo	Rest	Coaching Tip
Floor Bridge	2	12	Slow	0	
Floor Prone Cobra	2	12	Slow	0	
Single-Leg Balance Reach	2	12	Slow	0	
Squat Jump w/Stabilization	2	5	Slow	90 s.	Hold landing 3–5 seconds

SPEED, AGILITY, QUICKNESS

Exercise:	Sets	Reps	Rest	Coaching Tip
Optional				
Optional				

RESISTANCE

Exercise:		Sets	Reps	Tempo	Rest	Coaching Tip
Total Body	Ball Squat, Curl to Press	2	12	Slow	0	Vertical loading
Chest	Ball Dumbbell Chest Press	2	12	Slow	0	
Back	Standing Cable Row	2	12	Slow	0	
Shoulders	Single-Leg Dumbbell Scaption	2	12	Slow	0	
Biceps	Single-Leg Dumbbell Curl	2	12	Slow	0	
Triceps	Supine Ball Dumbbell Triceps Extensions	2	12	Slow	0	
Legs	Step-Up to Balance: Sagittal Plane	2	12	Slow	90 s.	

COOL-DOWN

Exercise:	Sets	Duration	Coaching Tip
Treadmill (optional)	1	5–10 min	Brisk walk; gradually reduce speed
SMR: Calves, IT-Band, Lats	1	30 s.	Hold each tender area for 30 sec
Static Stretch: Calves, Hip Flexors, Lats	1	30 s.	Hold each stretch for 30 sec

Coaching Tips:

National Academy of Sports Medicine

FIGURE 13.8   Completed resistance training section of the template.

REFERENCES

1. Fleck SJ, Schutt RC. Types of strength training. *Clin Sports Med.* 1985;4:159-167.

2. Stone MH, Collins D, Plisk S, Haff G, Stone ME. Training principles: evaluation of modes and methods of resistance training. *Strength Cond J.* 2000;22(3):65-76.

3. Tan B. Manipulating resistance training program variables to optimize maximum strength in men: a review. *J Strength Cond Res.* 1999;13(3):289-304.

4. Kraemer WJ, Nindl BC, Ratamess NA, et al. Changes in muscle hypertrophy in women with periodized resistance training. *Med Sci Sports Exerc.* 2004;36:697-708.

5. Kraemer WJ, Ratamess NA. Physiology of resistance training. *Orthop Phys Ther Clin North Am.* 2000;9(4):467-513.

6. Selye H. *The Stress of Life.* New York, NY: McGraw-Hill; 1976.

7. Cheung K, Hume P, Maxwell L. Delayed onset muscle soreness: treatment strategies and performance factors. *Sports Med.* 2003;33(2):145-164.

8. Kannus P. Structure of the tendon connective tissue. *Scand J Med Sci Sports.* 2000;10:312-320.

9. Meeusun R, Duclos M, Gleeson M, Rietjens G, Steinacker J, Urhausen A. Prevention, diagnosis and treatment of the Overtraining Syndrome: ECSS Position Statement 'Task Force.' *Eur J Sport Sci.* 2006;6(1):1-14.

10. Hakkinen K. Neuromuscular adaptation during strength training, aging, detraining and immobilization. *Crit Rev Phys Med.* 1994;6:161-198.

11. McEvoy KP, Newton RU. Baseball throwing speed and base running speed: the effects of ballistic resistance training. *J Strength Cond Res.* 1998;12(4):216-221.

12. Gabriel DA, Kamen G, Frost G. Neural adaptations to resistive exercise: mechanisms and recommendations for training practices. *Sports Med.* 2006;36:133-149.

13. Harmer AR, McKenna MJ, Sutton JR, et al. Skeletal muscle metabolic and ionic adaptations during intense exercise following sprint training in humans. *J Appl Physiol.* 2000;89(5):1793-1803.

14. Parra J, Cadefau JA, Rodas G, Amigó N, Cussó R. The distribution of rest periods affects performance and adaptations of energy metabolism induced by high-intensity training in human muscle. *Acta Physiol Scand.* 2000;169:157-165.

15. Ogita F, Stam RP, Tazawa HO, Toussaint HM, Hollander AP. Oxygen uptake in one-legged and two-legged exercise. *Med Sci Sports Exerc.* 2000;32(10):1737-1742.

16. Williford HN, Olson MS, Gauger S, Duey WJ, Blessing DL. Cardiovascular and metabolic costs of forward, backward, and lateral motion. *Med Sci Sports Med.* 1998;30(9):1419-1423.

17. Heus R, Wertheim AH, Havenith G. Human energy expenditure when walking on a moving platform. *Eur J Appl Physiol Occup Physiol.* 1998;77(4):388-394.

18. Lagally KM, Cordero J, Good J, Brown DD, McCaw ST. Physiologic and metabolic responses to a continuous functional resistance exercise workout. *J Strength Cond Res.* 2009;23(2):373-379.

19. Behm DG, Anderson K, Curnew RS. Muscle force and activation under stable and unstable conditions. *J Strength Cond Res.* 2002;16:416-422.

20. Cosio-Lima LM, Reynolds KL, Winter C, Paolone V, Jones MT. Effects of physioball and conventional floor exercises on early phase adaptations in back and abdominal core stability and balance in women. *J Strength Cond Res.* 2003;17:721-725.

21. Heitkamp HC, Horstmann T, Mayer F, Weller J, Dickhuth HH. Gain in strength and muscular balance after balance training. *Int J Sports Med.* 2001;22:285-290.

22. Bellew JW, Yates JW, Gater DR. The initial effects of low-volume strength training on balance in untrained older men and women. *J Strength Cond Res.* 2003;17:121-128.

23. Cressey EM, West CA, Tiberio DP, Kraemer WJ, Maresh CM. The effects of ten weeks of lower-body unstable surface training on markers of athletic performance. *J Strength Cond Res.* 2007;21:561-567.

24. Edgerton VR, Wolf SL, Levendowski DJ, Roy RR. Theoretical basis for patterning EMG amplitudes to assess muscle dysfunction. *Med Sci Sport Exerc.* 1996;28(6):744-751.

25. Campos GE, Luecke TJ, Wendeln HK, et al. Muscular adaptations in response to three different resistance-training regimens: specificity of repetition maximum training zones. *Eur J Appl Physiol.* 2002;88:50-60.

26. Marx JO, Ratamess NA, Nindl BC, et al. Low-volume circuit versus high-volume periodized resistance training in women. *Med Sci Sports Exerc.* 2001;33:635-643.

27. Rhea MR, Alvar BA, Burkett LN, Ball SD. A meta-analysis to determine the dose response for strength development. *Med Sci Sports Exerc.* 2003;35:456-464.

28. Kraemer WJ, Ratamess NA. Fundamentals of resistance training: progression and exercise prescription. *Med Sci Sports Exerc.* 2004;36:674-688.

29. Hass CJ, Garzarella L, de Hoyos D, Pollock ML. Single versus multiple sets in long-term recreational weightlifters. *Med Sci Sports Exerc.* 2000;32:235-242.

30. Abernathy PJ, Jürimäe J, Logan PA, Taylor AW, Thayer RE. Acute and chronic response of skeletal muscle to resistance exercise. *Sports Med.* 1994;17(1):22-38.

31. Kraemer WJ, Fleck SJ, Evans WJ. Strength and power training: physiological mechanisms of adaptation. *Exerc Sport Sci Rev.* 1996;24:363-397.

32. Mayhew TP, Rothstein JM, Finucane SD, Lamb RL. Muscular adaptation to concentric and eccentric exercise at equal power levels. *Med Sci Sport Exer.* 1995;27:868-873.

33. Staron RS, Karapondo DL, Kraemer WJ, et al. Skeletal muscle adaptations during early phase of heavy-resistance training in men and women. *J Appl Physiol.* 1994;76:1247-1255.

34. Brandenburg JP, Docherty D. The effects of accentuated eccentric loading on strength, muscle hypertrophy, and neural adaptations in trained individuals. *J Strength Cond Res.* 2002;16:25-32.

35. Häkkinen K, Alen M, Kraemer WJ, et al. Neuromuscular adaptations during concurrent strength and endurance training versus strength training. *Eur J Appl Physiol.* 2003;89:42-52.

36. Häkkinen K, Kraemer WJ, Newton RU, Alen M. Changes in electromyographic activity, muscle fibre and force production characteristics during heavy resistance/power strength training

in middle-aged and older men and women. *Acta Physiol Scand.* 2001;171:51-62.

37. McCall GE, Byrnes WC, Fleck SJ, Dickinson A, Kraemer WJ. Acute and chronic hormonal responses to resistance training designed to promote muscle hypertrophy. *Can J Appl Physiol.* 1999;24(1):96-107.

38. Moritani T, deVries HA. Neural factors versus hypertrophy in the time course of muscle strength gain. *Am J Phys Med.* 1979;58:115-130.

39. Gabriel DA, Kamen G, Frost G. Neural adaptations to resistive exercise: mechanisms and recommendations for training practices. *Sports Med.* 2006;36:133-149.

40. Coburn JW, Housh TJ, Malek MH, et al. Neuromuscular responses to three days of velocity-specific isokinetic training. *J Strength Cond Res.* 2006;20:892-898.

41. Finer JT, Simmons RM, Spudich JA. Single myosin molecule mechanics: piconewton forces and nanometre steps. *Nature.* 1994;368:113-119.

42. Sale DG. Neural adaptation to resistance training. *Med Sci Sports Exerc.* 1988;20(5 Suppl):S135-145.

43. Sale DG. Neural adaptation in strength and power training. In: Jones NL, McCartney N, McComas AJ, eds. *Human Muscle Power.* Champaign, IL: Human Kinetics; 1986:289-307.

44. McCall GE, Byrnes WC, Dickinson A, Pattany PM, Fleck SJ. Muscle fiber hypertrophy, hyperplasia, and capillary density in college men after resistance training. *J Appl Physiol.* 1996;81:2004-2012.

45. Kraemer WJ, Mazzetti SA, Nindl BC, et al. Effect of resistance training on women's strength/power and occupational performances. *Med Sci Sports Exerc.* 2001;33:1011-1025.

46. Chilibeck PD, Calder AW, Sale DG, Webber CE. A comparison of strength and muscle mass increases during resistance training in young women. *Eur J Appl Physiol Occup Physiol.* 1998;77:170-175.

47. Peterson MD, Rhea MR, Alvar BA. Maximizing strength development in athletes: a meta-analysis to determine the dose-response relationship. *J Strength Cond Res.* 2004;18:377-382.

48. Rhea MR, Alderman BL. A meta-analysis of periodized versus nonperiodized strength and power training programs. *Res Q Exerc Sport.* 2004;75:413-422.

49. Enoka RM. *Neuromechanics of Human Movement.* 3rd ed. Champaign, IL: Human Kinetics; 2002.

50. Bobbert MA, Van Soest AJ. Effects of muscle strengthening on vertical jump height: a simulation study. *Med Sci Sports Exerc.* 1994;26:1012-1020.

51. Newton RU, Kraemer WJ, Häkkinen K, Humphries BJ, Murphy AJ. Kinematics, kinetics, and muscle activation during explosive upper body movements. *J Appl Biomech.* 1996;12:31-43.

52. Cronin J, McNair PJ, Marshall RN. Force-velocity analysis of strength-training techniques and load: implications for training strategy and research. *J Strength Cond Res.* 2003;17:148-155.

53. Hoffman JR, Ratamess NA, Cooper JJ, Kang J, Chilakos A, Faigenbaum AD. Comparison of loaded and unloaded jump squat training on strength/power performance in college football players. *J Strength Cond Res.* 2005;19:810-815.

54. Newton RU, Häkkinen K, Häkkinen A, McCormick M, Volek J, Kraemer WJ. Mixed-methods resistance training increases power and strength of young and older men. *Med Sci Sports Exerc.* 2002;34:1367-1375.

55. Wilson GJ, Newton RU, Murphy AJ, Humphries BJ. The optimal training load for the development of dynamic athletic performance. *Med Sci Sports Exerc.* 1993;25:1279-1286.

56. Wilson GJ, Murphy AJ, Walshe AD. Performance benefits from weight and plyometric training: effects of initial strength level. *Coaching Sport Sci. J* 1997;2:3-8.

57. Ebben WP, Watts PB. A review of combined weight training and plyometric training modes: complex training. *Strength Cond.* 1998;20:18-27.

58. Sale DG, MacDougall JD, Upton AR, McComas AJ. Effect of strength training upon motoneuron excitability in man. *Med Sci Sports Exerc.* 1983;15(1):57-62.

59. Brown HS, Stein RB, Yemm R. Changes in firing rate of human motor units during linearly changing voluntary contractions. *J Physiol (Lond).* 1973;230:371-390.

60. Marx JO, Kraemer WJ, Nindl BC, et al. The effect of periodization and volume of resistance training in women (abstract). *Med Sci Sports Exerc.* 1998;30(5):S164.

61. Kraemer WJ, Ratamess N, Fry AC, et al. Influence of resistance training volume and periodization on physiological and performance adaptations in collegiate women tennis players. *Am J Sports Med.* 2000;28(5):626-633.

62. Starkey DB, Pollock ML, Ishida Y, et al. Effect of resistance training volume on strength and muscle thickness. *Med Sci Sports Exerc.* 1996;28:1311-1320.

63. Jacobson BH. Comparison of two progressive weight training techniques on knee extensor strength. *Athl Train.* 1986;21:315-319.

64. Reid CM, Yeater RA, Ullrich IH. Weight training and strength, cardiorespiratory functioning and body composition of men. *Br J Sports Med.* 1987;21:40-44.

65. [No authors listed] American College of Sports Medicine position stand. The recommended quantity and quality of exercise for developing and maintaining cardiorespiratory and muscular fitness in healthy adults. *Med Sci Sports Exerc.* 1990;22:265-274.

66. Stone MH, Plisk SS, Stone ME, Schilling BK, O'Bryant HS, Pierce KC. Athletic performance development: volume load—1 set vs. multiple sets, training velocity and training variation. *Strength Cond J.* 1998;20(6):22-31.

67. Rhea MR, Alvar BA, Ball SD, Burkett LN. Three sets of weight training superior to 1 set with equal intensity for eliciting strength. *J Strength Cond Res.* 2002;16:525-529.

68. Haltom RW, Kraemer R, Sloan R, Hebert EP, Frank K, Tryniecki JL. Circuit weight training and its effects on postexercise oxygen consumption. *Med Sci Sports Exerc.* 1999;31(11):1613-1618.

69. Harber MP, Fry AC, Rubin MR, Smith JC, Weiss LW. Skeletal muscle and hormonal adaptations to circuit weight training in untrained men. *Scand J Med Sci Sports.* 2004;14(3):176-185.

70. Fleck SJ, Kraemer WJ. *Designing Resistance Training Programs.* 2nd ed. Champaign, IL: Human Kinetics; 1997.

71. Ahtiainen JP, Pakarinen A, Alen M, Kraemer WJ, Häkkinen K. Short vs. long rest period between the sets in hypertrophic resistance training: influence on muscle strength, size, and hormonal adaptations in trained men. *J Strength Cond Res.* 2005;19:572-582.

72. Kraemer WJ. A series of studies—the physiological basis for strength training in American football: fact over philosophy. *J Strength Cond Res.* 1997;11:131-142.

73. Richmond SR, Godard MP. The effects of varied rest periods between sets to failure using the bench press in recreationally trained men. *J Strength Cond Res.* 2004;18:846-849.

74. Robinson JM, Stone MH, Johnson RL, et al. Effects of different weight training exercise/rest intervals on strength, power, and high intensity exercise endurance. *J Strength Cond Res.* 1995;9:216-221.

75. McCall GE, Byrnes WC, Fleck SJ, Dickinson A, Kraemer WJ. Acute and chronic hormonal responses to resistance training designed to promote muscle hypertrophy. *Can J Appl Physiol.* 1999;24:96-107.

76. Ratamess NA, Falvo MJ, Mangine GT, Hoffman JR, Faigenbaum AD, Kang J. The effect of rest interval length on metabolic responses to the bench press exercise. *Eur J Appl Physiol.* 2007;100:1-17.

Integrated Program Design and the Optimum Performance Training™ (OPT™) Model

After studying this chapter, you will be able to:

✔ Define and describe the acute training variables within the Optimum Performance Training (OPT) model.

✔ Describe the phases within the OPT model.

✔ Design programs for each phase of training.

Introduction to Program Design

Exercise training programs are often based largely on the past experiences of those designing them. For example, training programs designed by those with backgrounds in bodybuilding, powerlifting, or Olympic weightlifting tend to vary considerably from programs designed by those with group exercise or previous athletic experiences only. Although experience is always an important quality to have in any field, including personal training, it is not the only nor, in some cases, even the most important qualification to have. Designing safe and effective exercise training programs requires a variety of skills, including knowledge gained through education, personal interest in exercise, the ability to communicate effectively with clients, and experience in working with other, more experienced trainers, as well as past experiences.

Personal trainers need to develop the right blend of exercise training knowledge, experience, and skills to be competent at designing integrated training programs for a variety of clients. At a minimum, personal trainers should be able to answer the following questions with confidence for all their clients:

◆ What exercises are most appropriate for my client?
◆ What exercises are contraindicated for my client?

- What exercise intensities are appropriate for my client?
- How many exercises are appropriate for my client?
- How many sets and repetitions should I have my client perform?
- How many days per week should my client train?

Without possessing the appropriate knowledge and education to answer these questions, personal trainers may design inappropriate, ineffective, or even unsafe training programs for their clients. In an effort to help personal trainers, especially those new to the field, design safe and effective training programs based on the individual needs of clients, NASM recommends using a structured, scientifically based program design model. The training program should be a methodical approach to improve physical, physiologic, psychological and performance adaptations. The best way to achieve consistent, superior results is to follow a structured periodized training program (1–12). Evidence also exists that a multicomponent program that includes, but is not limited to, flexibility, core, balance, plyometrics, speed/agility/quickness, resistance, and cardiorespiratory training can decrease injury and improve performance (13–30).

Program Design

Program design A purposeful system or plan put together to help an individual achieve a specific goal.

Program design simply means creating a purposeful system or plan to achieve a specific goal. The purpose of a training program is to provide a pathway to help clients achieve their health and fitness goals. To be able to effectively create exercise training pathways that will lead to success for their clients, personal trainers need to understand the following key concepts:

Acute Variables

- What are they?
- How do they affect the desired adaptation?
- How do they affect the overall training program?

The OPT Model (Planned Fitness Training—Periodization)

- How and why must the physiologic, physical, and performance adaptations of stabilization, strength, and power take place in a planned, progressive manner to establish the proper foundation for each subsequent adaptation?

The Five Phases of Training in the OPT Model

- How do these phases promote specific adaptations?
- What are the acute variables for each of the phases?

Application

- How are the right exercises selected?
- How are the right acute variables selected?
- How are both applied in a systematic manner to different populations with different goals?

Program Design Using the OPT Model

NASM designed the Optimum Performance Training (OPT) model as a planned, systematic, periodized training program **Figure 14.1**. The OPT model was developed to concurrently improve all functional abilities, such as flexibility, core stabilization, balance, strength, power, and cardiorespiratory endurance. The OPT program has been

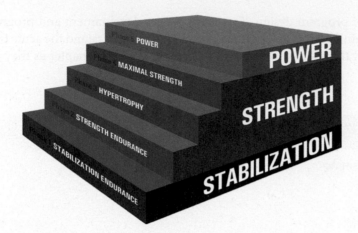

FIGURE 14.1

The OPT model.

extremely successful in helping clients from diverse populations to reduce their body fat, increase lean muscle mass and strength, and improve performance and overall health. This chapter presents detailed information on the following; what the acute variables of fitness training (or periodization) are and how they relate to the OPT model, what the five phases of the OPT model are, and how to apply the OPT program design model to specific goals or various clients.

SUMMARY

Personal trainers must be competent at designing training programs for a variety of clients, using acute variables and exercises in a structured, progressive manner. A structured, scientifically based program design model makes this process safer and more effective. The OPT model provides personal trainers with a proven system in which a client's information can simply be plugged in and a program designed. Program design is creating a purposeful system or plan to achieve a specific goal. To do so, the personal trainer must understand acute variables and the OPT model and its phases, as well as how to apply it all.

Acute Variables of Training

Acute variables are the most fundamental components of designing a training program. They determine the amount of stress placed on the body and, ultimately, what adaptations the body will incur.

The body will specifically adapt to the demands placed on it (known also as the principle of specificity). The acute variables applied during an exercise program will dictate these demands and the adaptations achieved. The OPT model provides a framework to help guide program design and allows for a planned, systematic progression by preassigning specific acute variables for each of the five phases of training to elicit the desired adaptation (2–5,7,9–12,31–40). Collectively, the acute variables are the

Acute variables
Important components that specify how each exercise is to be performed.

foundation of program design. To ensure proper development and progression of an integrated training program, personal trainers must understand the acute training variables. Each of the acute variables will be explained in this chapter as they relate to the OPT model.

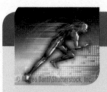

Memory Jogger

Acute Variables of Training

- Repetitions
- Sets
- Training intensity
- Repetition tempo
- Training volume
- Rest interval
- Training frequency
- Training duration
- Exercise selection

Repetitions

Repetition (or "rep")
One complete movement of a single exercise.

A **repetition** is one complete movement of a particular exercise. Most repetitions will involve the three muscle actions: concentric, isometric, and eccentric (not necessarily in that order) (41–43).

These muscle actions can be seen in the example of a biceps curl. A single repetition includes raising the dumbbell up against the direction of resistance (a concentric contraction), pausing for any specified amount of time (an isometric hold), and then lowering the dumbbell with the direction of resistance back to its starting position (an eccentric action).

Another example of these actions can be seen when performing a squat. Starting from a standing position, one repetition includes lowering the body (with the direction of resistance) toward the ground (eccentric), pausing for any specified amount of time (isometric), and then raising back up (against the direction of resistance) to the starting position (concentric).

Repetitions are simply a means to count the number of movements performed in a given amount of time. They can therefore be a means to count the time the muscles are under tension (*time under tension*). For instance, during the squat exercise, if the eccentric movement portion is performed at a 4-second pace, followed by a 2-second isometric pause and a 1-second concentric movement pace, the amount of time that the muscles are under tension would be equal to 7 seconds per repetition.

Each phase of training in the OPT model has specific goals and therefore requires a specific number of repetitions to achieve these goals. The number of repetitions performed in a given set is dependent on the client's work capacity, intensity of the exercise, and the specific phase of training. Personal trainers must keep in mind that all acute variables are interdependent. This means that the specific use of one will affect the others. For example, the more intense the exercise or heavier the load, the fewer the number of repetitions the individual can perform (39,44).

Research demonstrates that training in a specific repetition range yields specific adaptations. Therefore, depending on the goal of the individual and the phase of training, it is possible to define a specific repetition range (7,32,39,44–49).

◆ Muscular endurance and stabilization is best achieved by performing 12 to 20 repetitions at 50 to 70% of the one-repetition maximum (1RM).
◆ Hypertrophy (muscle growth) is best achieved using 6 to 12 repetitions at 75 to 85% of the 1RM.
◆ If maximal strength adaptations are desired, the repetition range is 1 to 5 at 85 to 100% of the 1RM.
◆ Power adaptations require 1 to 10 repetitions at 30 to 45% of 1RM, or approximately 10% of body weight.

The OPT model uses a specified repetition continuum to provide the desired adaptations in a systematic manner. The beginning phases consist of higher repetition schemes necessary to build proper connective tissue (tendons, ligaments) strength, stability, and muscular endurance, which is especially important for a beginning client. However, a common mistake of many advanced clients is to not use a planned training program that provides periods of low-repetition training alternated with periods of high-repetition training. Higher intensities of training can only be sustained for a short period without running the risk of overtraining (47,50). Using the OPT model enables the personal trainer to use a systematic training approach to prevent overtraining and yield specific results by using planned intervals of training.

Sets

A **set** is a group of consecutive repetitions (41–43). The quantities of the other acute variables (i.e., repetitions, training intensity, number of exercises, training level, and recoverability), as well as the training status of the client, determine the number of sets an individual performs (41,45–49,51).

Set A group of consecutive repetitions.

There is an inverse relationship between sets, repetitions, and intensity. The individual usually performs fewer sets when performing higher repetitions at a lower intensity (endurance adaptations) and more sets when performing lower repetitions at a higher intensity (strength and power adaptations) (42–49).

◆ Muscular endurance and stabilization is best developed with 1 to 3 sets of 12 to 20 repetitions at 50 to 70% of 1RM intensity.
◆ Hypertrophy adaptations are best stimulated by 3 to 5 sets of 6 to 12 repetitions at 75 to 85% of 1RM intensity level.
◆ For maximal strength adaptation, 4 to 6 sets of 1 and 5 repetitions at an intensity of 85 to 100% of 1RM are recommended.
◆ For power adaptations, 3 to 6 sets of between 1 and 10 repetitions at an intensity of 30 to 45% of 1RM (if using weights) or approximately 10% of body weight (if using medicine balls) are recommended.

Training Intensity

Training intensity is one of the most important acute variables to consider when designing an integrated training program. Training intensity is defined as an individual's level of effort compared with their maximal effort (7,39,42,43,45).

Training intensity An individual's level of effort, compared with their maximal effort, which is usually expressed as a percentage.

The specific training phase and an individual's training goal, as well as the training status of the client, will determine the number of sets and repetitions for an exercise. Intensity is then determined by the number of sets and repetitions to be performed, which is based on the individual's specific training goals.

- Muscular endurance and stabilization is best developed with a training intensity of 50 to 70% of 1RM.
- Hypertrophy is best achieved by training with 75 to 85% of 1RM.
- Maximal strength adaptations require training with 85 to 100% of 1RM.
- Power (high-velocity) adaptations are best attained with 30 to 45% of 1RM when using conventional weight training, or approximately 10% of body weight when using medicine balls.

Training in an unstable environment, as seen in the stabilization phases of the OPT model, can also increase the training intensity because it requires greater motor unit recruitment (52–55), which leads to greater energy expenditure per exercise (56–59) and allows for optimal development of neuromuscular efficiency. Changing other acute training variables such as rest periods and tempo also changes the training intensity. In short, intensity is a function of more than just external resistance. An integrated training program must focus on a holistic approach to force continued adaptations.

Repetition Tempo

Repetition tempo The speed with which each repetition is performed.

Repetition tempo refers to the speed with which each repetition is performed. This is an important variable that can be manipulated to achieve specific training objectives such as endurance, hypertrophy, strength, and power (39,41–43). Because movements occur at different velocities, to get the most appropriate results from training personal trainers must select the appropriate speed of movement (e.g., slower tempo for endurance and faster tempo for power) for the exercise.

- Muscular endurance and stabilization is best developed with a slow repetition tempo. One example of a slow tempo would be a 4-second eccentric action, 2-second isometric hold, and 1-second concentric contraction (4/2/1).
- Hypertrophy is best achieved with a moderate tempo. One example of a moderate tempo would be a 2-second eccentric action, 0-second isometric hold, and 2-second concentric contraction (2/0/2).
- Maximal strength adaptations are best achieved with a fast or explosive tempo that can be safely controlled. Keep in mind, because an individual will be using heavy loads when training for maximal strength, the actual velocity of the movement may be rather slow, but the individual will be exerting himself or herself with maximal effort.
- Power adaptations are best achieved with an fast or explosive tempo that can be safely controlled.

The OPT model places a major emphasis on the repetition tempo spectrum as it has a significant impact on the functional outcome of the stressed tissues. By emphasizing eccentric and isometric muscle actions at slower velocities during the initial stabilization phases of training, more demand is placed on the connective tissue (as well as the stabilizing muscles) and better prepares the nervous system for functional movements. This technique is important for building the appropriate structural and functional foundation for more specific forms of strength and power training that will follow.

Rest Interval

The **rest interval** is the time taken to recuperate between sets or exercises and has a dramatic effect on the outcome of the training program (39,41–43). Each exercise that is performed requires energy. The primary type of energy used during training depends on the training phase, intensity, exercise mode, and goal.

Rest interval The time taken to recuperate between sets.

♦ Muscular endurance and stabilization adaptations is best developed with relatively short rest periods; generally 0–90 seconds. However, the current work capacity of the client may dictate longer rest periods if needed (60).

♦ Hypertrophy is best achieved with relatively short rests periods often ranging from 0 to 60 seconds. However, the load, volume, and the current fitness level of the client may require longer rest periods (60).

♦ Maximal strength adaptations are best achieved with relatively long rest periods, generally 3–5 minutes, depending on the client's level of fitness and intensity of the exercises.

♦ Power adaptations also require relatively long rest periods, generally 3–5 minutes, depending on the client's level of fitness.

Dynamic resistance training, as well as isometric training, can significantly reduce adenosine triphosphate (ATP) and phosphocreatine (PC) supplies (61–63). The ability to replenish these supplies is crucial for optimal performance and the desired adaptation. By adjusting the rest interval, energy supplies can be regained according to the goal of the training program. Rest intervals of (64):

♦ 20 to 30 seconds will allow approximately 50% recovery of ATP and PC.
♦ 40 seconds will allow approximately 75% recovery of ATP and PC.
♦ 60 seconds will allow approximately 85 to 90% recovery of ATP and PC.
♦ 3 minutes will allow approximately 100% recovery of ATP and PC.

The rest interval between sets determines to what extent the energy resources are replenished before the next set (39,65). The shorter the rest interval, the less ATP and PC will be replenished and consequently less energy will be available for the next set (60). With new clients, this can result in fatigue, which can lead to decreased neuromuscular control, force production, and stabilization by decreasing motor unit recruitment (66). Therefore, inadequate rest intervals can decrease performance and could lead to altered movement patterns, and even injury. As the client advances, this can be used as a means to increase the intensity of the workout and promote better adaptations, especially for stability, endurance, and hypertrophy.

Conversely, if rest periods are too long between sets or exercises, the potential effects include decreased neuromuscular activity and decreased body temperature. If the beginner client is then asked to perform an intense bout of exercise, this could entail a potential increased risk of injury. For the advanced client, this may be necessary if heavy weight is being used repetitively. The goal of the training program should establish the appropriate rest periods (7,39,60). There are several factors to consider when prescribing appropriate rest intervals.

Individuals who are starting an exercise routine may respond better to longer rest periods until they adjust to the demands of their program. Longer rest periods also help to ensure proper exercise technique. By reducing the amount of fatigue experienced by the client, that individual may be able to perform each exercise with greater precision. Individuals who are at advanced levels of training or higher fitness levels may respond better to shorter rest periods, but it is still dependent on the phase of training and the client's goal.

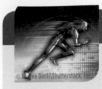

Memory Jogger

Factors for Appropriate Rest Intervals

- Training experience
- Training intensity
- Tolerance of short rest periods
- Muscle mass
- General fitness level
- Training goals
- Nutritional status
- Recoverability

Table 14.1 summarizes the appropriate acute variables (sets, reps, intensity, repetition tempo, rest periods) for muscular endurance, hypertrophy, maximal strength, and power adaptations.

Training Volume

Training volume Amount of physical training performed within a specified period.

Training volume is the total amount of work performed within a specified time (7,39,41). It is extremely important to plan and control training volume to prevent overtraining, as all training is cumulative. Training volume varies among individuals and is based on:

- Training phase
- Goals
- Age
- Work capacity or training status
- Recoverability
- Nutritional status
- Injury history
- Life stress

TABLE 14.1	**Program Design Continuum**					
Adaptation	**Reps**	**Sets**	**Intensity**	**Tempo**	**Rest Periods**
Muscular endurance/ stabilization	12–20	1–3	50–70% of 1RM	Slow (4/21)	0–90 s
Hypertrophy	6–12	3–5	75–85% of 1RM	Moderate (2/0/2)	0–60 s
Maximal strength	1–5	4–6	85–100% of 1RM	Fast/explosive	3–5 min
Power	1–10	3–6	30–45% of 1RM or ≤10% of body weight	Fast/explosive	3–5 min

© ilolab/ShutterStock, Inc.

For an individual to achieve optimal results from an integrated training program, the program must provide them with the appropriate planned training volume for extended periods. One of the most important training concepts to remember is that volume is always inversely related to intensity. In other words, an individual cannot safely perform high volumes of high-intensity exercises for any extended length of time (67,68). For example, when working with loads exceeding 90% of an individual's maximum, one rarely exceeds a workout volume of 30 repetitions (6 sets of 5 repetitions) per exercise. However, when working with loads of 60% of maximum, a client can easily perform a workout volume of 36 to 60 repetitions per exercise (3 sets of 12 to 20 repetitions). The exception is new clients who may only perform 12 to 20 total repetitions per exercise (1 set of each exercise).

The training phase and the training goal dictate the repetitions, sets, intensity, rest, and tempo, and these combined dictate the volume (7,32,39,43). Research demonstrates that higher volume training produces cellular (hypertrophy, fat loss) adaptations (Table 14.2) (39,43,48,49). Conversely, high-intensity training with low training volumes produces greater neurologic (maximal strength, power) adaptations Table 14.2 (39,44,50,53).

Training Frequency

Training frequency refers to the number of training sessions that are performed during a given period (usually 1 week). There is considerable debate concerning the adequate number of training sessions per body part per week necessary for optimal results. The number of training sessions per week per body part is determined by many factors, including training goals, age, general health, work capacity, nutritional status, recoverability, lifestyle, and other stressors (32,37,42,43).

New clients may begin by training their entire body two times a week. However, experienced bodybuilders with the specific goal of hypertrophy may have a training cycle in which they train with a split routine of six sessions per week, training each body part two times per week with a larger volume per session. The specific training goal dictates the program design. Research on training frequency indicates that the optimal training frequency for improvements in strength is three to five times per week (48). Other research indicates that training at least one to two times per week is sufficient to maintain the physical, physiologic, and performance improvements that were achieved during other phases of training (69–71).

Training frequency
The number of training sessions performed during a specified period (usually 1 week).

TABLE 14.2	Training Volume Adaptations

© ilolab/ShutterStock, Inc.

High Volume (Low/Moderate Intensity)	Low Volume (High Intensity)
Increased muscle cross-sectional area	Increased rate of force production
Improved blood lipid serum profile (improved cholesterol and triglycerides)	Increased motor unit recruitment
Increased metabolic rate	Increased motor unit synchronization

Training Duration

Training duration The timeframe of a workout or the length of time spent in one phase of training.

Training duration has two prominent meanings:

1. The timeframe from the start of the workout to the finish of the workout.
2. The length of time (number of weeks) spent in one phase (or period) of training.

The training duration for a workout is a function of the number of repetitions, number of sets, number of exercises, and the length of the rest intervals. Training programs that exceed 60 to 90 minutes (excluding warm-up/cool-down) are associated with rapidly declining energy levels. This causes alterations in hormonal and immune system responses that can have a negative effect on a training program and raise the risk of minor infections, especially upper respiratory infections (72–75).

The training duration for a phase of training is dictated by the client's level of physical ability, goal, and compliance to the program. Typically, a phase of training will last 4 weeks as this is the amount of time it generally takes for the body to adapt to a given stimulus. Afterward, the training stimulus will have to be raised to achieve further adaptations (76–78).

Exercise Selection

Exercise selection The process of choosing appropriate exercises for a client's program.

Exercise selection is the process of choosing exercises for program design that allow for the optimal achievement of the desired adaptation. It has a tremendous impact on the outcome of the training program (39,41). The human movement system is a highly adaptable system that readily adjusts to the imposed demands of training (principle of specificity). Therefore, exercises should be specific to the training goals Table 14.3 (75).

The OPT model uses exercises from all components (core, balance, plyometric, and resistance training), which are categorized by the adaptation for which they are primarily used. For example, exercises that are used in Phase 1 of the OPT model (stabilization) are termed *stabilization level* exercises because they are used and progressed for the stabilization adaptation. Similarly, the exercises used in Phases 2 to 4 are termed *strength level* exercises, and exercises used in Phase 5 are termed *power level* exercises (Table 14.3).

Exercises can be broken down simplistically into three different types on the basis of the number of joints used, movements performed, and adaptation desired Table 14.4 (75):

1. Single joint: These exercises focus on isolating one major muscle group or joint (e.g., biceps curls, triceps pushdowns, calf raises).
2. Multijoint: These exercises use the involvement of two or three joints (e.g., squats, lunges, step-ups, chest presses, rows).
3. Total body: These exercises include multiple joint movements (e.g., step-up balance to overhead press, squat to two-arm press, barbell clean).

TABLE 14.3	The Exercise Selection Continuum	
Training Adaptation	**Training Level**	**Exercise Selection**
Endurance / Stabilization	Stabilization level	Total body; multijoint or single joint; controlled unstable
Strength	Strength level	Total body; multijoint or single joint
Power	Power level	Total body; multijoint (explosive)

© Ilolab/ShutterStock, Inc.

TABLE 14.4	Exercise Selection—Examples		
Level	Total Body	Multijoint	Single Joint
Stabilization	Step-up, balance to overhead press	Ball dumbbell chest press Ball dumbbell row Standing overhead press	Single-leg dumbbell curl
Strength	Squat, curl to overhead press	Bench press Seated row machine Shoulder press machine	Standing two-arm dumbbell curl
Power	Two-arm push press	Two-arm medicine ball chest pass Ball medicine ball pullover throw Front Medicine ball oblique throw	N/A

© iiolab/ShutterStock. Inc.

The OPT model enables personal trainers to effectively select the appropriate exercise for each client. Completing a fitness assessment and reviewing the specific training goals will allow the fitness professional to implement these exercises into a properly planned, integrated training program.

For example, to develop optimal stability, traditional exercises can be *progressed* to a more unstable environment, such as standing up (two-leg, staggered-stance, single-leg) or from a stable environment to an unstable environment (foam pad, stability ball, BOSU ball, etc.). Research has shown that exercises performed in unstable environments produce superior results for the goal of stabilization and training the core stabilizing muscles (16,79,80). It is important to note, NASM only recommends training in a proprioceptive (unstable) environment that can be *safely* controlled based on the client's movement capabilities. Stabilization exercise examples include:

◆ Chest press on a stability ball
◆ Single-leg cable rows
◆ Single-leg dumbbell shoulder press on a ½ foam roll
◆ Single-leg squat

To develop optimal strength, the use of total-body and multijoint exercises has been shown to be most beneficial (81). Strength exercise examples include:

◆ Bench press
◆ Rows (machine, seated cable, barbell)
◆ Shoulder press (seated barbell, seated dumbbell, machine)
◆ Squats/leg press

To develop optimal power, plyometrics, and explosive strength-training exercises can be performed during functional movement patterns (82–94). Power exercise examples include:

◆ Overhead medicine ball throw
◆ Medicine ball chest pass
◆ Woodchop throw
◆ Squat jump
◆ Tuck jump
◆ Two-arm push press
◆ Barbell clean

All exercises, once selected, can be progressed or regressed in a systematic fashion Table 14.5.

Stabilization Continuum	Lower Body	Upper Body
TABLE 14.5 **The Progression Continuum** © ilolab/ShutterStock, Inc.		
Floor	Two-legs stable	Two-arm
↓	↓	↓
Sport beam	Staggered-stance stable	Alternating arms
↓	↓	↓
Half foam roll	Single-leg stable	Single-arm
↓	↓	↓
Foam pad[a]	Two-leg unstable	Single-arm with trunk rotation
↓	↓	
Balance disc[a]	Staggered-stance unstable	
↓	↓	
Wobble board[a]	Single-leg unstable	
↓		
BOSU Ball		

[a] These modalities come in many shapes and sizes that will dictate proper progression.

SUMMARY

Designing a safe and effective training program for clients is the primary function of a personal trainer. Programs should be individualized to meet the needs and goals of each client. Therefore, it is important that a scientifically based, systematic, and progressive model is used. The OPT model provides the fitness professional with all the necessary tools to properly use acute variables (repetitions, sets, and so forth), scientific concepts, and exercises to design programs.

Acute variables determine the amount of stress placed on the body and, ultimately, what adaptation the body will incur. The acute variables to consider when designing a program are as follows:

- Repetitions: The more intense the exercise, the fewer the number of repetitions that the individual should perform.
- Sets: The individual usually performs fewer sets when performing higher repetitions at a lower intensity (endurance adaptations) and more sets when performing lower repetitions at a higher intensity (strength and power adaptations).
- Training intensity: This should be determined after sets and reps. Altering other variables (such as environment stability, rest periods, and tempo) changes the training intensity.
- Repetition tempo: Different times under tension yield specific results. By emphasizing eccentric and isometric muscle actions at slower velocities, more demand is placed on the connective tissue.

◆ Rest interval: This has a dramatic effect on the outcome of the training program. By adjusting the rest interval, energy supplies can be regained according to the goal of the training program. The shorter the rest interval, the less ATP and PC will be replenished, and consequently less energy will be available for the next set. To avoid making rests too long or short, consider the following factors: training experience, training intensity, tolerance to short rest periods, general fitness level, training goals, nutritional status, and recoverability.

◆ Training volume: Plan and control training volume to prevent overtraining. Volume is always inversely related to intensity.

◆ Training frequency: Optimal training frequency for improvements in strength is three to five times per week. Training at least one to two times per week is sufficient to maintain improvements achieved during other phases of training.

◆ Training duration: Programs exceeding 60 to 90 minutes can have a negative effect on a training program and raise the risk of minor infections, especially upper respiratory infections. Typically, a phase of training will last 4 weeks.

◆ Exercise selection: Exercises should be specific to the training goals and based on the principles of the exercise selection continuum.

Periodization and the OPT Model (Planned Fitness Training)

Understanding the importance of designing safe and effective programs using acute variable manipulation is important fundamental information for all personal trainers and ultimately their success in the profession. The OPT model is based on the concepts of periodization. As discussed in chapter 13 (resistance training), periodization is a systematic approach to program design that uses the general adaptation syndrome and principle of specificity to vary the amount and type of stress placed on the body to produce adaptation and prevent injury. Periodization (or planned fitness training) varies the focus of a training program at regularly planned periods of time (weeks, months, and so forth) to produce optimal adaptation. Periodization involves two primary objectives:

1. Dividing the training program into distinct periods (or phases) of training.
2. Training different forms of strength in each period (or phase) to control the volume of training and to prevent injury (39,75,95).

Did You Know?

Undulating periodization allows the client to train at varying intensities during the course of a week, which allows for multiple adaptations once a level of fitness has been achieved. For example, the client may do a stabilization workout on Monday, a strength workout on Wednesday and a power workout on Friday. See the reference by Rhea et al. (11) for details.

Training Plans

To accomplish the objectives of periodization, training programs should be organized into a specific plan that involves using long-term and short-term goals and objectives. A **training plan** is a specific plan that a fitness professional uses to meet the client's goal. It will determine the forms of training to be used, how long it will take, how often

Training plan The specific outline, created by a fitness professional to meet a client's goals, that details the form of training, length of time, future changes, and specific exercises to be performed.

© ilolab/ShutterStock, Inc.

Annual plan Generalized training plan that spans 1 year to show when the client will progress between phases.

Monthly plan Generalized training plan that spans 1 month and shows which phases will be required each day of each week.

Weekly plan Training plan of specific workouts that spans 1 week and shows which exercises are required each day of the week.

it will change, and what specific exercises will be performed. The long-term portion of a training plan in the OPT model is known as an *annual plan*, whereas the short-term portions are termed *monthly and weekly plans*. By providing a training plan, clients will be able to see the future achievement of their goals in a timely, organized fashion.

An **annual plan** organizes the training program for a 1-year period **Figure 14.2**. The annual plan allows the health and fitness professional to provide the client with a blueprint (or map) that specifically shows how the OPT training program will progress for the long term, from month-to-month, to meet the desired goal. This gives the client a clear representation of how the personal trainer plans to get the client to his or her goal and how long it will take to get there. In Figure 14.2, the far left column represents the period or main strength adaptation and the second column shows the specific phases of the OPT model that make up each specific adaptation of training.

Each month within the annual plan is further broken down into periods of training called monthly plans **Figure 14.3**. The **monthly plan** details the specific days of each workout, showing the client exactly what phase of the OPT model (type of training) will be required each day of the week as well as when the reassessment will occur. The monthly plan also shows the client the necessary cardio requirements.

Each monthly plan also illustrates weekly plans, which are the specific workouts that the client will do for that week (Figure 14.3). The **weekly plan** gives the client a picture of exactly what phases will be used in his or her workout for that period.

FIGURE 14.2

Annual plan.

	PHASE	JAN	FEB	MAR	APR	MAY	JUN	JUL	AUG	SEP	OCT	NOV	DEC
Stabilization	1												
	2												
Strength	3												
	4												
Power	5												
Cardio														

FIGURE 14.3

The monthly or weekly plan.

Week			1							2							3							4				
Day	M	T	W	T	F	S	S	M	T	W	T	F	S	S	M	T	W	T	F	S	S	M	T	W	T	F	S	S
Phase 1																												
Phase 2																												
Phase 3																												
Phase 4																												
Phase 5																												
Cardio																												
Re-assess																												

FIGURE 14.4

Periodization cycles.

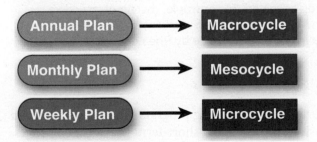

Annual Plan → Macrocycle

Monthly Plan → Mesocycle

Weekly Plan → Microcycle

Much of the literature regarding periodization refers to dividing the training program into specific cycles termed macrocycles, mesocycles, and microcycles **Figure 14.4**. For ease of understanding, a *macrocycle* is the largest cycle and, typically, covers a yearlong period of training (or annual plan). The macrocycle is divided into *mesocycles*, which are typically 1 to 3 months in length (or monthly plans). Each mesocycle in turn is divided into *microcycles*, which are usually a week in length (or weekly plans) (96).

Periodization has been shown to be an effective form of program design for many fitness-related goals, and yet, to date, it is not a common practice among all personal trainers. Periodization provides for the repeated use of different forms of training at specific times in an annual training program to elicit different adaptations in the body (stabilization, strength, and power). By intentionally cycling through different periods (or phases) of training, the acute variables are manipulated to adjust the volume of training. And by controlling the volume of training as a function of time in any given program, periodization allows for maximal levels of adaptation, while minimizing overtraining, which is a primary benefit of periodization, because overtraining will lead to fatigue and eventual injury (2–9,11,12,33,34,37,45).

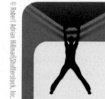

STRETCH Your Knowledge

What Is the Evidence to Support the Use of Planned, Periodized, Integrated Training Programs?

Making gradual increases in volume and decreases in intensity was the most effective program for increasing muscular endurance (1).

A 9-month periodized resistance-training program was superior for enhancing strength and motor performance in collegiate women tennis players (2).

Making program alterations on a daily basis was more effective in eliciting strength gains than doing so every 4 weeks (3).

Planned, integrated strength-training programs led to superior physical, physiologic, and performance improvements compared with nonperiodized training programs (4).

Planned variations in an integrated training program were essential because they enabled continuous adaptations to occur during a training period and prevented injury (5).

An evaluation of the body of research comparing periodized with nonperiodized training demonstrated a superior strength and power adaptation with periodized training (6).

REFERENCES

1. Rhea MR, Phillips WT, Burkett LN, et al. A comparison of linear and daily undulating periodized programs with equated volume and intensity for local muscular endurance. *J Strength Cond Res.* 2003;17:82-87.
2. Kraemer, WJ, Hakkinen K, Triplett-McBride NT, et al. Physiological changes with periodized resistance training in women tennis players. *Med Sci Sports Exerc.* 2003;35:157-168.
3. Rhea MR, Phillips WT, Burkett LN, Stone WJ, Ball SD. A comparison of daily and undulating periodized programs with equated volume and intensity for strength. *J Strength Cond Res.* 2002;16:250-255.
4. Kraemer WJ, Ratamess NA. Fundamentals of of resistance training: progression and exercise prescription. *Med Sci Sports Exerc.* 2004;36(4):674-688.
5. Tan B. Manipulating resistance training program variables to optimize maximum strength in men: a review. *J Strength Cond Res.* 1999;13:289-304.
6. Rhea MR, Alderman BL. A meta-analysis of periodized versus nonperiodized strength and power training programs. *Res Q Exerc Sport.* 2004;75:413-422.

SUMMARY

Planned fitness training (or periodization) shifts the focus of a training program at regularly planned intervals of time to vary stress placed on the body to produce adaptation and prevent injury. A training plan clarifies what forms of training will be used, how long it will take, how often it will change, and what specific exercises will be performed. An annual plan organizes the training program for a 1-year period to show when the client is in which phase. The annual plan is further broken down into periods of training called monthly plans, which detail the specific days of each workout, showing the client exactly what type of training will be required each day of the month. Weekly plans are the specific workouts and exercises that the client will do for that week.

The OPT Model

The different periods (or phases) of training seen in a traditional periodization model include a preparatory period (termed *anatomic adaptation*), a hypertrophy period, a maximal strength period, and a power period. The OPT model simplifies these phases into stabilization, strength, and power. The OPT model seen in a phase-specific model of training includes five different phases of training Table 14.6. These phases systematically progress all clients through the three main adaptations of stabilization, strength, and power. The OPT model should be thought of as a staircase guiding clients through different levels of adaptation. This journey will involve going up and down the stairs, stopping at different steps, and moving to various heights, depending on the client's goals, needs, and abilities. This section will detail the various phases of training in the OPT model.

Stabilization

The first level of training in the OPT model focuses on the main adaptation of stabilization (or anatomic adaptation) and is designed to prepare the body for the demands of higher levels of training that may follow. This period is crucial for all beginners. It is also necessary to cycle back through this level after periods of strength and power

TABLE 14.6   Summary Chart of OPT Model

© ilolab/ShutterStock, Inc.

Level	Specific Adaptation	Phases Used	Method of Progression
Stabilization	• Endurance • Stability	1	Proprioception (controlled unstable)
Strength	• Strength Endurance • Hypertrophy • Maximal Strength	2 3 4	Volume/load
Power	• Power	5	Speed/load

Chapter 14 – Integrated Program Design and the Optimum Performance Training™ (OPT™) Model   **369**

training to maintain a high degree of core and joint stability. In addition, it allows the body to actively rest from more intense bouts of training. The focus of stabilization training includes:

- Improving muscle imbalances
- Improving stabilization of the core musculature
- Preventing tissue overload by preparing muscles, tendons, ligaments, and joints for the upcoming imposed demands of training
- Improving overall cardiorespiratory and neuromuscular condition
- Establishing proper movement patterns and exercise technique

The above goals are accomplished through low-intensity, high-repetition training programs, emphasizing core and joint stabilization (as opposed to increasing the strength of the arms and legs), and will incorporate exercises that progressively challenge the body's stability requirements (or proprioception), as opposed to how much weight is being used.

The primary means of progressing (or increasing the intensity of training) in this period is by increasing the proprioceptive demands of the exercises. In other words, the exercises become progressively more unstable and challenge the client's ability to maintain proper balance and posture. This form of training has been shown to be extremely effective for increasing neuromuscular efficiency in the healthy (80), elderly (97), and unhealthy populations (98–101). Another important component of stabilization training is that it may help to ensure activity-specific strength adaptations (such as standing on one leg to kick a ball, climbing up stairs, or simply walking) (79).

The stabilization period of training in the OPT model consists of one phase of training: Stabilization Endurance Training.

Stabilization Endurance Training (Phase 1)

Stabilization Endurance Training is designed to create optimal levels of stabilization strength and postural control Table 14.7. Although this phase is the first phase of training in the OPT model, as previously stated, it will also be important to cycle back through this phase of training between periods of higher-intensity training seen in Phases 2 through 5. This will allow for proper recovery and maintenance of high levels of stability that will ensure optimal adaptations for strength, power, or both. The primary focus when progressing in this phase is on increasing the proprioception (controlled instability) of the exercises, rather than just the load. This phase of training focuses on:

- Increasing stability
- Increasing muscular endurance
- Increasing neuromuscular efficiency of the core musculature
- Improving intermuscular and intramuscular coordination

In addition to increasing proprioceptive demand, acute variables can be progressed by increasing the volume (sets, reps) and intensity (load, exercise selection, planes of motion), and by decreasing rest periods. A client in this category will generally stay in this phase of training for a 4-week duration. This period prepares clients for the demands of the Strength Endurance Phase (Phase 2).

TABLE 14.7	Phase 1: Stabilization Endurance Training							
	Reps	**Sets**	**Tempo**	**% Intensity**	**Rest Interval**	**Frequency**	**Duration**	**Exercise Selection**
Flexibility	1	1–3	30 s hold	N/A	N/A	3–7 times/wk	4–6 wk	SMR and static
Core	12–20	1–4	Slow 4/2/1	N/A	0–90 s	2–4 times/wk	4–6 wk	1–4 core-stabilization
Balance	12–20 6–10 (SL)	1–3	Slow 4/2/1	N/A	0–90 s	2–4 times/wk	4–6 wk	1–4 balance-stabilization
Plyometric*	5–8	1–3	3–5 s hold on landing	N/A	0–90 s	2–4 times/wk	4–6 wk	0–2 plyometric-stabilization
SAQ*	2–3	1–2	Moderate	N/A	0–90 s	2–4 times/wk	4–6 wk	4–6 drills with limited horizontal inertia and unpredictability
Resistance	12–20	1–3	4/2/1	50–70%	0–90 s	2–4 times/wk	4–6 wk	1–2 stabilization progression

*If a client does not have ample amounts of core stability and balance, plyometric exercises may not be included in this phase of training until these components are developed.

N/A = not applicable; SL = single leg; SMR = self-myofascial release.

Strength

The second level of training in the OPT model focuses on the main adaptation of strength, which includes strength endurance, hypertrophy, and maximal strength. It is designed to maintain stability while increasing the amount of stress placed on the body for increased muscle size and strength. This period of training is a necessary progression from stabilization for anyone who desires to increase caloric expenditure, muscle size, muscle strength, and bone mineral density. The focus of the strength period of training is to:

- Increase the ability of the core musculature to stabilize the pelvis and spine under heavier loads, through more complete ranges of motion
- Increase the load-bearing capabilities of muscles, tendons, ligaments, and joints
- Increase the volume of training
- Increase metabolic demand by taxing the ATP-PC and glycolysis energy systems to induce cellular changes in muscle (weight loss or hypertrophy)
- Increase motor unit recruitment, frequency of motor unit recruitment, and motor unit synchronization (maximal strength)

The strength period of training in the OPT model consists of three phases: Phase 2 (Strength Endurance Training), Phase 3 (Hypertrophy Training), and Phase 4 (Maximal Strength Training).

Professional's Name: Brian Sutton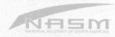

CLIENT'S NAME: JOHN SMITH	DATE: 5/01/13

GOAL: TOTAL BODY	PHASE: 1 STABILIZATION ENDURANCE

WARM-UP

Exercise:	Sets	Duration	Coaching Tip
SMR: Calves, IT-Band, Lats	1	30 s.	Hold each tender area for 30 sec
Static Stretch: Calves, Hip Flexors, Lats	1	30 s.	Hold each stretch for 30 sec
Treadmill	1	5 – 10 min	Brisk walk to slow jog

CORE / BALANCE / PLYOMETRIC

Exercise:	Sets	Reps	Tempo	Rest	Coaching Tip
Floor Bridge	2	15	Slow	0	
Floor Prone Cobra	2	15	Slow	0	
Single-Leg Balance Reach	2	8	Slow	0	8 reaches each leg
Squat Jump w/Stabilization	2	5	Slow	90 s.	Hold landing 3 – 5 seconds

SPEED, AGILITY, QUICKNESS

Exercise:	Sets	Reps	Rest	Coaching Tip
Optional				
Optional				

RESISTANCE

Exercise:		Sets	Reps	Tempo	Rest	Coaching Tip
Total Body	Ball Squat Curl to Press	2	15	Slow	0	Vertical loading
Chest	Push-Up	2	15	Slow	0	
Back	Standing Cable Row	2	15	Slow	0	
Shoulders	Single-Leg Scaption	2	15	Slow	0	
Biceps	Single-Leg Biceps Curl	2	15	Slow	0	
Triceps	Supine Ball DB Triceps Extensions	2	15	Slow	0	
Legs	Step-Up to Balance	2	15	Slow	90 s.	

COOL-DOWN

Exercise:	Sets	Duration	Coaching Tip
Treadmill (optional)	1	5 – 10 min	Brisk walk
SMR: Calves, IT-Band, Lats	1	30 s.	Hold each tender area for 30 sec
Static Stretch: Calves, Hip Flexors, Lats	1	30 s.	Hold each stretch for 30 sec

Coaching Tips:

National Academy of Sports Medicine

Strength Endurance Training (Phase 2)

Strength endurance is a hybrid form of training that promotes increased stabilization endurance, hypertrophy, and strength. This form of training entails the use of super-set techniques in which a more stable exercise (such as a bench press) is immediately followed with a stabilization exercise with similar biomechanical motions (such as a stability ball push-up). Thus, for every set of an exercise/body part performed according to the acute variables, there are actually two exercises or two sets being performed. High amounts of volume can be generated in this phase of training Table 14.8.

Similar to Phase 1, acute variables can be progressed by increasing proprioceptive demand, volume, (sets, reps), and intensity (load, exercise selection, planes of motion), and by decreasing rest periods. A client in this category will generally stay in this phase of training for a 4-week duration.

TABLE 14.8 **Phase 2: Strength Endurance Training**

	Reps	Sets	Tempo	% Intensity	Rest Interval	Frequency	Duration	Exercise Selection
Flexibility	5–10	1–2	1–2 s hold	N/A	N/A	3–7 times/wk	4 wk	SMR and active*
Core	8–12	2–3	Medium	N/A	0–60 s	2–4 times/wk	4 wk	1–3 core-strength
Balance	8–12	2–3	Medium	N/A	0–60 s	2–4 times/wk	4 wk	1–3 balance-strength
Plyometric	8–10	2–3	Repeating	N/A	0–60 s	2–4 times/wk	4 wk	1–3 plyometric-strength
SAQ†	3–5	3–4	Fast	N/A	0–60 s	2–4 times/wk	4 wk	6–8 drills allowing greater horizontal inertia but limited unpredictability
Resistance	8–12	2–4	(Str) 2/0/2 (Stab) 4/2/1	70–80%	0–60 s	2–4 times/wk	4 wk	1 strength superset with 1 stabilization

NOTE: Each resistance-training exercise is a superset of a strength level exercise immediately followed by a stabilization level exercise.
*Depending on the client, static stretching may still need to be used in this phase of training (followed by active-isolated stretching).
†SAQ may be optional in this phase of training (although recommended).
N/A = not applicable; SMR = self-myofascial release.

Professional's Name: Brian Sutton

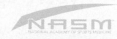

CLIENT'S NAME: JOHN SMITH	DATE: 5/01/13

GOAL: TOTAL BODY	PHASE: 2 STRENGTH ENDURANCE

WARM-UP

Exercise:	Sets	Duration	Coaching Tip
SMR: Calves, IT-Band, Lats	1	30 s.	Hold each tender area for 30 sec
Active Stretch: Calves, Hip Flexors, Lats	1	10 reps	Hold each stretch for 1–2 sec
Treadmill	1	5–10 min	Brisk walk to slow jog

CORE / BALANCE / PLYOMETRIC

Exercise:	Sets	Reps	Tempo	Rest	Coaching Tip
Ball Crunch	2	10	Medium	0	
Reverse Crunch	2	10	Medium	0	
Single-Leg Squat	2	10	Medium	0	
Squat Jump	2	10	Medium	60 s.	

SPEED, AGILITY, QUICKNESS

Exercise:	Sets	Reps	Rest	Coaching Tip
Optional				
Optional				

RESISTANCE

Exercise:		Sets	Reps	Tempo	Rest	Coaching Tip
Total Body	Optional					
Chest	Bench Press	2	12	Medium	0	Superset
	Push-Up		12	Slow	60 s.	
Back	Seated Cable Row	2	12	Medium	0	Superset
	Ball Dumbbell Row		12	Slow	60 s.	
Shoulders	Standing Dumbbell Should Press	2	12	Medium	0	Superset
	Single-Leg Scaption		12	Slow	60 s.	
Biceps	Optional					
Triceps	Optional					
Legs	Leg Press	2	12	Medium	0	Superset
	Step-Up to Balance		12	Slow	60 s.	

COOL-DOWN

Exercise:	Sets	Duration	Coaching Tip
Treadmill (optional)	1	5–10 min	Brisk walk
SMR: Calves, IT-Band, Lats	1	30 s.	Hold each tender area for 30 sec
Static Stretch: Calves, Hip Flexors, Lats	1	30 s.	Hold each stretch for 30 sec

Coaching Tips: Resistance program can be split into 2, 3, or 4-day workout routine. Ex. 3-day routine:
Day 1 (chest/back) Day 2 (legs) Day 3 (shoulders/biceps/triceps)

National Academy of Sports Medicine

© ilolab/ShutterStock, Inc.

Hypertrophy Training (Phase 3)

Hypertrophy training is specific for the adaptation of maximal muscle growth, focusing on high levels of volume with minimal rest periods to force cellular changes that result in an overall increase in muscle size Table 14.9.

Acute variables can be progressed if a client with the goal of increasing lean body mass and general performance has properly progressed through Phases 1 and 2 of the OPT model. Because the goal of this phase of training is primarily hypertrophy, the fitness professional will want to increase volume and intensity of the program. A client in this category will generally stay in this phase of training for a 4-week duration, before cycling back through Phase 1 or 2 or progressing on to Phase 4 or 5.

TABLE 14.9   Phase 3: Hypertrophy Training

© ilolab/ShutterStock, Inc.

	Reps	Sets	Tempo	% Intensity	Rest Interval	Frequency	Duration	Exercise Selection
Flexibility	5–10	1–2	1–2 s hold	N/A	N/A	3–7 times/wk	4 wk	SMR and active*
Core⁺	8–12	2–3	Medium	N/A	0–60 s	3–6 times/wk	4 wk	0–4 core-strength
Balance⁺	8–12	2–3	Medium	N/A	0–60 s	3–6 times/wk	4 wk	0–4 balance-strength
Plyometric⁺	8–10	2–3	Repeating	N/A	0–60 s	3–6 times/wk	4 wk	0–4 plyometric-strength
SAQ⁺	3–5	3–4	Fast	N/A	0–60 s	2–4 times/wk	4 wk	6–8 drills allowing greater horizontal inertia but limited unpredictability
Resistance	6–12	3–5	2/0/2	75–85%	0–60 s	3–6 times/wk	4 wk	2–4 strength level exercises/ body part

*Depending on the client, static stretching may still need to be used in this phase of training.
⁺Because the goal is muscle hypertrophy, core, balance, plyometric, and SAQ may be optional in this phase of training (although recommended). They can also be trained on nonresistance training days.
N/A = not applicable; SMR = self-myofascial release.

Professional's Name: Brian Sutton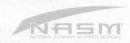

CLIENT'S NAME: JOHN SMITH	DATE: 5/01/13

GOAL: TOTAL BODY	PHASE: 3 HYPERTROPHY

WARM-UP

Exercise:	Sets	Duration	Coaching Tip
SMR: Calves, IT-Band, Lats	1	30 s.	Hold each tender area for 30 sec
Active Stretch: Calves, Hip Flexors, Lats	1	10 reps	Hold each stretch for 1–2 sec
Treadmill	1	5–10 min	Brisk walk to slow jog

CORE / BALANCE / PLYOMETRIC

Exercise:	Sets	Reps	Tempo	Rest	Coaching Tip
Ball Crunch	2	12	Medium	0	
Reverse Crunch	2	12	Medium	0	
Single-Leg Romanian Deadlift	2	12	Medium	0	
Squat Jump	2	10	Medium	60 s.	

SPEED, AGILITY, QUICKNESS

Exercise:	Sets	Reps	Rest	Coaching Tip
Optional				
Optional				

RESISTANCE

Exercise:		Sets	Reps	Tempo	Rest	Coaching Tip
Total Body	*Optional*					
Chest	Bench Press	3	10	Medium	60 s.	
Back	Lat Pulldown	3	10	Medium	60 s.	
Shoulders	Shoulder Press Machine	3	10	Medium	60 s.	
Biceps	Standing 2-arm Dumbbell Curl	3	10	Medium	60 s.	
Triceps	Cable Pressdown	3	10	Medium	60 s.	
Legs	Leg Press	3	10	Medium	60 s.	

COOL-DOWN

Exercise:	Sets	Duration	Coaching Tip
Treadmill (optional)	1	5–10 min	Brisk walk
SMR: Calves, IT-Band, Lats	1	30 s.	Hold each tender area for 30 sec
Static Stretch: Calves, Hip Flexors, Lats	1	30 s.	Hold each stretch for 30 sec

Coaching Tips: Resistance program can be split into 2, 3, or 4-day workout routine. Ex. 3-day routine:
Day 1 (chest/back) Day 2 (legs) Day 3 (shoulders/biceps/triceps)

National Academy of Sports Medicine

Maximal Strength Training (Phase 4)

The maximal strength training phase focuses on increasing the load placed on the tissues of the body Table 14.10. Maximal intensity improves:

- Recruitment of more motor units
- Rate of force production
- Motor unit synchronization

Maximal strength training has also been shown to help increase the benefits of power training used in Phase 5. Because the goal of this phase of training is primarily maximal strength, the personal trainer will want to increase intensity (load) and volume (sets). Rest periods may need to increase as the client trains with heavier loads. A client in this category will generally stay in this phase of training for a 4-week duration before cycling back through Phase 1 or 2 or progressing on to Phase 5.

TABLE 14.10 Phase 4: Maximal Strength Training

	Reps	Sets	Tempo	% Intensity	Rest Interval	Frequency	Duration	Exercise Selection
Flexibility	5–10	1–2	1–2 s hold	N/A	N/A	3–7 times/wk	4 wk	SMR and active*
Core⁺	8–12	2–3	Medium 1/1/1	N/A	0–60 s	2–4 times/wk	4 wk	0–3 core-strength
Balance⁺	8–12	2–3	Medium 1/1/1	N/A	0–60 s	2–4 times/wk	4 wk	0–3 balance-strength
Plyometric⁺	8–10	2–3	Repeating	N/A	0–60 s	2–4 times/wk	4 wk	0–3 plyometric-strength
SAQ⁺	3–5	3–4	Fast	N/A	0–60 s	2–4 times/wk	4 wk	6–8 drills allowing greater horizontal inertia but limited unpredictability
Resistance	1–5	4–6	X/X/X	85–100%	3–5 min	2–4 times/wk	4 wk	1–3 strength

*Depending on the client, static stretching may still need to be used in this phase of training.
⁺Because the goal is maximal strength, core, balance, plyometric, and SAQ may be optional in this phase of training (although recommended). They can also be trained on nonresistance training days.
N/A = not applicable; SMR = self-myofascial release; X/X/X = as fast as can be controlled.

Professional's Name: Brian Sutton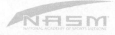

CLIENT'S NAME: JOHN SMITH			DATE: 5/01/13	

GOAL: TOTAL BODY			PHASE: 4 MAX STRENGTH	

WARM-UP

Exercise:	Sets	Duration	Coaching Tip
SMR: Calves, IT Band, Adductors	1	30 s.	Hold each tender area for 30 sec
Active Stretch: Calves, Hip Flexors, Lats	1	10 reps	Hold each stretch for 1–2 sec
Treadmill	1	5–10 min	Brisk walk to slow jog

CORE / BALANCE / PLYOMETRIC

Exercise:	Sets	Reps	Tempo	Rest	Coaching Tip
Cable Rotations	2	8	Medium	0	
Back Extension	2	8	Medium	0	
Step-Up to Balance	2	8	Medium	60 s.	

SPEED, AGILITY, QUICKNESS

Exercise:	Sets	Reps	Rest	Coaching Tip
Optional				
Optional				

RESISTANCE

Exercise:		Sets	Reps	Tempo	Rest	Coaching Tip
Total Body	Barbell Clean	4	5	Explosive	3 min	
Chest	Bench Press	4	5	Explosive	3 min	
Back	Lat Pulldown	4	5	Explosive	3 min	
Shoulders	Seated Dumbbell Shoulder Press	4	5	Explosive	3 min	
Biceps	Optional					
Triceps	Optional					
Legs	Barbell Squat	4	5	Explosive	3 min	

COOL-DOWN

Exercise:	Sets	Duration	Coaching Tip
Treadmill (optional)	1	5–10 min	Brisk walk
SMR: Calves, IT-Band, Lats	1	30 s.	Hold each tender area for 30 sec
Static Stretch: Calves, Hip Flexors, Lats	1	30 s.	Hold each stretch for 30 sec

Coaching Tips: Resistance program can be split into 2, 3, or 4-day workout routine. Ex. 3-day routine:
Day 1 (chest/back) Day 2 (legs) Day 3 (shoulders/biceps/triceps)

National Academy of Sports Medicine

Power

The third level of training, power, is designed to increase the rate of force production (or speed of muscle contraction). This form of training uses the adaptations of stabilization and strength acquired in the previous phases of training and applies them with more realistic speeds and forces that the body will encounter in everyday life and in sports.

Power training is usually not a common practice in the fitness environment, but has a very viable and purposeful place in a properly planned training program. Power is simply defined as force multiplied by velocity ($P = F \times V$). Therefore, any increase in either force or velocity will produce an increase in power. This is accomplished by either increasing the load (or force) as in progressive strength training, or increasing the speed with which you move a load (or velocity). The combined effect is a better rate of force production in daily activities and sporting events.

To develop optimal levels of power, individuals should train both with heavy loads (85 to 100%) and light loads (30 to 45%) at high speeds. The focus of power training is to increase the rate of force production by increasing the number of motor units activated, the synchrony between them, and the speed at which they are excited (29,102–105).

The power level of training in the OPT model consists of one phase of training: Phase 5 (Power Training).

Power Training (Phase 5)

The power training phase focuses on both high force and velocity to increase power Table 14.11. This is accomplished by combining a strength exercise with a power exercise for each body part (such as performing a barbell bench press superset with a medicine ball chest pass).

The range of training intensities is important to stimulate different physiologic changes. The 85 to 100% refers to the intensity for traditional strength training exercises. These exercises and loads increase power by increasing the *force* side of the power equation (force multiplied by velocity), whereas the 30 to 45% intensity range is used for "speed" exercises, such as speed squats in which the squats are performed as fast as possible with a lighter load. The 10% intensity is used as an indicator for medicine ball training that will require the throwing or release of a medicine ball. These last two forms of training affect the *velocity* side of the power equation (force multiplied by velocity). By using both heavy loads with explosive movement and low resistance with a high velocity, power outputs can be enhanced (93,102–105).

Because the goal of this phase of training is primarily power, the personal trainer will want to progress by increasing volume (sets), intensity (load), and velocity. A client in this category will generally stay in this phase of training for a 4-week duration before cycling back through Phase 1 or 2.

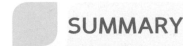

SUMMARY

The different levels of training seen in a traditional periodization model include anatomic adaptation, hypertrophy, maximal strength, and power. In the OPT model, these are simplified into stabilization, strength, and power. These are further broken down into five different phases of training.

The first level, stabilization, is crucial for all beginners as it is designed to prepare the body for the demands of higher levels of training. For advanced clients, this level allows for active rest from more intense bouts of training. It involves low-intensity,

TABLE 14.11								
Phase 5: Power								

	Reps	Sets	Tempo	% Intensity	Rest Interval	Frequency	Duration	Exercise Selection
Flexibility	10–15	1–2	Controlled	N/A	N/A	3–7 times/wk	4 wk	SMR and dynamic 3–10 exercises
Core*	8–12	2–3	X/X/X	N/A	0–60 s	2–4 times/wk	4 wk	0–2 core-power
Balance*	8–12	2–3	Controlled	N/A	0–60 s	2–4 times/wk	4 wk	0–2 balance-power
Plyometric*	8–12	2–3	X/X/X	N/A	0–60 s	2–4 times/wk	4 wk	0–2 plyometric-power
SAQ†	3–5	3–5	X/X/X	N/A	0–90 s	2–4 times/wk	4 wk	6–10 drills allowing maximal horizontal inertia and unpredictability
Resistance	1–5 (S) 8–10 (P)	3–5	X/X/X (S) X/X/X (P)	85–100% (Strength) up to 10% BW or 30–45% 1RM (Power)	1–2 min between pairs 3–5 min between circuits	2–4 times/wk	4 wk	1 strength superset with 1 power

*Because of the use of core-power, balance-power, and plyometric-power exercises in the resistance training portion of this program, it may not be necessary to perform these exercises before the resistance training portion of the program. They can be performed as part of a dynamic flexibility warm-up or performed on nonresistance training days.
†SAQ drills many be performed on nonresistance training days.
BW = body weight; N/A = not applicable; 1RM = 1 repetition maximum; SMR = self-myofascial release; X/X/X = as fast as can be controlled.

high-repetition training, emphasizing core and joint stabilization. Exercises in the stabilization level progressively challenge proprioception. The stabilization level consists of one phase of training: Phase 1 (Stabilization Endurance Training). This phase focuses on increasing core stability and endurance of all major muscles. The phase usually lasts 4 weeks.

The second level, strength, is designed to increase strength endurance, muscle size, and maximal strength. The strength period of training in the OPT model consists of three phases: Phase 2: Strength Endurance Training; Phase 3: Hypertrophy Training; and Phase 4: Maximal Strength Training. Phase 2 uses superset techniques

Professional's Name: Brian Sutton

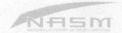

CLIENT'S NAME: JOHN SMITH		DATE: 5/01/13

GOAL: TOTAL BODY	PHASE: 5 POWER

WARM-UP

Exercise:	Sets	Duration	Coaching Tip
SMR: Calves, IT-Band, Lats	1	30 s.	Hold each tender area for 30 sec
Dynamic Stretch: Tube Walking, Multiplanar Lunges, Med Ball Lift and Chop	1	10 reps	

CORE / BALANCE / PLYOMETRIC

Exercise:	Sets	Reps	Tempo	Rest	Coaching Tip
Med Ball Rotation Chest Pass	2	8	Fast	0	
Single-Leg Hop with Stabilization	2	8	Medium	60 s.	

SPEED, AGILITY, QUICKNESS

Exercise:	Sets	Reps	Rest	Coaching Tip
Optional				
Optional				

RESISTANCE

Exercise:		Sets	Reps	Tempo	Rest	Coaching Tip
Total Body	*Optional*					
Chest	Bench Press Med Ball Chest Pass	4	5 10	Explosive	0 2 min	Superset
Back	Lat Pulldown Woodchop Throw	4	5 10	Explosive	0 2 min	Superset
Shoulders	Standing Dumbbell Should Press Med Ball Scoop Toss	4	5 10	Explosive	0 2 min	Superset
Biceps	*Optional*					
Triceps	*Optional*					
Legs	Barbell Squat Squat Jump	4	5 10	Explosive	0 2 min	Superset

COOL-DOWN

Exercise:	Sets	Duration	Coaching Tip
Treadmill (optional)	1	5–10 min	Brisk walk
SMR: Calves, IT-Band, Lats	1	30 s.	Hold each tender area for 30 sec
Static Stretch: Calves, Hip Flexors, Lats	1	30 s.	Hold each stretch for 30 sec

Coaching Tips:

(stabilization/strength) with high volume, for about 4 weeks. Phase 3 stresses maximal hypertrophy, focusing on high levels of volume with minimal rest periods, for about 4 weeks. Phase 4 focuses on increasing the load placed on the tissues of the body, for about 4 weeks.

The third level of training, power, is designed to increase the rate of force production. To develop optimal levels of power, it has been shown that individuals must train both with heavy loads and light loads at high speeds. The power level consists of one phase of training: Phase 5: Power Training. This phase focuses on both high force and velocity to increase power and lasts about 4 weeks.

Applying the OPT Model

The concepts of program design, periodization, and the OPT model have all been described. Program design was defined as creating a purposeful system or plan to achieve a goal. Periodization is the scientific basis that allows fitness professionals to strategically plan and design programs without the risk of placing improper stresses on the body.

The OPT model is a proven, easy-to-use system of periodization that can be used to create programs for clients with various goals. Although the understanding of these concepts is paramount, what matters most is the ability to apply the information in multiple situations to a variety of clients. This section will demonstrate how to specifically apply the OPT model for the goals of fat loss, increased lean body mass, and general sports performance.

Applying the OPT Model for the Goal of Body Fat Reduction

The goal of reducing body fat requires clients to follow the simple principle of burning more calories than they consume (see chapter 17, Nutrition). The best way to increase the calories burned is to move more. Weight training provides an extremely potent means to burn calories when it is combined with cardiorespiratory training by maintaining, or even increasing, lean muscle tissue. More activity and greater amounts of lean body mass result in more calories burned during exercise and throughout the day. Resistance training also provides the added benefit of increased muscle strength.

The following program is a general representation of how the OPT model is used for clients with the goal of body fat reduction. **Figure 14.5** shows a sample annual plan. Because the goal does not include maximal strength or power, the client only needs to be cycled through the first two phases of the OPT model, with Phase 3 as an optional phase (not illustrated). Phase 3, if the client desires, will help increase strength and lean

	PHASE	JAN	FEB	MAR	APR	MAY	JUN	JUL	AUG	SEP	OCT	NOV	DEC
Stabilization	1	X		X		X		X		X		X	
	2		X		X		X		X		X		X
Strength	3												
	4												
Power	5												
Cardio		X	X	X	X	X	X	X	X	X	X	X	X

FIGURE 14.5

Annual plan for the goal of body fat reduction.

body mass through a focus on muscle hypertrophy. Phase 3 might not be required for all weight-loss clients and should only be entered if clients desire to increase their lean muscle mass beyond what they have gained through the first two phases of training. The client will start in January in Phase 1, to ensure proper muscle balance and endurance of the stabilization muscles. He or she will remain there for approximately 4 weeks before moving on to Phase 2.

In addition, cardiorespiratory training will be used in conjunction with the OPT model to help weight-loss clients burn calories and improve health. Clients will progress through Stages I, II, and III (see chapter 8) as their fitness levels improve.

The remainder of the annual plan shows the client cycling back and forth between Phases 1 and 2 (Figure 14.5). Phase 2 will promote times of greater metabolic demand and more volume for increased caloric expenditure. Phase 1 will allow the client proper recovery time before entering back into Phase 2. Cardiorespiratory training can be performed each month. During Phase 1, the client may be inclined to do more cardiorespiratory work (in conjunction with weight training) to sustain good caloric expenditure without the higher intensity of weight training seen in Phase 2. This will also provide proper periodization of the client's cardiorespiratory training.

Figure 14.6 illustrates the monthly plan for January. This plan demonstrates a 3-day-per-week workout plan, with scheduled workouts on Mondays, Wednesdays, and Fridays. However, this monthly plan can easily be performed twice a week. Cardio can be done on the workout days (or any other day during the week, depending on the client's schedule).

Figure 14.7 illustrates the monthly plan for February. As with the previous month, this plan demonstrates a 3-day-per-week workout plan with scheduled workouts on Mondays, Wednesdays, and Fridays. Again, this monthly plan could easily be performed twice a week. Cardio can be done on the workout days (or any other day during the week depending on the client's schedule).

FIGURE 14.6

Monthly plan for the goal of body fat reduction, January— Phase 1: Stabilization Endurance.

Week	1							2							3							4						
Day	M	T	W	T	F	S	S	M	T	W	T	F	S	S	M	T	W	T	F	S	S	M	T	W	T	F	S	S
Phase 1	X		X		X			X		X		X			X		X		X			X		X		X		
Phase 2																												
Phase 3																												
Phase 4																												
Phase 5																												
Cardio	X		X		X			X		X		X			X		X		X			X		X		X		

FIGURE 14.7

Monthly plan for the goal of body fat reduction, February— Phase 2: Strength Endurance.

Week	1							2							3							4						
Day	M	T	W	T	F	S	S	M	T	W	T	F	S	S	M	T	W	T	F	S	S	M	T	W	T	F	S	S
Phase 1																												
Phase 2	X		X		X			X		X		X			X		X		X			X		X		X		
Phase 3																												
Phase 4																												
Phase 5																												
Cardio	X		X		X			X		X		X			X		X		X			X		X		X		

Applying the OPT Model for Increasing Lean Body Mass (Hypertrophy)

Muscle hypertrophy can be simply defined as the chronic enlargement of muscles. To accomplish this goal, training programs need to be progressed with higher volumes (more sets, reps, and intensity) to force muscles to regenerate their cellular makeup and produce increased size. The following program is a general representation of how the OPT model is used for clients with the goal of increased lean body mass. With the goal of hypertrophy the client can be cycled through the first four phases of the OPT model, depending on the needs and wants of the client.

Figure 14.8 shows the annual plan. The client will start January in Phase 1 to ensure proper muscle balance and endurance of the stabilization muscles. Clients will remain there for approximately 4 weeks before moving into Phase 2. Phase 1 is vital for this client, as it will prepare the connective tissues and muscles for the higher demands of training required for this goal. Without proper preparation, injury may be imminent. The remainder of the annual plan shows the client cycling through Phases 2 through 4. Phase 2 will promote greater strength endurance and more volume to prepare the client for the greater demands of Phases 3 and 4.

Phase 3 is specific for maximal hypertrophy and will place larger volumes of stress through the body to force cellular changes that result in muscle hypertrophy. Phase 4 is used to increase the strength capacity to allow the client to train with heavier weights in the future. This will equate to higher volumes of training and greater hypertrophy. Returning to Phase 1 will allow the client proper recovery time before entering back into Phases 2 through 4. Cardiorespiratory training can be performed each month to ensure the cardiorespiratory system is efficient and to promote optimal tissue recovery.

Figure 14.9 illustrates the monthly plan for January (Phase 1). This plan demonstrates a 3-day-per-week workout plan, with scheduled workouts on Mondays, Wednesdays, and Fridays. Cardio can be done on the workout days (or any other day during the week, depending on the client's schedule).

	PHASE	JAN	FEB	MAR	APR	MAY	JUN	JUL	AUG	SEP	OCT	NOV	DEC
Stabilization	1	X						X					
Strength	2		X		X				X				X
Strength	3			X		X				X		X	
Strength	4						X				X		
Power	5												
Cardio		X	X	X	X	X	X	X	X	X	X	X	X

FIGURE 14.8

Annual plan for the goal of muscle gain.

Week								1							2							3							4					
Day	M	T	W	T	F	S	S	M	T	W	T	F	S	S	M	T	W	T	F	S	S	M	T	W	T	F	S	S
Phase 1	X		X		X			X		X		X			X		X		X			X		X		X		
Phase 2																												
Phase 3																												
Phase 4																												
Phase 5																												
Cardio	X		X		X			X		X		X			X		X		X			X		X		X		

FIGURE 14.9

Monthly plan for the goal of muscle gain, January— Phase 1: Stabilization Endurance.

Figure 14.10 illustrates the monthly plan for February (Phase 2). As with the previous month, this plan demonstrates a 3-day-per-week workout plan, with scheduled workouts on Mondays, Wednesdays, and Fridays. This monthly plan could easily be performed four times per week, with a split routine for the body parts. Cardio can be done on the workout days (or any other day during the week, depending on the client's schedule).

Figure 14.11 illustrates the monthly plan for March (Phase 3). This plan demonstrates a 4-day-per-week workout plan (split routine) with scheduled workouts on Mondays, Tuesdays, Thursdays, and Fridays. Cardio can be done on the workout days (or any other day during the week, depending on the client's schedule).

During April and May the client will repeat Phases 2 and 3 respectively.

Figure 14.12 illustrates the monthly plan for June (Phase 4). This plan demonstrates a 4-day-per-week workout plan (split routine) with scheduled workouts on Mondays, Tuesdays, Thursdays, and Fridays. Cardio can be done on the workout days (or any other day during the week, depending on the client's schedule).

Applying the OPT Model for Improving General Sports Performance

The goal of improving general sports performance requires the client to increase overall proprioception, strength, and power output (or rate of force production). The training will need to be progressed from stabilization through power phases of training.

FIGURE 14.10

Monthly plan for the goal of muscle gain, February—Phase 2: Strength Endurance.

Week	1							2							3							4						
Day	M	T	W	T	F	S	S	M	T	W	T	F	S	S	M	T	W	T	F	S	S	M	T	W	T	F	S	S
Phase 1																												
Phase 2	X		X		X			X		X		X			X		X		X			X		X		X		
Phase 3																												
Phase 4																												
Phase 5																												
Cardio	X		X		X			X		X		X			X		X		X			X		X		X		

FIGURE 14.11

Monthly plan for the goal of muscle gain, March—Phase 3: Hypertrophy.

Week	1							2							3							4						
Day	M	T	W	T	F	S	S	M	T	W	T	F	S	S	M	T	W	T	F	S	S	M	T	W	T	F	S	S
Phase 1																												
Phase 2																												
Phase 3	X	X		X	X			X	X		X	X			X	X		X	X			X	X		X	X		
Phase 4																												
Phase 5																												
Cardio																												

FIGURE 14.12

Monthly plan for the goal of muscle gain, June—Phase 4: Maximal Strength.

Week	1							2							3							4						
Day	M	T	W	T	F	S	S	M	T	W	T	F	S	S	M	T	W	T	F	S	S	M	T	W	T	F	S	S
Phase 1																												
Phase 2																												
Phase 3																												
Phase 4	X	X		X	X			X	X		X	X			X	X		X	X			X	X		X	X		
Phase 5																												
Cardio																												

The following program is a general representation of how the OPT model is used for clients with the goal of improving general performance. The client can be cycled through the entire OPT model, depending on the needs and wants of the client. However, for the typical client, Phases 1, 2, and 5 will be the most important. Because Phase 3 is dedicated to maximal hypertrophy, it will not be necessary for the goal of general performance. Phase 4 can be used in moderation to help increase the initial strength levels required to optimize the adaptation in Phase 5, if necessary.

Figure 14.13 shows the annual plan. The client will start January in Phase 1 to ensure proper muscle balance and endurance of the stabilization muscles. Clients will remain there for approximately 4 weeks before moving on to Phase 2. Phase 1 is vital for this client, as it will prepare the connective tissues and muscles for the higher demands of training to follow. Without proper preparation, injury will be imminent for the athletic client. The remainder of the annual plan shows the client cycling through Phases 1, 2, and 5. Phase 2 will promote greater overall strength endurance to prepare the client for the greater demands of Phase 5. As previously mentioned, Phase 4 can be used to increase the strength capacity of the client, but is not vitally necessary for general performance.

From March on, Phases 1 or 2 and 5 are used in the same month and week. This is a hybrid form of periodization known as *undulating periodization.* Undulating periodization allows the client to train at various intensities during the course of a week, eliciting multiple adaptations once a certain level of fitness is achieved (106). In this program, stabilization (Phase 1), strength (Phase 2), and power (Phase 5) are all being trained together. Cardio can be done on the workout days (or any other day during the week, depending on the client's schedule). It is important not to perform high-intensity cardiorespiratory exercise the same day as a high-intensity OPT workout. Rather a high-intensity OPT workout (Phase 5) should be paired with a low-intensity cardio program (Stage 1). Conversely, a high-intensity cardio program (Stage III) should be paired with a low-intensity OPT workout (Phase 1).

Figure 14.14 illustrates the monthly plan for January. This plan demonstrates a 3-day-per-week workout plan with scheduled workouts on Mondays, Wednesdays, and Fridays. Cardio can be done on the workout days (or any other day during the week, depending on the client's schedule).

	PHASE	JAN	FEB	MAR	APR	MAY	JUN	JUL	AUG	SEP	OCT	NOV	DEC
Stabilization	1	X		X		X		X		X		X	
	2		X	X	X	X	X	X	X	X	X	X	X
Strength	3												
	4												
Power	5			X	X	X	X	X	X	X	X	X	X
Cardio		X	X	X	X	X	X	X	X	X	X	X	X

FIGURE 14.13

Annual plan for the goal of general performance.

Week			1							2							3							4				
Day	M	T	W	T	F	S	S	M	T	W	T	F	S	S	M	T	W	T	F	S	S	M	T	W	T	F	S	S
Phase 1	X		X		X			X		X		X			X		X		X			X		X		X		
Phase 2																												
Phase 3																												
Phase 4																												
Phase 5																												
Cardio	X		X		X			X		X		X			X		X		X			X		X		X		

FIGURE 14.14

Monthly plan for the goal of general performance, January—Phase 1: Stabilization Endurance.

Figure 14.15 illustrates the monthly plan for February. As with the previous month, this plan demonstrates a 3-day-per-week workout plan with scheduled workouts on Mondays, Wednesdays, and Fridays. This monthly plan could easily be four times a week, with a split routine for the body parts. Cardio can be done on the workout days (or any other day during the week, depending on the client's schedule).

Figure 14.16 illustrates the monthly plan for March. As with the previous month, this plan demonstrates a 3-day-per-week workout plan with scheduled workouts on Mondays, Wednesdays, and Fridays. In this month, however, Phases 1, 2, and 5 are all used in the same week. This helps to introduce power training at a slower, more moderate pace, with low weekly volumes, while ensuring optimal levels of stabilization and strength necessary to increase power. Cardio can be done on the workout days (or any other day during the week, depending on the client's schedule).

Filling in the Template

Now that all the necessary components of the OPT template have been discussed, the resistance-training section of the template can be completed. The importance of the OPT system is that it provides a systematic format to follow. When filling in the resistance-training portion of the OPT template, just simply choose which phase of training the client will work in. In this manner, all of the major acute variables are already predetermined. Therefore, *sets, reps, intensity, tempo,* and *rest intervals* are already given. In the *exercises* box, simply choose an exercise that fits the desired body part as well as the guidelines of the specific phase of training. For example, Phase 2, strength endurance, consists of a strength exercise, followed by a stabilization exercise. Thus, in the *chest* section, a bench press followed by a stability ball push-up would be appropriate exercise selections.

Using information from chapter 13 (resistance training), the fitness professional can choose a particular system of training (such as using a circuit-training or vertical-loading method) to increase the intensity of the workout. If the client works out 2 to 6 days a week, a split routine may be used with varying body parts. Essentially, the possibilities are endless and only limited by creativity. The most important thing, however, is to follow the physiologic guidelines of the OPT model.

FIGURE 14.15

Monthly plan for the goal of general performance, February—Phase 2: Strength Endurance.

Week		1							2							3							4					
Day	M	T	W	T	F	S	S	M	T	W	T	F	S	S	M	T	W	T	F	S	S	M	T	W	T	F	S	S
Phase 1																												
Phase 2	X		X		X			X		X		X			X		X		X			X		X		X		
Phase 3																												
Phase 4																												
Phase 5																												
Cardio	X		X		X			X		X		X			X		X		X			X		X		X		

FIGURE 14.16

Monthly plan for the goal of general performance, March—hybrid Phases 1, 2, and 5.

Week		1							2							3							4					
Day	M	T	W	T	F	S	S	M	T	W	T	F	S	S	M	T	W	T	F	S	S	M	T	W	T	F	S	S
Phase 1			X							X							X							X				
Phase 2	X							X							X							X						
Phase 3																												
Phase 4																												
Phase 5					X							X							X							X		
Cardio	X		X		X			X		X		X			X		X		X			X		X		X		

Refer to the Appendix for sample program templates for the goals of body fat reduction, lean body mass gain, and general performance.

SUMMARY

The OPT model is a planned fitness training system that can be used to create programs for clients with various goals. Personal trainers must be able to apply the information in multiple situations to a variety of clients. The OPT model can be used to reduce body fat, increase lean body mass, and improve general performance.

To reduce body fat, clients must burn more calories than they consume. The client will work in Phase 1 for 4 weeks to ensure proper muscle balance and endurance of the stabilization muscles. The remainder of the annual plan shows the client cycling back and forth between Phases 1 and 2 (metabolic demand and more volume for increased caloric expenditure). Phase 3 is optional for fat-loss clients. Cardiorespiratory training should be performed each month to improve cardiorespiratory system efficiency and increase caloric expenditure.

To increase lean body mass, clients must work with higher volumes to increase muscle size. Clients will work in Phase 1 for 4 weeks to ensure proper muscle balance and endurance of the stabilization muscles. The remainder of the annual plan shows the client cycling through Phase 1 (recovery time), Phase 2 (greater strength endurance and more volume), Phase 3 (larger volumes of stress for hypertrophy), and Phase 4 (increased strength capacity with even higher volumes of training and more hypertrophy). Cardiorespiratory training can be performed each month to ensure the cardiorespiratory system is efficient and promoting optimal tissue recoverability.

To improve general performance, clients must increase overall proprioception, strength, and rate of force production. The training will use the entire OPT model, although for the typical client, Phases 1, 2, and 5 will be the most important. The client will work in Phase 1 for 4 weeks to ensure proper muscle balance and endurance of the stabilization muscles. The remainder of the annual plan shows the client cycling through Phases 1, 2, and 5. After the first 4 months, undulating periodization is used, and stabilization (Phase 1), strength (Phase 2), and power (Phase 5) are used in the same month and week. Cardiorespiratory training can be performed each month as well.

REFERENCES

1. Hakkinen K, Kraemer WJ, Newton RU, Alen M. Changes in electromyographic activity, muscle fibre and force production characteristics during heavy resistance/power strength training in middle-aged and older men and women. *Acta Physiol Scand.* 2001;171:51-62.

2. Hakkinen K, Pakarinen A, Hannonen P, et al. Effects of strength training on muscle strength, cross-sectional area, maximal electromyographic activity, and serum hormones in pre-menopausal women with fibromyalgia. *J Rheumatol.* 2002;29:1287-1295.

3. Hass CJ, Garzarella L, de Hoyos D, Pollock ML. Single versus multiple sets in long-term recreational weightlifters. *Med Sci Sports Exerc* 2000;32:235-242.

4. Izquierdo M, Hakkinen K, Ibanez J, et al. Effects of strength training on muscle power and serum hormones in middle-aged and older men. *J Appl Physiol.* 2001;90:1497-1507.

5. Kraemer WJ, Hakkinen K, Triplett-Mcbride NT, et al. Physiological changes with periodized resistance training in women tennis players. *Med Sci Sports Exerc.* 2003;35:157-168.

6. Kraemer WJ, Mazzetti SA, Nindl BC. Effect of resistance training on women's strength/power and occupational performances. *Med Sci Sports Exerc.* 2001;33:1011-1025.

7. Kraemer WJ, Ratamess N, Fry AC, et al. Influence of resistance training volume and periodization on physiological and performance adaptations in collegiate women tennis players. *Am J Sports Med.* 2000;28:626-633.

8. Kraemer WJ, Ratamess NA. Fundamentals of resistance training: progression and exercise prescription. *Med Sci Sports Exerc.* 2004;36:674-688.

9. Mazzetti SA, Kraemer WJ, Volek JS, et al. The influence of direct supervision of resistance training on strength performance. *Med Sci Sports Exerc.* 2000;32:1175-1184.

10. Rhea MR, Alvar BA, Ball SD, Burkett LN. Three sets of weight training superior to 1 set with equal intensity for eliciting strength. *J Strength Cond Res.* 2002;16:525-529.

11. Rhea MR, Ball SD, Phillips WT, Burkett LN. A comparison of linear and daily undulating periodized programs with equated volume and intensity for strength. *J Strength Cond Res.* 2002;16:250-255.

12. Rhea MR, Phillips WT, Burkett LN, et al. A comparison of linear and daily undulating periodized programs with equated volume and intensity for local muscular endurance. *J Strength Cond Res.* 2003;17:82-87.

13. Baker D. Improving vertical jump performance through general, special and specific strength training: a brief review. *J Strength Cond Res.* 1996;10:131-136.

14. Bruhn S, Kullmann N, Gollhofer A. The effects of a sensorimotor training and a strength training on postural stabilisation, maximum isometric contraction and jump performance. *Int J Sports Med.* 2004;25:56-60.

15. Caraffa A, Cerulli G, Projetti M, Aisa G, Rizzo A. Prevention of anterior cruciate ligament injuries in soccer. A prospective controlled study of proprioceptive training. *Knee Surg Sports Traumatol Arthrosc.* 1996;4:19-21.

16. Cosio-Lima LM, Reynolds KL, Winter C, Paolone V, Jones MT. Effects of physioball and conventional floor exercises on early phase adaptations in back and abdominal core stability and balance in women. *J Strength Cond Res.* 2003;17:721-725.

17. Hanten WP, Olson SL, Butts NL, Nowicki AL. Effectiveness of a home program of ischemic pressure followed by sustained stretch for treatment of myofascial trigger points. *Phys Ther.* 2000;80:997-1003.

18. Hewett TE, Lindenfeld TN, Riccobene JV, Noyes FR. The effect of neuromuscular training on the incidence of knee injury in female athletes. A prospective study. *Am J Sports Med.* 1999;27:699-706.

19. Junge A, Rosch D, Peterson L, Graf-Baumann T, Dvorak J. Prevention of soccer injuries: a prospective intervention study in youth amateur players. *Am J Sports Med.* 2002;30:652-659.

20. Kokkonen J, Nelson AG, Eldredge C, Winchester JB. Chronic static stretching improves exercise performance. *Med Sci Sports Exerc.* 2007;39:1825-1831.

21. Luebbers PE, Potteiger JA, Hulver MW, Thyfault JP, Carper MJ, Lockwood RH. Effects of plyometric training and recovery on vertical jump performance and anaerobic power. *J Strength Cond Res.* 2003;17:704-709.

22. Mandelbaum BR, Silvers HJ, Wantanabe DS, et al. Effectiveness of a neuromuscular and proprioception training program in preventing anterior cruciate ligament injuries in female athletes: a 2-year follow-up. *Am J Sports Med.* 2005;33:1003-1110.

23. Myer GD, Ford KR, Brent JL, Hewett TE. The effects of plyometric vs. dynamic stabilization and balance training on power, balance, and landing force in female athletes. *J Strength Cond Res.* 2006;20:345-353.

24. Paterno MV, Myer GD, Ford KR, Hewett TE. Neuromuscular training improves single-limb stability in young female athletes. *J Orthop Sports Phys Ther.* 2004;34:305-316.

25. Rimmer E, Sleivert G. Effects of a plyometrics intervention program on sprint performance. *J Strength Cond Res.* 2000; 14:295-301.

26. Thompson CJ, Cobb KM, Blackwell J. Functional training improves club head speed and functional fitness in older golfers. *J Strength Cond Res.* 2007;21:131-137.

27. Vera-Garcia FJ, Grenier SG, McGill SM. Abdominal muscle response during curl-ups on both stable and labile surfaces. *Phys Ther.* 2000;80:564-569.

28. Willson JD, Ireland ML, Davis I. Core strength and lower extremity alignment during single leg squats. *Med Sci Sports Exerc.* 2006;38:945-952.

29. Wilson GD, Murphy AJ, Giorgi A. Weight and plyometric training: effects on eccentric and concentric force production. *Can J Appl Physiol.* 1996:301–315.

30. Witvrouw E, Danneels L, Asselman P, D'Have T, Cambier D. Muscle flexibility as a risk factor for developing muscle injuries in male professional soccer players. A prospective study. *Am J Sports Med.* 2003;31:41-46.

31. Blazevich AJ, Gill ND, Bronks R, Newton RU. Training-specific muscle architecture adaptation after 5-wk training in athletes. *Med Sci Sports Exerc.* 2003;35:2013–2022.

32. Campos GE, Luecke TJ, Wendeln HK, et al. Muscular adaptations in response to three different resistance-training regimens: specificity of repetition maximum training zones. *Eur J Appl Physiol.* 2002;88:50-60.

33. Hakkinen A, Sokka T, Kotaniemi A, Hannonen P. A randomized two-year study of the effects of dynamic strength training on muscle strength, disease activity, functional capacity, and bone mineral density in early rheumatoid arthritis. *Arthritis Rheum.* 2001;44:515-522.

34. Hakkinen K, Alen M, Kraemer WJ, et al. Neuromuscular adaptations during concurrent strength and endurance training versus strength training. *Eur J Appl Physiol.* 2003;89:42-52.

35. Harber MP, Fry AC, Rubin MR, Smith JC, Weiss LW. Skeletal muscle and hormonal adaptations to circuit weight training in untrained men. *Scand J Med Sci Sports.* 2004;14:176-185.

36. Kraemer WJ, Nindl BC, Ratamess NA, et al. Changes in muscle hypertrophy in women with periodized resistance training. *Med Sci Sports Exerc.* 2004;36:697-708.

37. Marx JO, Ratamess NA, Nindl BC, et al. Low-volume circuit versus high-volume periodized resistance training in women. *Med Sci Sports Exerc.* 2001;33:635-643.

38. McCall GE, Byrnes WC, Fleck SJ, Dickinson A, Kraemer WJ. Acute and chronic hormonal responses to resistance training designed to promote muscle hypertrophy. *Can J Appl Physiol.* 1999;24:96-107.

39. Tan B. Manipulating resistance training program variables to optimize maximum strength in men: a review. *J Strength Cond Res.* 1999;13:289-304.

40. Willardson JM. A brief review: factors affecting the length of the rest interval between resistance exercise sets. *J Strength Cond Res.* 2006;20:978-984.

41. Fleck SJ, Kraemer WJ. *Designing Resistance Training Programs.* 2nd ed. Champaign, IL: Human Kinetics; 1997.

42. Kraemer WJ, Adams K, Cafarelli E, et al. American College of Sports Medicine position stand. Progression models in resistance training for healthy adults. *Med Sci Sports Exerc.* 2002;34:364-380.

43. Spiering BA, Kraemer WJ. Resistance exercise prescription. In: Chandler TJ, Brown LE, eds. *Conditioning for Strength*

and Human Performance. Baltimore, MD: Wolters Kluwer, Lippincott Willams & Wilkins, 2008:273-291.

44. Baker D, Wilson G, Carlyon R. Periodization: the effects on strength of manipulating volume and intensity. *J Strength Cond Res*. 1994;8:235-242.

45. Rhea MR, Alvar BA, Burkett LN, Ball SD. A meta-analysis to determine the dose response relationship for strength development. *Med Sci Sports Exerc*. 2003;35:456-464.

46. Rhea MR, Alvar BA, Burkett LN. Single versus multiple sets for strength: a meta-analysis to address the controversy. *Res Q Exerc Sport*. 2002;73:485-488.

47. Peterson MD, Rhea MR, Alvar BA. Maximizing strength development in athletes: a meta-analysis to determine the dose-response relationship. *J Strength Cond Res*. 2004;18:377-382.

48. Krieger JW. Single versus multiple sets of resistance exercise: a meta-regression. *J Strength Cond Res*. 2009;23:1890-1901.

49. Krieger JW. Single vs. multiple sets of resistance exercise for muscle hypertrophy: a meta-analysis. *J Strength Cond Res*. 2010;24:1150-1159.

50. Hakkinen K, Pakarinen A, Alen M. Neuromuscular and hormonal responses in elite athletes to two successive strength training sessions in one day. *Eur J Appl Physiol*. 1988;57:133-139.

51. Bompa TO. Variations of periodization of strength. *Strength Cond J*. 1996;18:58-61.

52. Anderson K, Behm DG. The impact of instability resistance training on balance and stability. *Sports Med*. 2005;35:43-53.

53. Behm DG. Neuromuscular implications and applications of resistance training. *J Strength Cond Res*. 1995;9:264-274.

54. Behm DG, Anderson KG. The role of instability with resistance training. *J Strength Cond Res*. 2006;20:716-722.

55. Kornecki, S., Kebel A, Siemieński A. Muscular co-operation during joint stabilisation, as reflected by EMG. *Eur J Appl Physiol*. 2001;84:453-461.

56. Ogita F, Stam RP, Tazawa HO, Toussaint HM, Hollander AP. Oxygen uptake in one-legged and two-legged exercise. *Med Sci Sports Exerc*. 2000;32:1737-1742.

57. Williford HN, Olson MS, Gauger S, Duey WJ, Blessing DL. Cardiovascular and metabolic costs of forward, backward, and lateral motion. *Med Sci Sports Exerc*. 1998;30:1419-1423.

58. Cressey EM, West CA, Tiberio DP, Kraemer WJ, Maresh CM. The effects of ten weeks of lower-body unstable surface training on markers of athletic performance. *J Strength Cond Res*. 2007;21:561-567.

59. Lagally KM, Cordero J, Good J, Brown DD, McCaw ST. Physiologic and metabolic responses to a continuous functional resistance exercise workout. *J Strength Cond Res*. 2009;23:373-379.

60. Willardson JM, Burkett LN. The effect of rest interval length on the sustainability of squat and bench press repetitions. *J Strength Cond Res*. 2006;20:400-403.

61. Baker JS, Graham MR, Davies B. Metabolic consequences of resistive force selection during cycle ergometry exercise. *Res Sports Med*. 2007;15:1-11.

62. Chandler TJ, Arnold CE. Bioenergetics. In: Chandler TJ, Brown LE, eds. *Conditioning for Strength and Human Performance*. Baltimore, MD: Wolters Kluwer, Lippincott Williams & Wilkiins; 2008:3-19.

63. Tesch PA, Karlsson J. Lactate in fast and slow twitch skeletal muscle fibres of man during isometric contraction. *Acta Physiol Scand*. 1977;99:230-236.

64. Harris RC, Edwards RH, Hultman E, Nordesjö LO, Nylind B, Sahlin K. The time course of phosphorylcreatine resynthesis during recovery of the quadriceps muscle in man. *Pflugers Archiv*. 1976;367:137-142.

65. Brooks GA, Fahey TD, White TP. *Exercise Physiology: Human Bioenergetics and its Application*. Mountain View, CA: Mayfield Publishing Company; 1996.

66. Fitts RH. Cellular mechanisms of muscle fatigue. *Physiol Rev*. 1994;74:49-94.

67. Hakkinen K. Neuromuscular adaptation during strength training, aging, detraining and immobilization. *Crit Rev Phys Med*. 1994;6:161-198.

68. Kaneko M, Ito A, Fuchimoto T, Toyooka J. Effects of running speed on the mechanical power and efficiency of sprint- and distance-runners. *Nippon Seirigaku Zasshi*. 1983;45:711-713.

69. Hickson RC, Rosenkoetter MA. Reduced training frequencies and maintenance of increased aerobic power. *Med Sci Sports Exerc*. 1981;13:13-16.

70. Mujika I, Padilla S. Detraining: loss of training-induced physiological and performance adaptations. Part I: Short term insufficient training stimulus. *Sports Med*. 2000;30:79-87.

71. Mujika I, Padilla S. Detraining: loss of training-induced physiological and performance adaptations. Part II: Long term insufficient training stimulus. *Sports Med*. 2000;30:145-154.

72. Kraemer WJ, Fleck SJ, Callister R, et al. Training responses of plasma beta-endorphin, adrenocorticotropin, and cortisol. *Med Sci Sports Exerc*. 1989;21:146-153.

73. Kraemer WJ, Marchitelli L, Gordon SE, et al. Hormonal growth factor responses to heavy resistance protocols. *J Appl Physiol*. 1990;69:1442-1450.

74. Kraemer WJ, Patton JF, Gordon SE, et al. Compatibility of high-intensity strength and endurance training on hormonal and skeletal muscle adaptations. *J Appl Physiol*. 1995;78:976-989.

75. Kraemer WJ, Ratamess NA. Physiology of resistance training. *Orthop Clin J North Am*. 2000;9:467-513.

76. Bompa TO. *Periodization of Strength: The New Wave in Strength Training*. Toronto, ON: Verita Publishing, Inc; 1993.

77. Enoka RM. Muscle strength and its development: new perspectives. *Sports Med*. 1988;6:146-168.

78. Sale DG. Neural adaptation to resistance training. *Med Sci Sports Exerc*. 1988;20(Suppl):S135-145.

79. Behm DG, Anderson K, Curnew RS. Muscle force and activation under stable and unstable conditions. *J Strength Cond Res*. 2002;16:416-422.

80. Heitkamp HC, Horstmann T, Mayer F, Weller J, Dickhuth HH. Gain in strength and muscular balance after balance training. *Int J Sports Med*. 2001;22:285-290.

81. Azegami M, Ohira M, Miyoshi K, et al. Effect of single and multi-joint lower extremity muscle strength on the functional capacity and ADL/IADL status in Japanese community-dwelling older adults. *Nurs Health Sci*. 2007;9:168-176.

82. Carter AB, Kaminski TW, Douex AT Jr, Knight CA, Richards JG. Effects of high volume upper extremity plyometric training on throwing velocity and functional strength ratios of the shoulder rotators in collegiate baseball players. *J Strength Cond Res*. 2007;21:208-215.

83. Chimera NJ, Swanik KA, Swanik CB, Straub SJ. Effects of plyometric training on muscle-activation strategies and performance in female athletes. *J Athl Train*. 2004;39:24-31.

84. Hoffman JR, Ratamess NA, Cooper JJ, Kang J, Chilakos A, Faigenbaum AD. Comparison of loaded and unloaded jump squat training on strength/power performance in college football players. *J Strength Cond Res.* 2005;19:810-815.

85. Markovic G. Does plyometric training improve vertical jump height? A meta-analytical review. *Br J Sports Med.* 2007;41:349-355.

86. Markovic G, Jukic I, Milanovic D, Metikos D. Effects of sprint and plyometric training on muscle function and athletic performance. *J Strength Cond Res.* 2007;21:543-549.

87. Matavulj D, Kukolj M, Ugarkovic D, Tihanyi J, Jaric S. Effects of plyometric training on jumping performance in junior basketball players. *J Sports Med Phys Fitness.* 2001;41:159-164.

88. Newton RU, Kraemer WJ, Häkkinen K. Effects of ballistic training on preseason preparation of elite volleyball players. *Med Sci Sports Exerc.* 1999;31:323-330.

89. Saunders PU, Telford RD, Pyne DB, et al. Short-term plyometric training improves running economy in highly trained middle and long distance runners. *J Strength Cond Res.* 2006;20:947-954.

90. Spurrs RW, Murphy AJ, Watsford ML. The effect of plyometric training on distance running performance. *Eur J Appl Physiol.* 2003;89:1-7.

91. Stemm JD, Jacobson BH. Comparison of land- and aquatic-based plyometric training on vertical jump performance. *J Strength Cond Res.* 2007;21:568-571.

92. Toumi H, Best TM, Martin A, F'Guyer S, Poumarat G. Effects of eccentric phase velocity of plyometric training on the vertical jump. *Int J Sports Med.* 2004;25:391-398.

93. Wilson GJ, Newton RU, Murphy AJ, Humphries BJ. The optimal training load for the development of dynamic athletic performance. *Med Sci Sports Exerc.* 1993:1279-1286.

94. Young WB, Wilson GJ, Byrne C. A comparison of drop jump training methods: effects on leg extensor strength qualities and jumping performance. *Int J Sports Med.* 1999;20:295-303.

95. Plisk SS, Stone MH. Periodization strategies. *Strength Cond J.* 2003;25:19-37.

96. Graham J. Periodization research adn an example application. *Strength Cond J.* 2002;24:62-70.

97. Wolf B, Feys H, Weerdt D, et al. Effect of a physical therapeutic intervention for balance problems in the elderly: a single-blind, randomized, controlled multicentre trial. *Clin Rehab.* 2001:15:624-636.

98. Fitzgerald GK, Childs JD, Ridge TM, Irrgang JJ. Agility and perturbation training for a physically active individual with knee osteoarthritis. *Phys Ther.* 2002;82:372-382.

99. Luoto S, Aalto H, Taimela S, Hurri H, Pyykko I, Alaranta H. One footed and externally disturbed two footed postural control in patients with chronic low back pain and health control subjects. A controlled study with follow-up. *Spine.* 1998;23:2081-2089.

100. Borsa PA, Lephart SM, Kocher MS, Lephart SP. Functional assessment and rehabilitation of shoulder proprioception for glenohumeral instability. *J Sports Rehab.* 1994;3:84-104.

101. Hirsch M, Toole T, Maitland CG, Rider RA. The effects of balance training and high-intensity resistance training on persons with idiopathic Parkinson's disease. *Arch Phys Med Rehab.* 2003;84:1109-1117.

102. Ebben WP, Blackard DO. Complex training with combined explosive weight and plyometric exercises. *Olympic Coach.* 1997;7:11-12.

103. Newton RU, Hakkinen K, Hakkinen A, McCormick M, Volek J, Kraemer WJ. Mixed-methods resistance training increases power and strength of young and older men. *Med Sci Sports Exerc.* 2002;34:1367-1375.

104. Schmidtbleicher D. Training for power events. In: Chem PV, ed. *Strength and Power in Sports.* Boston: Backwell Scientific; 1992:381-96.

105. Crewther B, Cronin J, Keogh J. Possible stimuli for strength and power adaptation: acute mechanical responses. *Sports Med.* 2005;35:967-989.

106. Herrick AB, Stone WJ. The effects of periodization versus progressive resistance exercise on upper and lower body strength in women. *J Strength Cond Res.* 1996;10:72-76.

Introduction to Exercise Modalities

After studying this chapter, you will be able to:

✔ Define and describe the safe and effective use of selected exercise training methods, including various forms of resistance and proprioceptive modalities.

✔ Describe how these exercise training modalities can safely and effectively be incorporated into a training program for a variety of clients.

✔ Describe how these exercise training modalities can be systematically used within the Optimum Performance Training™ (OPT™) model.

Introduction to Resistance-Training Modalities

Personal trainers, their clients, and health club members alike are always searching for newer or more effective ways to train and stay motivated. Thus it is important for personal trainers to learn how to effectively incorporate the use of various resistance-training modalities into new or existing programs in an effort to help clients stay motivated and achieve their personal health and fitness goals. A more detailed discussion of resistance training, including additional resistance-training exercises, can be found in chapter 13.

There are a variety of resistance-training modalities that can be used to develop strength. The most common form of resistance used in strength-training programs is actual load in the form of free weights (dumbbells, barbells), body weight, and selectorized machines and cable apparatuses. Resistance can also come in the form of elasticity through the use of tubing and bands. This section presents basic information on popular resistance-training modalities, their benefits, and what phases of training these modalities would be most used in the OPT model.

Strength-Training Machines

Strength-training machines are popular in fitness facilities and are often a good resistance-training method for new clients. The majority of strength-training machines are fairly self-explanatory and are often less intimidating than dumbbells or barbells. Because most novice exercisers lack resistance-training experience, strength-training machines offer those new to exercise a safer and effective option to free weights. Machines tend to keep the individual in a fixed plane of motion, which limits excessive ranges of motion that may result in unnecessary musculoskeletal stress. Strength-training machines may also be the strength modality of choice for those who lack stability or have other functional limitations, such as the elderly. Another advantage of most strength-training machines is that they offer the client the ability to change the load rather quickly with a simple pull of a pin or turn of the dial. Thus, strength-training machines are commonly used by novice lifters to perform supersets and circuit-training workouts. Lastly, strength-training machines have the ability to perform many resistance exercises without the need of a spotter.

Although strength-training machines are sometimes less intimidating, they do have their share of disadvantages. Strength machines are generally regarded as inferior to free weights for improving core stability and neuromuscular efficiency (proper movement patterns) because they offer artificial support versus one's core musculature providing the stability (1). Machines oftentimes fail to accommodate multijoint movements that can incorporate the use of both the upper and lower extremities simultaneously (1). Not all strength-training machines are designed to fit all body types and thus can limit the effectiveness of the exercise and possibly create more stress to joints. Lastly, machines primarily work in one plane of motion and can limit one's ability to develop strength in all planes of motion (1).

During the initial stages of training, the use of strength machines by apparently healthy adults may be necessary to offer a less intimidating environment and to provide a strength-training option that meets their current physical capabilities. Eventually, through proper instruction and education, personal trainers should strive to progress individuals into a more proprioceptively enriched environment (e.g., using dumbbells in supine, prone, and standing positions) while emphasizing multiple planes of motion to improve overall stability and multiplanar neuromuscular coordination to be better accustomed to handle the movement demands experienced in everyday life. For example, a client may begin by performing a chest press machine during their initial week of training to become acclimated to resistance exercise before progressing to a dumbbell chest press **Figure 15.1**. This puts the individual in a new position (supine), and the use of dumbbells forces the individual to have to stabilize himself or herself on the bench through his or her core muscles as well as creating greater demand on shoulder stability to handle the load. The next progression may be a stability ball dumbbell chest press (Figure 15.1). The stability ball creates an even greater demand on the core musculature while stabilizing the dumbbells. It must be stressed the exercise modality used must be specific to the client's goals, needs, and abilities. The pros and cons of strength-training machines are illustrated in **Table 15.1**.

Because strength-training machines can be used for many goals and by varied populations, they can be effectively used in all phases (Phases 1–5) of the OPT model. However, during Phase 1 of the OPT model, personal trainers should strive to progress clients from strength-training machines to more proprioceptively enriched environments.

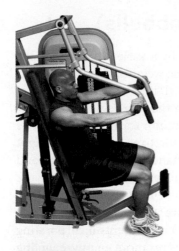
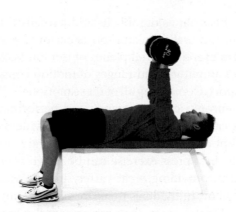
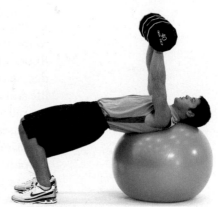

FIGURE 15.1 Progression from chest press machine.

TABLE 15.1

Pros and Cons of Strength Machines and Free Weights

© ilolab/ShutterStock, Inc.

	Pros	Cons
Machines	May be less intimidating for certain individuals	Many machines do not allow the user to perform total-body exercises
	Can emphasize certain muscle groups for rehabilitation or bodybuilding purposes	Moves primarily in one plane of motion
	Various intensities (load) provided in one weight stack	Does little to provide challenge to the core stabilization system
	Does not require a spotter	May not be ideal for improving athletic performance
	Provides extra support for special-needs clients	Machines do not fit all body types (short, tall, or obese clients may have a hard time adjusting the machine)
	Keeps the individual in a fixed plane of motion, which may limit excessive ranges of motion	Expensive in comparison to other strength-training modalities
Free Weights	Can be used to emphasize certain muscle groups, *or* target multiple muscle groups	May require a spotter
	Can improve athletic performance	May be too difficult for beginning clients to perform until exercise technique is mastered
	Can challenge the core stabilization system	Requires multiple dumbbells or barbells to change intensity (load)
	May improve dynamic joint stabilization and proprioception	Potentially more dangerous
	Allows individuals to move in multiple planes of motion	Intimidating for certain individuals

Free Weights (Barbells and Dumbbells)

Free weights such as dumbbells and barbells can be used by a variety of populations to meet fitness, wellness, and sports performance goals. Free weights allow individuals to perform exercises in all planes of motion (sagittal, frontal, transverse) with various degrees of amplitude and ranges of motion consistent with those experienced in daily life and sport. Combining all of these motions will enhance motor learning and improve overall neuromuscular efficiency and performance (1). Moreover, many free-weight exercises can be easily progressed to provide greater demands on core stability and proprioception by progressing from bilateral to unilateral movements. For example, the dumbbell chest press exercise can be progressed from two-arms, to alternating-arms, to one-arm, providing great variety in one exercise **Figure 15.2**. Lastly, free-weight exercises allow individuals to perform multijoint (complex) movements incorporating the entire kinetic chain. Performing complex exercises requires more energy, enabling individuals to expend more calories in a shorter period (1). This is ideal for individuals seeking alterations in body composition.

Although free weights can offer many benefits such as improving postural stability, strength, and muscle size and power, they can be potentially dangerous for novice exercisers until proper exercise technique (control and stability) is mastered. If certain exercises are too difficult to perform using free weights, one may need to regress to a strength-training machine until baseline levels of strength and coordination are met. After this period, free-weight exercises can be reintroduced into the exercise program to further enhance stability, strength, and power. In addition, many free-weight exercises, especially overhead lifts, often require a spotter to ensure proper exercise technique and safety. The pros and cons of free weights are illustrated in Table 15.1. Because free

© Eky Studio/ShutterStock, Inc.

Did You Know?

Spotting Techniques

Personal trainers must be competent and skilled in various spotting techniques to ensure that all resistance-training sessions are both safe and effective for their clients. Research has shown strength training–related injuries can be reduced through greater education, equipment warnings, and proper spotting technique (2). The following is a checklist for proper spotting technique.

- Determine how many repetitions the client is going to perform before the initiation of the set.
- The spotter should never take the weight away from the client (unless they are in immediate danger of dropping or losing control of the weight). A proficient spotter provides just enough assistance for the client to successfully complete the lift.
- Spot at the client's wrists instead of the elbows, especially if the client is using dumbbells. Spotting at the elbows does not prevent the elbows from flexing and caving inward (particularly during the dumbbell chest press, incline dumbbell chest press, and dumbbell overhead press).
- Spotters should provide enough assistance for clients to successfully complete a lift through the "sticking point."
- Never spot a machine-based exercise by placing your hands underneath the weight stack.

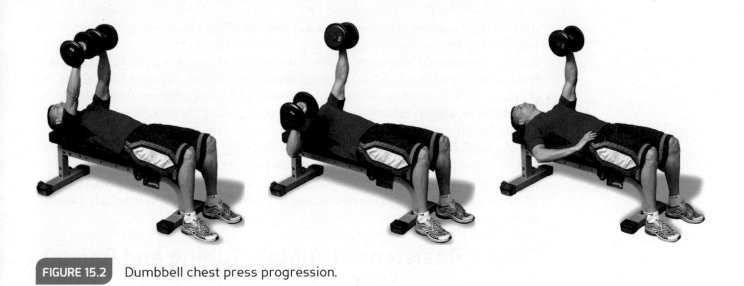

FIGURE 15.2   Dumbbell chest press progression.

weights can be used in a variety of fashions, for many goals, and by virtually all populations, they can be effectively used in all phases (Phases 1–5) of the OPT model.

Cable Machines

Cable machines offer a variety of fitness and sports performance benefits because they allow similar freedom of movement as free weights, yet most exercises do not require a spotter. Cable machines can be adapted to offer resistance for all body parts and are effective for developing stability, muscular endurance, hypertrophy, strength, and power. When using a cable machine it is important to align the line of pull of the cable with the line of pull of the muscle being worked. Remember that joint motion is caused by muscles pulling on bones; muscles cannot actively push. Therefore each cable exercise must match the muscle's natural line of pull. For example, when performing a biceps curl (elbow flexion), the cable should be positioned to offer resistance in a vertical motion against elbow flexion (pulling the elbow into extension; **Figure 15.3**. The opposite is true of a standing triceps extension exercise **Figure 15.4**, in which now

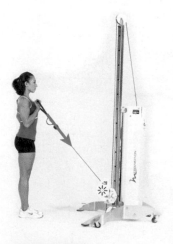

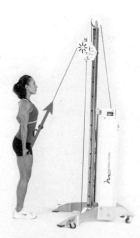

FIGURE 15.3   Cable biceps curl.   FIGURE 15.4   Standing triceps extension.

the resistance must be placed in such a way to resist elbow extension (pulling the elbow into flexion). During a standing cable row (shoulder extension and scapular retraction), the resistance should be positioned to resist shoulder extension and scapular retraction (pulling the shoulders into flexion and scapular protraction; **Figure 15.5**. During the standing cable chest press (shoulder horizontal adduction), the resistance should be positioned to resist shoulder horizontal adduction (pulling the shoulder into horizontal abduction; **Figure 15.6**.

Because cable machines can be used in a variety of fashions similar to free weights and by virtually all populations, they can be effectively used in all phases (Phases 1–5) of the OPT model. Cable machines are also an excellent option to challenge the core while having individuals perform exercises in a standing position versus seated as seen in many machine exercises.

Elastic Resistance (Rubber Tubing and Bands)

Elastic resistance training is an inexpensive alternative to training with resistance. Various forms of elastic resistance training can be used to help improve proprioceptive demands, muscular endurance, and joint stabilization. Elastic resistance training may not be ideal for improving maximal strength, but it has been shown to be very beneficial in helping to improve muscular strength and endurance for fitness and rehabilitative purposes (3,4).

Elastic resistance-training techniques allow clients to move in multiple planes of motion and oftentimes achieve a greater range of motion (ROM) during training (as opposed to a strength-training machine that works in one plane of motion). Clients can also adjust the angle of the resistance (line of pull) by moving the fixed point higher or lower, and combine several exercises seamlessly. Elastic bands and tubing also allow clients to perform resisted exercises that mimic sport-specific movements such as a golf swing or tennis forehand.

Elastic bands come in a variety of colors, shapes, and thicknesses. A color-coding system is used to identify differences in the thickness of rubber, and thus the resistance of elastic tubing and bands. Elastic resistance works like a rubber band—the greater the thickness of the tubing, the more resistant it will be to stretch, thus greater force will be required to stretch it. Rarely should the elastic band be stretched longer than 250% of

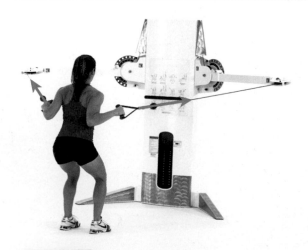

FIGURE 15.5   Standing cable row.

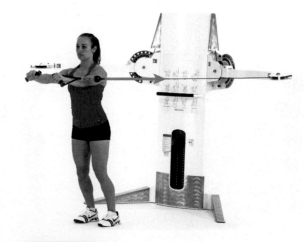

FIGURE 15.6   Standing cable chest press.

its resting length (5). If the resistance provided by the elastic band is not sufficient, then the individual will need to progress to either a thicker band or use two pieces of tubing of the same medium resistance. It is important to note that thicker tubing will reach its elastic limit sooner in the movement than thinner or medium thickness tubing. This can affect one's ability to perform the movement in a full range of motion. This may also cause too much stress at certain joint positions. Thus, in some cases using two pieces of medium resistance may be a better solution as a progression.

One of the problems with elastic tubing or bands is the tension (resistance) in rubber changes as it is being stretched through a full range of motion. For example, the amount of tension (resistance) from the start of a tubing biceps curl compared with the end of a tubing biceps curl can vary significantly, meaning the tension (resistance) is not constant **Figure 15.7**. The mechanical stretch properties of elastic tubing vary according to its thickness, age, how often it is used, and how quickly the rubber is stretched. Thus, it is difficult to know exactly what the resistance is of each elastic tube or band used. Although precise quantification of resistance using color-coded bands is not possible in a fitness setting, research studies have accurately developed linear equations to predict force at different stages of elongation (6). It should be noted that each manufacturer of elastic tubing and bands uses different color-coding systems, so it is important to review the color-coding system when using different brands of elastic resistance-training equipment to ensure the correct resistance is selected.

Because elastic resistance is so versatile, health and fitness professionals frequently use elastic resistance with their clients in a variety of settings, including health clubs, boot camps, athletic performance centers, and rehabilitation clinics. In addition to its versatility, one of the greatest advantages of elastic resistance over free weights is its low cost and portability. Elastic resistance bands are lightweight and can be taken anywhere. For example, traveling business men and women, vacationers, and in-home personal trainers can all benefit from the rewards elastic resistance offers.

Elastic resistance can be used in a variety of fashions, similar to cable machines, and by virtually all populations. They can be effectively used in Phases 1, 2, and 5 of the OPT model. As stated earlier, elastic resistance may not be the ideal modality for individuals seeking hypertrophy (Phase 3) or maximal strength (Phase 4), in which high intensities (heavy loads) are required to overload the musculoskeletal system. In Phase 5 of the OPT model elastic tubing can provide resistance during power exercises requiring explosive movement, such as a tubing speed squat **Figure 15.8**.

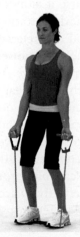
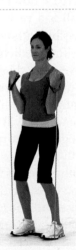

FIGURE 15.7

Tubing biceps curl.

Tubing speed squat.

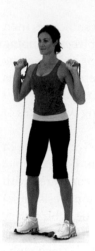
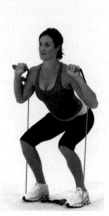
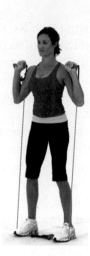

Medicine Balls

Medicine balls are weighted balls that come in an assortment of weights and sizes, and they are made with a variety of materials. They are one of the oldest means of resistance training dating back to the Greeks and Egyptians nearly 3,000 years ago. The name medicine ball came from early use by physicians who used them in the rehabilitation process. For hundreds of years medicine balls have been considered one of the "Four Horsemen of Fitness" next to the Indian club, the dumbbell, and the wand (7). Medicine balls are still popular today because they can be thrown, caught, and used to provide resistance for a variety of movements, in a variety of planes of motion, and at a variety of velocities. Medicine balls can be used similar to any other resistance implement to add load, such as the medicine ball squat **Figure 15.9**, or instability to an exercise, such as the medicine ball push-up **Figure 15.10**.

Medicine balls can be used with a variety of populations as part of a program to increase muscular strength, endurance, and power, or in some cases, to help rehabilitate from injury (7–9). Personal training clients enjoy the versatility of medicine balls whereas athletes often benefit from the dynamic power opportunities afforded by their ability to be thrown and caught. The ability to develop explosive power is one of the unique benefits of training with medicine balls because velocity of movement is critical to developing power. In an ideal training environment, maximal movement velocity should be attained to increase power capabilities, particularly for sports performance (10,11). The medicine ball is a very useful modality because it allows movements to occur as explosively as possible without the need for eccentric deceleration. For example, when performing a kneeling medicine ball chest pass, you can release the medicine ball at the end of the movement, thus allowing for full concentric power development **Figure 15.11**. Most free-weight exercises performed in an explosive fashion (such as a speed bench press) require the individual to decelerate the load near the end of the movement (otherwise the weight will fly through the air) and thus do not allow for full expression of power through the entire range of motion. Explosive medicine ball movements in conjunction with resistance training have been found effective in improving movement velocity and other factors influencing sports performance (10–13).

When using medicine balls for their explosive power capabilities, it is important to assess their intended use and chose one that safely and effectively accomplishes the desired goal. Medicine balls can be made of hard rubber, leather, or other leatherlike material. They often weigh between 1 and 30 pounds. High-velocity movements will

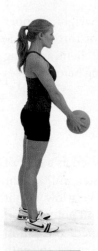 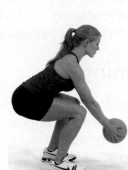 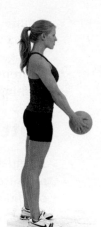

FIGURE 15.9   Medicine ball squat.

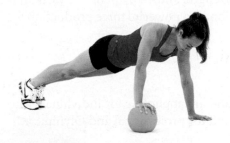 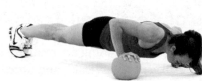

FIGURE 15.10   Medicine ball push-up.

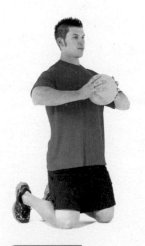 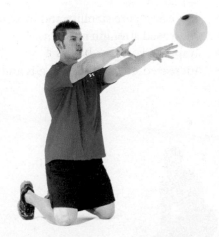

FIGURE 15.11   Kneeling medicine ball chest pass.

require a lighter ball, generally less than 10% an individual's body weight. Rubber medicine balls are best used for rebound activities such as bouncing or throwing the ball against a wall. It is important for personal trainers to assess their client, training environment, and their own level of expertise with medicine ball training before implementing programs in which medicine balls are thrown and caught.

Kettlebell Training

A kettlebell is a flat-bottomed cast iron ball with a handle. It was first used as a unit of measurement on market and farming scales, and later used in the Russian military for conditioning and strength. The *giyra*, Russian for kettlebell, ranges from very low weight (4 kg), over 8 pounds, to competition style weight (64 kg), more than 140 pounds, and higher weights exist. A kettlebell differs from a dumbbell, barbell, or medicine ball in that the center of mass is away from the handle, which may require more strength and coordination, as well as increased recruitment from stabilizers and prime movers simultaneously during particular movements. This is especially true of, but not limited to, swing type movements, the foundation for all kettlebell training **Figure 15.12**. Whether using a two-handed, single-arm, hand-to-hand grip, or release-and-catch movement, the variety of positions and movement options allows for increased skill, coordination, neuromuscular control, dynamic strength, and enjoyment. All variations allow the user to transform dynamic force reduction into powerful force production for a fun, challenging, and effective workout.

Benefits of Kettlebell Training

The benefits of kettlebell training are numerous and are applicable for individuals who wish to increase all aspects of health and fitness and for professional and Olympic athletes. Such benefits include (14–18):

◆ Enhanced athleticism, coordination, and balance
◆ Increased mental focus and physical stamina
◆ Increased oxygen uptake
◆ Increased total body conditioning as opposed to isolation training
◆ Recruitment of the posterior chain (calves, hamstring complex, gluteal muscles, spinal erectors)
◆ Increased core stability and muscular endurance
◆ Increased strength and power
◆ Improved grip strength
◆ Increased metabolic demands and caloric expenditure

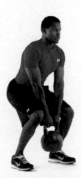
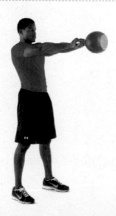

FIGURE 15.12

Kettlebell swing: two-arm.

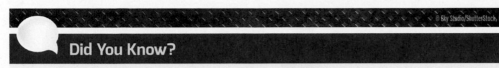

Did You Know?

Kettlebell Training Improves Stamina

The high metabolic cost of throwing, catching, decelerating, and accelerating kettlebells can develop unprecedented stamina. By working many fitness components at the same time, workout demands are intensely increased, equating to further caloric expenditure. This cardiovascular demand can be felt during the foundational swing exercise.

Kettlebell Program Design Strategies

As with any training method, proper form and technique must be mastered to avoid injury. The skill required for kettlebell training requires meticulous focused practice, starting with instruction from a qualified kettlebell instructor. Most kettlebell exercises incorporate multiple joint motions and muscle groups when done correctly. From stabilizers to prime movers, there is a symphony and synchronicity used, equating to muscular endurance and mental fortitude. Without inward focus and conscious attention to technique, injury may occur. Honing all skills with exquisite technique per exercise is mandatory. The emphasis on the posterior chain, working from the ground up and keeping perfect form throughout each repetition, must be top priority. Practicing appropriate skills of gluteal and latissimus dorsi contraction along with abdominal hollowing and bracing must be continued and progressed carefully. Thus, one must be qualified to perform many kettlebell movements, and this modality may not be appropriate for all populations.

Moreover, as with all exercises, quality should always come before quantity or weight progression, and the five kinetic chain checkpoints should be monitored **Figure 15.13**:

1. *Feet:* approximately shoulders-width apart and pointing straight ahead
2. *Knees:* in line with the second and third toes (avoid valgus or varus motions)
3. *Hips:* level with lumbar spine in a neutral position
4. *Shoulders:* depressed and slightly retracted to activate scapulae stabilizers
5. *Head:* cervical spine in a neutral position (chin tuck)

Additional guidelines for further safety and proper form include using a good quality chalk to protect the hands, having plenty of space available with rubber flooring or using an outdoor area, and excluding the use of gloves.

Kettlebells can be effectively integrated into the OPT model, particularly Phases 1, 2, and 5. For example, a kettlebell exercise that can be used in Phase 1 to improve stability is a renegade row **Figure 15.14**. In Phase 2, you can superset the renegade row with a seated cable row **Figure 15.15**. In Phase 5, you may superset a squat to overhead press with a kettlebell snatch **Figure 15.16**. Sample OPT programs using a kettlebell can be found in Appendix B.

Body Weight Training

Body weight exercises are exercises that do not require additional load such as dumbbells, barbells, or strength-training machines. An individual's own body weight along with gravity provides the resistance for the movement. Common body weight strength exercises include push-ups, pull-ups, body weight squats, and sit-ups. Body weight exercises are often used for core, balance, and plyometric training as well (see chapters 9–11).

FIGURE 15.13

Kettlebell five kinetic chain checkpoints.

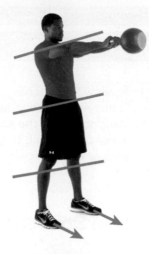

FIGURE 15.14

Kettlebell renegade row.

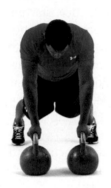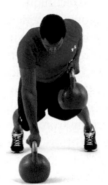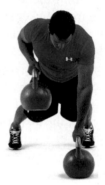

FIGURE 15.15

Cable row superset with kettlebell renegade row.

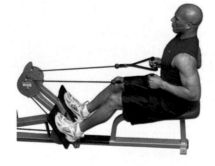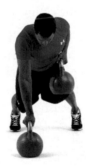

FIGURE 15.16

Squat to overhead press superset with kettlebell snatch.

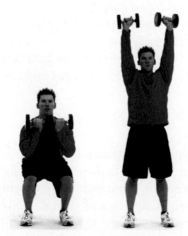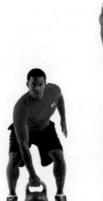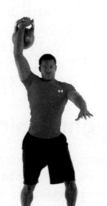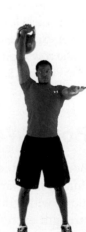

By performing body-weight training exercises, individuals can learn how to train in all planes of motion and may acquire greater kinesthetic awareness. This is partially true because most body-weight training exercises are closed-chain exercises. Closed-chain exercises may result in greater motor unit activation and synchronization when compared with open-chain exercises (19,20). Moreover, body-weight training makes workouts portable, an added benefit for people who travel frequently or for those who do not enjoy the health club environment.

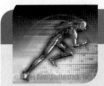

Memory Jogger

Closed-chain exercises involve movements in which the distal extremities (hands or feet) are in a constant fixed position and thus the force applied by an individual is not great enough to overcome the resistance (such as the ground or immovable object). Examples of closed-chain exercises include push-ups, pull-ups, and squats.

Open-chain exercises involve movements in which the distal extremities (hands or feet) are not in a fixed position and the force applied by the body is great enough to overcome the resistance (such as barbells or dumbbells). Examples of open-chain exercises include the bench press, lat pulldown, and the machine leg extension exercise.

Suspension Body-Weight Training

Suspension trainers are an innovative approach to body-weight fitness training that uses a system of ropes and webbing that allows the user to work against their own body weight while performing various exercises. Suspension trainers are a unique training concept in that it allows personal trainers to modify exercises to meet the needs of virtually any client. Suspension movements are distinguished from traditional exercises in that either the user's hands or feet are supported by a single anchor point while the opposite end of the body is in contact with the ground, enabling the loading and unloading of movements to meet individual needs and goals **Figure 15.17**. They allow individuals to manipulate body position and stability to provide multiplanar, multijoint exercises in a proprioceptively enriched environment.

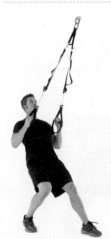
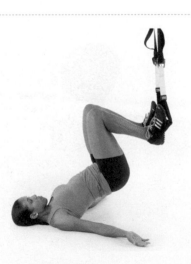

FIGURE 15.17

TRX suspension trainer.

Benefits of Suspension Body-Weight Training

Some of the physiologic benefits that come with suspension body-weight training include (21–25):

◆ Increased muscle activation
◆ Low compressive loads to the spine
◆ Increased performance
◆ Potential increase in caloric expenditure
◆ Improvements in cardiovascular fitness

When the personal trainer is properly educated on how to safely set up and instruct clients, suspension body-weight exercises become a powerful way to teach proper movement patterns, enhance stability and core strength, and gain metabolic benefits. Because of the stabilization requirements of the mode of training, suspension body-weight exercises are ideal in Phases 1 and 2 of the OPT model. For example, in Phase 1 you may use a suspension push-up as your chest-stabilization exercise **Figure 15.18**. In Phase 2, you may superset this same exercise after performing a barbell bench press **Figure 15.19**. Sample suspension body-weight programs incorporating NASM's OPT model can be found in Appendix B.

FIGURE 15.18

TRX Suspension push-up.

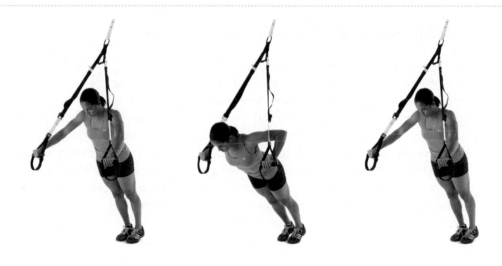

FIGURE 15.19

Bench press superset with TRX suspension push-up.

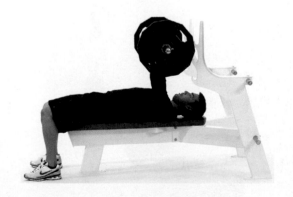
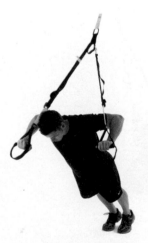

SUMMARY

There are a variety of resistance-training modalities that can be used to develop endurance, strength, and power. The main difference between different types of strength-training methods is the type of resistance being used. Although the most common form of resistance used in strength-training programs is actual weight, including free weights (barbells and dumbbells) or weight machines, resistance can come in a variety of other forms including resistance bands and tubing, medicine balls, and kettlebells, and an individual's own body weight can also provide the resistance necessary to develop strength.

Introduction to Proprioceptive Modalities

Proprioception is defined as the cumulative sensory input to the central nervous system from all mechanoreceptors, which sense body position and limb movements. In other words, proprioception is information that the nervous system receives to make an individual aware of his or her body position and body movements. Improving the speed and quality of this information enhances motor learning and improves movement patterns and overall performance. Popular proprioceptive modalities used within the fitness industry include stability balls, BOSU balls, and whole-body vibration. Other proprioceptive devices are reviewed in chapter 10.

Stability Balls

Stability balls, also known as Swiss balls, are frequently used in a variety of training facilities with a wide range of populations. The stability ball was popularized by Swiss physical therapist Dr. Susanne Klein-Vogleback for adults with a variety of ortho-pedic problems (26). American physical therapists began to observe and apply these techniques, referring to the training implements as "Swiss balls" (27). These balls are most often made of soft polyvinylchloride (PVC) and can come in a variety of sizes Table 15.2. They are primarily used to increase the demand for stability in an exercise, but can also be used to reinforce proper posture during squatting movements.

TABLE 15.2	Stability Ball Size Chart
Height	**Suggested Size[a]**
≤5'0" tall	45 cm
5'1" to 5'7"	55 cm
5'8" to 6'	65 cm
>6'	75 cm

© ilolab/ShutterStock, Inc.

[a]These are *suggested* sizes. Individuals should select a ball size with which they can comfortably sit on top of the ball with their knees bent at a 90° angle and their feet flat on the floor.

Proper use of stability balls allows for increases in strength and stability of the core musculature when substituted for more stable surfaces such as exercise benches, chairs, and the floor (28–30). The spherical shape of the ball creates an unstable base of support, forcing users to constantly adjust their body position to the subtle movements of the ball. The most popular use of stability balls involves using it in place of traditional benches during the performance of a variety of prone **Figure 15.20** and supine exercises **Figure 15.21**. Stability balls can also be used for reinforcing postural awareness during seated exercises **Figure 15.22**. However, stability balls can be dangerous if one does not possess good balance or control, so it is important to evaluate the risk versus reward for the individual involved and follow all safety guidelines **Table 15.3**. Standing on a stability ball is never recommended.

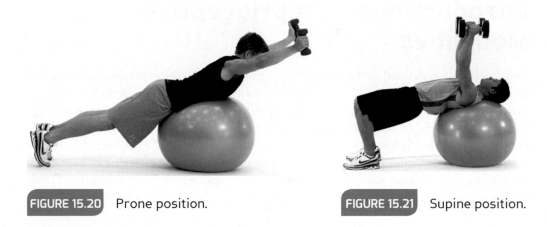

FIGURE 15.20 Prone position.

FIGURE 15.21 Supine position.

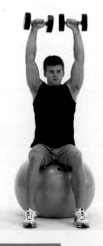

FIGURE 15.22 Seated position.

TABLE 15.3	Stability Ball Safety Guidelines	
Inspection process before use	Inspect stability ball for any damage, tears, worn spots, etc.	
	Make sure the stability ball is fully inflated (should feel "firm").	
	Opt for a burst-resistant stability ball.	
	Inspect and do not exceed suggested weight capacity.	
Proper use of stability ball	Only use a stability ball in an open space away from exercise machines, furniture, or other equipment.	
	Keep the ball away from direct heat sources such as prolonged sun exposure, heaters, and fireplaces.	
	Do not wear sharp objects that could puncture the ball such as jewelry.	
	Do not perform any standing exercises on the stability ball.	
	For first-time users, personal trainers may need to hold the ball for added stability to ensure proper exercise technique and relieve user apprehension of falling.	
	Children should only use a stability ball with proper adult supervision.	
	Maintain proper posture (five kinetic chain checkpoints) during all exercises.	

Stability balls are best used with clients who demonstrate a need for increased overload of stability. As with any exercise technique a proper progression from stable to unstable surfaces should be observed. For example, if a client can hold a prone iso-ab (plank) on a stable surface such as the floor or bench, a stability ball can increase the intensity and difficulty of the exercise Figure 15.23. Moreover, because of the spherical shape of a stability ball, greater ranges of motion can occur during certain exercises, such as the stability ball crunch versus the traditional floor crunch exercise Figure 15.24. Because of the contour of the ball, performing crunches on the ball allows one to go further into spinal extension in comparison with performing this exercise on the floor, thus increasing abdominal strength through a greater range of motion (29). For clients with orthopedic limitations such as low-back pain, the contouring nature of the ball allows for greater comfort and support during upright activities, most notably observed during ball wall squats Figure 15.25. Performing a ball wall squat can help individuals learn proper movement patterns and gain the necessary stability and strength required for squatting motions.

Unless there is an orthopedic limitation that using the stability ball would alleviate, it is recommended that novice exercisers with poor balance first attain proficiency at performing exercises on a stable surface and progress to a more unstable environment such as a stability ball particularly during Phase 1 of the OPT model. As mentioned earlier, the unstable nature of the ball can create a falling hazard for individuals with poor balance or proprioception. In addition, using a stability ball as a base of support is not recommended for individuals aiming to create maximal force during an exercise; thus, stability ball training is not recommended during maximal lifts using heavy loads (85–100% of 1RM) (31).

FIGURE 15.23

Stability ball prone iso-ab.

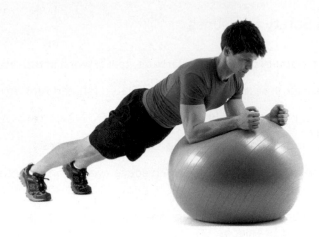

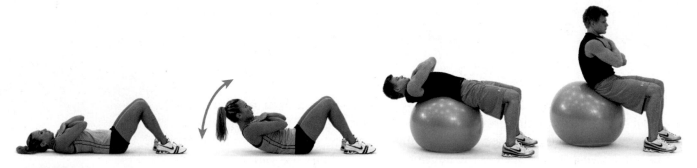

FIGURE 15.24 Floor crunch vs. stability ball crunch.

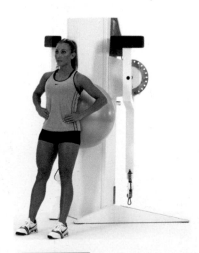
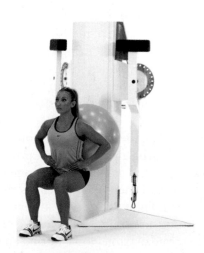
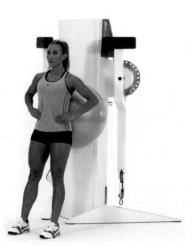
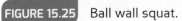

FIGURE 15.25 Ball wall squat.

BOSU Balls

The BOSU ball is an inflated rubber hemisphere attached to a solid plastic surface. It looks like a stability ball cut in half. The name is an acronym for "Both Sides Up" referring to the ability to use the device with either side up. When the flat side is down, the dome offers a surface similar to a stability ball, providing a stability challenge, yet stable enough to stand on **Figure 15.26**. When the dome is down, the hemisphere on the ground provides an unstable surface with the flat bottom on top offering a platform on which the hands can be placed to perform upper body exercises **Figure 15.27**.

Training with the BOSU ball offers the ability to increase the intensity of an exercise by decreasing the stability. Unlike the stability ball, the BOSU ball is relatively safe to stand on, so it is a practical device to train with to target lower limb balance and stability. Training while standing on an unstable surface has been found to increase neuromuscular activity when compared with standing on a stable surface, which can have implications for increasing balance, stability, and strength, particularly for injury prevention and during rehabilitation (31–33). Because of the BOSU ball's unique shape and functionality, it offers a wide variety of exercises that can be performed by a wide range of clients. Like using a stability ball, proper progression from a stable, supported environment to the more unstable BOSU ball should be observed to ensure safety.

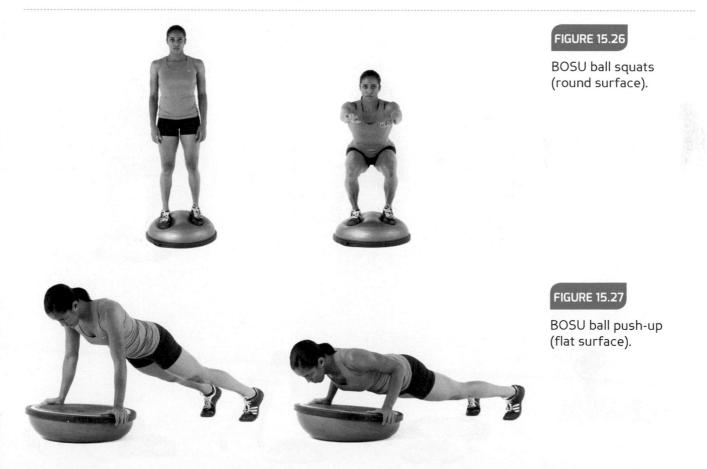

FIGURE 15.26

BOSU ball squats (round surface).

FIGURE 15.27

BOSU ball push-up (flat surface).

Because of its stabilization demands, BOSU balls are ideal modalities to use in Phases 1 and 2 of the OPT model. In addition, certain plyometric exercises performed on a BOSU ball can be used in Phase 5 (Power Training). For example, in Phase 1, you may use a BOSU ball overhead press as your shoulder-stabilization exercise **Figure 15.28**. In Phase 2, you may superset a leg press with a BOSU ball squat **Figure 15.29**. In Phase 5, a bench press can be superset with a BOSU ball plyometric push-up **Figure 15.30**.

FIGURE 15.28

BOSU ball shoulder press.

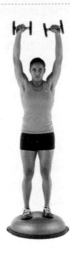

FIGURE 15.29

Leg press superset with BOSU ball squat.

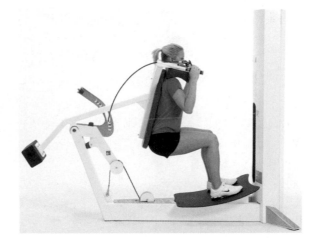
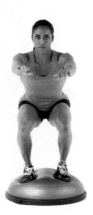

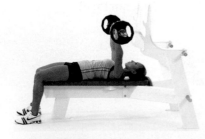
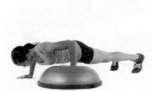
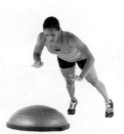

FIGURE 15.30   Bench press superset with BOSU ball plyometric push-up.

Vibration Training

Vibration training, more commonly referred to as whole-body vibration (WBV), was developed by a Russian scientist who used it in the training of cosmonauts in an effort to decrease the loss of muscle and bone mass while in space. Knowing that a lack of gravity during long-term exposure to space causes a loss of muscular strength and bone density, Soviet aerospace engineers discovered that exposing cosmonauts to vibration training before their departure to space increased their bone density and muscular strength and helped prevent some of the harmful effects of space flight. Vibration training has now become a popular form of training in the fitness industry owing to its reported beneficial effects on stimulating greater muscle fiber involvement during exercise, leading to greater increases in lean body mass, weight loss, and changes in body composition.

Vibration training is typically performed on a platform **Figure 15.31** that generates (mainly) vertical sinusoidal vibrations (a smooth repetitive oscillation) that stimulate muscle contractions that are comparable to the tonic vibration reflex. Studies have shown that training on a vibration platform results in strength increase similar to that of conventional resistance training (34–36). The manipulation of frequency (rate of vibration) and amplitude (size of movement) creates what is known as acceleration, which can be compared with gravitational (or g-) forces on Earth. For example, our bodies are accustomed to, and respond to, the gravity on Earth, which is defined as one g-force. The force of gravity the body experiences is dependent on mass (weight), so by increasing mass (such as lifting a barbell or dumbbell), your body builds strength to cope with the increase in force. Vibration training manipulates acceleration, therefore creating an environment in which the body is stimulated to increase strength as a result of higher g-forces, without the need for additional loads being placed on the musculoskeletal system.

However, not every form of vibration elicits the same effects. One study in particular showed that there is a certain minimal amplitude necessary to stimulate the body to adjust, which is not surprising because any form of training needs to be delivered at a level of intensity high enough to stimulate the body to adapt (34). How the body reacts to the stimulation of vibration training follows the same principles as conventional strength and power training. Positioning the body on the vibrating platform in a standing, kneeling, or lying position, or when using the accessory cables **Figure 15.32**, causes a set of chain reactions at different biologic and physical levels. The different

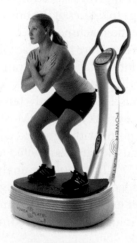

FIGURE 15.31

Power Plate vibration platform.

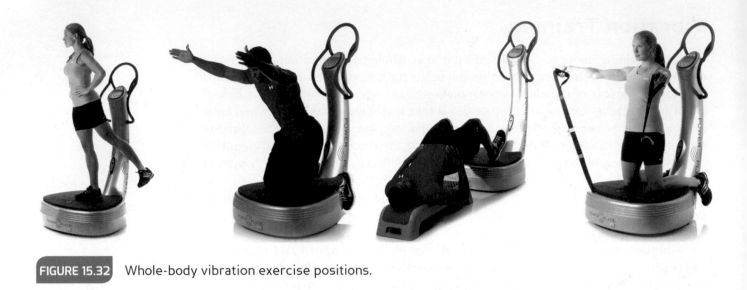

FIGURE 15.32 Whole-body vibration exercise positions.

systems involved in these responses are the bone and connective tissue, neuromuscular, vascular, and hormonal systems. These complex systems interact to provide the necessary reactions to the training environment (36).

The Benefits of Vibration Training

Several research studies have demonstrated favorable adaptations for individuals involved with vibration. Some of these benefits include (35,37–52):

◆ Improving circulation and cardiovascular function
◆ Alleviation of muscle soreness
◆ Weight reduction and increased metabolism
◆ Increasing bone density
◆ Increasing flexibility and range of motion
◆ Improving overall well-being and potentially reducing the symptoms of Parkinson disease, multiple sclerosis, and fibromyalgia

Program Design Strategies

As with every form of training, the correct use of equipment, intensity, and protocol will determine the benefits and effects of applying vibration training, while at the same time reducing the risk of injury or damage to tissues of the body. Vibration training is not just about the level of g-forces; the way the machine is used is equally important. Research supports the theory that prolonged exposure to intense vibration could be a risk factor, for example, for those working in industries such as transportation, construction, and the military (53–56). However, body posture and muscle tension are important contributing factors as well. When muscles are already tensed, they will tend to absorb vibrations better and thus result in less risk of injury. Most vibration-training programs require people to be active (e.g., standing with semiflexed knees on the platform) versus stationary, which means that the muscles are contracted and will therefore limit transmission as a result of dampening (57). This could be analogous to lifting heavy objects in occupational situations versus specific forms of strength training. During strength training, focus is directed on proper exercise technique and appropriate acute variables (e.g., sets and reps) to minimize injury risk and maximize performance and fitness adaptations. One study stated that the risk is negligible when performing vibration training for a maximum of 30 minutes per session, three times a week (58).

Vibration training should be used starting with low-intensity, low-frequency settings and short sessions. The body should be gently stimulated in a way that will create adjustment but will not overwork the system. With time, the intensity and duration can be increased in the same manner as other progressive training programs. Once the body has adapted to the stimulus, the training needs to be changed or intensified to keep improving performance, whether the goal is to improve overall wellness, body composition, or sports performance. WBV training can be incorporated in most phases of the OPT model. For example, in Phase 1 you may perform a prone iso-ab (core-stabilization exercise) with your arms on the vibration platform **Figure 15.33**. In Phase 2, you may perform a barbell squat superset with a step up to balance on to the vibration platform **Figure 15.34**. In Phase 5 you might perform a row using the platforms cables superset with a soccer throw **Figure 15.35**. Sample WBV programs incorporating NASM's OPT model (Phases 1, 2, 3, and 5) can be found in Appendix B.

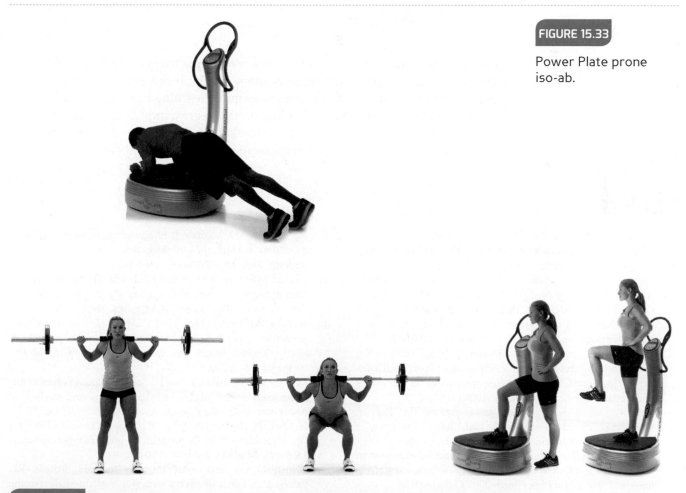

FIGURE 15.33

Power Plate prone iso-ab.

FIGURE 15.34 Barbell squat superset with Power Plate step-up to balance.

© ilolah/ShutterStock, Inc.

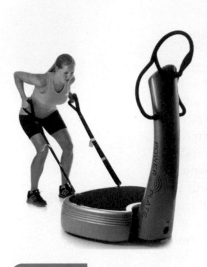
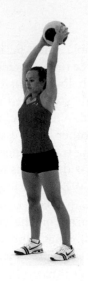
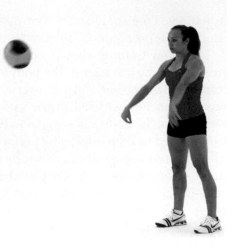

FIGURE 15.35 Power Plate row superset with medicine ball soccer throw.

SUMMARY

Proprioception is defined as the cumulative sensory input to the central nervous system from all mechanoreceptors that sense position and limb movements. Improving the speed and quality of this information enhances motor learning and improves movement patterns and overall performance. Popular proprioceptive modalities used within the fitness industry include stability balls, BOSU balls, and whole-body vibration platforms. All of these modalities can be easily implemented into the OPT model.

REFERENCES

1. Stone M, Plisk S, Collins D. Training principles: evaluation of modes and methods of resistance training—a coaching perspective. *Sports Biomech.* 2002;1(1):79-103.
2. Lombardi VP, Troxel RK. U.S. injuries and deaths associated with weight training. *Med Sci Sports Exerc.* 2003;35(5):S203.
3. Colado JC, Garcia-Masso X, Pellicer M, Alakhdar Y, Benavent J, Cabeza-Ruiz R. A comparison of elastic tubing and isotonic resistance exercises. *Int J Sports Med.* 2010;31(11):810-817.
4. Andersen LL, Andersen CH, Mortensen OS, Poulsen OM, Bjørnlund IB, Zebis MK. Muscle activation and perceived loading during rehabilitation exercises: comparison of dumbbells and elastic resistance. *Phys Ther.* 2010;90(4):538-549.
5. Page P. Dosing of elastic resistance exercise. In: Page P, Ellenbecker TS, eds. *The Scientific and Clinical Application of Elastic Resistance.* Champaign, IL: Human Kinetics; 2003. p. 21-36.
6. Thomas M, Müller T, Busse MW. Quantification of tension in Thera-Band and Cando tubing at different strains and starting lengths. *J Sports Med Phys Fitness.* 2005;45(2):188-198.
7. Jespersen, M, Potvin AN. *The Great Medicine Ball Handbook: The Quick Reference Guide to Medicine Ball Exercises.* Surrey, B.C.: Productive Fitness Products; 2002.
8. Faigenbaum AD, Mediate P. Effects of medicine ball training on fitness performance of high-school physical education students. *Phys Educ.* 2006;63(3):160-167.
9. Paterno MV, Myer GD, Ford KR, Hewett TE. Neuromuscular training improves single-limb stability in young female athletes. *J Orthop Sports Phys Ther.* 2004;34(6):305-316.
10. McBride JM, Triplett-McBride T, Davie A, Newton RU. A comparison of strength and power characteristics between power lifters, Olympic lifters, and sprinters. *J Strength Cond Res.* 1999;13(1):58-66.
11. Kaneko M, Fuchimoto T, Toji H, Suei K. Training effect of different loads on the force-velocity relationship and mechanical power output in human muscle. *Scand J Sports Sci.* 1983;5:50-55.
12. Fletcher IM, Hartwell M. Effect of an 8-week combined weights and plyometrics training program on golf drive performance. *J Strength Cond Res.* 2004;18(1):59-62.
13. Szymanski DJ, Szymanksi JM, Bradford TJ, Schade RL, Pascoe DD. Effect of twelve weeks of medicine ball training on high school baseball players [published correction appears in *J Strength Cond Res* 2007;21(4):1002]. *J Strength Cond Res.* 2007;21(3):894-901.

14. Manocchia P, Spierer DK, Minichiello J, Braut S, Castro J, Markowitz R. Transference of kettlebell training to traditional Olympic weight lifting and muscular endurance. *J Strength Cond Res.* 2010;24:1.

15. Tichonov VF, Sukovey AV, Leonov DV. *Basic Weight Sport.* Moscow: Russian Sport; 2009.

16. Jay K. *Viking Warrior Conditioning.* St. Paul, MN: Dragon Door Publication, Inc; 2009.

17. Castellano J. Metabolic demand of a kettlebell workout routine. *Med Sci Sports Exerc.* 2009;41(5):137-138.

18. Tsatsouline P. *Enter the Kettlebell! Strength Secret of The Soviet Supermen.* St. Paul, MN: Dragon Door Publication, Inc; 2006.

19. Augustsson J, Esko A, Thomeé R, Svantesson U. Weight training of the thigh muscles using closed vs. open kinetic chain exercises: A comparison of performance enhancement. *J Orthop Sports Phys Ther.* 1998;27(1):3-8.

20. Brindle TJ, Nyland J, Ford K, Coppola A, Shapiro R. Electromyographic comparison of standard and modified closed-chain isometric knee extension exercises. *J Strength Cond Res.* 2002;16(1):129-134.

21. Beach TA, Howarth SJ, Callaghan JP. Muscular contribution to low-back loading and stiffness during standard and suspended push-ups. *Hum Mov Sci.* 2008;27(3):457-472.

22. Fenwick CM, Brown SH, McGill SM. Comparison of different rowing exercises: trunk muscle activation and lumbar spine motion, load, and stiffness. *J Strength Cond Res.* 2009;23(2): 350-358.

23. Aartun J, Ervin M, Halewood Z, et al. An evaluation of the TRX Suspension Training System. Presented at the American College of Sports Medicine. Seattle, WA; 2009.

24. Dudgeon WD, Aartun JD, Herrin J, Thomas DD, Scheett TP. Metabolic responses during and following a suspension training workout. *Med Sci Sports Exerc.* 2010;42(5 Suppl):695-696.

25. Scheett TP, Aartun JD, Thomas DD, Herrin J, Dudgeon WD. Physiological markers as a gauge of intensity for suspension training exercise. *Med Sci Sports Exerc.* 2010;42(5 Suppl):696.

26. Klein-Vogelback S. *Functional Kinetics: Observing, Analyzing, and Teaching Human Movement.* Heidelberg: Springer-Verlag; 1990.

27. Carrière B. *The Swiss Ball: Theory, Basic Exercises and Clinical Application.* New York, NY: Springer-Verlag; 1998.

28. Carter JM, Beam WC, McMahan SG, Barr ML, Brown LE. The effects of stability ball training on spinal stability in sedentary individuals. *J Strength Cond Res.* 2006;20(2):429-435.

29. Sternlicht E, Rugg S, Fujii LL, Tomomitsu KF, Seki MM. Electromyographic comparison of a stability ball crunch with a traditional crunch. *J Strength Cond Res.* 2007;21(2): 506-509.

30. Vera-Garcia FJ, Grenier SG, McGill SM. Abdominal muscle response during curl ups on both stable and labile surfaces. *Phys Ther.* 2000;80(6):564-569.

31. Anderson KG, Behm DG. Maintenance of EMG activity and loss of force output with instability. *J Strength Cond Res.* 2005;19(3):193-201.

32. Fitzgerald GK, Axe MJ, Snyder-Mackler L. The efficacy of perturbation training in nonoperative anterior cruciate ligament rehabilitation programs for physical active Individuals. *Phys Ther.* 2000;80(2):128-140.

33. Myer GD, Ford KR, McLean SG, Hewett TE. The effects of plyometric versus dynamic stabilization and balance training on lower extremity biomechanics. *Am J Sports Med.* 2006;34(3):445-455.

34. Delecluse C, Roelants M, Verschueren S. Strength increase after whole-body vibration compared with resistance training. *Med Sci Sports Exerc.* 2003;35(6):1033-1041.

35. Roelants M, Delecluse C, Goris M, Verschueren S. Effects of 24 weeks of whole body vibration training on body composition and muscle strength in untrained females. *Int J Sports Med.* 2004;25(1):1-5.

36. Prisby RD, Lafage-Proust MH, Malaval L, Belli A, Vico L. Effects of whole body vibration on the skeleton and other organ systems in man and animal models: what we know and what we need to know. *Ageing Res Rev.* 2008;7(4):319-329.

37. Lohman EB 3rd, Petrofsky JS, Maloney-Hinds C, Betts-Schwab H, Thorpe D. The effect of whole body vibration on lower extremity skin blood flow in normal subjects. *Med Sci Monit.* 2007;13(2):CR71-6.

38. Maloney-Hinds C, Petrofsky JS, Zimmerman G. The effect of 30 Hz vs. 50 Hz passive vibration and duration of vibration on skin blood flow in the arm. *Med Sci Monit.* 2008;14(3):CR112-116.

39. Bakhtiary AH, Safavi-Farokhi Z, Aminian-Far A. Influence of vibration on delayed onset of muscle soreness following eccentric exercise. *Br J Sports Med.* 2007;41(3):145-148.

40. Fjeldstad C, Palmer IJ, Bemben MG, Bemben DA. Whole-body vibration augments resistance training effects on body composition in postmenopausal women. *Maturitas.* 2009;63(1):79-83.

41. Vissers D, Verrijken A, Mertens I, et al. Effect of long-term whole body vibration training on visceral adipose tissue: a preliminary report. *Obes Facts.* 2010;3(2):93-100.

42. Stengel SV, Kemmler W, Bebenek M, Engelke K, Kalender WA. Effects of whole body vibration training on different devices on bone mineral density. *Med Sci Sports Exerc.* 2010 Oct 26 [Epub ahead of print].

43. Slatkovska L, Alibhai SM, Beyene J, Cheung AM. Effect of whole-body vibration on BMD: a systematic review and meta-analysis. *Osteoporos Int.* 2010;21(12):1969-1980.

44. Humphries B, Fenning A, Dugan E, Guinane J, MacRae K. Whole-body vibration effects on bone mineral density in women with or without resistance training. *Aviat Space Environ Med.* 2009;80(12):1025-1031.

45. Di Giminiani R, Manno R, Scrimaglio R, Sementilli G, Tihanyi J. Effects of individualized whole-body vibration on muscle flexibility and mechanical power. *J Sports Med Phys Fitness.* 2010;50(2):139-151.

46. Feland JB, Hawks M, Hopkins JT, Hunter I, Johnson AW, Eggett DL. Whole body vibration as an adjunct to static stretching. *Int J Sports Med.* 2010;31(8):584-589.

47. Jacobs PL, Burns P. Acute enhancement of lower-extremity dynamic strength and flexibility with whole-body vibration. *J Strength Cond Res.* 2009;23(1):51-57.

48. Dolny DG, Reyes GF. Whole body vibration exercise: training and benefits. *Curr Sports Med Rep.* 2008;7(3):152-157.

49. King LK, Almeida QJ, Ahonen H. Short-term effects of vibration therapy on motor impairments in Parkinson's disease. *NeuroRehabilitation.* 2009;25(4):297-306.

50. Wunderer K, Schabrun SM, Chipchase LS. Effects of whole body vibration on strength and functional mobility in multiple sclerosis. *Physiother Theory Pract.* 2010;26(6):374-384.

51. Schuhfried O, Mittermaier C, Jovanovic T, Pieber K, Paternostro-Sluga T. Effects of whole-body vibration in patients with multiple sclerosis: a pilot study. *Clin Rehabil.* 2005;19(8):834-842.

52. Sañudo B, de Hoyo M, Carrasco L, et al. The effect of 6-weeks exercise programme and whole body vibration on strength and quality of life in women with fibromyalgia: a randomised study. *Clin Exp Rheumatol.* 2010 Nov 24 [Epub ahead of print].

53. Coggins MA, Van Lente E, McCallig M, Paddan G, Moore K. Evaluation of hand-arm and whole-body vibrations in construction and property management. *Ann Occup Hyg.* 2010;54(8):904-914.

54. Viikari-Juntura E, Riihimäki H, Tola S, Videman T, Mutanen P. Neck trouble in machine operating, dynamic physical work and sedentary work: a prospective study on occupational and individual risk factors. *J Clin Epidemiol.* 1994;47(12): 1411-1422.

55. Rozali A, Rampal KG, Shamsul Bahri MT, et al. Low back pain and association with whole body vibration among military armoured vehicle drivers in Malaysia. *Med J Malaysia.* 2009;64(3):197-204.

56. Miyashita K, Morioka I, Tanabe T, Iwata H, Takeda S. Symptoms of construction workers exposed to whole body vibration and local vibration. *Int Arch Occup Environ Health.* 1992;64(5): 347-351.

57. Roelants M. Effect of vibration training on muscle performance and velocity-related mechanical muscle characteristics [thesis]. Katholieke Universiteit Leuven, Leuven, Belgium; 2006.

58. Issurin VB, Liebermann DG, Tenenbaum G. Effect of vibratory stimulation training on maximal force and flexibility. *J Sports Sci.* 1994;12(6):561-566.

Chronic Health Conditions and Physical or Functional Limitations

After studying this chapter, you will be able to:

✔ Define and describe the cause and symptoms of selected chronic health conditions.

✔ Describe the characteristics of selected health and age-related physical and functional limitations to exercise.

✔ Recognize how the conditions discussed in this chapter affect exercise training variables within the OPT™ model.

✔ Recognize how acute and chronic responses to exercise vary in clients with chronic health conditions or physical or functional limitations compared with apparently healthy clients.

✔ Describe how to modify program design for clients with chronic health and physical or functional limitations.

OBJECTIVES

The information presented to this point has focused on exercise considerations for apparently healthy adults. This chapter covers important information and recommendations for assessing and designing exercise programs for clients with selected chronic health conditions and physical or functional limitations. It is important to note that as you begin reading and studying the material in this chapter that exercise training principles for apparently healthy adults will often be different or modified for clients with chronic health conditions and physical or functional limitations. For example, exercise training principles typically require significant modifications for individuals with known coronary heart disease but require little if any modifications for otherwise apparently healthy elderly clients.

This chapter provides a brief overview of selected chronic health conditions and physical or functional limitations common in clients seeking personal training services.

The conditions discussed in this chapter are not inclusive. There are considerably more chronic health conditions and physical or functional limitations that are not addressed in this chapter that may require modifications to standard exercise assessment and prescription procedures, for example, clients with neuromuscular disease or those with mental disabilities. Other more comprehensive resources on exercise considerations for individuals with chronic health conditions and physical or functional limitations are available elsewhere (1–3).

Age Considerations

Youth fitness programs and services, including personal training, is one of the fastest growing segments of the health club industry. The term youth refers to children and adolescents between the ages of 6 and 20. Although a group of children or adolescents may be the same age, their response to exercise can vary considerably as a result of individual differences in growth, development, and physical maturation. Published guidelines on youth fitness and exercise have previously focused primarily on sport-specific training. However, given the alarming increase in childhood obesity and diabetes, current youth fitness guidelines focus on promoting healthy lifestyles and health-related physical fitness (4). Current recommendations state that children and adolescents should get 60 minutes (1 hour) or more of physical activity daily. Children and adolescents should engage in aerobic, muscle-strengthening, and bone-strengthening activities daily to improve their health and reduce their risk of developing chronic disease. In response to the growing problem of obesity and diabetes in American children, the National Association for Sport and Physical Education (NASPE) has revised their statement on physical activity and now also recommends that children ages 5 to 12 get up to 60 minutes of exercise and up to several hours of physical activity daily (5). Additional resources are available on exercise testing and training guidelines for youth (6,7).

Physiologic Differences Between Children and Adults

It is important to understand that there are fundamental physiologic differences between children and adults. Although youth may experience similar effects of exercise training as adults, they do not respond, adapt, or progress the same as adults do. Despite differences in the way youths and adults respond and adapt to exercise, the OPT model for training purposes is still used with youths, but their progress is specific to their physiologic capabilities. Personal trainers should be aware of important physiologic differences between children and adults that impact their response and adaptation to exercise. These include Table 16.1 (8):

♦ Peak oxygen uptake: Because children do not typically exhibit a plateau in oxygen uptake at maximal exercise, the term "peak oxygen uptake" is a more appropriate term than $\dot{V}o_2$max or maximal oxygen uptake. Adjusted for body weight, peak oxygen consumption is similar for young and mature males, and slightly higher for young females (compared with mature females). A similar relationship also exists for force production, or strength.

♦ Submaximal oxygen demand (or economy of movement): Children are less efficient and tend to exercise at a higher percentage of their peak oxygen uptake during submaximal exercise compared with adults.

TABLE 16.1	Physiologic and Training Considerations for Youth		
Physiologic Considerations	**Implication of Exercise Compared with Adult**	**Considerations for Health and Fitness**	**Considerations in Sport and Athletic Training**
"$\dot{V}o_2$ peak" is similar to adult when adjusted for body weight	Able to perform endurance tasks relatively well	Physical activity of 60 minutes on most or all days of the week for elementary school children, emphasizing developmentally appropriate activities (5)	Progression of aerobic training volume should not exceed 10% per period of adaptation (if weekly training volume was 200 minutes per week, increase to 220 minutes before further increases in intensity)
Submaximal oxygen demand is higher compared with adults for walking and running	Greater chance of fatigue and heat production in sustained higher-intensity tasks	Moderate to vigorous physical activity for adolescents, for a total of 60 minutes 3 or more days of the week or 3 days per week if vigorous	Intensive anaerobic exercise exceeding 10 seconds is not well tolerated (if using stage II or III training, provide sufficient rest and recovery intervals between intense bouts of training)
Glycolytic enzymes are lower than adult	Decreased ability to perform longer-duration (10–90 seconds), high-intensity tasks	Resistance exercise for muscular fitness: 1–2 sets of 8–10 exercises 8–12 reps per exercise	Resistance exercise should emphasize proprioception, skill, and controlled movements Repetitions should not exceed 6–8 per set for strength development or 20 for enhanced muscular endurance
Sweating rate	Decreased tolerance to environmental extremes, particularly heat and humidity	2–3 days per week, duration of 30 minutes, with added time for warm-up and cool-down	2–3 days per week, with increases in overload occurring through increases in reps first, then resistance

$\dot{V}o_2$, oxygen consumption.

- Children do not produce sufficient levels of glycolytic enzymes to be able to sustain bouts of high-intensity exercise.
- Children have immature thermoregulatory systems, including both a delayed response and limited ability to sweat in response to hot, humid environments.

Because of their relatively high peak oxygen uptake levels, children can perform endurance activities fairly well, which enables them to train in the stabilization level of the OPT model (phase 1). However, children do not tolerate exercise in hot, humid environments because they have higher submaximal oxygen demands and a lower absolute sweating rate when compared with adults. Vigorous exercise in hot, humid environments should be restricted for children to less than 30 minutes, including frequent rest periods. And as with adults, adequate hydration before, during, and after exercise is very important for youths. And unlike with sustained low-intensity endurance activities, children are at a distinct disadvantage when participating in short-duration (10 to 90 seconds) high-intensity anaerobic activities because they produce less glycolytic enzymes that are required to support sustained anaerobic power. For safety and training considerations, children should have planned rest intervals when training at high-intensity levels.

Resistance Training for Youth

Research has clearly demonstrated that resistance training is both safe and effective in children and adolescents (9). Resistance training for health and fitness conditioning in youth also results in a lower risk of injury when compared with many popular sports (including soccer, football, and basketball) (10,11). The most common injuries associated with resistance training in youth are sprains (injury to ligament) and strains (injury to tendon or muscle), which are usually attributable to a lack of qualified supervision, poor technique, and improper progression. Injuries can and do occur in youth participating in any activity or sport, including resistance training; however, no injuries have ever been reported in well-designed scientific studies looking at the effect of resistance training in youth (9). Furthermore, the majority of published research on the subject has reported that both children and adolescents can gain significant levels of strength as a result of resistance training beyond that normally associated with growth and development (12,13).

A recent review of the literature suggests that untrained children can improve their strength by an average of 30 to 40% after 8 weeks of progressive resistance training (9). Resistance training in youth has also been shown to improve motor skills such as sprinting and jumping, body composition, and bone mineral density (9,12,13). Improvements in strength and performance after a resistance training program in youth appear to be owing to neural adaptations versus muscular hypertrophy (9). A variety of guidelines and recommendations, as well as books, has been published on how to design resistance training programs for children and adolescents (9,14).

When designing an exercise training program for a youth client, it is important to assess for any movement deficiencies, using a variety of movement assessments discussed in chapter 6. Information from the movement assessments will help the fitness professional design an individualized phase 1 Stabilization Endurance program. Progression into phases 2 through 5 should be decided on the basis of maturity level, dynamic postural control (flexibility and stability), and how they have responded to training up to this point. One of the most important aspects to consider when designing and implementing exercise training programs for youth is to make it safe and fun. Recommendations for youth fitness training are presented in Table 16.1 and Table 16.2.

Seniors

By the middle of this century, it is estimated that 87 million people or roughly 21% of the entire U.S. population will be 65 years of age or older (15). As America's population ages, we are faced with dealing with issues such as mortality, longevity, and quality of life. The upward drift in average age has significant implications for personal trainers as well. As the role of exercise in helping to improve and maintain functional independence becomes more widely known and accepted, opportunities for personal trainers will continue to increase.

Unfortunately, aging has become synonymous with degeneration and loss of functional ability in older adults, which is a mistake (15). Typical forms of degeneration associated with aging include osteoporosis, arthritis (osteoarthritis) (16,17), low-back pain (LBP) (18,19), and obesity (20). Although special considerations for those chronic conditions associated with aging will be addressed in subsequent modules, considerations for apparently healthy older adults help provide the personal trainer with the fundamental knowledge to effectively evaluate and design programs for this population.

TABLE 16.2	Basic Exercise Guidelines for Youth Training
Mode	Walking, jogging, running, games, activities, sports, water activity, resistance training
Frequency	5 to 7 days of the week
Intensity	Moderate to vigorous cardiorespiratory exercise training
Duration	60 minutes per day
Movement assessment	Overhead squats 10 push-ups (if 10 cannot be performed, do as many as can be tolerated Single-leg stance (if can tolerate, perform 3–5 single-leg squats per leg)
Flexibility	Follow the flexibility continuum specific for each phase of training
Resistance training	1–2 sets of 8–12 repetitions at 40–70% on 2–3 days per week Phase 1 of OPT model should be mastered before moving on Phases 2–5 should be reserved for mature adolescents on the basis of dynamic postural control and a licensed physician's recommendation
Special considerations	Progression for the youth population should be based on postural control and not on the amount of weight that can be used. Make exercising fun!

It is vital to note that various physiologic changes are considered normal with aging and some are considered pathologic, meaning related to disease. For example, blood pressure tends to be higher at rest and during exercise, which can be the result of either natural causes, as a result of disease, or a combination of both. **Arteriosclerosis** is a normal physiologic process of aging that results in arteries that are less elastic and pliable, which in turn leads to greater resistance to blood flow and thus higher blood pressure. On the other hand, **atherosclerosis**, which is caused largely by poor lifestyle choices (smoking, obesity, sedentary lifestyle, etc.), restricts blood flow as the result of plaque buildup within the walls of arteries and thus leads to increased resistance and blood pressure.

Another disease-related cause of hypertension is called **peripheral vascular disease**, which refers to plaques that form in any peripheral artery, typically those of the lower leg. Individuals with blood pressure levels between 120/80 mm Hg and 139/89 mm Hg are considered prehypertensive and should be carefully monitored and referred to a physician if their blood pressure continues to rise or if they have other risk factors for heart disease. All individuals regardless of their age who have a blood pressure reading of 140/90 mm Hg or higher should be referred to a physician for further evaluation.

Despite the normal decline in physiologic functioning associated with aging, older adults with and without other chronic health conditions can and do respond to exercise much in the same manner as apparently healthy younger adults. Some of the normal physiologic and functional changes associated with aging include reductions in the following:

- Maximal attainable heart rate
- Cardiac output
- Muscle mass
- Balance
- Coordination (neuromuscular efficiency)

Arteriosclerosis A general term that refers to hardening (and loss of elasticity) of arteries.

Atherosclerosis Buildup of fatty plaques in arteries that leads to narrowing and reduced blood flow.

Peripheral vascular disease A group of diseases in which blood vessels become restricted or blocked, typically as a result of atherosclerosis.

- ◆ Connective tissue elasticity
- ◆ Bone mineral density

Both normal physiologic as well as abnormal pathologic changes associated with aging affect the response to exercise training. Degenerative processes associated with aging can lead to a decrease in the functional capacity of older adults, including potentially significant reductions in muscular strength and endurance, cardiorespiratory fitness, and proprioceptive neural responses (1,21). One of the most important and fundamental functional activities affected with degenerative aging is walking. The decreased ability to move freely in one's own environment not only reduces the physical and emotional independence of an individual, it also can lead to an increase in the degenerative cycle (22). The ability or inability to perform normal activities of daily living (ADLs) such as bathing, eating, housekeeping, and leisure activities can be measured to help determine the functional status of an individual.

Individuals with one or more of these degenerative conditions may tend to avoid engaging in activities such as resistance or aerobic training because of a fear of injury or feelings of inadequacy (23). However, research has shown that musculoskeletal degeneration may not be entirely age-related and that certain measures can be taken to prevent loss of muscle strength and functional immobility with aging (24–26). It has also been demonstrated that many of the structural deficits responsible for decreased functional capacity in older adults, including loss of muscle strength and neural proprioception, can be slowed and even reversed through participating in routine physical activity and exercise.

By adhering to the OPT model, personal trainers can make a dramatic impact on the overall health and well-being of older adults. Before initiating any exercise training, older adults must complete a Physical Activity Readiness Questionnaire (PAR-Q) and movement assessment such as the overhead squat assessment, sitting and standing from a seated position, or a single-leg stance. Assessments such as those included in the Senior Fitness Test help provide information about an individual's quality of movement as well as the ability to perform activities of daily living. Flexibility assessment and training is also an important consideration with older adults because they tend to lose the elasticity of their connective tissue, which reduces movement and increases the risk of injury. Self-myofascial release and static stretching are advised for this population, provided there is sufficient ability to perform the necessary movements. Otherwise, simple forms of active or dynamic stretching can be recommended to help get the client to start moving their joints during the warm-up period.

Stages I and II will be appropriate levels of cardiorespiratory training for this population. However, older adults taking certain prescribed medications and those with other chronic health conditions must be carefully monitored and progressed slowly. Phase 1 of the OPT model will be applicable for this population and should be progressed slowly, with an emphasis on stabilization training (core, balance, and progression to standing resistance exercises) before moving on to phases 2 through 5. When designing an exercise program for seniors, the personal trainer must take specialized care in ensuring safety for the participants. The better a personal trainer can match exercises appropriate to the clients' capabilities, the more safe and effective the program will be. All exercises should be performed with precise technique and kinetic chain control to minimize risk of injury. As always, personal trainers are encouraged to consult with a licensed physician whenever questions arise regarding older adult clients.

Physiologic considerations and their implications for training in apparently healthy older adults are listed in Table 16.3 and Table 16.4. Additional resources are available that provide greater detail on the normal physiologic changes associated with aging and their implications for exercise training (1).

TABLE 16.3	Physiologic and Training Considerations for Seniors

Physiologic Considerations	Implications of Health and Fitness Training
Maximal oxygen uptake, maximal exercise heart rate, and measures of pulmonary function will all decrease with increasing age	Initial exercise workloads should be low and progressed more gradually to 3–5 days per week Duration = 20–45 minutes Intensity = 45–80% of peak
Percentage of body fat will increase, and both bone mass and lean body mass will decrease with increasing age	Resistance exercise is recommended, with lower initial weights and slower progression (for example, 1–3 sets of 8–10 exercises, 8–20 reps, session length = 20–30 minutes)
Balance, gait, and neuromuscular coordination may be impaired	Exercise modalities should be chosen and progressed to safeguard against falls and foot problems Cardio options include stationary or recumbent cycling, aquatic exercise, or treadmill with handrail support Resistance options include seated machines, progressing to standing exercises
There is a higher rate of both diagnosed and undetected heart disease in the elderly	Knowledge of pulse assessment during exercise is critical, as is monitoring for chronic disease signs and symptoms
Pulse irregularity is more frequent	Careful analysis of medication use and possible exercise effects

TABLE 16.4	Basic Exercise Guidelines for Seniors

Mode	Stationary or recumbent cycling, aquatic exercise, or treadmill with handrail support
Frequency	3–5 days per week of moderate-intensity activities or 3 days per week of vigorous-intensity activities
Intensity	40–85% of $\dot{V}O_2$ peak
Duration	30–60 minutes per day or 8- to 10-minute bouts
Movement assessment	Push, pull, OH squat, or Sitting and standing into a chair Single-leg balance
Flexibility	Self-myofascial release and static stretching
Resistance training	1–3 sets of 8–20 repetitions at 40–80% on 3–5 days per week Phase 1 of OPT model should be mastered before moving on Phases 2–5 should be based on dynamic postural control and a licensed physician's recommendation
Special considerations	Progression should be slow, well monitored, and based on postural control Exercises should be progressed if possible toward free sitting (no support) or standing Make sure client is breathing in normal manner and avoid holding breath as in a Valsalva maneuver If client cannot tolerate SMR or static stretches because of other conditions, perform slow rhythmic active or dynamic stretches

SMR, self-myofascial release; OH, overhead squats; $\dot{V}O_2$, oxygen consumption.

SUMMARY

Both children and adolescents are encouraged to get 60 minutes of moderate to vigorous physical activity daily. Children tend to have lower peak oxygen uptake levels, sweating rates, and tolerance for temperature extremes compared with adults. High-intensity or volume aerobic or anaerobic training should be discouraged in children. Youth fitness training should focus on physiologic adaptations that are developed through a combination of physical activity and resistance and aerobic training that emphasizes skill and controlled movements.

Regarding older adults, it is important to remember that many reductions in normal physiologic functioning with aging are normal and predictable. Older adults may have elevated resting and exercise blood pressures and reduced maximal heart rates and cardiac outputs. Resistance training for older clients is recommended 3 to 5 days per week, using lighter weights and slower progressions.

Obesity

Obesity The condition of subcutaneous fat exceeding the amount of lean body mass.

Obesity is the fastest growing health problem in America as well as in all other industrialized countries. At present 66% of Americans older than the age of 20 are overweight. Approximately 34% of Americans are obese, which equates to approximately 72 million Americans (20). Obesity is a complex disease and is associated with a variety of chronic health conditions as well as emotional and social problems.

Body Mass Index

Body mass index (BMI) is used to estimate healthy body weight ranges based on a person's height. Because it is simple to measure and calculate, it is the most widely used assessment tool to identify individuals who are underweight, overweight, and obese. BMI is defined as total body weight in kilograms divided by the height in meters squared. For example, a client with a body weight of 200 pounds (91 kg) and height of 70 inches (178 cm, or 3.16 m^2) would have a BMI of 28.79 (91 kg/3.16 m^2). Because BMI does not actually measure body composition, other techniques such as skin-fold or circumference measurements may be performed to assist in developing realistic weight loss goals and to help provide feedback to clients. However, these techniques may need to be avoided for obese individuals because assessing body fat using skinfold calipers can be a sensitive situation. Although BMI is not a perfect measurement, it does provide reliable values for comparison and for reasonable goal setting. For example, once BMI is calculated, realistic goals can be set to achieve a weight associated with a lower BMI. A BMI of 18.5 to 24.9 is considered within normal limits, 25 to 29.9 is considered overweight, and a BMI of 30 or greater is obese. An estimated two thirds of adults in the United States have a BMI of 25 or greater and one third have a BMI of 30 or greater. The risk of chronic disease increases in proportion to the rise in BMI in both adults and adolescents.

Causes of Obesity

Although the causes of obesity are complex and varied, few disagree that the primary problem is energy balance (too many calories consumed and too few expended). Because obesity is such a complex medical problem, it is important for personal trainers to either work closely with or refer their obese clients to a registered dietician (or other qualified licensed professional) who can provide accurate and achievable dietary recommendations.

It has been suggested that adults who remain sedentary throughout their life span will lose approximately 5 pounds of muscle per decade, while simultaneously adding 15 pounds of fat per decade (27). In addition to the facts stated above, the average adult will experience a 15% reduction in fat-free mass (FFM) between the ages of 30 and 80. When age-related fat gain was investigated, it was determined that body fat is not an age-related problem, but instead relates to the number of hours individuals spend exercising per week (28). It has also been shown in sedentary individuals that daily-activity levels account for more than 75% of the variability of body-fat storage in men (29).

Obesity and Exercise Training

Regular physical activity and exercise is one of the most important factors related to long-term successful weight loss. It is important to note that obese and morbidly obese clients have unique problems associated with exercise. For example, research has also shown a correlation between body weight and the mechanics of their gait. In one study involving more than 200 75-year-old women, the relationship between balance, muscular strength, and gait was such that heavier individuals exhibited worse balance, slower gait velocity, and shorter steps, regardless of their level of muscular strength (30). Exercise training for obese clients should focus primarily on energy expenditure, balance, and proprioceptive training to help them expend calories and improve their balance and gait mechanics. By performing exercises in a proprioceptively enriched environment (controlled, unstable), the body is forced to recruit more muscles to stabilize itself. In doing so, more calories are potentially expended (31,32).

For effective weight loss, obese clients should expend 200 to 300 kcal (calories) per exercise session, with a minimum weekly goal of 1,250 kcal of energy expenditure from combined physical activity and exercise. The initial exercise energy expenditure goal should be progressively increased to 2,000 kcal per week. Resistance training can gradually be added to any exercise program designed to promote weight loss, but sustained long-term aerobic endurance activities will always remain a priority. Research suggests circuit-style resistance training, when compared with walking at a fast pace, produces nearly identical caloric expenditure rates in the same given time span (33). Resistance training is an important component of any weight-loss program because it helps increase lean body mass, which eventually results in a higher metabolic rate and improved body composition. The same exercise training guidelines for apparently healthy adults can be used when designing aerobic and resistance training programs for obese clients. Health and movement assessments should always be performed to establish initial program design goals and parameters. Assessing obese clients can be challenging, but there are some excellent resources available on fitness testing of obese individuals (1). Some of the fitness assessments presented in chapter 6 can be used with this population, for example, using pushing, pulling, and squatting assessments.

Resistance training exercises for assessment or training may be best performed with cables, exercise tubing, or body weight from a standing or seated position for obese clients. In addition, using a single-leg balance assessment may be more appropriate than a single-leg squat for this population. Flexibility exercises should also be performed from a standing or seated position. For example, using the standing hip flexor (rather than the kneeling hip flexor stretch), standing hamstring stretch, wall calf stretch, and seated adductor stretch would be advised. Self-myofascial release should be used with caution and may need to be avoided or performed at home (see Psychosocial Aspects of Working with Obese Clients).

Core and balance training is also important for this population because they lack balance and walking speed, both of which are important to exercise. Personal trainers must use caution when placing an obese client in a prone or supine position because these obese individuals are prone to both hypotensive and hypertensive responses to exercise. Having obese clients perform exercises in a standing position may be more appropriate and more comfortable for them. For example, performing prone iso-abs (planks) on an incline **Figure 16.1** or a standing medicine ball rotation **Figure 16.2** may be best suited for certain obese clients versus supine crunches. Resistance training exercises may need to be started in a seated position and progressed to a standing position.

Phases 1 and 2 of the OPT model will be appropriate for the obese population. Personal trainers should ensure that the client is breathing correctly during resistance training exercises and avoids straining during exercise or squeezing exercise bars too tightly, which can cause an increase in blood pressure.

Psychosocial Aspects of Working with Obese Clients

Obesity is a unique chronic disease because it also affects a person's sense of emotional well-being and self-esteem (34). Obesity can alter the emotional and social aspects of a person's life as much as it does the physical aspects. Personal trainers must be very aware of the psychosocial aspects of obesity when training obese clients to ensure that the client feels socially and emotionally safe. Such attention to their emotional as well

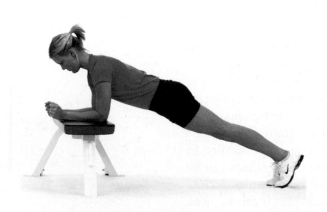

FIGURE 16.1 Incline prone iso-abs.

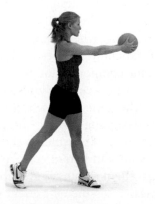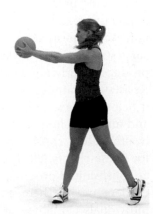

FIGURE 16.2 Standing medicine ball rotations.

as their physical well-being will help to create trust between the client and professional and assist the client in adhering to a weight-loss and exercise program.

Proper exercise selections and positions are very important to the client's sense of well-being. For example, machines are often not designed for obese individuals and may require a significant amount of mobility to get in and out. Dumbbells, cables, or exercise tubing exercises work quite well instead of machines. The use of self-myofascial release should be done with caution as many obese clients will not feel comfortable rolling or lying on the floor. It may be a good idea to recommend that certain exercises be performed in the privacy of their own home or in a location within a health club that offers privacy. In addition, it is recommended that obese clients engage in weight-supported exercise (such as cycling or swimming) to decrease orthopedic stress. However, walking is often both a preferred activity for many obese clients and one that is easily engaged in and adhered to. Thus, if the benefits of walking, particularly adherence, exceed the observed or perceived risk of an orthopedic injury, walking may be a primary exercise recommendation. When working with this population, personal trainers must make sure of all the situations in which the obese client will exercise, including positions, locations in the training facility that offer greater privacy, and choice of exercise equipment. Exercise considerations for obese clients are given in Table 16.5 and Table 16.6.

TABLE 16.5	Physiologic and Training Considerations for Individuals Who Are Overweight or Obese
Physiologic Considerations	**Considerations for Health and Fitness**
May have other comorbidities (diagnosed or undiagnosed), including hypertension, cardiovascular disease, or diabetes	Initial screening should clarify the presence of potential undiagnosed comorbidities
Maximal oxygen uptake and ventilatory (anaerobic) threshold is typically reduced	Consider testing and training modalities that are weight-supported (such as cycle ergometer, swimming). If a client does not have these limitations, consider a walking program to improve compliance
Coexisting diets may hamper exercise ability and result in significant loss of lean body mass	Initial programming should emphasize low intensity, with a progression in exercise duration (up to 60 minutes as tolerable) and frequency (5–7 days per week), before increases are made in intensity of exercise Exercise intensity should be no greater than 60–80% of work capacity, with weekly caloric volume a minimum of 1,250 kcal per week and a progression to 2,000, as tolerable
Measures of body composition (hydrostatic weighing, skin-fold calipers) may not accurately reflect degree of overweight or obesity	BMI, scale weight, or circumference measurements are recommended measures of weight loss

TABLE 16.6	Basic Exercise Guidelines for Individuals Who Are Overweight or Obese
Mode	Low-impact or step aerobics (such as treadmill walking, rowing, stationary cycling, and water activity)
Frequency	At least 5 days per week
Intensity	60–80% of maximum heart rate. Use the Talk Test[a] to determine exertion Stage I cardiorespiratory training progressing to stage II (intensities may be altered to 40–70% of maximal heart rate if needed)
Duration	40–60 minutes per day, or 20- to 30-minute sessions twice each day
Assessment	Push, pull, squat Single-leg balance (if tolerated)
Flexibility	SMR (only if comfortable to client) Flexibility continuum
Resistance training	1–3 sets of 10–15 repetitions on 2–3 days per week Phases 1 and 2 will be appropriate performed in a circuit-training manner (higher repetitions such as 20 may be used)
Special considerations	Make sure client is comfortable—be aware of positions and locations in the facility your client is in Exercises should be performed in a standing or seated position May have other chronic diseases; in such cases a medical release should be obtained from the individual's physician

[a]The "Talk Test" is a method of measuring intensity if the health and fitness professional is unable to assess intensity via heart rate. If the client can comfortably carry on a conversation while exercising, he or she is probably at the lower ranges of training heart rate. If he or she is having difficulty finishing a sentence, the client is probably at the high range. Depending on the individual's response and exercise status, adjust intensity accordingly.
SMR, self-myofascial release.

SUMMARY

Obesity is the fastest growing health problem in the United States. Personal trainers must be prepared and willing to work with obese clients. Once BMI is determined, realistic weight-loss and exercise goals can be discussed. When designing programs for overweight and obese clients, adherence to the type and amount of exercise should be considered. Walking is often recommended if the risk of orthopedic injury is low. For effective weight loss, a reasonable energy expenditure goal using aerobic exercise should be 200 to 300 kcal per session, with a minimum weekly goal of 1,250 kcal combined exercise and physical activity. In addition, resistance training should be part of any exercise regimen to promote weight loss. Although resistance training typically burns fewer calories than aerobic exercise, it preserves lean body mass, which is important for maintaining metabolism and improving body composition. Similar resistance training guidelines used for adults of normal weight should be used in the obese population, focusing on correct form and breathing and technique.

Diabetes

Diabetes is a metabolic disorder in which the body does not produce enough insulin (type 1) or the body cannot respond normally to the insulin that is made (type 2). An estimated 23.6 million children and adults in the United States (7.8% of the population) have diabetes, and 1.6 million new cases are diagnosed each year (35). Diabetes is the seventh leading cause of death in the United States, and is associated with a greater risk for heart disease, hypertension, and adult-onset blindness (35). It has been shown that people who develop diabetes before the age of 30 are 20 times more likely to die by age 40 than those who do not have diabetes (30).

There are two primary forms of diabetes: type 1 (insulin-dependent diabetes) and type 2 (non–insulin-dependent diabetes). Although type 2 is referred to as non–insulin-dependent diabetes, some individuals with type 2 diabetes cannot manage their blood glucose levels and do require additional insulin. Type 2 diabetes is strongly associated with an increase in childhood and adult-onset obesity.

Type 1 diabetes is typically diagnosed in children, teenagers, or young adults. With type 1 diabetes, specialized cells in the pancreas called beta cells stop producing insulin, causing blood sugar levels to rise, resulting in *hyperglycemia* (high levels of blood sugar). To control this high level of blood sugar, the individual with type 1 diabetes must inject insulin to compensate for what the pancreas cannot produce. Exercise increases the rate at which cells utilize glucose, which may mean that insulin levels may need to be adjusted with exercise. If the individual with type 1 diabetes does not control his or her blood glucose levels (via insulin injections and dietary carbohydrates) before, during, and after exercise, blood sugar levels can drop rapidly and cause a condition called *hypoglycemia* (low blood sugar), leading to weakness, dizziness, and fainting. Although insulin, proper diet, and exercise are the primary components prescribed for individuals with type 1 diabetes, these individuals must still be monitored throughout exercise to ensure safety.

Type 2 diabetes is associated with obesity, particularly abdominal obesity. The incidence and prevalence of adult type 2 diabetes in the United States has increased sharply in recent years. There is a significant public health concern about the rising incidence of type 2 diabetes in children, associated with both the increase in abdominal obesity and decrease in voluntary physical activity. Individuals with type 2 diabetes usually produce adequate amounts of insulin; however, their cells are resistant to the insulin (the insulin present cannot transfer adequate amounts of blood sugar into the cell). This condition can lead to *hyperglycemia* (high blood sugar). Chronic hyperglycemia is associated with a number of diseases associated with damage to the kidneys, heart, nerves, eyes, and circulatory system. Although individuals with type 2 diabetes do not experience the same fluctuations in blood sugar as those with type 1, it is still important to be aware of the symptoms, particularly for individuals with type 2 diabetes who use insulin medications.

> **Diabetes** Chronic metabolic disorder, caused by insulin deficiency, which impairs carbohydrate usage and enhances usage of fat and protein.

Exercise and Diabetes

The most important goals of exercise for individuals with either type of diabetes are glucose control and for those with type 2 diabetes, weight loss. Exercise training is effective with both goals because it has a similar action to insulin by enhancing the uptake of circulating glucose by exercising skeletal muscle. Research has shown that exercise improves a variety of glucose measures, including tissue sensitivity, improved glucose tolerance, and even a decrease in insulin requirements (1,36).

Thus, exercise has been shown to have a substantial positive effect on the prevention of type 2 diabetes.

There are specific exercise guidelines and recommendations to follow when working with a diabetic population, including strategies to prevent hypoglycemic and hypergly-cemic events during or after exercise as well as when to defer exercise based on resting blood glucose levels or symptoms. In most cases, excluding other health-related problems, the exercise management goals for individuals with diabetes are similar to those for physical inactivity and excess body weight. In contrast to walking being a highly preferred form of exercise for obese clients, care must be taken when recommending walking to clients with diabetes to prevent blisters and foot microtrauma that could result in foot infection. Special care should also be taken with respect to giving advice to clients with diabetes regarding carbohydrate intake and insulin use, not only before exercise but afterward, to reduce the risk of a hypoglycemic or hyperglycemic event.

Exercise guidelines for clients with diabetes are similar to those advised for obese adults, as many clients with type 2 diabetes are obese. In such case, daily exercise is recommended for more stable glucose management and maximal caloric expenditure Table 16.7 and Table 16.8. Low-impact exercise activities can reduce the risk of injury, whereas resistance training is advised as part of an overall exercise plan for

---

TABLE 16.7

Physiologic and Training Considerations for Individuals with Diabetes

© ilolab/ShutterStock, Inc.

Physiologic Considerations	Considerations for Health and Fitness	Considerations in Sport and Athletic Training
Frequently associated with comorbidities (including cardiovascular disease, obesity, and hypertension)	Type 2 diabetes, program should target weekly caloric goal of 1,000–2,000 kcal, progressing as tolerable, to maximize weight loss and cardio protection	Screening for comorbidities is important
Exercise exerts an effect similar to that of insulin	Increased risk of exercise-induced hypoglycemia	Be aware of signs and symptoms of hypoglycemia
Hypoglycemia may occur several hours after exercise, as well as during exercise	For those recently diagnosed, glucose should be measured before, during, and after exercise	Restoration of glucose after the event may be necessary to prevent nocturnal hypoglycemia
Clients taking β-blocking medications may be unable to recognize signs and symptoms of hypoglycemia	Some reduction in insulin and increase in carbohydrate intake may be necessary and proportionate to exercise intensity and duration	Substantial insulin dose reduction may be necessary before exercise Carbohydrate intake before and during exercise may be necessary
Exercise in excessive heat may mask signs of hypoglycemia	Postexercise carbohydrate consumption is advisable	Initial exercise prescription should emphasize low intensity, with a progression in exercise duration (up 60 minutes as tolerable) and frequency (5–7 days per week), for consistent glucose control. Intensity should be no greater than 50–90% of work capacity to start with

Physiologic Considerations	Considerations for Health and Fitness	Considerations in Sport and Athletic Training
Increased risk for retinopathy	Be cognizant of signs and symptoms of hypoglycemia	Resistance training guidelines may follow those for normal weight healthy adults (e.g., 1–3 sets of 8–10 exercises, 10–15 reps per set, 2–3 days per week)
Peripheral neuropathy may increase risk for gait abnormalities and infection from foot blisters that may go unnoticed	Use weight-bearing exercise cautiously and wear appropriate footwear	Check daily for blisters or skin injury and appropriate footwear

TABLE 16.8   Basic Exercise Guidelines for Individuals With Diabetes

Mode	Low-impact activities (such as cycling, treadmill walking, low-impact or step aerobics)
Frequency	4–7 days per week
Intensity	50–90% of maximum heart rate
	Stage I cardiorespiratory training (may be adjusted to 40–70% of maximal heart rate if needed) progressing to stages II and III based on a physician's approval
Duration	20–60 minutes
Assessment	Push, pull, OH squat
	Single-leg balance or single-leg squat
Flexibility	Flexibility continuum
Resistance training	1–3 sets of 10–15 repetitions 2–3 days a week
	Phases 1 and 2 of the OPT model (higher repetitions such as 20 may be used)
Special considerations	Make sure client has appropriate footwear and have client or physician check feet for blisters or abnormal wear patterns
	Advise client or class participant to keep a snack (quick source of carbohydrate) available during exercise, to avoid sudden hypoglycemia
	Use SMR with special care and licensed physician's advice
	Avoid excessive plyometric training, and higher-intensity training is not recommended for typical client

SMR, self-myofascial release; OH, overhead squat.

health and fitness. Assessment procedures should follow those outlined in chapter 6. Flexibility exercises can be used as suggested; however, special care should be given to self-myofascial release, and this may be contraindicated for anyone with peripheral neuropathy (loss of protective sensation in feet and legs). Obtain the advice of a licensed physician concerning self-myofascial release (foam rolling) as well as from a licensed diabetes educator if clients are under the care of one. Phases 1 and 2 of the OPT model are appropriate for this population; however, the use of plyometric training may be inappropriate.

SUMMARY

Diabetes impairs the body's ability to either produce or use insulin effectively. Type 1 diabetes (insulin-dependent diabetes) is typically found in younger individuals. If individuals with type 1 diabetes do not control their blood glucose levels (via insulin injections and dietary carbohydrates) before, during, and after exercise, blood sugar levels can rise or fall rapidly and cause hyperglycemia and hypoglycemia, with the latter leading to weakness, dizziness, and fainting. Type 2 diabetes (non–insulin-dependent diabetes) is associated with obesity, particularly abdominal obesity. Individuals with type 2 diabetes usually produce adequate amounts of insulin; however, their cells are resistant to the insulin, which can lead to hyperglycemia.

Exercise is effective for glucose control and weight loss. Exercise recommendations generally follow those advised for obese adults, as many clients with type 2 diabetes are obese, and daily exercise is recommended for more stable glucose management and caloric expenditure. Weight-bearing activities may need to be avoided at least initially to prevent blisters and foot microtrauma that could result in foot infections. Carbohydrate intake or insulin use should be stressed before exercise as well as afterward to reduce the risk of postexercise hyperglycemic or hypoglycemic events.

Follow exercise guidelines for obese adults, using lower-impact exercise modalities. Special care should be given to self-myofascial release, and this may be contraindicated for anyone with a loss of protective sensation in the feet and legs. Phases 1 and 2 of the OPT model are appropriate for this population, but plyometric training may be inappropriate.

Hypertension

Hypertension
Consistently elevated arterial blood pressure, which, if sustained at a high enough level, is likely to induce cardiovascular or end-organ damage.

Blood pressure is defined as the pressure exerted by the blood against the walls of the blood vessels, especially the arteries. It varies with the strength of the heartbeat, the elasticity of the arterial walls, the volume and viscosity of the blood, and a person's health, age, and physical condition. **Hypertension**, or high blood pressure, is a common medical disorder in which arterial blood pressure remains abnormally high (resting systolic ≥140 or diastolic ≥90 mm Hg). A client is considered to have hypertension (HTN) if they have had two or more resting blood pressure measurements made on separate days that are ≥140 or ≥90 mm Hg or if they are currently taking medication to control blood pressure. Recent guidelines state that individuals with resting blood pressure measurements between 120/80 and 135/85 mm Hg are considered to be prehypertensive and should be encouraged to lower their blood pressure through appropriate lifestyle modifications. Most people think that normal blood pressure is 120/80 mm Hg, but new guidelines published by the American Heart Association have changed the definition of normal blood pressure to "less than 120 and 80 mm Hg." Some of the most common causes of hypertension include smoking, a diet high in fat (particularly saturated fat), and excess weight. The health risks of hypertension are well known and include increased risk for stroke, cardiovascular disease, chronic heart failure, and kidney failure.

One of the most common and traditional methods of controlling hypertension is through antihypertensive medications. Although medications have been proven to be highly effective, comprehensive lifestyle changes, including regular physical activity, diet, and smoking cessation, have also been shown to reduce blood pressure, potentially eliminating the need for medications.

Research has shown that exercise can have a modest impact on lowering elevated blood pressure by an average of 10 mm Hg for both systolic and diastolic blood pressure (37–39). Exercise may help the body to produce more appropriate responses to physical activity or other physiologic stressors. The changes appear modest, but any lowering of pressure conveys a lowered overall health risk and is important. Low to moderately intense cardiorespiratory exercise has been shown to be just as effective as high-intensity activity in reducing blood pressure. This is important for elderly or obese individuals with high blood pressure and who are not physically capable of performing high-intensity cardiorespiratory exercise.

It is also important to emphasize the importance of an overall plan to reduce blood pressure that includes exercise, diet, weight loss (if appropriate), and, most important, compliance with any medical treatment plans if clients are under the care of a physician. Personal trainers are encouraged to stress the importance of taking any prescribed medications with all of their clients.

Personal trainers should evaluate their client's heart rate response to exercise, as measured during a submaximal exercise test or even during a simple assessment of heart rate during a comfortable exercise load. Individuals with hypertension frequently take medications that can alter the heart rate response to exercise, in most cases blunting the heart rate response to exercise, thus invalidating prediction equations or estimates of training heart rate. Personal trainers are also encouraged to learn how to accurately assess both resting and exercise blood pressure with all of their clients, but especially those clients with hypertension. Classes to learn how to take blood pressure measurements are available through local organizations such as the American Heart Association and the American Red Cross, or through local hospitals.

It is important to monitor the body position of clients with hypertension at all times throughout an exercise training session. As with obese and diabetic clients, body position can have a dramatic effect on blood pressure response before, during, and after exercise in clients with hypertension. Supine or prone positions (especially when the head is lower in elevation than the heart) can often increase blood pressure, and, as such, these positions may be contraindicated. For example, a standing cable hip extension **Figure 16.3** exercise may be more appropriate than a floor bridge **Figure 16.4** for

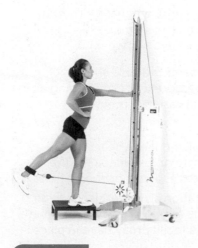

FIGURE 16.3   Standing cable hip extension.

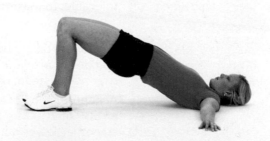

FIGURE 16.4   Floor bridge.

strengthening the gluteals. It is important to note that both hypotensive and hypertensive responses to exercise are possible in clients with hypertension, especially when taking into account the effects of medication, body position, and exercise selection.

When assessing clients with hypertension, personal trainers should follow the guidelines in chapter 6. Use of a single-leg balance (or squat) assessment can also be beneficial, if tolerated by the client. If possible, all other exercises should be performed in a seated or standing position Table 16.9 and Table 16.10. Clients may use the full flexibility continuum; however, static and active stretching may be the easiest and safest. Foam rolling may be contraindicated as it requires lying down. Cardiorespiratory endurance training should focus on stage I and progress only after a physician's approval.

Core exercises in the standing position are preferred over supine core exercises. Some examples include performing standing torso cable iso-rotation Figure 16.5, or cobras in a standing position Figure 16.6. Use plyometric training with care for this population.

Resistance training should be performed in a seated or standing position as well. Phases 1 and 2 of the OPT model will be appropriate for this population, but should be progressed slowly. The programs should be performed in a circuit-style or Peripheral Heart Action (PHA) training system (see chapter 13) to distribute blood flow between the upper and lower extremities. Personal trainers should always ensure that clients with hypertension try and breathe normally and avoid the **Valsalva maneuver** or overgripping

Valsalva maneuver
A maneuver in which a person tries to exhale forcibly with a closed glottis (windpipe) so that no air exits through the mouth or nose as, for example, in lifting a heavy weight. The Valsalva maneuver impedes the return of venous blood to the heart.

TABLE 16.9   Physiologic and Training Considerations for Individuals with Hypertension

© Itolab/ShutterStock, Inc.

Physiologic Considerations	Considerations for Health and Fitness, Sport and Athletic Training
Blood pressure response to exercise may be variable and exaggerated, depending on the mode and level of intensity	A program of continuous, lower-intensity (50–85% of work capacity) aerobic exercise is initially recommended. Frequency and duration parameters should be at a minimum 3–5 days per week, 20–45 minutes per day, with additional increases in overall volume of exercise if weight loss is also desired
Despite medication, clients may arrive with preexercise hypertension	Resistance exercise should consist of a Peripheral Heart Action or circuit-training style Avoid Valsalva maneuvers (holding breath), emphasize rhythmic breathing and a program design for muscular fitness (e.g., 1–3 sets of 8–10 exercises, 10–20 reps, 2–3 days per week)
Hypertension frequently is associated with other comorbidities, including obesity, cardiovascular disease, and diabetes	Screening for comorbidities is important. Exercise should target a weekly caloric goal of 1,500–2,000 kcal, progressing as tolerable, to maximize weight loss and cardio protection
Some medications, such as β-blockers, for hypertension will attenuate the heart rate at rest and its response to exercise	For clients taking medications that will influence heart rate, do not use predicted maximal heart rate or estimates for the exercise. Instead, use actual heart rate response or the Talk Test. Accepted blood pressure contraindications for exercise include an SBP of 200 mm Hg and a DBP of 115 mm Hg. Always check with any other lower guidelines the fitness facility may have in place.

SBP, systolic blood pressure; DBP, diastolic blood pressure.

TABLE 16.10	Basic Exercise Guidelines for Individuals with Hypertension
Mode	Stationary cycling, treadmill walking, rowers
Frequency	3–7 days per week
Intensity	50–85% of maximal heart rate Stage I cardiorespiratory training progressing to stage II (intensities may be altered to 40–70% of maximal heart rate if needed)
Duration	30–60 minutes
Assessment	Push, pull, OH squat Single-leg balance (squat if tolerated)
Flexibility	Static and active in a standing or seated position
Resistance training	1–3 sets of 10–20 repetitions 2–3 days per week Phases 1 and 2 of the OPT model Tempo should not exceed 1 second for isometric and concentric portions (e.g., 4/1/1 instead of 4/2/1) Use circuit or PHA weight training as an option, with appropriate rest intervals
Special considerations	Avoid heavy lifting and Valsalva maneuvers—make sure client breathes normally Do not let client overgrip weights or clench fists when training Modify tempo to avoid extended isometric and concentric muscle action Perform exercises in a standing or seated position Allow client to stand up slowly to avoid possible dizziness Progress client slowly

OH, overhead squats; PHA, Peripheral Heart Action.

(squeezing too tightly) when using exercise equipment as this can dramatically increase blood pressure. Personal trainers should also monitor clients with hypertension carefully when rising from a seated or lying position as they may experience dizziness.

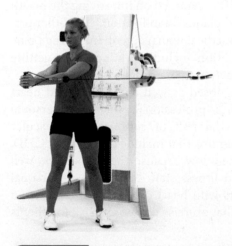

FIGURE 16.5 Standing torso cable iso-rotation.

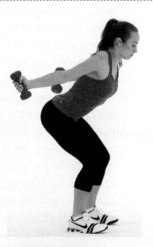

FIGURE 16.6 Standing cobra.

SUMMARY

A normal blood pressure is considered ≤120/80 mm Hg. Hypertension is defined as a blood pressure ≥140/90 mm Hg, whereas a blood pressure between 120/80 and 135/85 mm Hg is considered prehypertensive. Hypertension can be controlled through cardiorespiratory exercise, diet, and other lifestyle changes; however, clients are encouraged to take all prescribed medications as directed by their physician.

Individuals with hypertension should engage in low-intensity aerobic exercise, and may want to avoid high-intensity, high-volume resistance training. Personal trainers are encouraged to measure and pay close attention to the heart rate response to exercise of clients with hypertension, instead of relying on estimates or equations.

Monitoring body position is very important as well when working with this population; supine or prone positions (especially when the head is lower in elevation than the heart) may be contraindicated. The majority of exercises for clients with hypertension should be performed in a seated or standing position. The full flexibility continuum can be used, but static and active stretching may be easiest and safest. Self-myofascial release may be contraindicated depending on body position. Cardiorespiratory training should focus on stage I and progress only with a physician's approval. Plyometric training should be used with care for this population. Resistance training should be performed in a seated or standing position as well. Phases 1 and 2 of the OPT model are appropriate. Programs should be performed in a circuit style or using the Peripheral Heart Action (PHA) training system.

Coronary Heart Disease

Coronary heart disease (CHD) remains the leading cause of death and disability for both men and women despite a significant (29.2%) reduction in death rates from CHD between 1996 and 2006. CHD is caused by atherosclerosis (plaque formation), which leads to narrowing of the coronary arteries and ultimately angina pectoris (chest pain), myocardial infarction (heart attack), or both (40). The primary cause of CHD is poor lifestyle choices, primarily cigarette smoking, poor diet, and physical inactivity. From a medical standpoint, the emphasis on treating CHD is centered on improving the health of the internal lining of the coronary artery, called plaque "stabilization." The other primary focus on the treatment of CHD is through medical management, including pharmaceuticals, as well as aggressive lifestyle intervention, including eating better, getting more exercise, smoking cessation, and stress reduction, to name a few.

Increasing numbers of individuals with diagnosed as well as undiagnosed heart disease are seeking the advice of health and fitness professionals, including personal trainers, to get advice on exercise training. The risk of serious cardiovascular complications, even death, is low in exercise programs that include clients with CHD. The risk of exercise for clients with CHD is likely low because they should be well screened and monitored by their physician and fitness staff. Nonetheless, personal trainers must be aware of the presence of clients with heart disease and help design effective exercise programs with the knowledge that exercise *can* pose a risk for clients with heart disease **Table 16.11**.

In some cases, clients with CHD will begin a fitness program after completing a cardiac rehabilitation program. Regardless of whether a client with CHD has completed a

TABLE 16.11	Physiologic and Training Considerations for Individuals with Coronary Heart Disease

Physiologic Considerations	Considerations for Health and Fitness, Sport and Athletic Training
The nature of heart disease may result in a specific level of exercise, above which it is dangerous to perform	The upper safe limit of exercise, preferably by heart rate, must be obtained Heart rate should never be estimated from existing prediction formulas for clients with heart disease. Consult their physician
Clients with heart disease may not have angina (chest pain equivalent) or other warning signs	Clients must be able to monitor pulse rate or use an accurate monitor to stay below the upper safe limit of exercise
Between the underlying disease and medication use, the heart rate response to exercise will nearly always vary considerably from age-predicted formulas, and will almost always be lower	Although symptoms should always supersede anything else as a sign to decrease or stop exercising, some clients may not have this warning system, so monitoring of heart rate becomes increasingly important
Clients may have other comorbidities (such as diabetes, hypertension, peripheral vascular disease, or obesity)	Screening for comorbidities is important and modifications to exercise may be made based on these diagnoses
Peak oxygen uptake (as well as ventilatory threshold) is often reduced because of the compromised cardiac pump and peripheral muscle deconditioning	The exercise prescription should be low intensity, to start, and based on recommendations provided by a certified exercise physiologist or physical therapist with specialty training Aerobic training guidelines should follow, at minimum, 20–30 minutes 3–5 days per week at 40–85% of maximal capacity, but below the upper safe limits prescribed by the physician A weekly caloric goal of 1,500–2,000 kcal is usually recommended, progressing as tolerable, to maximize cardio protection Resistance training may be started after the patient has been exercising asymptomatically and comfortably for >3 months in the aerobic exercise program A circuit-training format is recommended, 8–10 exercises, 1–3 sets of 10–20 reps per exercise, emphasizing breathing control and rest as needed between sets

cardiac rehabilitation program or not, personal trainers must have a clear understanding about the client's disease, medication use, and most importantly, the upper safe limit of exercise—and any other restrictions—imposed by the client's physician. Personal trainers must not compromise on obtaining this information, and client participation must not proceed until the information is received. In many cases, the client can facilitate obtaining this information.

Clients must be able to find and monitor their own pulse rate or use an accurate monitor to stay below their safe upper limit of exercise. It is important to note that the heart rate response to exercise in this population can vary considerably from age-predicted formulas, and will often be lower. Although signs and symptoms should always supersede all else as a sign to decrease or stop exercising, signs and symptoms vary greatly among individuals with CHD, so careful monitoring of heart rate, rating of perceived exertion (RPE), and signs of worsening CHD like angina become increasingly important. Using rate of perceived exertion to assess exercise intensity **Table 16.12**, which allows personal trainers to gauge the intensity of the exercise without having to assess heart rate, is another useful tool.

Clients with stable coronary artery disease (and especially those who have participated in a cardiac rehabilitation program) should know or be taught information on the importance and benefits of exercise, which include a lower risk of mortality (death), increased exercise tolerance, muscle strength, reduction in angina and heart failure symptoms, and improved psychological status and social adjustment. There is also evidence that heart disease may be slowed (or even reversed) when a multifactor intervention program of intensive education, exercise, counseling, and lipid-lowering medications are used, as appropriate (41,42).

Personal trainers must be careful to not overstate the benefits of exercise as a singular intervention and must emphasize to clients the importance of a multidisciplinary approach to heart disease. However, exercise is critically important and can be safely

TABLE 16.12 Rating of Perceived Exertion

Original Scale		Category–Ratio Scale		
6		0.0	Nothing at all	No intensity
7	Very, very light	0.3		
8		0.5	Extremely weak	Just noticeable
9	Very light	0.7		
10		1.0	Very weak	
11	Fairly light	1.5		
12		2.0	Weak	Light
13	Somewhat hard	2.5		
14		3.0	Moderate	
15	Hard	4.0		
16		5.0	Strong	Heavy
17	Very hard	6.0		
18		7.0	Very strong	
19	Very, very hard	8.0		
20		9.0		
		10.0	Extremely strong	Strongest intensity
		11.0		
			Absolute maximum	Highest possible

conducted in most health and fitness settings Table 16.13. Personal trainers should follow the guidelines in chapter 6 for assessment of these clients with CHD. Use of a single-leg balance (or squat) exercise can also be beneficial, if tolerated by the client. If possible, all other exercises should be performed in a seated or standing position. Clients should stay with static and active stretching in a standing or seated position because they may be the easiest and safest to perform. Consult with a licensed physician for specific recommendations concerning self-myofascial release. Cardiorespiratory training should focus on stage I and only progress with the physician's advice.

Core exercises in the standing position are preferred. Some examples include performing prone iso-abs (planks) on an incline, standing torso cable iso-rotation, or cobras in a standing position (two-leg or single-leg). Plyometric training would not be recommended for this population in the initial months of training.

Resistance training should be performed in a seated or standing position, as well. Phases 1 and 2 of the OPT model will be appropriate for this population. The programs should be performed in a circuit-style or PHA training system (see chapter 13). The health and fitness professional should always ensure that the client is breathing normally and is not straining to exercise or overgripping (squeezing too tightly) the exercise equipment, as this can increase blood pressure.

TABLE 16.13	Basic Exercise Guidelines for Individuals with Coronary Heart Disease
Mode	Large muscle group activities, such as stationary cycling, treadmill walking, or rowing
Frequency	3–5 days/week
Intensity	40–85% of maximal heart rate reserve
	The Talk Test may also be more appropriate as medications may affect heart rate
	Stage I cardiorespiratory training
Duration	5–10 minutes warm-up, followed by 20–40 minutes of exercise, followed by a 5- to 10-minute cool-down
Assessment	Push, pull, OH squat
	Single-leg balance (squat if tolerated)
Flexibility	Static and active in a standing or seated position
Resistance training	1–3 sets of 10–20 repetitions 2–3 days per week
	Phases 1 and 2 of the OPT model
	Tempo should not exceed 1 second for isometric and concentric portions (e.g., 4/1/1 instead of 4/2/1)
	Use circuit or PHA weight training as an option, with appropriate rest intervals
Specific considerations	Be aware that clients may have other diseases to consider as well, such as diabetes, hypertension, peripheral vascular disease, or obesity
	Modify tempo to avoid extended isometric and concentric muscle action
	Avoid heavy lifting and Valsalva maneuvers—make sure client breathes normally
	Do not let client overgrip weights or clench fists when training
	Perform exercises in a standing or seated position
	Progress exercise slowly

OH, overhead squat; PHA, Peripheral Heart Action.

SUMMARY

The leading cause of death and disability for both men and women is coronary heart disease. CHD is caused by atherosclerosis (plaque formation) which leads to narrowing of the coronary arteries and ultimately angina pectoris (chest pain), myocardial infarction (heart attack), or both. The cardiovascular complication rate is low in exercise programs; however, personal trainers must be aware of the presence of clients with heart disease and help design effective exercise programs with the knowledge that exercise *can* pose a risk for clients with heart disease.

Personal trainers must have a clear understanding about a client's disease, medication use, and upper safe limit of exercise imposed by the client's physician. Participation must not proceed until the information is received. Aerobic low-intensity exercise is recommended, with a weekly caloric expenditure goal of 1,500 to 2,000 kcal. Resistance training should not be started until the client has been exercising without any problems for at least 3 months. Most exercises should be performed in a seated or standing position. Flexibility exercises should be limited to static and active stretching in a seated or standing position. Self-myofascial release should be preapproved by a physician. Cardiorespiratory training should focus on stage I and progress only with the physician's approval. Plyometric training would not be recommended for this population in the initial months of training. Resistance training should be performed in a seated or standing position as well. Phases 1 and 2 of the OPT model are appropriate. Programs should be performed in a circuit style or using the PHA training system.

Osteoporosis

Osteopenia A decrease in the calcification or density of bone as well as reduced bone mass.

Osteoporosis Condition in which there is a decrease in bone mass and density as well as an increase in the space between bones, resulting in porosity and fragility.

Osteopenia is a condition in which bone mineral density (BMD) is lower than normal and is considered a precursor to osteoporosis, whereas **osteoporosis** is a disease of bones in which BMD is reduced, bone microstructure is disrupted, and the actual proteins in bone are altered. There are two types or classes of osteoporosis: type 1 (primary) and type 2 (secondary). Primary osteoporosis is associated with normal aging and is attributable to a lower production of estrogen and progesterone, both of which are involved with regulating the rate at which bone is lost. Secondary osteoporosis is caused by certain medical conditions or medications that can disrupt normal bone reformation, including alcohol abuse, smoking, certain diseases, or certain medications. Both types of osteoporosis are treatable and can occur in both men and women. Personal trainers are encountering an increase in the number of clients with osteopenia and osteoporosis as they seek out help in trying to slow or reverse the effects of these conditions through exercise. Although the vast majority of clients will be women, men can, in fact, have either of these diseases.

Type 1 osteoporosis is most prevalent in postmenopausal women because of a deficiency in estrogen (usually secondary to menopause). The disease is characterized by an increase in bone resorption (removal of old bone) with a decrease in bone remodeling (formation of new bone), which leads to a decrease in bone mineral density.

Osteoporosis commonly affects the neck of the femur and the lumbar vertebrae. These structures are considered part of the core and are located in the region of the body where the majority of all forces come together. Thus, a decrease in bone mineral density places the core in a weakened state and, thus, more susceptible to injury, such as a fracture. Research has shown that the risk of hip fractures doubles every 5 years in postmenopausal women older than the age of 50 (43). In the United States today, an estimated 10 million individuals already have the disease and nearly 34 million are estimated to have low bone mass, placing them at increased risk for developing osteoporosis in the future. Furthermore, osteoporosis affects more than 25 million people each year, resulting in approximately 1.5 million hip fractures. Of these 1.5 million hip fractures, only 20% of the patients return to a normal functional status (43,44).

There are a variety of risk factors that influence osteoporosis. One of the most important is peak bone mass (or density). Peak bone mass is the highest amount of bone mass a person is able to achieve during his or her lifetime. New bone formation (remodeling) occurs as the result of stress placed on the musculoskeletal system. To maintain consistent bone remodeling, people must remain active enough to ensure adequate stress is being placed on their bodies. This is especially important for adolescents and young adults trying to reach peak bone mass.

Other risk factors include a lack of physical activity, smoking, excess alcohol consumption, and low dietary calcium intake. The key for personal trainers is to recognize that these factors can be positively influenced through a comprehensive health and fitness program Table 16.14. In addition to exercise programs, clients should be encouraged to increase dietary intake of calcium, decrease alcohol intake, and to cease smoking.

With respect to physical activity, whether a client has osteopenia or osteoporosis, it is important to determine to what degree the client may engage in weight-bearing activities (walking, jogging, dancing, stair climbing, etc.) or resistance training. For example, there is a balance between the benefit of providing exercises that are designed

TABLE 16.14	Physiologic and Training Considerations for Individuals with Osteoporosis

© ilolab/ShutterStock, Inc.

Physiologic Considerations	Considerations for Health and Fitness, Sport and Athletic Training
Maximal oxygen uptake and ventilatory threshold is frequently lower, as a result of chronic deconditioning	Typical exercise loads prescribed are consistent with fitness standards: 40–70% of maximum work capacity, 3–5 days per week, approximately 20–30 minutes per session
Gait and balance may be negatively affected	Physiologic and physical limitations point to low-intensity, weight-supported exercise programs that emphasize balance training
Chronic vertebral fractures may result in significant lower-back pain	For clients with osteopenia (and no contraindications to exercise), resistance training is recommended to build bone mass Loads >75% of 1RM have been shown to improve bone density, but clients must be properly progressed to be able to handle these loads A circuit-training format is recommended, 8–10 exercises, 1 set of 8–12 reps per exercise, with rest as needed between sets
Age, disease, physical stature, and deconditioning may place the client at risk for falls	For clients with severe osteoporosis, exercise modality should be shifted to water exercise to reduce risk of loading fracture. If aquatic exercise is not feasible, use other weight-supported exercise, such as cycling, and monitor signs and symptoms Reinforce other lifestyle behaviors that will optimize bone health, including smoking cessation, reduced alcohol intake, and increased dietary calcium intake

1RM, one repetition maximum.

to increase bone through the provision of bone stress (weight-bearing exercise or heavier resistance exercises) and the risk of fracture that might be precipitated by advanced osteoporosis. It has been demonstrated that individuals who participate in resistance training have a higher bone mineral density than those who do not (45). Resistance training, however, has been shown to improve bone mineral density by no more than 5%, and some researchers believe that this does not represent a high enough increase to prevent fractures from occurring (45). In fact, it has been estimated that a 20% increase in bone mineral density is necessary to offset fractures. Thus, it has been suggested that training that focuses on the prevention of falls, rather than strength alone, is more advantageous for the elderly. Therefore, exercise regimens that combine resistance training to increase bone mineral density with flexibility, core, and balance training to enhance proprioception (as seen in the OPT model) might better facilitate the needs of this population Table 16.15.

When using the OPT model with this population, personal trainers must follow some precautionary measures; for example, if the client demonstrates the ability to move fairly well without assistance, the movement assessments may be followed (Overhead Squat, Single-Leg Squat or Balance, Push, Pull). If the client is not able to get around very well, it is a good idea to use more stable, machine-based equipment during the assessment process and oftentimes during the exercise program. Follow the kinetic chain checkpoints as closely as possible with this population, but realize that there may be degenerative changes in their posture that cannot be corrected. Try and get clients to their own ideal position, not a general ideal position, and remember to have clients from this population exercise while seated or in a standing position.

Flexibility should be limited to static and active stretching. The use of self-myofascial release may be contraindicated for this population. Cardiorespiratory training should

TABLE 16.15	Basic Exercise Guidelines for Individuals with Osteoporosis
	© ilolab/ShutterStock, Inc.
Mode	Treadmill with handrail support
Frequency	2–5 days per week
Intensity	50–90% of maximal heart rate Stage I cardiorespiratory training progressing to stage II
Duration	20–60 minutes per day or 8- to 10-minute bouts
Assessment	Push, pull, overhead squat, or sitting and standing into a chair (if tolerated)
Flexibility	Static and active stretching
Resistance training	1–3 sets of 8–20 repetitions at up to 85% on 2–3 days per week Phases 1 and 2 of OPT model should be mastered before moving on
Special considerations	Progression should be slow, well monitored, and based on postural control Exercises should be progressed if possible toward free sitting (no support) or standing Focus exercises on hips, thighs, back, and arms Avoid excessive spinal loading on squat and leg press exercises Make sure client is breathing in normal manner and avoid holding breath as in a Valsalva maneuver

$\dot{V}o_2$, oxygen consumption.

begin in stage I (with a walking program, if tolerated). Weight-bearing activities may be more beneficial to increasing bone mineral density. Progression to stage II cardiorespiratory training should be based on physician's advice and client's ability.

Example core exercises in the standing position would include performing prone iso-abs on an incline, or cobras in a standing position. Other examples include performing a standing cable torso iso-rotation or medicine ball rotations. Care should be taken with crunches or movements with a lot of spinal flexion. Monitor range of motion and check with a licensed physician. Plyometric training is not typically recommended for this population.

Resistance training should be performed in a seated or standing position, as well. Phases 1 and 2 of the OPT model will be appropriate for this population. Research has indicated that higher intensities (75–85%) are needed to stimulate bone formation. Furthermore, it appears that the load (rather than the number of repetitions) is the determining factor in bone formation (45). However, to ensure proper kinetic chain preparation for these higher intensities, the health and fitness professional should progress clients through the OPT model. Stabilization training is also important to counter a lack of balance that can lead to falls and hip fractures. It generally takes about 6 months of consistent exercise at relatively high intensities before any effect on bone mass is realized. If clients within this population are not progressed appropriately (following the OPT model), they may get injured and have a setback in their progress. Exercise training programs for clients in this population may be performed in a circuit-style or PHA training system (see chapter 13), focusing on hips, thighs, back, and arms. Progressing exercises to the standing position will help increase stress to the hips, thighs, and back as well as increase the demand for balance. Both components are necessary to overcome the effects of osteoporosis.

SUMMARY

Osteopenia is a condition in which bone mineral density is lower than normal and is considered a precursor to osteoporosis, whereas osteoporosis is a disease of bones in which bone mineral density is reduced, bone microstructure is disrupted, and the actual proteins in bone are altered. Physical inactivity, smoking, excess alcohol consumption, and low dietary calcium intake are factors that contribute to the risk of osteoporosis. In addition to exercise, clients should be encouraged to increase dietary intake of calcium, lower alcohol intake, and quit smoking.

If a client has a diagnosis of osteoporosis, a physician must dictate to what degree he or she can engage in weight-bearing activities or resistance training. Exercise is designed to increase bone density and reduce the potential risk of future fractures. Exercise training programs that combine resistance training to increase bone mineral density with flexibility, core, and balance training to enhance proprioception are highly recommended for this population as long as they have been cleared by their physician and the preassessment indicates they can.

Clients in this population, who can move fairly well without assistance, can perform many of the movement assessments discussed in chapter 6 (overhead squat, single-leg squat, pushing, pulling). Those not able to get around very well should use more stable, machine-based equipment to assess movement quality and often during the exercise program. Kinetic chain checkpoints should be followed, taking into consideration that degenerative deformations in posture may not be able to be corrected. Exercises should be performed in a seated or standing position.

Flexibility exercises should be limited to static and active stretching in a seated or standing position. Self-myofascial release may be contraindicated for this population. Cardiorespiratory training should focus on stage I (with a walking program, if tolerated). Progression to stage II cardiorespiratory training should be based on a physician's advice and client's ability. Care should be taken with crunches or movements with a lot of spinal flexion. Plyometric training would not be recommended for this population. Resistance training should be performed in a seated or standing position. Phases 1 and 2 of the OPT model are appropriate. Six months of consistent exercise at high intensities, progressed appropriately, will be required for training to have an effect on bone mass. This means that the client will be making a long-term commitment to the exercise program. Programs should be performed in a circuit style or using the PHA training system, focusing on hips, thighs, back, and arms and progressing exercises to the standing position.

Arthritis

Arthritis Chronic inflammation of the joints.

Osteoarthritis Arthritis in which cartilage becomes soft, frayed, or thins out, as a result of trauma or other conditions.

Rheumatoid arthritis Arthritis primarily affecting connective tissues, in which there is a thickening of articular soft tissue, and extension of synovial tissue over articular cartilages that have become eroded.

Arthritis is an inflammatory condition that mainly affects the joints of the body. Arthritis is the leading cause of disability among U.S. adults, and is also associated with significant activity limitation, work disability, reduced quality of life, and high health-care costs. Currently an estimated 21.6% of the adult U.S. population (46.4 million individuals) have arthritis (46). Two of the most common types of arthritis are *osteoarthritis* and *rheumatoid arthritis*.

Osteoarthritis is caused by degeneration of cartilage within joints. This lack of cartilage creates a wearing on the surfaces of articulating bones, causing inflammation and pain at the joint. Some of the most commonly affected joints are in the hands, knees, hips, and spine.

Rheumatoid arthritis is a degenerative joint disease in which the body's immune system mistakenly attacks its own tissue (in this case, tissue in the joint or organs). This can cause an inflammatory response in multiple joints, leading to pain and stiffness. The condition is systemic and may affect both a variety of joints and organ systems. Joints most commonly affected by this condition include the hands, feet, wrists, and knees. It is usually characterized by morning stiffness, lasting more than a half hour, which can be both acute and chronic, with eventual loss of joint integrity.

It is important for personal trainers to understand the difference between rheumatoid arthritis and osteoarthritis, and be aware of the signs and symptoms of an acute rheumatoid arthritis exacerbation. In the presence of an arthritic flare-up, even flexibility exercises may need to be postponed Table 16.16.

Personal trainers should also monitor the progress of clients with arthritis to assess the effects of the exercise program on joint pain. Pain persisting for more than 1 hour after exercise is an indication that the exercise should be modified or eliminated from the routine. Moreover, exercises of higher intensity or involving high repetitions are to be avoided to decrease joint aggravation. In that regard, a low-volume circuit program or multiple session format is suitable for clients with arthritis Table 16.17.

Health and fitness professionals need to be aware of the medications being taken by clients with arthritis. Clients taking oral corticosteroids, particularly over time, may have osteoporosis, increased body mass, and, if there is a history of gastrointestinal bleeding, anemia. Steroids also increase fracture risk. Research indicates that people exhibiting osteoarthritis have a decrease in strength and proprioception. Research has shown that individuals with arthritis have a decreased ability to balance while

TABLE 16.16 Physiologic and Training Considerations for Individuals with Arthritis	
Physiologic Considerations	**Considerations for Health and Fitness, Sport and Athletic Training**
Maximal oxygen uptake and ventilatory threshold are frequently lower as a result of decreased exercise associated with pain and joint inflammation	Multiple sessions or a circuit format, using treadmill, elliptical trainer, or arm and leg cycles, are a better alternative than higher-intensity, single-modality exercise formats. The usual principles for aerobic exercise training apply (60–80% peak work capacity, 3–5 days per week). Duration of exercise should be an accumulated 30 minutes, following an intermittent or circuit format, 3–5 days per week
Medications may significantly influence bone and muscle health	Incorporate functional activities in the exercise program whenever possible
Tolerance to exercise may be influenced by acute arthritic flare-ups	Awareness of the signs and symptoms that may be associated with acute arthritic flare-ups should dictate a cessation or alteration of training, and joint pain persisting for more than 1 hour should result in an altered exercise format
Rheumatoid arthritis results, in particular, in early morning stiffness	Avoid early morning exercise for clients with rheumatoid arthritis
Evaluate for presence of comorbidities, particularly osteoporosis	Resistive exercise training is recommended, as tolerable, using pain as a guide. Start with very low number of repetitions and gradually increase to the number usually associated with improved muscular fitness (e.g., 10–12 reps, before increasing weight, 1 set of 8–10 exercises, 2–3 days per week)

standing and that a loss in knee-extensor strength is a strong predictor of osteoarthritis (47,48). Furthermore, researchers have shown that patients with osteoarthritis exhibit increased muscle inhibition of knee extensors and were not able to effectively activate their knee-extensor musculature to optimal levels (49,50). Balance (or proprioception) and muscle strength are vital components of walking, and therefore any deficit in these areas could potentially have a negative effect on one's ability to exercise and perform activities of daily living. This claim was supported by a study that showed a significant decrease in dynamic balance for elderly people who had a history of falling (51).

It used to be common practice for arthritic patients to avoid strenuous exercise; however, research on the effects of training on the symptoms of arthritis has led to a shift in that thinking (52,53). One study showed that a 12-week strength-training program provided relief from arthritic symptoms (53), whereas another demonstrated that a 4-week training regimen (including proprioceptive training) decreased muscle inhibition and increased muscle strength in patients with moderate muscle inhibition (49). Therefore, individuals with arthritis are advised to participate in a regular exercise program that follows the OPT methodology for increasing stabilization and strength, while also increasing activities of daily living. In spite of the risks associated with exercise in clients with arthritis, it is very important in restoring functional mobility and endurance in a deconditioned client who has joint limitations secondary to arthritis. Symptoms of arthritis (such as joint pain and stiffness) are heightened through inactivity as a result of muscle atrophy and lack of tissue flexibility. Progressing exercises

TABLE 16.17	Basic Exercise Guidelines for Individuals with Arthritis
Mode	Treadmill walking, stationary cycling, rowers, and low-impact or step aerobics
Frequency	3–5 days per week
Intensity	60–80% of maximal heart rate Stage I cardiorespiratory training progressing to stage II (may be reduced to 40–70% of maximal heart rate if needed)
Duration	30 minutes
Assessment	Push, pull, overhead squat Single-leg balance or single-leg squat (if tolerated)
Flexibility	SMR and static and active stretching
Resistance training	1–3 sets of 10–12 repetitions 2–3 days per week Phase 1 of OPT model with reduced repetitions (10–12) May use a circuit or PHA training system
Special considerations	Avoid heavy lifting and high repetitions Stay in pain-free ranges of motion Only use SMR if tolerated by the client There may be a need to start out with only 5 minutes of exercise and progressively increase, depending on the severity of conditions

SMR, self-myofascial release; PHA, Peripheral Heart Action.

so that they are performed in the seated position (without support) and standing position will increase functional capacity and balance of clients.

A methodical approach is important in the assessment and activity recommendations to reduce symptoms of flare-ups. Follow the guidelines for assessment in chapter 6 and note the pain-free range of motion that clients exhibit during these assessments. Improving muscle strength and enhancing flexibility through exercise can assist in decreasing symptoms associated with arthritis. Static and active forms of stretching can be used and may be better tolerated from a seated or standing position. The use of self-myofascial release can be used if tolerated. Cardiorespiratory training should begin in stage I and may progress to stage II or stage III, depending on the client's capabilities and a physician's advice. Core and balance exercises will be very important for this population to increase levels of joint stability and balance. Plyometric training is not recommended for arthritic clients. Phase 1 of the OPT model will be used for this population with modified repetitions (10 to 12) to avoid heavy, repetitive joint loading that increases stress to the affected joints.

SUMMARY

Arthritis is an inflammatory condition that mainly affects the joints of the body. Two of the most common types of arthritis are *osteoarthritis* and *rheumatoid arthritis*.

Osteoarthritis is caused by degeneration of cartilage in joints. Rheumatoid arthritis is a systemic, degenerative joint disease in which the body's immune system mistakenly attacks its own tissues in the joint or organs, causing an inflammatory response leading to pain and stiffness. Improving muscle strength and enhancing flexibility through exercise can decrease arthritis symptoms. However, health and fitness professionals must be aware of the signs and symptoms of an acute rheumatoid arthritis flare-up. In the case of an arthritic flare-up, even flexibility exercises may not be able to be performed. In addition, exercises that cause pain to persist for more than 1 hour after exercise should be modified or eliminated from the routine. Personal trainers need to be aware of the medications being taken by clients, especially oral corticosteroids and steroids.

Clients with osteoarthritis have a decrease in strength and proprioception and a loss of knee-extensor strength in some cases. Symptoms of arthritis (such as joint pain and stiffness) are heightened through inactivity as a result of muscle atrophy and lack of tissue flexibility. Functional capacity and balance can be increased by progressing exercises so that they are performed in the seated position (without support) to a standing position.

Flexibility exercises should improve muscle strength and enhance flexibility. Static and active forms of stretching can be used and may be better tolerated from a seated or standing position. The use of self-myofascial release can be used, if tolerated. Cardiorespiratory training should begin in stage I and may progress to stage II or stage III, depending on the client's capabilities and a physician's advice. Core and balance exercises will be very important. Plyometric training is not recommended. Phase 1 will be used for this population with modified repetitions (10 to 12) to avoid heavy, repetitive joint loading that increases stress to the affected joints.

Cancer

Cancer is the second leading cause of death in the United States with more than one-half million deaths annually, behind cardiovascular disease. It has been estimated that American men have about a 44% probability and women have a 38% probability of developing cancer during their lifetime (54).

Because of better detection and treatment strategies, those living with cancer have improved quality of life and life spans. In recent years there has been a variety of studies that have documented the positive benefits of exercise in the treatment of cancer, including improved aerobic and muscular fitness, retention of lean body mass, less fatigue, improved quality of life, and positive effects on mood and self-concept (1). Because cancer is not a single disease, but a collection of diseases that share the same description (with respect to cell division, accumulation, and death), its signs and symptoms vary widely. This section is only meant to serve as a brief overview of the role of exercise in the prevention and treatment of cancer. There are several excellent and descriptive resources that can be reviewed for more information (1).

Medications used by clients with cancer can result in substantial adverse effects, including peripheral nerve damage, cardiac and pulmonary problems, skeletal muscle myopathy (muscle weakness and wasting), and anemia, as well as frequent nausea. In addition, the combination of the disease and its treatments frequently result in a diminished quality of life. Personal trainers must have knowledge of and appreciation for the varied adverse effects of the treatments for cancer, as they can be substantially greater than the treatments prescribed for most other chronic diseases **Table 16.18**.

Cancer Any of various types of malignant neoplasms, most of which invade surrounding tissues, may metastasize to several sites, and are likely to recur after attempted removal and to cause death of the patient unless adequately treated.

TABLE 16.18	Physiologic and Training Considerations for Individuals with Cancer
Physiologic Considerations	**Considerations for Health and Fitness, Sport and Athletic Training**
Fatigue and weakness is common	Aerobic exercise should be done at low-moderate intensity (40–50% of peak capacity), 3–5 days per week, using typical aerobic modes (treadmill, elliptical trainer, cycle, depending on patient preference) In particular, avoid higher-intensity training during periods of cancer treatment
Excessive fatigue may result in overall diminished activity	Use intermittent bouts of exercise to accumulate 20–30 minutes of total aerobic exercise
Diminished immune function	Resistance training can be performed (1 set of 8–10 exercises, 10–15 repetitions to fatigue, 2–3 days per week)
Decreased lean muscle mass	Assess and provide intervention for decreased range of motion and balance

Exercise is an important intervention for clients recovering from cancer. It can improve exercise tolerance, reduce the cellular risks associated with cancer, and also improve quality of life. Specifically, exercise at low to moderate intensities for moderate durations appears to have a more positive effect on the immune system (when compared with higher intensities for longer durations) (55). However, research also indicates that moderate to high levels of physical activity seem to be associated with decreased incidence and mortality rates for certain forms of cancer (56).

Exercise programs for this population should follow the OPT model Table 16.19. Assessment procedures for individual with cancer can follow the guidelines in chapter 6. The specific push, pull, and overhead squat assessments should be representative of the client's ability level. A single-leg balance assessment would also be advised if a single-leg squat cannot be performed by the client. Flexibility should include static and active stretching. Self-myofascial release can be used if no complications exist that would prevent its use. Check with a physician if there is any question. Self-myofascial release is not recommended for clients receiving chemotherapy or radiation treatments. Cardiorespiratory training for this population is very important, but may have to start with 5 minutes of stage I training, progressing up to 30 minutes, 3 to 5 days per week. Stage II or stage III training may be used on agreement of the client's physician.

Core and balance exercises will be essential for this population. These exercises will help in regaining stabilization necessary for activities of daily living that may have been lost (as a result of the lack of activity caused by treatments). Clients should be progressed slowly using the stabilization, strength, and power continuums. Plyometric training is not recommended until the client has sufficiently progressed to performing three complete phase 1 workouts per week. Resistance training for this population will include phases 1 and 2 of the OPT model. Other phases may be used as the client progresses and are approved by his or her physician.

TABLE 16.19	Basic Exercise Guidelines for Individuals with Cancer
Mode	Treadmill walking, stationary cycling, rowers, low-impact or step aerobics
Frequency	3–5 days per week
Intensity	50–70% of maximal heart rate reserve Stage I cardiorespiratory training progressing to stage II (may be reduced to 40–70% of maximal heart rate if needed)
Duration	15–30 minutes per session (may only start with 5 minutes)
Assessment	Push, pull, overhead squat Single-leg balance (if tolerated)
Flexibility	SMR and static and active stretching
Resistance training	1–3 sets of 10–15 repetitions 2–3 days per week Phases 1 and 2 of OPT model May use a circuit or PHA training system
Special considerations	Avoid heavy lifting in initial stages of training Allow for adequate rest intervals and progress client slowly Only use SMR if tolerated by the client—avoid SMR for clients undergoing chemotherapy or radiation treatments There may be a need to start with only 5 minutes of exercise and progressively increase, depending on the severity of conditions and fatigue

SMR, self-myofascial release; PHA, Peripheral Heart Action.

SUMMARY

Cancer is the second leading cause of death in the United States, although the number of individuals living with cancer has increased substantially. There are several positive benefits of exercise in the treatment of cancer. Exercise is an important intervention in terms of improving exercise tolerance, reducing cellular risks associated with cancer, and improving quality of life. Medications used by clients with cancer can result in substantial adverse effects. In addition, the combination of the disease and its treatments frequently result in a diminished quality of life. The adverse effects of the treatments for cancer can be substantially greater than the treatments prescribed for most other chronic diseases.

For clients recovering from cancer, exercise that follows the OPT model at low to moderate intensities for moderate durations has a positive effect on the immune system. Research indicates that moderate to high levels of physical activity seem to be associated with decreased incidence and mortality rates for certain forms of cancer.

Assessment procedures for the individual with cancer can follow fitness assessment guidelines described in chapter 6. The specific push, pull, and overhead squat assessments should be representative of the client's ability level. A single-leg balance assessment would also be advised, if the client is capable. Flexibility should include static and active stretching. Self-myofascial release can be used if no complications exist that would prevent its use such as chemotherapy or radiation treatments. Cardiorespiratory training for this population is very important, but may have to start with 5 minutes of stage I training, progressing up to 30 minutes, 3 to 5 days per week. Stage II or stage III training may be used on agreement of the client's physician. Core and balance exercises are essential for this population. Plyometric training is not recommended until the client has progressed to three phase 1 workouts per week. Resistance training for this population will include phases 1 and 2 of the OPT model. Other phases may be used as the client progresses and are approved by his or her physician.

Exercise and Pregnancy

The physiologic differences during exercise between men and women have been well documented. The majority of observed disparities in athletic performance between men and women are explained by differences in body structure, muscle mass, lean to fat body mass ratio, and, to a lesser extent, blood chemistry. When measures are adjusted for body composition, both physiologic and performance parameters narrow considerably or completely vanish **Table 16.20**.

There has been substantial research documenting the beneficial effects of exercise during pregnancy on the physiology and health of both the mother and developing fetus. Fears that the fetus may be harmed by increased blood circulation, thermoregulatory changes, or decreased oxygen supply can be minimized with appropriate precautions. The general consensus is that most recreational pursuits are appropriate for all pregnant women. Those already engaged in an exercise program before pregnancy may continue with moderate levels of exercise until the third trimester, when a logical reduction in activity is recommended (57).

The gradual growth of the fetus can alter the posture of pregnant women, making flexibility and core training important, particularly core-stabilization exercises to improve strength of the pelvic floor musculature. As the mother-to-be progresses to the more advanced stages of pregnancy (second and third trimesters, or after 12 weeks), performing exercises in a prone (on stomach) or supine (on back) position, as well as uncontrolled twisting motions of the torso, is not advised. Moreover, certain resistance exercises such as hip abduction and hip adduction machines are not advised. Changes also occur in the cardiovascular system, decreasing work capacity and leading to necessary alterations in the cardiorespiratory program and the increased importance of proper hydration during aerobic activity. Lastly, personal trainers should be aware that women in the childbearing period are vulnerable to nausea, dizziness, and fainting. Pregnant women should immediately stop exercising if they experience any of these symptoms along with any abdominal pain (or contractions), excessive shortness of breath, or bleeding or leakage of amniotic fluid (57).

During the postpartum period, there may be a tendency to rush an exercise program in an effort to return to pre-pregnancy physiologic and morphologic status. Personal trainers must be careful to advise clients that the changes that occurred during

TABLE 16.20	Physiologic and Training Considerations for Women and Pregnancy

Physiologic Considerations	Considerations for Health and Fitness, Sport and Athletic Training
Contraindications include persistent bleeding 2nd to 3rd trimester, medical documentation of incompetent cervix or intrauterine growth retardation, pregnancy-induced hypertension, preterm rupture of membrane, or preterm labor during current or prior pregnancy	Screen carefully for potential contraindications to exercise
Decreased oxygen available for aerobic exercise	Low-moderate intensity aerobic exercise (40–50% of peak work capacity) should be performed 3–5 days per week, emphasizing non–weight-bearing exercise (e.g., swimming, cycling), although certain treadmill or elliptical training modes may be preferred and are appropriate
Posture can affect blood flow to uterus during vigorous exercise	Avoid supine exercise, particularly after the first trimester
Even in the absence of exercise, pregnancy may increase metabolic demand by 300 kcal per day to maintain energy balance	Advise adequate caloric intake to offset exercise effect
High-risk pregnancy considerations include individuals older than the age of 35, history of miscarriage, diabetes, thyroid disorder, anemia, obesity, and a sedentary lifestyle	There are no published guidelines for resistance, flexibility, or balance training specific to pregnancy exercise. Provided exercise intensity is below the aerobic prescription of 40–50% of peak work capacity, with careful attention to special considerations and contraindications described, adding these components may be helpful. For resistance training, if cleared by the physician, a circuit-training format is recommended, 1–3 sets of 12–15 reps per exercise, emphasizing breathing control and rest, as needed, between sets Advise clothing that will dissipate heat easily during exercise Postpartum exercise should be similar to pregnancy guidelines, as physiologic changes that occur during pregnancy may persist for up to 6 weeks

pregnancy may persist for a month to a month and a half. Ideally, postnatal women should be encouraged to reeducate posture, joint alignment, muscle imbalances, stability, motor skills, and recruitment of the deep core stabilizers such as the transverse abdominis, internal oblique, and pelvic floor musculature. A return to a more vigorous program should be deferred and entered into gradually.

Personal trainers should follow the assessment guidelines in chapter 6, using seated and standing assessments **Table 16.21**. A single-leg squat assessment may be performed as well, if a woman is capable. If not, a single-leg balance assessment may be more appropriate. Flexibility exercises should be performed in seated and standing

TABLE 16.21	Basic Exercise Guidelines for Women and Pregnancy
Mode	Low-impact or step aerobics that avoid jarring motions, treadmill walking, stationary cycling, and water activity
Frequency	3–5 days per week
Intensity	Stage I and only enter stage II on a physician's advice
Duration	15–30 minutes per day. There may be a need to start out with only 5 minutes of exercise and progressively increase to 30 minutes, depending on the severity of conditions
Assessment	Push, pull, overhead squat Single-leg squat or balance
Flexibility	Static, active stretching and SMR
Resistance training	2–3 days per week, using light loads at 12–15 repetitions Phases 1 and 2 of the OPT model are advised (use only phase 1 after first trimester)
Special considerations	Avoid exercises in a prone (on stomach) or supine (on back) position after 12 weeks of pregnancy Avoid SMR on varicose veins and areas of swelling Plyometric training is not advised in the second and third trimesters

SMR, self-myofascial release.

positions, especially in the second and third trimesters. Static and active stretching should be used, and self-myofascial release may also be used as tolerated. However, self-myofascial release should not be performed on varicose veins that are sore, or on areas where there is swelling (such as the calves). During more advanced stages of pregnancy (second and third trimesters), performing self-myofascial release exercises in prone or supine positions is not advised. Cardiorespiratory training should consist primarily of stage I and only enter stage II on a physician's advice. Women who have not exercised before pregnancy can begin with 15 minutes of continuous aerobic activity and gradually progress to 30 minutes of low to moderate aerobic activity. Plyometric training is not advised for this population after the first trimester. Phases 1 and 2 of the OPT model may be used in the first trimester; however, in the second and third trimesters the use of only phase 1 is advised.

SUMMARY

Appropriate precautions can minimize the risks of exercise during pregnancy, including increased blood circulation, thermoregulatory changes, or decreased oxygen supply. Most recreational pursuits are appropriate for all pregnant women, and moderate levels of exercise are encouraged until the third trimester. In the postpartum period, a return to a more vigorous program should be entered into gradually.

Personal trainers should follow the assessment guidelines in chapter 6, using seated or standing assessments. A single-leg squat assessment may be performed depending on the trimester. In the second and third trimester, a single-leg balance assessment may be more appropriate. Flexibility exercises should be performed in the seated or standing position, especially in the second and third trimesters. Static and active stretching should be used. Self-myofascial release can be used as long as the client avoids using the foam roll on varicose veins or anywhere there is swelling. Cardiorespiratory training should consist primarily of stage I. Plyometric training is not advised for this population in the second and third trimesters. Phases 1 and 2 of the OPT model may be used in the first trimester. In the second and third trimesters only phase 1 is advised.

Chronic Lung Disease

Smoking has progressively declined during the last few decades; however, it is still one of the leading preventable causes of death and a primary risk factor for the development of chronic lung diseases. Chronic lung disease is largely broken into two major categories, obstructive and restrictive. In **restrictive lung disease** or disorders, lung tissue may be fibrotic and, thus, dysfunctional (as in the case of pulmonary fibrosis or asbestosis). In restrictive lung disease the ability to expand the lungs may be decreased as a result of any number of causes (such as fractured ribs, a neuromuscular disease, or even obesity). In **chronic obstructive lung disease**, the lung tissue may be normal, but airflow is restricted. The major obstructive lung diseases include asthma, chronic bronchitis, and emphysema. These diseases are characterized by chronic inflammation (caused primarily by smoking, although in the case of asthma may be caused by environmental irritants) and airway obstruction via mucus production. Cystic fibrosis is another disease that is characterized by excessive mucus production, but is instead a genetic disorder.

Restrictive lung disease The condition of a fibrous lung tissue, which results in a decreased ability to expand the lungs.

Chronic obstructive lung disease The condition of altered airflow through the lungs, generally caused by airway obstruction as a result of mucus production.

The impairments during exercise are similar with regard to both restrictive and obstructive lung disease Table 16.22. Problems include decreased ventilation and decreased gas exchange ability (resulting in decreased aerobic capacity and endurance and in oxygen desaturation). Clients with lung disease experience fatigue at low levels of exercise and often have shortness of breath (or *dyspnea*). Those with emphysema are frequently underweight and may exhibit overall muscle wasting with hypertrophied neck muscles (which are excessively used to assist in labored breathing). Those with chronic bronchitis may be the opposite: overweight and barrel-chested.

In general, exercise for these clients is similar to what would be appropriate for the general population Table 16.23. Exercise can improve functional capacity and decrease the symptoms of dyspnea in this population, among many other physiologic and psychological benefits (58). The use of lower body cardiorespiratory and resistance training exercises seem to be best tolerated. Upper extremity exercises place an increased stress on the secondary respiratory muscles that are involved in stabilizing the upper extremities during exercise (59). Therefore, caution should be used when designing programs for this population to ensure adequate rest intervals. The use of the Peripheral Heart Action (PHA) training system would be advised.

TABLE 16.22	Physiologic and Training Considerations for Individuals with Lung Disease
Physiologic Considerations	**Considerations for Health and Fitness, Sport and Athletic Training**
Lung disease frequently is associated with other comorbidities, including cardiovascular disease	Screen for presence of other comorbidities
A decrease in the ability to exchange gas in the lungs may result in oxygen desaturation and marked dyspnea at low workloads	If possible and properly trained, ascertain the level of oxygen saturation using a pulse oximeter Pulse oximetry values should be above 90% and certainly above 85%. Values below this level are a contraindication to continued exercise, regardless of symptoms
Chronic deconditioning results in low aerobic fitness and decreased muscular performance	The aerobic exercise prescription should be guided by the client's shortness of breath. Workloads of 40–60% of peak work capacity, 3–5 days per week, 20–45 minutes as tolerable, may be achievable. Intermittent exercise with frequent rest breaks may be necessary to achieve sufficient overall exercise duration
Upper extremity exercise may result in earlier onset of dyspnea and fatigue than expected, when compared with lower extremity exercise	Upper extremity exercise should be programmed carefully and modified, based on fatigue Resistance training can be helpful; use conservative guidelines Circuit training in a PHA format is recommended (8–10 exercises, 1 set of 8–15 reps per exercise), emphasizing breathing control and rest as needed between sets
Clients may have significant muscle wasting and be of low body weight (with a BMI <18)	If the client is very thin, be certain to recommend adequate caloric intake to offset exercise effects
Clients may be using supplemental oxygen	Trainers may not adjust oxygen flow during exercise; it is considered a medication. If a client experiences unusual dyspnea or has evidence of oxygen desaturation during exercise, stop exercise and consult with the client's physician

BMI, body mass index; PHA, Peripheral Heart Action.

In some clients, inspiratory muscle training can specifically improve the work associated with breathing. Health and fitness professionals working with clients who have lung disease should inquire about this intervention to see whether it might augment the general exercise program. For more information, read the comprehensive guidelines regarding the exercise assessment and training of individuals with lung disease published by the American Association of Cardiovascular and Pulmonary Rehabilitation (59).

TABLE 16.23	Basic Exercise Guidelines for Individuals with Lung Disease
Mode	Treadmill walking, stationary cycling, steppers, and elliptical trainers
Frequency	3–5 days per week
Intensity	40–60% of peak work capacity Stage I
Duration	Work up to 20–45 minutes
Assessment	Push, pull, overhead squat Single-leg squat or balance
Flexibility	Static and active stretching and SMR
Resistance training	1 set of 8–15 repetitions 2–3 days per week Phase 1 of the OPT model is advised PHA training system is recommended
Special considerations	Upper body exercises cause increased dyspnea and must be monitored Allow for sufficient rest between exercises

SMR, self-myofascial release; PHA, Peripheral Heart Action.

SUMMARY

Chronic lung disease is largely broken into two major categories, *obstructive* and *restrictive*. In restrictive disease or disorders, lung tissue may be fibrotic and the ability to expand the lungs may be decreased owing to any number of causes. In obstructive lung disease, the lung tissue may be normal, but airflow is restricted. Both types cause decreased ventilation and decreased gas exchange ability.

Clients with lung disease are often short of breath (*dyspnea*) and fatigue at low levels of exercise. Exercise can improve functional capacity and decrease the symptoms of dyspnea. In some clients, inspiratory muscle training can specifically improve the work associated with breathing.

In general, exercise for this population is similar to what would be appropriate for the general population. Lower body cardiorespiratory and resistance training exercises seem to be best tolerated. Adequate rest intervals need to be maintained. The Peripheral Heart Action training system is advised.

Intermittent Claudication/Peripheral Arterial Disease

Intermittent claudication The manifestation of the symptoms caused by peripheral arterial disease.

Peripheral arterial disease A condition characterized by narrowing of the major arteries that are responsible for supplying blood to the lower extremities.

Intermittent claudication is the name for the manifestation of the symptoms caused by peripheral arterial disease (PAD). (The term *peripheral vascular disease* is also commonly used to describe the activity-induced symptoms that characterize this disease.) Essentially, intermittent claudication is characterized by limping, lameness, or pain in the lower leg during mild exercise resulting from a decrease in blood supply (oxygen) to the lower extremities. **Peripheral arterial disease** is characterized by narrowing of the major arteries that are responsible for supplying blood to the lower extremities.

The primary limiting factor for exercise in the client with PAD is leg pain. One of the problems facing personal trainers is the ability to differentiate between those who are limited by symptoms of true intermittent claudication versus similar leg complaints (such as tightness, cramping, and pain) that might simply be associated with deconditioning Table 16.24. If the client has a diagnosis of PAD, the symptoms are likely to

TABLE 16.24	Physiologic and Training Considerations for Individuals with Intermittent Claudication or PAD
Physiologic Considerations	**Considerations for Health and Fitness, Sport and Athletic Training**
PAD patients frequently have coexisting coronary artery disease or diabetes	For clients with coexisting coronary artery disease, do not exceed established heart rate upper limit (usually, this limit is established from a walking test, in which leg pain is the limiting factor)
	Switching modalities so that leg pain will not limit exercise may result in a higher—and possibly inappropriate—cardiac workload
	If possible, a continuous format of exercise using walking is preferred
	Exercise duration should strive to be 20–30 total minutes, with continuous bouts of 10 minutes or greater, 3–5 days per week working up to every day
Smoking significantly worsens PAD and exercise tolerance	Strongly recommend smoking cessation. If a client continues to smoke, do not allow smoking for at least 1 hour before exercise
PAD frequently results in decreased aerobic capacity and endurance	Focus on aerobic exercise activities, with an emphasis on walking
Resistance training may improve overall physical function, but may not address limitations of PAD	Resistance exercise should be complementary to but not substituted for aerobic exercise
	A circuit-training format is recommended (e.g., 8–10 exercises, 1–3 sets of 8–12 reps per exercise, progressing up to 12–20 reps)
	An intermittent format of exercise may be necessary, with intensity guided by pain tolerance
	Typical guidelines suggest exercise into moderate to severe discomfort, rest until subsided, and repeat until total exercise time is achieved (20–30 minutes)
	Always screen for comorbidities

PAD, peripheral arterial disease.

be accurate for intermittent claudication, although they still could be associated with deconditioning (60). Consult with the client's physician concerning the condition. If pain continues during exercise, the personal trainer must refer the client to a licensed physician immediately.

Although experience will improve the ability of the personal trainer to differentiate between disease and deconditioning, in many respects it does not really matter. The personal trainer should still develop a training regimen that attempts to improve physical function in the face of limiting factors (60). In the case of peripheral vascular disease or deconditioning, the use of an intermittent format of exercise, with rest as necessary between exercise bouts, is similar Table 16.25. Because PAD is associated with coronary heart disease and diabetes, health and fitness professionals should be aware of other existing comorbidities and be suspicious that these comorbidities may still exist, undiagnosed. Thus, physician clearance for exercise is necessary for the client with PAD.

Exercise programming should follow the OPT methodology, using the suggested assessment process in chapter 6. The number of repetitions for movement assessments may have to be decreased depending on the client's abilities. It will be important to make clients feel comfortable and competent with this process to ensure compliance. Static and active stretching should be used for this population. Guidelines for self-myofascial release are not known at this time, and it is suggested that it not be used in this population, unless approved by a licensed physician. Phase 1 of the OPT model is suggested. Repetitions may need to start at 8 to 12 (lower than indicated by these phases) and slowly progress to 12 to 20. Exercise bouts may initially start with 5 to 10 minutes of activity and progress slowly to 20 to 30 minutes.

TABLE 16.25	Basic Exercise Guidelines for Individuals with Intermittent Claudication/PAD
Mode	Treadmill walking is preferred, also stationary cycling, steppers, and elliptical trainers
Frequency	3–5 days per week working up to every day
Intensity	50–85% of maximal heart rate
Duration	Work up to 20–30 minutes
Assessment	Push, pull, overhead squat Single-leg squat or balance
Flexibility	Static and active stretching
Resistance training	1–3 sets of 8–12 repetitions 2–3 days per week, and slowly increasing up to 12–20 reps Phase 1 of the OPT model is advised
Special considerations	Allow for sufficient rest between exercises Workout may start with 5–10 minutes of activity Slowly progress client

SUMMARY

Intermittent claudication is the name for the manifestation of the symptoms caused by PAD. When there is increased activity of the leg muscles, PAD results in symptoms in which oxygen supply does not meet demand. Exercise for PAD should *induce* symptoms, causing a stimulus that increases local circulation. The primary limiting factor is leg pain. The health and fitness professional must differentiate between true intermittent claudication versus similar leg complaints associated with deconditioning. If the client has a diagnosis of PAD, the symptoms are likely to be accurate for intermittent claudication, although they still could be associated with deconditioning.

Exercise in an intermittent format, with rest as necessary between exercise bouts, is recommended. Physician clearance for exercise is necessary for the client with PAD. Exercise programming should follow the OPT methodology, using the fitness assessments discussed in chapter 6. The number of repetitions for movement assessments may have to be decreased depending on the client's abilities. Static and active stretching should be used for this population. However, self-myofascial release is not recommended. Phase 1 of the OPT model should be used. Repetitions may need to start at 8 to 1 2 and slowly progress to 12 to 20. Exercise bouts may initially start with 5 to 10 minutes of activity and progress slowly to 20 to 30 minutes.

REFERENCES

1. *ACSM's Exercise Management for Persons with Chronic Diseases and Disabilities.* 3rd ed. Champaign, IL: Human Kinetics; 2009.
2. *ACSM's Resource Manual for Guidelines for Graded Exercise and Prescription.* 6th ed. Philadelphia: Lippincott Williams & Wilkins; 2010.
3. *ACSM's Resources for Clinical Exercise Physiology.* 2nd ed. Philadelphia: Lippincott Williams & Wilkins; 2009.
4. US Department of Health and Human Services (USDHHS). *2008 Physical Activity Guidelines for Americans.* Washington, DC: USDHHS; 2008.
5. Corbin C, Pangrazi R. *Physical Activity for Children: A Statement of Guidelines for Children Ages 5-12.* Reston VA: National Association for Sport and Physical Education; 2004.
6. Shaping America's Youth. Childhood, Teenage, and Youth Obesity, Nutrition, Health and Exercise Statistics and Grants. Available at: http://www.shapingamericasyouth.com. Accessed October 20, 2010.
7. *ACSM's Guidelines for Graded Exercise and Prescription.* 8th ed. Philadelphia: Lippincott Williams & Wilkins; 2009.
8. Saltarelli W. Children. In: Ehrman JK, Gordon PM, Visich PS, Keteyian SJ, eds. *Clinical Exercise Physiology.* 2nd ed. Champaign, IL: Human Kinetics; 2009:111-134.
9. Faigenbaum AD, Kraemer WJ, Blimkie CJ, et al. Youth resistance training: updated position statement paper from the National Strength And Conditioning Association. *J Strength Cond Res.* 2009;23(5 Suppl):S60-79.
10. US Consumer Product Safety Commission. *National Electronic Injury Surveillance System.* Washington, DC: Director of Epidemiology, National Injury Information Clearinghouse; 1987.
11. Haff GG. Roundtable discussion: youth resistance training. *Strength Cond J.* 2003;25(1):49-64.
12. Falk B, Tenenbaum G. The effectiveness of resistance training in children: a meta-analysis. *Sports Med.* 1996;22:176-186.
13. Payne V, Morrow J, Johnson L. Resistance training in children and youth: a meta-analysis. *Res Q Exerc Sport.* 1997;68:80-89.
14. Roberts S, Ciapponi T, Lytle R. *Developing Strength in Children and Adolescents.* Reston, VA: National Association for Sport and Physical Education; 2008.
15. Federal Interagency Forum on Aging-Related Statistics. *Older Americans 2008: Key Indicators of Well-Being.* Federal Interagency Forum on Aging-Related Statistics, Washington, DC: US Government Printing Office; March 2008.
16. CDC. *Targeting Arthritis: Reducing Disability for 43 Million Americans: at a Glance 2006.* Atlanta, GA: US Department of Health and Human Services, CDC; 2006.
17. Hootman J, Helmick C. Projections of US prevalence of arthritis and associated activity limitations. *Arthritis Rheum.* 2006;54:226-229.
18. National Center for Health Statistics. Chartbook on Trends in the Health of Americans, 2006; Special Feature: Pain. Available at http://www.ncbi.nlm.nih.gov/bookshelf/br.fcgi?book=healthus06&part=A43. Accessed October 20, 2010.

19. Chronic low-back pain on the rise: study finds "alarming increase" in prevalence. *ScienceDaily.* Feb 18, 2009.

20. Ogden CL, Carroll MD, McDowell MA, Flegal KM. *Obesity Among Adults in the United States—No Statistically Significant Change Since 2003-2004.* NCHS data brief no 1. Hyattsville, MD: National Center for Health Statistics; 2007.

21. Goble DJ, Coxon JP, Wenderoth N, Van Impe A, Swinnen, SP. Proprioceptive sensibility in the elderly: degeneration, functional consequences and plastic-adaptive processes. *Neurosci Biobehav Rev.* 2009;33(3):271-278.

22. Hertling D, Kessler RM. *Management of Common Musculoskeletal Disorders: Physical Therapy Principles and Methods.* Baltimore, MD: Lippincott, Williams & Wilkins; 2006.

23. Wescott WL, Baechle TR. *Strength Training for Seniors.* Champaign, IL: Human Kinetics; 1999:1-2.

24. Humphries BD. Strength training for bone, muscle and hormones. ACSM Current Comment. Available at: http://www.acsm.org/AM/Template.cfm?Section=current_comments1&Template=/CM/ContentDisplay.cfm&ContentID=8654. Accessed October 20, 2010.

25. Johnston AP, De Lisio M, Parise G. Resistance training, sarcopenia, and the mitochondrial theory of aging. *Appl Physiol Nutr Metab.* 2008;33(1):191-199.

26. Roth SM, Ferrell RF, Hurley BF. Strength training for the prevention and treatment of sarcopenia. *J Nutr Health Aging.* 2000;4(3):143-155.

27. Evans W, Rosenberg I. *Biomarkers.* New York: Simon and Schuster; 1992.

28. Meredith CN, Zackin MJ, Frontera WR, Evans WJ. Body composition and aerobic capacity in young and middle-aged endurance-trained men. *Med Sci Sports Exerc.* 1987;19:557-563.

29. Drewnowski A, Darmon N. The economics of obesity: dietary energy density and energy cost. *Am J Clin Nutr.* 2005;82 (1 Suppl):265S-73S.

30. Slemenda C, Heilman DK, Brandt KD, et al. Reduced quadriceps strength relative to body weight. A risk factor for knee osteoarthritis in women? *Arthritis Rheum.* 1998;41:1951-1959.

31. Ogita F, Stam RP, Tazawa HO, Toussaint HM, Hollander AP. Oxygen uptake in one-legged and two-legged exercise. *Med Sci Sports Exerc.* 2000;32(10):1737-1742.

32. Lagally KM, Cordero J, Good J, Brown DD, McCaw ST. Physiologic and metabolic responses to a continuous functional resistance exercise workout. *J Strength Cond Res.* 2009;23(2):373-379.

33. Catenacci VA, Ogden LG, Stuht J, et al. Physical activity patterns in the National Weight Control Registry. *Obesity.* 2008;16:153-161.

34. Vaidya V. Psychosocial aspects of obesity. *Adv Psychosom Med.* 2006;27:73-85.

35. American Diabetes Association. Diabetes statistics. Available at: http://www.diabetes.org/diabetes-basics/diabetes-statistics. Accessed October 20, 2010.

36. American Diabetes Association. Diabetes mellitus and exercise. *Diabetes Care.* 2002;25(Suppl 1):s64.

37. Joint National Committee of Prevention, Detection, Evaluation, and Treatment of High Blood Pressure. The sixth report of the Joint National Committee of Prevention, Detection,

Evaluation, and Treatment of High Blood Pressure. *Arch Int Med.* 1997;157:2413-2446.

38. Tsai JC, Yang HY, Wang WH, et al. The beneficial effect of regular endurance exercise training on blood pressure and quality of life in patients with hypertension. *Clin Exp Hypertens.* 2004;26(3):255-265.

39. Ketelhut RG, Franz IW, Scholze J. Regular exercise as an effective approach in antihypertensive therapy. *Med Sci Sports Exerc.* 2004;36(1):4-8.

40. American Heart Association. *Heart Disease and Stroke Statistics 2007 update. Dallas,* Tx: American Heart Association; 2007.

41. Ornish D, Scherwitz L, Billings J, et al. Intensive lifestyle changes for reversal of coronary heart disease: five-year follow-up of the Lifestyle Heart Trial. *JAMA.* 1998;280:2001-2007.

42. Pischke CR, Weidner G, Scherwitz L, Ornish D. Long-term effects of lifestyle changes on well-being and cardiac variables among CHD patients. *Health Psychol.* 2008;27(5):584-592.

43. Banks E, Reeves G, Beral V, Balkwill A, Liu B, Roddam A. Hip fracture incidence in relation to age, menopausal status, and age at menopause: prospective analysis. *PLoS Med.* 2009;6(11):e1000181.

44. The National Osteoporosis Foundation. Fast Facts on Osteoporosis. Available at: http://www.nof.org/node/40 Accessed October 20, 2010.

45. Layne JE, Nelson ME. The effects of progressive resistance training on bone density: a review. *Med Sci Sports Exerc.* 1999;31(1):25-30.

46. Centers for Disease Control and Prevention (CDC). Prevalence of doctor-diagnosed arthritis and arthritis-attributable activity limitation—United States, 2003-2005. *MMWR Morb Mortal Wkly Rep.* 2006;55(40):1089-1092.

47. Slemenda C, Heilman DK, Brandt KD, et al. Reduced quadriceps strength relative to body weight. A risk factor for knee osteoarthritis in women? *Arthritis Rheum.* 1998;41:1951-1959.

48. Slemenda C, Brandt KD, Heilman DK, et al. Quadriceps weakness and osteoarthritis of the knee. *Ann Int Med.* 1997;17:97-104.

49. Hurley MV, Scott DL, Rees J, Newham DJ. Sensorimotor changes and functional performance in patients with knee osteoarthritis. *Ann Rheum Disord.* 1997;56:641-648.

50. O'Reilly SC, Jones A, Muir KR, Doherty M. Quadriceps weakness in knee osteoarthritis: the effect on pain and disability. *Ann Rheum Disord.* 1998;57:588-594.

51. Pai YC, Rogers MW, Patton J, Cain TD, Hanke TA. Static versus dynamic predictions of protective stepping following waist-pull perturbations in young and older adults. *J Biomech.* 1998;31(12):1111-1118.

52. Hurley MV, Jones DW, Newham DJ. Arthrogenic quadriceps inhibition and rehabilitation of patients with extensive traumatic knee injuries. *Clin Sci.* 1994;86:305-310.

53. [Anonymous] Never too late to build up your muscle. *Tufts Univ Diet Nutr Lett.* 1994;12(September):6-7.

54. American Cancer Society. *Cancer Facts and Figures 2010.* Atlanta, GA: American Cancer Society; 2010.

55. Woods JA, Davis JM, Smith JA, Nieman DC. Exercise and cellular innate immune function. *Med Sci Sports Exerc.* 1999;31:57-66.

56. Segal R, Johnson D, Smith J, et al. Structured exercise improves physical functioning in women with stages I and II breast cancer: results of a randomized controlled trial. *J Clin Oncol.* 2001;19(3):657-665.

57. The American College of Obstetricians and Gynecologists. *Exercise During Pregnancy.* Washington, DC: The American College of Obstetricians and Gynecologists; 2003.

58. Ries AL, Carlin BW, Carrieri-Kohlman V, et al. Pulmonary rehabilitation: joint ACCP/AACVPR evidence-based guidelines. *Chest.* 1997;112:1363-1396.

59. *American Association of Cardiovascular and Pulmonary Rehabilitation Guidelines for Pulmonary Rehabilitation Programs.* 3rd ed. Champaign, IL: Human Kinetics; 2004.

60. Greenland PG. Clinical significance, detection, and medical treatment for peripheral arterial disease. *J Cardiopulm Rehabil.* 2002;22(2):73-79.

Nutrition and Supplementation

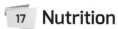

Nutrition

OBJECTIVES

After studying this chapter, you will be able to:

✔ Describe the macronutrients and their functions.

✔ Describe how the macronutrient composition of an individual's food intake can affect satiety, compliance, daily energy expenditure, and weight control.

✔ Provide basic nutritional recommendations for optimizing health.

✔ Answer questions, handle issues, and dispel myths regarding the relationship of macronutrients to the successful alteration of body composition.

Introduction to Nutrition

Knowledge of basic nutrition concepts and applications is important in understanding how the human movement system functions properly and for personal trainers to be able to design individualized integrated exercise programs for their clients. NASM recognizes the importance of developing a fundamental knowledge of basic nutrition concepts and applications as being an important and vital characteristic for all personal trainers. This chapter is a review of basic nutritional concepts and how they relate to the human movement system, especially during and after exercise. The information presented in this chapter will further enable the personal trainer to provide a scientific rationalization when providing nutritional recommendations or guidance to their clients.

Nutrition The process by which a living organism assimilates food and uses it for growth and repair of tissues.

Definition

Nutrition is defined as the sum of the processes by which an animal or plant takes in and uses food substances for growth and repair of tissues (1). This very basic definition does not begin to illuminate the role that diet plays in the health, appearance, performance, and well-being of an individual. A basic understanding of nutrition is vital to the safety and success of a personal trainer's clients. An individually planned nutrition strategy can enhance the results from the stimulus of exercise, improve health and athletic performance, reduce the risk of disease and illness, increase energy levels, and favorably alter body composition in clients. The information presented in this chapter provides an understanding of the basics of nutrition and how nutrition can help apparently healthy clients achieve their personal health and fitness goals. The information provided throughout this chapter is *not* intended to provide the knowledge or skills necessary to counsel high-risk clients or to treat medical or health-related illnesses or diseases. It is important that personal trainers have a network of qualified health-care professionals (physicians, dieticians, eating-disorder specialists, and other health-care professionals) in their area to which they can refer clients with health or medical-related problems. Such an arrangement can be mutually beneficial as these same health-care professionals often need to refer their clients to qualified personal trainers for exercise guidance.

Standards of Practice and Scope of Practice: Personal Trainers Versus Licensed Dieticians

Personal trainers should be familiar with the concepts of nutrition. Integrating nutritional strategies with exercise will help clients achieve their desired outcomes. It is important, however, to recognize and respect the scope of practice of each professional field. The professional, legally qualified to practice in the field of nutrition, is a Registered Dietician (RD). The Registered Dietician is a specialized food and nutrition expert with extensive training who meets specified criteria. Table 17.1 describes the RD's educational and professional requirements. RD can be recognized by the use of the "RD" credential.

TABLE 17.1	Educational and Professional Requirements for the RD
Bachelor's Degree	RD's receive their degrees at an accredited college or university with course work approved by the Commission on Accreditation for Dietetics Education (CADE).
Supervised Practice Program	RD's then complete a CADE-accredited program, typically 6 to 12 months in length, with focused practice and study in clinical and community nutrition, and food-service management. Graduate study is often combined.
National Examination	After completing the supervised practice program, candidates must pass the national examination to receive their RD credential.
Continuing Education	Individuals must complete continuing education requirements to maintain an active RD credential.

RD, registered dietician.

The practice of nutrition, more formally called dietetics, is governed by national credentialing programs and state licensing laws. Currently, 46 states have specific laws that explicitly define the scope of practice for nutrition and dietetics professionals, and performing these duties without a license could be considered illegal. Some health-care professionals (other than Registered Dieticians) often make nutrition recommendations; however; they are usually licensed by the state as a nurse or physician and are thus protected regarding state laws and regulations. Personal trainers are not licensed health-care professionals (unless they have additional training and education) but often give nutrition advice to their clients. Thus, it is important for all personal trainers to be aware of the standards of practice and scope of practice guidelines that pertain to them.

A general understanding of basic nutrition and weight management should exist to educate clients and provide general guidance in this area. It is likely that a personal trainer will be the first person approached with nutrition questions, so being confident about the nature of the relationship between nutrition, fitness, and weight control is essential. However, providing individual nutrition assessment, meal plans, or recommendations for nutritional therapy are best left to an RD or other qualified licensed professionals. The skills and abilities required to calculate, counsel, or prescribe an individualized nutrition or weight-management plan exceeds the training and expertise of the personal trainer (2). This becomes especially important if the client has health and medical concerns such as obesity, diabetes, heart disease, allergies, or hypertension. Table 17.2 offers examples of nutrition topics that the personal trainer should be prepared to discuss with clients.

Energy and Body Composition

By 2015, public health experts expect that 75% of all US adults will be either overweight or obese (3). The desire for a quick solution for weight loss has fostered numerous myths about exercise and diet and has led to the overcommercialization of quick weight-loss methods, fad diets, and ineffective exercise programs and devices (4–6). It is important for personal trainers to understand what the common myths and inaccuracies about weight loss and diets are, and to be able to educate clients regarding safe and effective diet and weight-loss methods. The majority of common diet and weight-loss myths usually hinder more than help a client's progress and may result in serious negative health consequences if they are not dispelled.

TABLE 17.2	Examples of Nutrition Topics of Discussion for the Fitness Professional © Ilolab/ShutterStock, Inc.
Food preparation methods	Food guidance systems, i.e., food guide pyramid, MyPlate
Healthy snacks	Carbohydrate, protein, and fat basics
Statistical information on the relationship between chronic disease and the excesses or deficiencies of specific nutrients	Nutrients contained in foods or supplements
Vitamins and minerals as essential nutrients	Importance of water and hydration status

The facts about weight loss and gain are quite simple. Eat fewer calories than are expended and there will be a reduction in weight. Conversely, consume more calories than are expended and there will be an increase in weight (7,8). However, there are many factors that can affect both scenarios. The environment in which we live today provides a constant supply of palatable food (increasing energy intake) while promoting a sedentary lifestyle (reducing energy expenditure), which when viewed collectively, have played a significant role in the rising obesity rates in the United States (9).

The following sections address daily energy needs, macronutrients (protein, carbohydrate, and fat), their uses, and recommendations, and will explore many common myths associated with diet, weight loss, and exercise. These topics will be addressed as they relate to the common goals of favorably altering body composition and increasing athletic performance.

SUMMARY

Diet plays an important role in a person's health, appearance, energy, athletic performance, and response to exercise, as well as overall well-being. Personal trainers should not give individualized dietary advice or counsel their clients regarding nutrition therapy, especially with respect to treating illness in high-risk clients; rather, they should refer these clients to a qualified health-care professional. Personal trainers are, however, encouraged to help educate their clients with respect to making healthy food choices. The majority of clients seeking personal training services often have numerous misconceptions about diet, nutrition, and weight loss. It is vital that personal trainers help educate them by providing factual information on safe and effective diet, weight-loss, and nutritional methods.

Daily Energy Needs

A **calorie** (lower case *c*) is a unit of energy and is defined as the amount of heat energy required to raise the temperature of 1 gram of water 1 degree Celsius. A **Calorie** (upper case *C*) or **kilocalorie** (kcal) is equal to 1,000 calories. Although not technically correct, calorie, Calorie, and kilocalorie are used interchangeably in nonscientific, everyday language. The term *calorie* is used throughout this chapter.

Estimated total energy expenditure (TEE), also referred to as total daily energy expenditure (TDEE), is defined as the amount of energy (calories) spent, on average, in a typical day. TEE is actually the sum total of three different energy components:

◆ *Resting metabolic rate (RMR)*: The amount of energy expended while at rest; represents the minimal amount of energy required to sustain vital bodily functions such as blood circulation, respiration, and temperature regulation. RMR typically accounts for 70% of TEE.

◆ *Thermic effect of food (TEF)*: The amount of energy expended above RMR as a result of the processing of food (digestion) for storage and use. TEF typically accounts for approximately 6–10% of TEE.

◆ *Energy expended during physical activity*: The amount of energy expended above RMR and TEF associated with physical activity. Physical activity accounts for approximately 20% of TEE.

calorie The amount of heat energy required to raise the temperature of 1 gram of water 1°C.

Calorie A unit of expression of energy equal to 1,000 calories. The amount of heat energy required to raise the temperature of 1 kilogram or liter of water 1°C.

Kilocalorie A unit of expression of energy equal to 1,000 calories. The amount of heat energy required to raise the temperature of 1 kilogram or liter of water 1°C.

© ilolab/ShutterStock, Inc.

Resting Metabolic Rate

RMR accounts for approximately 70% of total daily energy expenditure in the sedentary person, although it may vary among individuals. RMR can be affected by a wide variety of factors including age, sex, genetics, hormonal changes, body size, body composition, temperature, altitude, illness, medication, food and caffeine intake, and cigarette smoking. Constant factors that cannot be altered are age, sex, and genetics. Slight increases in fat-free mass can have a gradual increase in RMR; thus, exercise is said to have a positive effect on RMR indirectly if fat-free mass (FFM) is increased or decreased. Factors that temporarily alter RMR include hormonal changes, exercise, environmental temperature, altitude, caffeine intake, and cigarette smoking.

Chronic or acute illness as well as hormonal changes and certain types of medications can influence RMR as well. Hormonal changes can increase or decrease RMR (10). For example, thyroid hormones influence many metabolic functions throughout the body, including fat and carbohydrate metabolism and growth. Thyroid hormones have a constant effect on energy expenditure and affect every cell in the body. High concentrations of thyroid hormones tend to cause an increase in RMR, whereas lower than normal levels tend to cause a decrease in RMR. According to the American Association of Clinical Endocrinologists (AACE), 27 million Americans have thyroid-related disorders, but more than half remain undiagnosed (11). Another endocrine disorder, diabetes, is the seventh leading cause of death in the United States. The total cost of diagnosed diabetes in the United States in 2007 was $174 billion (12). Because of this fact, fitness professionals should remain cautious when providing nutritional advice and refer clients to a Registered Dietician and qualified health-care professionals.

Certain medications have also been shown to alter RMR. For example, certain cardiovascular medications can reduce RMR from 4% to 12%, chemotherapy can reduce RMR 6% to 11%, long-term use of human growth hormone has been shown to increase RMR by 12%, and thyroid medications used in hypothyroidism can increase RMR as much as 17% (13,14). It is important for personal trainers to be aware of any long-term medications their clients may be taking that can potentially affect the individual's metabolic rate. Regarding the effect of exercise on RMR, several studies have demonstrated the following (13–16):

- Energy expenditure can be elevated between 10 and 90 minutes after exercise depending on the intensity and duration.
- Regular chronic exercise may affect RMR slightly.
- Changes in FFM from exercise training can increase or decrease RMR.

To avoid declines in resting metabolism individuals should be encouraged to avoid starvation diets that could lead to wasting of skeletal muscle and instead be encouraged to build and maintain muscle for active living. Maintaining muscle mass is particularly important during aging because some of the decline in RMR associated with age is caused by a decline of muscle (17).

Did You Know?

Resting metabolic rate (RMR) and basal metabolic rate (BMR) are often used interchangeably, but BMR is different. BMR is the term used when the measurements are taken after the subject has spent the night in a metabolic ward or chamber and has fasted for 12 hours. RMR is measured after the subject spends the night at home and is driven to the research laboratory for measurement. BMR and RMR usually differ by less than 10%.

The Thermic Effect of Food

When food is consumed it is mechanically digested and moved through the digestive tract. Nutrients are transported from the gut to the blood, where they are distributed throughout the body. All of these processes require energy that can be measured after the meal is consumed. This increase in energy expenditure after the meal is called the thermic effect of food (TEF) and comprises approximately 6% to 10% of total energy expenditure depending on the frequency and energy content of the meal.

Energy Expended During Physical Activity

Any physical activity requires energy expenditure above resting metabolism. Even sedentary people who only engage in modest daily physical activities consisting of personal care and other necessary daily movement expend energy above their RMR. Participating in sports and exercise can significantly increase energy expenditure above that of resting metabolism. Physical activity can account for 20% or more of an individual's TEE, although the exact percentage can vary greatly depending on an individual's current fitness level and the type, intensity, and duration of physical activity or exercise engaged in. Physical activity can be influenced more dramatically than RMR and TEF, which for the most part are relatively constant.

Estimating Total Daily Energy Expenditure

One of the most common ways to estimate total energy expenditure is to first estimate RMR, then multiply RMR by an appropriate activity factor. There are several different prediction equations used to estimate RMR. Such simplified equations can provide a reasonable estimate of TEE in most cases. The following is an example of a simplified TEE calculation:

Step 1. Weight (lbs) × 10 = RMR
Step 2. RMR × activity factor (see **Table 17.3**) = TEE
Example: Heavily active 180-pound man
- Step 1. 180 (lb) × 10 = 1,800 RMR
- Step 2. 1,800 (RMR) × 2.1 (activity factor) = 3,780 calories expended per day (TEE)

TABLE 17.3	Physical Activity Factors for Various Levels of Activity for Adults of Average Size 19 Years or Older	
Very Light	Seated and standing activities, office work, driving, cooking; no vigorous activity	1.2–1.3
Low Active	In addition to the activities of a sedentary lifestyle, 30 minutes of moderate activity equivalent of walking 2 miles in 30 minutes; most office workers with additional planned exercise routines	1.5–1.6
Active	In addition to the activities of a low active lifestyle, an additional 3 hours of activity such as bicycle 10–12 miles an hour, walk 4.5 miles an hour	1.6–1.7
Heavy	Planned vigorous activities, physical labor, full-time athletes, hard-labor professions such as steel or road workers	1.9–2.1

Adapted from the Food and Nutrition Board. Dietary Reference Intakes for Energy, Carbohydrates, Fiber, Fat, Protein, and Amino Acids (Macronutrients). Washington, DC: National Academy of Sciences; 2002.

Even the most commonly used formulas can have up to a 20% variance in overestimating or underestimating resting metabolism and total energy expenditure. Thus caution should be used when applying a prediction equation to calculate RMR. Other options for personal trainers to help estimate TEE are online calculators such as the one provided by the US Department of Agriculture at www.choosemyplate.gov or seeking the guidance of a Registered Dietician.

Moreover, it is important to note that calorie requirements change with life stage, activity level, and illness, and proper weight management for most individuals should include regularly monitoring weight status with weekly or monthly weigh-ins or body composition assessments. In doing so, any unwanted weight gain can be immediately addressed, which consequently prevents creeping obesity and related health complications.

Protein

Protein Amino acids linked by peptide bonds.

The primary function of **protein** is to build and repair body tissues and structures. It is also involved in the synthesis of hormones, enzymes, and other regulatory peptides. Additionally, protein can be used for energy if calories or carbohydrate are insufficient in the diet (18).

The Structure of Protein

Proteins are made up of amino acids linked together by peptide bonds. The body uses approximately 20 amino acids to build its many different proteins (19). Just as specific words are formed by certain sequences of letters, arranging the amino acids in different sequences yields the body's myriad of proteins (from a muscle protein like actin to proteins that make up the lens of the eye).

There are two general classes of amino acids: *essential* and *nonessential* Table 17.4. Essential amino acids cannot be manufactured in the body (or are manufactured in

TABLE 17.4 Amino Acids		
Essential	**Nonessential**	**Semiessential**
Isoleucine	Alanine	Arginine
Leucine	Asparagine	Histidine
Lysine	Aspartic acid	
Methionine	Cysteine	
Phenylalanine	Glutamic acid	
Threonine	Glutamine	
Tryptophan	Glycine	
Valine	Proline	
	Serine	
	Tyrosine	

insufficient amounts); therefore, they must be obtained from the food supply or some other exogenous source. There are eight essential amino acids. The second group of amino acids is termed nonessential because the body is able to manufacture them from dietary nitrogen and fragments of carbohydrate and fat (18). Because of their rate of synthesis within the body, arginine and histidine are considered semiessential amino acids. It appears that these amino acids cannot be manufactured by the body at a rate that will support growth (especially in children).

Digestion, Absorption, and Utilization

Proteins must be broken down into the constituent amino acids before the body can use them to build or repair tissue or as an energy substrate. The fate of the amino acids after digestion and absorption by the intestines depends on the body's homeostatic needs, which can range from tissue replacement or tissue addition to a need for energy. **Figure 17.1** depicts the digestion, absorption, and synthesis sequence.

As ingested proteins enter the stomach, they encounter hydrochloric acid (HCl), which uncoils (or *denatures*) the protein so that digestive enzymes can begin dismantling the peptide bonds. In addition, the enzyme pepsin begins to cleave the protein strand into smaller polypeptides (strands of several amino acids) and single amino acids. As these protein fragments leave the stomach and enter the small intestine, pancreatic and intestinal proteases (or protein enzymes) continue to dismantle the protein fragments.

The resulting dipeptides, tripeptides, and single amino acids are then absorbed through the intestinal wall into the enterocytes and released into the blood supply to the liver **Figure 17.2**. Once in the bloodstream, the free-form amino acids have several

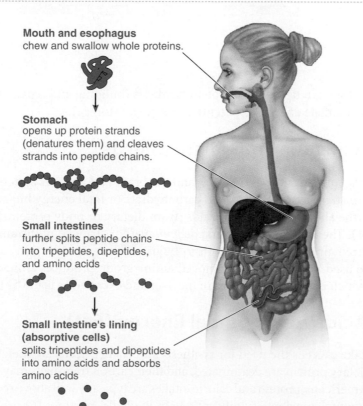

Mouth and esophagus
chew and swallow whole proteins.

Stomach
opens up protein strands
(denatures them) and cleaves
strands into peptide chains.

Small intestines
further splits peptide chains
into tripeptides, dipeptides,
and amino acids

**Small intestine's lining
(absorptive cells)**
splits tripeptides and dipeptides
into amino acids and absorbs
amino acids

FIGURE 17.1

Protein digestion, absorption, and endogenous synthesis.

FIGURE 17.2

Amino acid absorption.

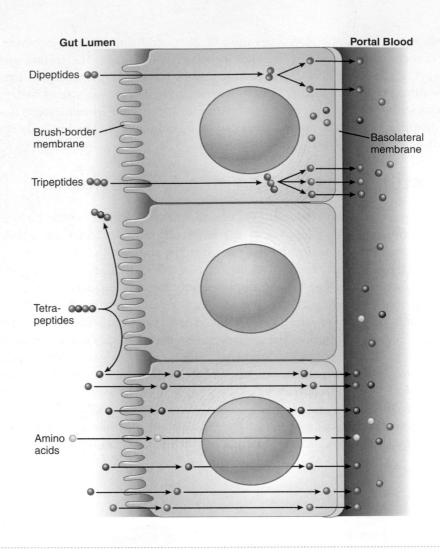

possible fates: they can be used for protein synthesis (building and repairing tissues or structures), immediate energy, or potential energy (fat storage).

Amino Acids for Immediate Energy

The body has a constant need for energy, and the brain and nervous system, in particular, have a constant need for glucose. If carbohydrate or total energy intake is too low, the body has the ability to use amino acids (from dietary or body proteins) to provide energy (20,21). The amino acids are first *deaminated* (or stripped of the amine group), allowing the remaining carbon skeleton to be used for the production of glucose or ketones to be used for energy. The removed amine group produces ammonia, a toxic compound, which is converted to urea in the liver and excreted as urine by the kidneys.

Amino Acids for Potential Energy (Fat)

If protein intake exceeds the need for synthesis and energy needs are met, then amino acids from dietary protein are deaminated, and their carbon fragments may be stored as fat. Among Americans, protein and caloric intakes are typically well above requirements, allowing protein to contribute significantly to individuals' fat stores (6).

Protein in Foods

Dietary protein is the delivery vehicle for amino acids. Meats, fruits, vegetables, grains, dairy products, and even supplements supply us with the valuable building blocks of protein we need. If a food supplies all of the essential amino acids in appropriate ratios, it is called a *complete protein*. If a food source is low or lacking in one or more essential amino acids, it is called an *incomplete protein*. The essential amino acid that is missing or present in the smallest amount is called the *limiting factor* of that protein. Because the process of protein synthesis works on an all-or-none principle, all amino acids must be present at the site of protein manufacture, or synthesis will be reduced to the point at which the cell runs out of the limiting amino acid (22).

The ability of a protein to satisfy these essential amino acid requirements can be quantified in several ways. Terms used to rate dietary protein include protein efficiency ratio (PER), net protein utilization (NPU), and biologic value (BV) (18). BV is a measure frequently used when discussing protein sources in popular media and by supplement manufacturers. Essentially, BV is a measure of protein quality, or how well it satisfies the body's essential amino acid needs. A protein source with a higher score provides an amino acid profile that is more closely related to the needs of the human body. BV is a concept that is often misused, especially by marketers of protein supplements. One is led to believe that consuming specially prepared high-BV proteins will allow an individual who is already consuming adequate protein to build muscle to a greater degree, or more quickly. However, consuming protein above requirements will not force the body to unleash a previously untapped muscle-building capacity (23,24). Instead, if individuals exclusively consume very high BV proteins, their amino acid requirements would be met with less protein. Conversely, if individuals choose a diet composed of mostly lower BV protein sources, the total protein requirements will increase **Figure 17.3**.

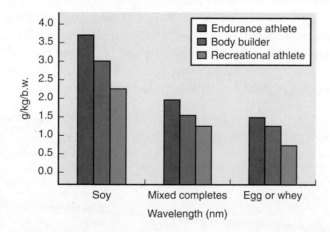

FIGURE 17.3 Adaptation-phase protein requirements. This graph illustrates the approximate amounts of different types of protein necessary to supply the ideal pattern of amino acids needed to satisfy the body's maintenance and growth needs. Protein consumption beyond these amounts does not result in strength or size increases, presuming total energy requirements are met through dietary carbohydrates and fat. When you exceed the amount of protein needed for growth, maintenance, or repair, your body will store it as fat or glycogen, use it for energy, or convert it to other nitrogenous compounds.

The major sources of complete proteins are animal sources, dairy and meats Table 17.5. Sources of incomplete protein include grains, legumes, nuts, seeds, and other vegetables. Barley, cornmeal, oats, buckwheat, pasta, rye, wheat, beans, lentils, dried peas, peanuts, chickpeas, soy products, sesame seeds, sunflower seeds, walnuts, cashews, pumpkin seeds, and other nuts are the main sources of incomplete proteins. Incomplete proteins can be combined to make available all of the essential amino acids and form a complete protein (Table 17.5).

Protein quality improves when a small amount of complete protein like a dairy food is combined with plant-based foods and when incomplete proteins from plant-based foods such as rice and beans are mixed together.

Factors Affecting Protein Requirements

There are several factors that affect protein requirements, including an individual's daily exercise and physical activity levels, daily caloric consumption, body-composition goals, and sports-performance goals.

Exercise

Both anaerobic and aerobic exercise can affect protein requirements in different ways. Exercise increases the oxidation of amino acids as well as the rate of protein turnover in lean body mass during recovery. Because different types of exercise have specific effects, an individual participating in both types of exercise may have a need for protein greater than someone involved in only one (25,26).

Caloric Intake

Because protein can be used for tissue repair and synthesis as well as for energy, protein requirements will increase as total energy intake decreases (27,28). As total caloric intake is reduced, energy needs may no longer be satisfied by carbohydrate and fat intake alone, necessitating that protein be used to provide energy. The goal is to satisfy the majority of energy needs with carbohydrate and fat, saving protein for tissue repair and growth. This is why carbohydrates are often referred to as protein sparing. If one does not eat adequate amounts of carbohydrate and fat (as is often seen in low-calorie

TABLE 17.5	Complete Protein Food Sources
Whole egg	Yogurt and granola
Milk and milk products	Oatmeal with milk
Meat and poultry	Lentils and bread
Fish	Tortillas with beans or bean burritos
Rice and beans	Macaroni and cheese
Peanut butter on whole-wheat bread	Hummus (chickpeas and sesame paste) with bread
Sunflower seeds and peanuts	Bean soup with whole-grain crackers

or low-carbohydrate diets or during physique-competition preparation), more protein will be used for energy by default. Individuals interested in general fat loss or muscle hypertrophy have erroneously mimicked the acceptable use of a high-protein diet by a physique competitor. However, under the proper circumstances, these diets, when used temporarily, can be effective.

Negative Energy Balance

For clients pursuing body-fat reduction, body-fat loss goals require that a caloric deficit be maintained until the goal is reached. During a negative energy balance, amino acids are used to assist in energy production, a term referred to as *gluconeogenesis*. Anaerobic or aerobic exercise depletes glycogen, increasing gluconeogenesis. The increase in gluconeogenesis is supported by the release of branched-chain and other amino acids from structural proteins to maintain glucose homeostasis during exercise (29–32). A hypocaloric diet establishes less-than-optimal glycogen stores, and when this is combined with increased glycogen demand during exercise, protein's energy utilization is increased (33,34). The amount of lean body mass lost in persons in a negative energy balance can be reduced by increasing the amount of protein in the diet, leading to a more rapid return to nitrogen balance. A number of studies show that an increase in protein utilization during a hypocaloric diet will produce effects that can be exacerbated by exercise (28,35–40).

Protein and the Bodybuilder

Bodybuilders during positive energy balance (off-season) should follow the same protein recommendations as strength athletes. However, during negative energy balance (used to create competition-level body-fat percentages), protein requirements may dramatically increase. To reach competitive body-fat levels, calorie intake is continually lowered while exercise (such as cardiorespiratory training, weight training, and posing) is increased.

Competitive levels of body fat are generally unhealthy and impossible to maintain for prolonged periods. Each component of this regimen may have additive effects on protein requirements. The body's survival mechanisms, related to increases in energy expenditure and decreases in food supply, are probably highly active during this period, forcing a continued reduction in food intake to achieve the goal (41,42). However, because of its anabolic requirements, protein intake cannot be lowered. In fact, protein intake may have to be increased in the final weeks before competition. During this period, the body must have the option to use available food either for energy or muscle support. The body does not have a choice with dietary carbohydrate or fat, making them the only dispensable calories. Therefore, protein intake could be dramatically increased to theoretically lessen the obligatory loss of lean tissue during drastic training measures (28–40).

It is quite common to see clients consuming the majority of their calories from protein in the final weeks before competition. However, during the off-season, athletes return to normal food intake (or protein at anabolic requirements and energy needs met primarily with carbohydrates and fats) and normal energy balance. This return to normal eating habits enables greater muscular gains than would be achieved by maintaining a high-protein intake year-round (43–45). In fact, it appears that carbohydrate (1 g/kg or 0.5 gram per pound), not protein, consumed within an hour after heavy resistance training inhibits muscle-protein breakdown, resulting in a positive protein balance (44).

How much protein is required to build muscle (46)?

◆ Skeletal muscle is approximately 72% water, 22% protein, and 6% fat, glycogen, and minerals, and 1 pound of muscle tissue contains approximately 100 grams of protein.

◆ Theoretically, an athlete would have to ingest an extra 14 grams of protein per day, although most experts believe the single most important factor in gaining lean mass (along with resistance training, of course) is consuming adequate calories.

◆ Therefore, to ensure the body has sufficient energy for lean mass accretion, consume an additional 200 to 400 calories daily (3 to 5 calories per kg or 1.5 to 2.5 calories per pound per day) above maintenance requirements in addition to consuming a little extra protein (approximately 2 ounces of lean meat).

Protein's Effect on Satiety

In addition to the above factors, protein intake may be adjusted to aid in *satiety* (the feeling of fullness). Protein's role in satiety is an important consideration. As with all macronutrients, protein activates specific satiety mechanisms and may be more satiating than fat and carbohydrate. Protein-induced suppression of food intake in animals and humans is greater than its energy content alone, which suggests that protein has a direct effect on satiety (47). In studies of rats and humans, a preload of protein suppressed their food intake for several hours and to a greater extent than a similar energy load of fat and carbohydrate (48–52). Individuals seeking fat loss may benefit from the satiating properties of protein to feel full and energized throughout the day. This can assist clients in program adherence (53,54).

Protein-Intake Recommendations

The Recommended Dietary Allowance (RDA) for protein is 0.8 g/kg per day. The Acceptable Macronutrient Distribution Range for protein intake for an adult is 10% to 35% of total caloric intake (55). Table 17.6 lists the appropriate recommendations for most athletes and exercisers (56).

These protein recommendations range from 10% to 35% of total caloric intake, which allows not only for differences in goals and activity but also for bioindividuality in terms of satiety and performance. Some people respond better to slightly higher or lower protein intakes, which may help with adherence to the amount of calories required to reach and maintain goals. Individuals eating lower amounts of protein may need supplementation. Whatever the percentage of protein ends up being, in

TABLE 17.6	Recommended Protein Intakes
Activity Level	**Grams of Protein per kg Body Weight per Day**
Sedentary (adult)	0.8 (0.4 g/lb)
Strength athletes	1.2–1.7 (0.5–0.8 g/lb)
Endurance athletes	1.2–1.4 (0.5–0.6 g/lb)

relation to total caloric intake, the protein intake should still fall approximately within the above ranges of grams per kilogram. In other words, a small person losing fat (or hypocaloric) and exercising using strength and aerobic training may have a high percentage of protein (around 25%) but still fall in the appropriate range of absolute protein (1.2 to 1.7 g/kg per day).

Negative Side Effects Associated with Chronic Use of High-Protein Diets

A high-protein diet is typically defined as one that consists of more than 35% of total caloric intake from protein, or three times the protein RDA for athletes. Chronic consumption of a high-protein diet is generally associated with a higher intake of saturated fat and low fiber intake, both of which are risk factors for heart disease and some types of cancer (57,58). In addition, because the kidneys are required to work harder to eliminate the increased urea produced, caution should always be taken when recommending high-protein intakes to people with a history of kidney problems such as renal insufficiency or kidney stones.

The effects of high-protein diets on bone health have been debated in the literature with reports that a high-protein intake can increase urinary calcium losses. Early researchers in this area speculated that bone was the source of elevated urinary calcium excretion during a high-protein diet. Kerstetter et al. (59) found that consuming a low-protein diet (0.7 g/kg) caused an increase in two hormones that work together to increase blood calcium levels. The elevated hormone levels suggest that a low-protein diet may decrease calcium absorption. However, a follow-up evaluation showed that 18% of calcium consumed is absorbed during a low-protein diet (0.7 g/kg), and absorption increases to 26% during a high-protein (2.1 g/kg) diet (60). Therefore, it appears that an increase in intestinal calcium absorption as people follow a high-protein diet likely accounts for a majority of observed increases in calcium (60–62).

In addition, there is a need for greater fluid consumption when consuming large quantities of protein. Protein requires approximately seven times the water for metabolism than carbohydrate or fat (63). Low-carbohydrate consumption typically accompanies high-protein diets (especially for weight loss), which can lead to decreased glycogen stores, inhibition of performance, and possible dehydration. Therefore, the main concern with high-protein diets is dehydration because the urea nitrogen cycle processes dietary nitrogen and water is eliminated via the urinary system. Because dehydration of as little as 3% can impair performance, athletes and active individuals ingesting extra protein should weigh themselves regularly to ensure they are properly hydrated.

Review of Properties of Protein

One gram of protein yields 4 calories. Protein must be broken down completely (into constituent amino acids) before it can be used.

Amino acids from protein are used by the body for the following:

- Synthesizing body-tissue protein
- Providing glucose for energy (many can be converted to glucose)
- Providing nitrogen in the form of amine groups to build nonessential amino acids
- Contributing to fat stores

Amino acids are not used to build protein under the following conditions:

- Not enough available energy from carbohydrate and fat
- Consistently low or lacking essential dietary amino acids owing to the exclusive consumption of incomplete proteins
- An excess of necessary protein

The following conditions are necessary for the body to synthesize endogenous protein:

- Availability of all essential and nonessential amino acids in proper amounts
- An adequate supply of exogenous protein (supplying amine groups, which synthesize the nonessential amino acids)
- Adequate energy-yielding carbohydrate and fat (sparing the protein)

Recommended protein intake for athletes and exercisers:

- 1.2 to 1.7 g/kg depending on goal, activity, protein source, and total caloric intake
- Typically falls in a range of 10 to 35% of total caloric intake

Chronic high-protein intake (greater than three times the RDA) diets can lead to:

- Higher intake of saturated fat and low fiber intake
- Increased urea production
- Decreased glycogen stores
- Possible dehydration

SUMMARY

Protein requirements can be affected by anaerobic and aerobic exercise, total energy intake, caloric intake, and carbohydrate intake. During a negative energy balance (or caloric deficit), amino acids are used to assist in energy production (or gluconeogenesis), wherein protein requirements may dramatically increase. Protein intake may also be adjusted to aid in satiety in individuals seeking fat loss, who may benefit from protein by feeling full and energized throughout the day. The recommended dietary allowance for protein is 0.8 g/kg per day. However, this may vary among athletes from 1.2 to 1.7 g/kg per day.

Protein supplementation is not typically recommended in general use among athletes. No substantial evidence exists that either using protein supplements to replace food or increasing protein intake above requirements will enhance performance or adult skeletal muscle hypertrophy. However, supplemental protein may be useful:

- To quickly get amino acids into the blood before and after weight training
- To replace whole-food proteins for weight loss
- In situations when whole food is not available
- For bodybuilders, wrestlers, or other weight-conscious athletes preparing for competition

Carbohydrates

Carbohydrates are compounds containing carbon, hydrogen, and oxygen and are generally classified as sugars (simple), starches (complex), and fiber. The definition of sugar, as it would appear on a food label, is any monosaccharide or disaccharide (64).

A *monosaccharide* is a single sugar unit, many of which are connected to make starches (the storage form of carbohydrates in plants) and glycogen (the storage form of carbohydrates in humans). Monosaccharides include glucose (commonly referred to as blood sugar), fructose (or fruit sugar), and galactose. *Disaccharides* (two sugar units) include sucrose (or common sugar), lactose (or milk sugar), and maltose.

Polysaccharides are long chains of monosaccharide units linked together and found in foods that contain starch and fiber. These foods are often called complex carbohydrates and include starch found in plants, seed, and roots. Complex carbohydrates are primarily starch and fiber, and the starch is digested to glucose. Dietary fiber is a part of the plant that cannot be digested by human gut enzymes and passes through the small intestine and colon, where it is expelled as fecal material or fermented and used as food by the gut bacteria (65).

Carbohydrates are a chief source of energy for all body functions and muscular exertion. This fact leads to a rapid depletion of available and stored carbohydrates and creates a continual craving for this macronutrient. Carbohydrates also help regulate the digestion and utilization of protein and fat (66,67).

Carbohydrates Neutral compounds of carbon, hydrogen, and oxygen (such as sugars, starches, and celluloses).

Digestion, Absorption, and Utilization

The principal carbohydrates present in food occur in the form of simple sugars, starches, and cellulose. Simple sugars, such as those in honey and fruits, are very easily digested. Double sugars, such as table sugar, require some digestive action but are not nearly as complex as starches, such as those found in whole grain. Starches require prolonged enzymatic action to be broken down into simple sugars (i.e., glucose) for utilization. Cellulose, commonly found in the skins of fruits and vegetables, is largely indigestible by humans and contributes little energy value to the diet. It does, however, provide the bulk necessary for intestinal motility and aids in elimination (68,69).

The rate at which ingested carbohydrate raises blood sugar and its accompanying effect on insulin release is referred to as the *glycemic index* (GI) Table 17.7. The GI for a food is determined when the particular food is consumed by itself on an empty stomach. Mixed meals of protein, other carbohydrate, and fat can alter the glycemic effect of single foods (70). One can see in Table 17.8 that foods lower on the glycemic index are good sources of complex carbohydrates, as well as being high in fiber and overall nutritional value.

TABLE 17.7 Glycemic Index	
High	>70
Moderate	56–69
Low	>55

© ilolab/ShutterStock, Inc.

TABLE 17.8	Glycemic Index (GI) for Assorted Foods					

© ilolab/ShutterStock, Inc.

Low		Moderate		High	
Food	**GI**	**Food**	**GI**	**Food**	**GI**
Peanuts	14	Apple juice	40	Life Savers	70
Plain yogurt	14	Snickers	41	White bread	70
Soy beans	18	Peach	42	Bagel	72
Peas	22	Carrots	47	Watermelon	72
Cherries	22	Brown rice	50	Popcorn	72
Barley	25	Strawberry jam	51	Graham crackers	74
Grapefruit	25	PowerBar	53	French fries	75
Link sausage	28	Orange juice	53	Grape-Nuts	75
Black beans	30	Honey	55	Shredded wheat	75
Lentils	30	Pita bread	57	Gatorade	78
Skim milk	32	Oatmeal plain	58	Corn flakes	81
Fettuccine	32	Pineapple	59	Rice cakes	82
Chickpeas	33	Sweet potato	61	Pretzels	83
Chocolate milk	32	Coca Cola	63	Baked white potato	85
Whole-wheat spaghetti	37	Raisins	64	Instant rice	87
Apple	38	Cantaloupe	65	Gluten-free bread	90
Pinto beans	39	Whole-wheat bread	67	Dates	103

Through the processes of digestion and absorption, all disaccharides and polysaccharides are ultimately converted into simple sugars such as glucose or fructose **Figure 17.4**. However, fructose must be converted to glucose in the liver before it can be used for energy. Some of the glucose (or blood sugar) is used as fuel by tissues of the brain, nervous system, and muscles. Because humans are periodic eaters, a small portion of the glucose is converted to glycogen after a meal and stored within the liver and muscles. Any excess is converted to fat and stored throughout the body as a reserve source of energy. When total caloric intake exceeds output, any excess carbohydrate, dietary fat, or protein may be stored as body fat until energy expenditure once again exceeds energy input.

Role of Fiber in Health

One of the greatest contributions made by dietary complex carbohydrate is fiber. Higher intakes of dietary fiber are associated with lower incidence of heart disease and certain types of cancer (71,72). Fiber is an indigestible carbohydrate. There are two types

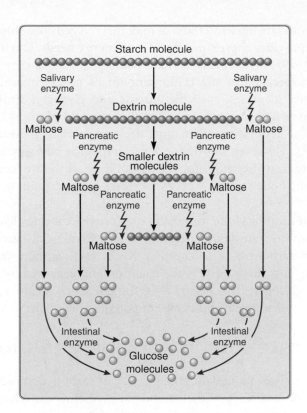

FIGURE 17.4

Gradual breakdown of large starch molecules by enzymes in digestion.

of dietary fiber, soluble and insoluble. Soluble fiber is dissolved by water and forms a gel-like substance in the digestive tract. Soluble fiber has many benefits, including moderating blood glucose levels and lowering cholesterol. Good sources of soluble fiber include oats and oatmeal, legumes (peas, beans, lentils), barley, and many uncooked fruits and vegetables (especially oranges, apples, and carrots).

Insoluble fiber does not absorb or dissolve in water. It passes through the digestive tract close to its original form. Insoluble fiber offers many benefits to intestinal health, including a reduction in the risk and occurrence of colorectal cancer, hemorrhoids, and constipation. Most of insoluble fibers come from the bran layers of cereal grains. The recommended intake of fiber is set at 38 g per day and 25 g per day for young men and women, respectively (73). Additional benefits of fiber include (72–77):

- Provides bulk in the diet, thus increasing the satiety value of foods.
- Some fibers also delay the emptying of the stomach, further increasing satiety (78).
- Prevents constipation and establishes regular bowel movements.
- May reduce the risks of heart and artery disease by lowering blood cholesterol.
- Regulates the body's absorption of glucose (diabetics included), perhaps because fiber is believed to be capable of controlling the rate of digestion and assimilation of carbohydrates.
- High-fiber meals have been shown to exert regulatory effects on blood glucose levels for up to 5 hours after eating.

Carbohydrate and Performance

Carbohydrate availability is vital for maximal sports performance. When performing high-intensity, short-duration activity (anaerobic), muscular demand for energy is provided for and dependent on muscle glycogen. During endurance exercise (aerobic) performed at a moderate intensity (60% of maximal oxygen consumption [$\dot{V}o_2$ max]), muscle glycogen provides approximately 50% of energy needs. During high-intensity aerobic exercise (>79% of $\dot{V}o_2$ max), it yields nearly all of the energy needs (79).

Duration of exercise also affects the amount of glycogen used for energy. As duration of activity increases, available glucose and glycogen diminish, increasing the reliance on fat as a fuel source. In addition, one could presume that if there is an appreciable increase in duration, there must also be a decrease in intensity, decreasing the use of glycogen. However, this does not mean that the best way to lose body fat is to perform low-intensity activities for a long duration. If the workout contributes to a caloric deficit, the body will draw on its fat stores at some point to make up for the deficit (80).

Ultimately, the limiting factor for exercise performance is carbohydrate availability: "Fat burns in a carbohydrate flame." That is to say, maximal fat utilization cannot occur without sufficient carbohydrate to continue Krebs cycle activity (66,67). When an endurance athlete "hits the wall," it is the result of fatigue caused by severely lowered liver and muscle glycogen. This occurs even though there is sufficient oxygen being delivered to the muscles and an abundance of potential energy from fat stores (81).

Carbohydrate-Intake Recommendations

A diet containing between 6 and 10 g/kg per day of carbohydrate (2.7 to 4.5 g/lb), is recommended (56). According to the Institute of Medicine, the Acceptable Macronutrient Distribution Range for carbohydrate intake for an adult is 45 to 65% of total caloric intake (55). Complex carbohydrates (such as whole grains and fresh fruits and vegetables) should constitute the majority of calories because of their nutrient-dense (providing B vitamins, iron, and fiber) nature.

The amount of carbohydrate in the diet can affect performance. High-carbohydrate diets increase the use of glycogen as fuel, whereas a high-fat diet increases the use of fat as fuel (80). However, a high-fat diet results in lower glycogen synthesis (82,83). This is of particular concern if the individual is consuming a reduced-energy diet (84). For the endurance athlete, a carbohydrate-rich diet will build glycogen stores and aid in performance and recovery (85,86). Although some studies show an increase in performance associated with the consumption of a high-fat diet, these improvements are seen in exercise performed at a relatively low intensity (less than 70% of $\dot{V}o_2$ max) (83,87). As the intensity of exercise increases, performance of high-intensity exercise will ultimately be impaired (88–90).

Before Exercise

It is recommended that the individual consume a high-carbohydrate meal 2 to 4 hours before exercising for more than an hour. This will allow time for appropriate gastric emptying before exercise. This is especially helpful for morning workouts when glycogen stores are lowered by as much as 80% (80). If this is not feasible because of time constraints, a liquid meal such as a meal-replacement formula may be used. One advantage to such formulas is their quick gastric emptying time. Some research recommends a carbohydrate intake of 1 to 4.5 g/kg, between 1 and 4 hours before exercise, respectively (91). In this study, the group ingesting 4.5 g/kg of carbohydrate 4 hours before exercise saw performance improved by 15% (91). To avoid gastrointestinal distress, smaller meals should be consumed closer to the exercise session.

Carbohydrate Loading

In endurance exercise of greater than a 90-minute duration (e.g., marathon running), muscle-glycogen stores become depleted. This depletion limits the performance of endurance exercise. Carbohydrate loading, also called glycogen supercompensation, is a technique used to increase muscle glycogen before an endurance event. This practice can nearly double muscle glycogen stores, increasing endurance potential (92).

Historically, the weeklong program includes 4 days of glycogen depletion (through a low-carbohydrate diet that is approximately 10% of calories and exhaustive exercise), followed by 3 days of rest and a high-carbohydrate diet (approximately 90% of calories). This method has many drawbacks, including periods of hypoglycemia, irritability, increased susceptibility to injury, and difficulty in compliance. In 1981, one study proposed a revised method Table 17.9 that accomplishes the same goal with greater ease of compliance and fewer side effects (93).

Although maximizing muscle glycogen before an event may improve power, performance, output, and speed by postponing muscle glycogen depletion, glycogen loading before exercise does not always improve performance. Some athletes experience extreme gastrointestinal distress including diarrhea when attempting glycogen loading. Thus, meals should contain familiar foods that are relatively low in fat and fiber to minimize gastrointestinal distress. Because leg muscles become heavier with the addition of glycogen and water, many athletes complain they feel heavy and sluggish, and they can experience a slight weight gain. Athletes should experiment with glycogen loading before using it for competition.

During Exercise

For exercise lasting more than 1 hour, carbohydrate feedings during exercise can help supply glucose to working muscles whose glycogen stores are dwindling. This technique also maintains blood glucose levels, increasing time to exhaustion by 20 to 60 minutes (94–97). It is recommended that endurance athletes consume between 30 and 60 g of carbohydrate every hour to accomplish this. Popular sports beverages are perfect for this goal and have the added benefit of replacing fluid losses, also benefiting performance. The replacement of carbohydrate and water has individual benefits that together are additive.

TABLE 17.9 Glycogen-Loading Schedule[a]

Days Before the Event	Exercise Intensity and Duration	Carbohydrate Intake
6 days out	70–75% of $\dot{V}_{O_2}$ max, for 90 min	4 g/kg of body weight
4–5 days out	70–75% of $\dot{V}_{O_2}$ max, for 40 min	4 g/kg of body weight
2–3 days out	70–75% of $\dot{V}_{O_2}$ max, for 20 min	10 g/kg of body weight
1 day out	Rest	10 g/kg of body weight

[a]Athletes with diabetes or high triglycerides should consult a physician before using this plan.
$\dot{V}_{O_2}$ max, maximal oxygen consumption.

One study showed that performance during 1 hour of intense cycling was improved by 12% with the consumption of 1,330 mL (53 oz) of water containing 79 g of carbohydrate (98). Sports beverages including potassium and sodium help replace electrolytes, whereas carbohydrates provide energy. Sports beverages containing 6% to 8% carbohydrate are recommended for exercise lasting longer than 1 hour (56).

After Exercise

Repeated days of strenuous exercise take a toll on an individual's glycogen stores. A high-carbohydrate intake helps to replenish glycogen stores; however, the timing of carbohydrate ingestion can also be important to maximizing recovery. Consuming 1.5 g per kg of carbohydrate within 30 minutes of completing exercise is recommended to maximize glycogen replenishment (99). Delaying carbohydrate intake by even 2 hours can decrease total muscle glycogen synthesis by 66% (100). The postworkout environment may hasten glycogen repletion as a result of increased blood flow to the muscles and an increased sensitivity of the cells to the effects of insulin (80). Additional meals of 1.5 g per kg of carbohydrate every 2 hours are recommended to completely restore muscle glycogen (99).

For Altering Body Composition

Carbohydrate should generally make up the highest percentage of macronutrient calories when one is attempting fat loss or muscle gain. Carbohydrates provide variety, valuable nutrients, and volume to the diet. The satiating value of complex carbohydrate is especially important when one is in a caloric deficit for the goal of fat loss (100–102). For most moderately active adults, a carbohydrate intake of between 45 and 65% is recommended, which will provide sufficient food volume and the fuel necessary for energy and productive workouts (55).

Despite the popularity of low-carbohydrate diets and the perpetuation of erroneous claims regarding type or time of carbohydrate intake, there is no need for one to reduce carbohydrate percentage to lose fat (see Carbohydrate and Weight Gain section). However, there is recent evidence from examining the glycemic response to specific foods, suggesting that a diet that is centered around low glycemic index carbohydrates may be useful in the prevention of obesity, coronary artery disease, colon cancer, and breast cancer (71,72).

Weight loss or gain is primarily related to total caloric intake, not the macronutrient profile of the diet. The weight lost on a low-carbohydrate diet can be attributed to two factors: low caloric intake and loss of fat-free mass (FFM) (103). If an individual begins dropping carbohydrate-rich foods from his or her diet, it is inevitable that caloric intake will drop as a result. Added to the caloric reduction are dwindling glycogen stores. For every gram of glucose taken out of glycogen, it brings with it 2.7 g of water (104). This loss of muscle glycogen (including water) can be quite significant in the first week of a low-carbohydrate diet, and adds to the pounds lost on the scale. This is how low-carbohydrate fad diets can promise dramatic weight loss in such a short period. Long-term success in weight loss is associated with a realistic eating style, not one that severely limits or omits one of the macronutrients (105).

Carbohydrate and Weight Gain: The Facts

A significant amount of time, energy, and resources is spent investigating the link between carbohydrate intake and the increased prevalence of obesity in Americans.

The accusations are familiar: "carbohydrates make you fat," and "Americans are getting fatter, despite lower fat intakes."

Data available from the Third National Health and Nutrition Examination Survey (NHANES III), which summarizes Americans' nutrition patterns for the years 1988 through 1991, show that percentage of calories consumed from fat has indeed dropped, from 36% (NHANES II 1976–1980) to 34% of total energy intake (106). However, when total fat intake (grams per person per day) is measured, and not simply the percentage contributed, the data show that fat intake has remained quite constant for the past several years (107). Additionally, these data may not accurately reflect fat consumption in America, as many people underreport fat consumption owing to its negative health connotations (64). The data from NHANES III also show an increase in total energy intake. This would support the relationship of excessive energy intake leading to increased fat stores.

When reviewing the data on Americans' food intake, it is interesting to note that in the early 1900s, the percentage of carbohydrates consumed as energy intake was higher and consumption of fat lower than it is today, without the prevalence of obesity we now experience (108). Only during the last two decades has there been a significant increase in obesity. The data support two primary variables responsible for this dramatic rise in obesity: an increased energy intake and a reduction in energy expenditure (108,109). It is estimated that more than 75% of the American adult population does not partake, on a daily basis, in 30 minutes of low-to-moderate physical activity (110).

At the turn of the century, carbohydrate intake as a percentage of total energy was higher, fat as a percentage was lower, and obesity was not the problem it is today. Currently, total fat intake is higher, carbohydrate is lower, and obesity has reached epidemic proportions (111,112). In addition, energy intake has increased and energy expenditure has decreased. The facts are very clear: America's increasing problem of obesity is not a direct result of carbohydrate intake, but rather of energy imbalance.

Review of the Properties of Carbohydrates

One gram of carbohydrate yields 4 calories. Carbohydrates provide the body with:

- Nutrition that fat and protein cannot (from complex carbohydrates)
- Satiety by keeping glycogen stores full and adding bulk to the diet
- Proper cellular fluid balance, maximizing cellular efficiency
- Proper blood sugar levels, if there is a consistent intake of low-glycemic carbohydrates
- Spare protein for building muscle

The body needs carbohydrates because:

- They are the perfect and preferred form of energy
- They constantly need to be replaced, causing a craving that must be satisfied
- Parts of the central nervous system rely exclusively on carbohydrate
- They efficiently burn and use fat and protein

Recommended carbohydrate intake:

- Daily diet should include 25 to 38 g of fiber.
- Carbohydrate intake typically should be between 45 and 65% of total caloric intake according to preference, performance, and satiety.

- ◆ Carbohydrate recommendations should be estimated after protein and fat requirements are met.
- ◆ Fruits, whole grains, and vegetables are all excellent sources of fiber.

SUMMARY

Carbohydrates are a chief source of energy for all body functions and muscular exertion. They are compounds containing carbon, hydrogen, and oxygen and are generally classified as sugars (simple), starches (complex), and fiber. A monosaccharide is a single sugar unit (such as glucose, fructose, or galactose), many of which are connected to make starches and glycogen. Disaccharides (two sugar units) include sucrose, lactose, and maltose. Polysaccharides are foods that contain starch and fiber. These foods are often called complex carbohydrates. Carbohydrates help to regulate the digestion and utilization of protein and fat.

GI is the rate at which ingested carbohydrate raises blood sugar and affects insulin release. Foods lower on the glycemic index are good sources of complex carbohydrates, as well as being high in fiber and overall nutritional value. When total caloric intake exceeds output, any excess carbohydrate, dietary fat, or protein may be stored as body fat until needed.

Fiber is one of the greatest contributions made by dietary complex carbohydrate. Higher intakes of dietary fiber are associated with lower incidence of heart disease and certain types of cancer. In addition, fiber provides many other benefits including satiety, intestinal health, and regulation of the body's absorption of glucose.

The availability of carbohydrate is vital for fitness enthusiasts and optimal sports performance because the demand for energy is provided for and dependent on muscle glycogen. Duration and intensity of exercise affects the amount of glycogen used for energy. Maximal fat utilization cannot occur without sufficient carbohydrate. A diet containing between 6 and 10 g/kg/day of carbohydrate (2.7 to 4.5 g per pounds) is recommended. Complex carbohydrates (such as whole grains and fresh fruits and vegetables) should constitute the majority of calories because of their nutrient-dense (providing B vitamins, iron, and fiber) nature.

It is recommended that the individual consume a high-carbohydrate meal 2 to 4 hours before exercising for more than an hour. In endurance exercise of greater than a 90-minute duration, carbohydrate loading can be used to increase muscle glycogen before an endurance event. For exercise lasting more than 1 hour, endurance athletes should consume between 30 and 60 g of carbohydrate every hour (which may consist of sports beverages). After exercise, consuming 1.5 g per kg of carbohydrate within 30 minutes is recommended. Additional meals of 1.5 g per kg of carbohydrate every 2 hours are recommended to completely restore muscle glycogen.

For fat loss or muscle gain, carbohydrates should generally make up the highest percentage of macronutrient calories. According to the Institute of Medicine the Acceptable Macronutrient Distribution Range for carbohydrate intake for an adult is 45 to 65% of total caloric intake. There is no need to reduce carbohydrate percentage and carbohydrate-rich whole foods to lose fat. America's increasing problem of obesity is not a direct result of carbohydrate intake, but rather one of energy imbalance.

Lipids

Lipids are a group of compounds that include *triglycerides* (fats and oils), *phospholipids,* and *sterols*. Of the lipids contained in food, 95% are fats and oils. In the body, 99% of the stored lipids are also triglycerides (113). Structurally, triglycerides are three fatty acids attached to a glycerol backbone **Figure 17.5**.

Lipids A group of compounds that includes triglycerides (fats and oils), phospholipids, and sterols.

Fatty Acids

Fatty acids may be *saturated* or *unsaturated* **Figure 17.6**. Unsaturated fatty acids may be further classified according to their degree of unsaturation. If the fatty acid has one double bond in its carbon chain, it is called a *monounsaturated* fatty acid. If there is more than one point of unsaturation, it is classified as a *polyunsaturated* fatty acid.

Polyunsaturated fatty acids provide important essential fatty acids (or fats that cannot be manufactured by the body but are essential for proper health and functioning) (114). Saturated fatty acids are implicated as a risk factor for heart disease because they raise bad cholesterol levels (low-density lipoproteins; LDL), whereas unsaturated fats are associated with increases in good cholesterol (high-density lipoproteins; HDL) and decreased risk of heart disease (115,116). Monounsaturated fatty acids (found in olive and canola oils) and polyunsaturated fatty acids such as omega-3 fatty acids (found in cold-water fish, such as salmon) are considered to have favorable effects on blood

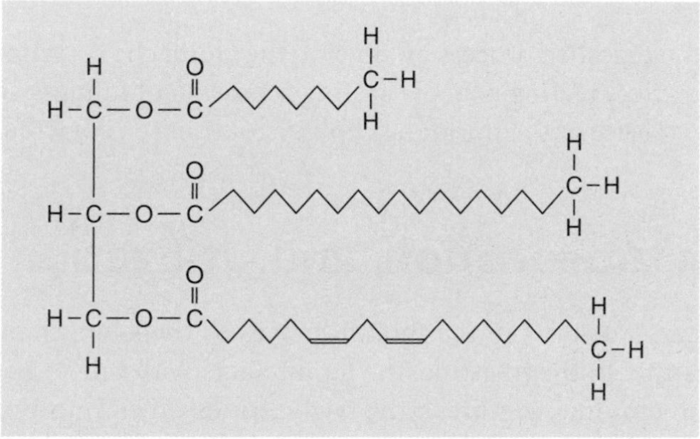

FIGURE 17.5

The triglyceride molecule.

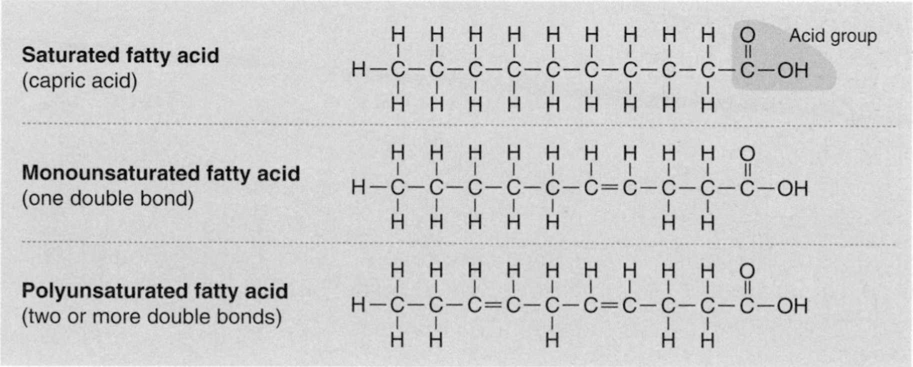

FIGURE 17.6

Fatty acids.

lipid profiles and may play a role in the treatment and prevention of heart disease, hypertension, arthritis, and cancer (115,116) **Table 17.10**. Another prevalent fatty acid in today's food supply is trans-fatty acids, the result of *hydrogenation* (or the process of adding hydrogen to unsaturated fatty acids to make them harder at room temperature and increase food shelf-life). Trans-fatty acids have been shown to increase LDL cholesterol and decrease HDL cholesterol, much like saturated fats (117–119).

The Function of Lipids

Lipids (or fats) are the most concentrated source of energy in the diet. One gram of fat yields approximately 9 calories when oxidized, furnishing more than twice the calories per gram of carbohydrates or proteins. In addition to providing energy, fats act as carriers for the fat-soluble vitamins A, D, E, and K. Vitamin D aids in the absorption of calcium, making it available to body tissues, particularly to the bones and teeth. Fats are also important for the conversion of carotene to vitamin A (120). Fats are involved in the following (120):

♦ Cellular membrane structure and function
♦ Precursors to hormones
♦ Cellular signals
♦ Regulation and excretion of nutrients in the cells
♦ Surrounding, protecting, and holding in place organs, such as the kidneys, heart, and liver
♦ Insulating the body from environmental temperature changes and preserving body heat
♦ Prolonging the digestive process by slowing the stomach's secretions of hydrochloric acid, creating a longer-lasting sensation of fullness after a meal
♦ Initiating the release of the hormone cholecystokinin (CCK), which contributes to satiety

Digestion, Absorption, and Utilization

Digestion of dietary fat starts in the mouth, moves to the stomach, and is completed in the small intestine. In the intestine, the fat interacts with bile to become emulsified so that pancreatic enzymes can break the triglycerides down into two fatty acids and a monoglyceride. Absorption of these constituents occurs through the intestinal wall

---

TABLE 17.10 Food Sources and Types of Fats

Monounsaturated Fats	Polyunsaturated Fats	Saturated Fats	Trans-Fats
Olive oil, canola oil, peanut oil, avocados, peanuts, almonds, pistachios	Vegetable oils: safflower, soy, corn, and sunflower oils Omega-3 fatty acids: herring, mackerel, salmon, sardines, flaxseeds Most nuts and seeds	Meat, poultry, lard, butter, cheese, cream, eggs, whole milk Tropical oils: coconut oil, palm, and palm kernel oil Many baked goods	Stick margarine, shortening Fried foods: fried chicken, doughnuts Fast food Many baked goods and pastries

into the blood. In the intestinal wall, they are reassembled into triglycerides that are then released into the lymph in the form of a lipoprotein called *chylomicron*. Chylomicrons from the lymph move to the blood. The triglyceride content of chylomicron is removed by the action of the enzyme lipoprotein lipase (LPL), and the released fatty acids are taken up by the tissues. Throughout the day, triglycerides are constantly cycled in and out of tissues, including muscles, organs, and adipose.

Recommendations

Clients must be satiated by the amount of calories necessary to allow fat loss or energy balance or they will eventually overeat. The goal is to keep the client's diet within the guidelines for health. According to the Institute of Medicine, the Acceptable Macronutrient Distribution Range for fat intake for an adult is 20 to 35% of total caloric intake (55). Athletes are recommended to consume 20 to 25% of total calories from fat, but there appears to be no health or performance benefit to consuming less than 15% of energy from fat (56). Conversely, higher-fat diets are not conducive to successful weight loss or maintenance and appear to increase the ease with which the body converts ingested calories to body fat (121–123).

Fat has a lower *thermic effect* than other macronutrients (124). The thermic effect of a food (TEF) is the rise in metabolic rate that occurs after the food is ingested. Typically, TEF amounts to 10% of ingested calories (114). As fat percentage in the diet increases, the amount of heat given off (TEF) decreases. Conversely, as carbohydrate percentage in the diet increases, so does the TEF. It is metabolically inexpensive to convert dietary fat to body-fat stores. Only 3% of the calories in fat are required to store it as fat. In contrast, it takes 23% of the calories in carbohydrate to convert it to body fat (124).

Fat and Satiety

Dietary fats stimulate the release of CCK, a hormone that signals satiety. Additionally, fats slow the digestion of foods (and thus the nutrient content in the bloodstream), assisting in blood sugar stabilization. Reducing blood sugar fluctuations can contribute to satiety. However, diets containing more than 35% of calories from fat lose the volume of food provided by higher-carbohydrate diets. In other words, both a tablespoon of oil and a large salad with nonfat dressing may contain the same amount of calories. Because satiety is achieved by more than just total caloric intake, this low-volume, high-calorie contribution of fat may not satisfy other peripheral satiation mechanisms (chewing, swallowing, stomach distention), leading to *hyperphagia* (or overeating) (125).

Fat Supplementation During Exercise

In general, fat is digested and absorbed quite slowly. Long-chain triglycerides (LCT), which make up the majority of dietary fatty acids (16 to 18 carbons), must go through the process of digestion and absorption described earlier before they can be utilized. Medium-chain triglycerides (MCT), however, are more rapidly absorbed. Additionally, they do not require incorporation into chylomicrons for transport, but can enter the systemic circulation directly through the portal vein, providing a readily available, concentrated source of energy (114). It has been suggested that MCT could benefit endurance performance by supplying an exogenous energy source in addition to carbohydrate during exercise and increase plasma free fatty acids (FFA), sparing muscle glycogen (126,127). However, several studies of well-trained endurance athletes have found that MCT ingestion does not alter fat metabolism, spare muscle glycogen, or improve performance (128,129). Goedecke et al. (130) found that ingestion of MCT with ultraendurance cyclists actually compromised performance. The impaired performance may have been related to the gastrointestinal upset from the MCT solution.

Insulin Resistance and Obesity

Proponents of high-protein, low-carbohydrate diets have profited from the erroneous assertion that carbohydrates are to blame for the increasing prevalence of metabolic syndrome (or syndrome X) and therefore lead to weight gain. Metabolic syndrome is a cluster of symptoms characterized by obesity, insulin resistance, hypertension, and dyslipidemia, leading to an increased risk of cardiovascular disease. Syndrome X is usually associated with obesity (especially abdominal), a high-fat diet, and a sedentary lifestyle (131–134).

A common denominator associated with these factors is high levels of circulating free fatty acids (FFA). In the presence of high FFA concentrations, the body will favor their use as energy, decreasing glucose oxidation and glycogen synthesis and inhibiting glucose transport (131). The result is chronically elevated levels of blood sugar levels, a condition called hyperglycemia. During states of hyperglycemia, insulin will also be elevated, leading to the conversion of the excess blood sugar to other products such as glycoproteins and fatty acids.

These facts alone seem to bolster the idea that carbohydrates lead to health problems. The truth is that a healthy person would need to eat an extremely high percentage of simple carbohydrates (such as sucrose) and fat, maintain a constant energy excess, or be overweight to have chronically elevated blood sugar. Although there is some evidence that there may be a genetic component that contributes to insulin resistance (IR), the condition itself will not allow for weight gain without an energy intake in excess of expenditure (7,135,136). In fact, obesity itself is a risk factor for development of IR, not the other way around (137).

So, what is the common cause of IR? If one constantly overeats, excess calories are stored as fat, which causes fat cells to increase in size. The growing fat cell itself becomes insulin resistant, and the resulting prevalence of FFA will cause the body to favor the use of fat for energy at the expense of glucose (138). This becomes a vicious cycle, with the overweight condition leading to IR, which in turn leads to impaired glucose use. Blood sugar levels rise, insulin levels rise, and cholesterol, triglycerides, and blood pressure rise as well. To make matters worse, the impaired ability of glucose to enter muscle cells keeps glycogen stores lower, which can increase appetite, motivating the individual to eat more, increasing fat stores, exacerbating IR, and so on.

As numerous studies point out, high-fat diets are strongly associated with obesity, and thus insulin resistance and diabetes (138–140). It should be noted that eating fat does not make one fat (the same applies to carbohydrate) unless it is consumed in excess of energy requirements. However, it is easier to consume excess energy (or be hyperphagic) on a high-fat diet, owing to fat's high caloric density. When large quantities of high-caloric-dense foods are consumed in combination with excess calories and a sedentary lifestyle, it is easy to envision an abundance of fatty acids floating around in the bloodstream.

It is much more likely that a high-fat diet leads to excess consumption of calories, obesity, IR, and eventually non–insulin-dependent diabetes mellitus than it is that carbohydrates cause IR and, as a result, obesity. The only solution is a diet containing the appropriate amount of energy, high in fibrous vegetables or starchy carbohydrates, and exercise.

In fact, a study of type 2 diabetics, those with IR, and people of normal weight found that 3 weeks of a high-carbohydrate, low-fat diet and an exercise program significantly lowered insulin levels (141).

Perhaps it is convenient to place blame on carbohydrates; with obesity continuing to rise, a simple solution to the problem of America's weight gain would be welcomed. Our current environment has created a society that encourages the growth of the human organism. Highly palatable and caloric-rich food is available to most, and today's work and recreational demands do not call for much physical movement. On the surface, the cure for obesity is simple: move more and eat less. However, the influence of societal, psychological, and physiologic factors can make putting this simple plan into action very difficult. Be that as it may, any solution will ultimately provide a way to increase energy expenditure, decrease energy consumption, or a combination of both.

Review of the Properties of Lipids

One gram of fat yields 9 calories. Fat is generally insoluble in water. Fat is present in all cells: high in adipose and nerve tissue, low in epithelial and muscle tissue. Fatty acids can be saturated, polyunsaturated, and monounsaturated. The body needs fats for:

- Energy
- Structure and membrane function
- Precursors to hormones
- Cellular signals
- Regulation of uptake and excretion of nutrients in the cells

Recommended fat intake:

- The Acceptable Macronutrient Distribution Range for fat intake for an adult is 20 to 35% of total caloric intake (20 to 25% for athletes).
- There appears to be no health or performance benefit to consuming less than 15% of energy from fat.
- A high polyunsaturated-to-saturated fat ratio is desirable.
- More than 35% leads to overeating (lack of food volume) and often slows metabolism.

SUMMARY

Lipids are a group of compounds that include triglycerides (fats and oils), phospholipids, and sterols. Most lipids in food and in the body are triglycerides, which are three fatty acids (saturated or unsaturated) attached to a glycerol backbone. Polyunsaturated fatty acids provide important essential fatty acids. Saturated fatty acids and trans-fatty acids are implicated as a risk factor for heart disease because they raise bad cholesterol levels (LDL), whereas unsaturated fats are associated with increases in good cholesterol (HDL) and decreased risk of heart disease.

Lipids are the most concentrated source of energy in the diet. One gram of fat yields approximately 9 calories. Lipids also regulate and excrete nutrients and act as carriers for vitamins A, D (which aids in the absorption of calcium), E, and K. Fats have many other benefits, including cellular membrane structure and function, body insulation, aid in the digestive process, and satiety. Digestion of dietary fat starts in the mouth, moves to the stomach, and is completed in the small intestine. Throughout the day, triglycerides are constantly cycled in and out of tissues. The Acceptable Macronutrient Distribution Range for fat intake for an adult is 20 to 35% of total caloric intake. Fat has a lower thermic effect than other macronutrients, only taking 3% of its calories to store it in the body as fat. Fat is digested and absorbed quite slowly. Thus, medium-chain triglycerides are not recommended as supplements for the goal of improving endurance exercise.

Metabolic syndrome is a cluster of symptoms characterized by obesity and insulin resistance. However, insulin resistance alone will not allow for weight gain without an energy intake in excess of expenditure. Obesity itself is a risk factor for development of insulin resistance, not the other way around.

Water

Sedentary men and women should consume on average 3.0 L (approximately 13 cups) and 2.2 L (approximately 9 cups) of water per day, respectively (55). Those participating in a fat-loss program should drink an additional 8 ounces of water for every 25 pounds they carry above their ideal weight. Water intake should also be increased if an individual is exercising briskly or residing in a hot climate.

The Importance of Water

Water is vital to life itself; it constitutes approximately 60% of the adult human body by weight. Whereas deficiencies of nutrients such as the macronutrients, vitamins, and minerals may take weeks or even years to develop, one can only survive for a few days without water. Consuming an adequate amount of water will benefit the body in the following ways (142):

- Endocrine gland function improves.
- Fluid retention is alleviated.
- Liver functions improve, increasing the percentage of fat used for energy.
- Natural thirst returns.
- Metabolic functions improve.
- Nutrients are distributed throughout the body.
- Body-temperature regulation improves.
- Blood volume is maintained.

Water and Performance

The importance of proper hydration cannot be stressed enough. The body cannot adapt to dehydration, which impairs every physiologic function. Table 17.11 shows the effects of dehydration. Studies have shown that a fluid loss of even 2% of body weight will adversely affect circulatory functions and decrease performance levels (143–146). However, if a fairly regular daily pattern of exercise and water and food consumption is followed, average body weight will provide a very good index of the body's state of hydration. Realizing this, the organizers of certain ultradistance running events make it mandatory for competitors to weigh themselves at stations along the course and require each runner to consume enough fluid to regain a predetermined body weight before being allowed to continue.

Thirst alone is a poor indicator of how much water is needed. Athletes consistently consume inadequate fluid volume, managing to replace approximately 50% of sweat

TABLE 17.11	Effects of Dehydration	
Decreased blood volume	Increased heart rate
Decreased performance	Sodium retention
Decreased blood pressure	Decreased cardiac output
Decreased sweat rate	Decreased blood flow to the skin
Increased core temperature	Increased perceived exertion
Water retention	Increased use of muscle glycogen

losses (143). A good way to keep track of how much one needs to drink is to first determine his or her average daily weight. Use this number as the standard for the person's *euhydrated* (or normal) state. Do not begin a practice session or endurance competition until the body is at, or slightly above, its standard weight. Drink enough water, juice, or sports drinks during exercise to maintain the starting weight.

Guidelines for fluid replacement in the athlete are as follows (56):

◆ Consume 14 to 22 ounces (1.75 to 2.75 cups) of fluid 2 hours before exercise.
◆ Drink 6 to 12 ounces of fluid for every 15 to 20 minutes of exercise.
◆ Fluids should be cold because of more rapid gastric emptying.
◆ If exercise exceeds 60 minutes, use of a sports drink (containing up to 8% carbohydrate) can replace both fluid and dwindling muscle glycogen stores.
◆ When exercising for less than 60 minutes, water is the experts' choice for fluid replacement.
◆ The goal is to replace sweat and urine losses.
◆ Ingest 16 to 24 ounces of fluid for every pound of body weight lost after an exercise bout, especially if rapid rehydration is necessary, as in twice-a-day training.

SUMMARY

Sedentary men and women should consume on average 3.0 L (approximately 13 cups) and 2.2 L (approximately 9 cups) of water per day, respectively. Those on fat-loss programs should drink an additional 8 ounces of water for every 25 pounds carried above ideal weight. Water intake should also be increased if an individual is exercising briskly or residing in a hot climate. The body cannot adapt to dehydration, which impairs every physiologic function. A fluid loss of even 2% of body weight will adversely affect circulatory functions and decrease performance levels.

Consuming an adequate amount of water will improve body temperature regulation, metabolic function, and endocrine gland and liver function. In addition, nutrients are distributed throughout the body, blood volume is maintained, and fluid retention is alleviated. Thirst alone is a poor indicator of how much water is needed. Instead, determine average daily weight and use this number as the standard for a euhydrated state. Consume 14 to 22 ounces of fluid 2 hours before exercise and drink 6 to 12 ounces of fluid for every 15 to 20 minutes of exercise. Finally, ingest 16 to 24 ounces of fluid for every pound of body weight lost after an exercise bout.

Altering Body Composition

Basic Nutritional Guidelines for Altering Body Composition (55,56,147)

For Fat Loss

◆ Make small decreases in food and beverage calories and increase physical activity.
◆ Distribute protein, carbohydrate, and fat throughout the day and at each meal.
◆ Consume less than 10% of calories from saturated fat.
◆ Choose whole grains and fiber-rich fruits and vegetables over refined grains and simple sugars (as the fiber and complexity of the starch will aid in hunger control).
◆ Limit alcohol consumption.
◆ Schedule no fewer than four and as many as six meals a day. This helps to control hunger, minimize blood sugar fluctuations, and increase energy levels throughout the day.
◆ Avoid empty calories and highly processed foods, which contain many calories and do little to provide satiety.
◆ Drink plenty of water (minimum of 9 to 13 cups per day).
◆ Have clients weigh and measure food for at least 1 week. This will make them more aware of caloric values and serving sizes, as well as decrease the likelihood of underreporting calories.

For Lean Body Mass Gain

◆ Eat four to six meals a day. Insulin response to a meal stimulates protein synthesis.
◆ Spread protein intake throughout the day to take advantage of the previous tip.
◆ Keep in mind the postworkout window of opportunity. Ingestion of protein and carbohydrate within 90 minutes of a workout will increase recovery and protein synthesis, maximizing gains. This may be most easily accomplished with a liquid meal-replacement formula that can be absorbed quickly owing to being predigested. Food may take several hours to digest and absorb, missing the window.
◆ Do not neglect the importance of carbohydrate and fat. It takes more than protein to increase lean body mass.

Frequently Asked Questions

Do Carbohydrates Make Me Fat?

The answer is no. Carbohydrates are necessary nutrients. They provide energy for the body, metabolism of fats, spare muscle proteins, and provide essential fiber, vitamins, and minerals. Excess intake of any nutrient, carbohydrate, fat, protein, or alcohol over daily calorie needs will cause weight gain.

Selecting carbohydrates that are moderate- to low-glycemic foods and high in fiber can help with satiety, blood sugar regulation, and energy balance indirectly. Overconsumption of sugar, refined processed carbohydrates, and high-glycemic foods could lead to uncontrolled spikes in blood sugar, low energy, and increased appetite. Therefore, to avoid hunger, it is advised to choose unprocessed, whole-food carbohydrate sources such as vegetables, starchy vegetables, whole fruit, and grains to provide fiber, vitamins, and minerals for healthy weight loss. In addition, carbohydrate is imperative to glycogen repletion before, during and after exercise for strength, power, aerobic and anaerobic performance, and conditioning. The Acceptable Macronutrient Distribution Range for carbohydrate intake for an adult is 45 to 65% of total caloric intake. Table 17.12 illustrates carbohydrate content of several popular diets.

Does Eating at Night Make Me Fat?

Weight gain is a result of eating more calories than you burn on a regular basis, not when you eat. Because of their preference or schedule, many people eat later in the evening, before bed, or even wake up in the middle of the night to take in calories. If one gains weight doing this, it is because of excess calorie intake, not the timing.

The body does not have an enzyme with a watch that after 7 P.M. preferentially stores items, especially carbohydrates, as fat. We all have a certain number of calories that we can consume without gaining weight. As long as we do not exceed that number, weight gain will not occur. Imagine this scenario: at your height, weight, and activity level, you know that you burn 2,750 calories in a 24-hour period. You have had a busy day, and since your 350-calorie breakfast, you have not had the opportunity to eat. You get home late after a long day and you are starving. At 9 P.M. you eat an enormous 1,000-calorie meal. Added to the 350-calorie breakfast, this brings your total calories consumed for the day to 1,350 calories. After your late meal you are exhausted and promptly go to bed. Will you gain weight? Simply put, no. You have burned 1,400 calories more than you consumed. So, the moral here is to figure out how many calories you can have during the day to lose or maintain weight and distribute those calories and foods in a manner that makes you feel your best and prevents hunger.

TABLE 17.12   Carbohydrate Content of Several Popular Diets

Percent Carbohydrate	Diet
<21% Very low	• Atkins diet • Protein power plan • Ketogenic diet
21–42% Low	• Zone diet • Carbohydrate addicts diet • Abs diet • South Beach diet • Sugar busters • Testosterone diet
43–50% Moderate	• Average American diet
51–60% Moderately high	• RDA food pyramid • Flat belly diet • Mediterranean diet
>60% High	• Dean Ornish • Pritikin diet

Adapted from Haff GG, Whitley A. Low carbohydrate diets and high intensity anaerobic exercise. *Strength Cond.* 2002;24(4):42–53; and *Essentials and Sports Nutrition and Supplementation.* Totowa, NJ: Humana Press; 2008:282.

Which Is Superior for Weight Loss, a Low-Fat and High-Carbohydrate or a High-Protein and Low-Carbohydrate Diet?

Neither a low-fat and high-carbohydrate or a high-protein and low-carbohydrate diet is superior for weight loss. Weight loss is achieved when calories consumed are less than calories expended. Numerous studies have examined and compared popular weight-loss diets. One study examined weight loss in obese subjects using four popular weight-loss diets (148): the Atkins diet, the Zone, Weight Watchers, and the Ornish plan. The weight-loss average among subjects was the same after 1 year regardless of the diet program. The more restrictive diets such as the Atkins very low carbohydrate, high-fat, and high-protein diet and the Ornish plan high-carbohydrate and very low fat diet had higher dropout rates. For those who completed the study, weight loss after a year was approximately 5 to 7 pounds regardless of the diet plan. The more restricted the diet, e.g., Atkins and Ornish, the harder it was for subjects to adhere to (i.e., the higher the dropout rate) (148).

According to research, people initially lose weight faster on a low-carbohydrate and high-protein diet when compared with energy equivalent low-fat and high-carbohydrate diets. But after 12 months, the total weight loss is similar (149).

Because of individual responses, it is not appropriate to recommend "one" weight-loss plan for the entire population. The primary goal in weight loss is to improve health by lowering body fat while maintaining or increasing the proportion of FFM and muscle tissue. If FFM and muscle can be increased during weight loss, it is easier to maintain RMR and fat loss. Maintaining muscle is also important to strength and the ability to perform physical activities of daily living.

Can I Eat Whatever I Want as Long as I Exercise?

The majority of daily caloric expenditure is not in the time spent exercising but in the total energy expenditure during 24 hours. Approximately 3,500 calories equals a pound of body fat, so to lose 1 to 2 pounds per week, a client must maintain an average caloric deficit of 500 to 1,000 calories per day. However, a person may burn 250 calories from exercise and spend the rest of the day participating in sedentary activities. Calories that are not used for energy production are stored as fat. Therefore, a person can eat 100 calories a day more than what their body needs to maintain, and in the course of 35 days, theoretically they will gain a pound of fat. Even a mere 10 extra calories a day over daily maintenance needs could add up to a 1 pound of weight gain over 350 days!

What Are the Risks of Starvation (Very Low Calorie) Diets?

This chapter has reviewed the physiology of weight loss, and established that an energy deficit must be created for weight loss to occur. However, personal trainers should caution their clients against going too low. Most nutrition experts do not recommend an energy intake any lower than 1,200 calories and even that may be too low for an active or very large person.

Very low calorie diets (VLCD) should be followed only under the supervision of a medical professional. A VLCD is a doctor-supervised diet that typically uses commercially prepared formulas to promote rapid weight loss in patients who are obese. These formulas, usually liquid shakes or bars, replace all food intake for several weeks or months. VLCD formulas need to contain appropriate levels of vitamins and micronutrients to ensure that patients meet their nutritional requirements. People on a VLCD consume about 800 calories per day or less (150).

VLCD formulas are not the same as the meal replacements sold at grocery stores or pharmacies, which are meant to substitute for one or two meals a day. Over-the-counter meal replacements such as bars, entrees, or shakes should account for only part of one's daily calories. There is a good amount of evidence, including a recent meta-analysis, that supports the use of meal replacements for weight loss and maintenance (151).

When used under proper medical supervision, VLCDs may produce significant short-term weight loss in patients who are moderately to extremely obese. VLCDs should be part of a comprehensive weight-loss treatment program that includes behavioral therapy, nutrition counseling, and physical activity. Additionally, long-term maintenance of weight lost with VLCDs is poor and no better than other forms of obesity treatment. Incorporation of behavioral therapy and physical activity in VLCD treatment programs seems to improve weight-loss maintenance (149).

Some of the risks of following an overly restrictive diet include:

◆ Increased risk of malnutrition
◆ Poor energy and inability to complete the essential fitness program
◆ A behavioral "pendulum" swing—an inability to reintroduce "forbidden foods" in a moderate manner
◆ Many patients on a VLCD for 4 to 16 weeks report minor side effects such as fatigue, constipation, nausea, or diarrhea. The most common serious side effect is gallstone formation. People who are obese, especially women, are at a higher risk of getting gallstones, and they are even more common during rapid weight loss (151).

Fitness professionals should discourage overly restrictive programs advocating less than 1,000 to 1,200 calories per day, and support safe, maintainable weight loss by means of more healthful eating, smaller portions, and increased activity.

Is Consuming a High-Protein Diet Superior for Muscle Gain?

The body needs the correct amount of protein, carbohydrate, and fat to grow, maintain, and repair itself, including the growth of lean body mass. Amino acids, the component blocks of proteins, are used as building materials for the body. Whether "building" a hormone, an antibody, an enzyme, or a biceps muscle, the body relies on its reserve of amino acids to build proteins as needed. Resistance training, and to a certain extent all exercise, increases the body's need for repair material. Therefore, an active individual needs more protein than a sedentary individual. Although gym lore places recommendations as high as 2 grams of protein per pound of body weight, the scientifically based recommendation for strength athletes range from 0.5 to 0.8 grams of protein per pound (1.2 to 1.7 g per kg) (56).

Why do bodybuilders think they need massive amounts of protein? Perhaps this legend derives from the fact that many ferociously strong animals are carnivores, or perhaps it is as simple as the association between muscle and the material from which muscle is made. Regardless, the right amount of protein (and the obligatory resistance training) will support hypertrophy, and an excess of protein above total calorie needs will be stored as body fat.

SUMMARY

Personal trainers are in an excellent position to "demystify" the world of nutrition and exercise for weight loss. By using academic resources and authoritative recommendations from credentialed sources, personal trainers can educate their clients and empower them to make healthful behavior changes. This chapter addresses some of the more common myths heard in exercise environments, but tomorrow will bring new myths and fads. It is the responsibility of the health and fitness professional to read current research, investigate and dispel new falsehoods as they develop, and help "digest" the science for their clients.

REFERENCES

1. *Webster's Ninth New Collegiate Dictionary*. Springfield, MA: Merriam-Webster Inc; 1991.
2. Sass C, Eickhoff-Shemek JM, Manore MM, Kruskall, LJ. Crossing the line: understanding the scope of practice between registered dietitians and health/fitness professionals. *ACSM Health Fitness J*. 2007;11(3):12-19.
3. Wang Y, Beydoun MA. The obesity epidemic in the United States—gender, age, socioeconomic, racial/ethnic, and geographic characteristics: a systematic review and meta-regression analysis. *Epidemiol Rev*. 2007;29:6-28.
4. [No authors listed] Clinical guidelines on the identification, evaluation, and treatment of overweight and obesity in adults—the evidence report. National Institutes of Health [published correction appears in *Obes Res* 1998;6(6):464]. *Obes Res*. 1998;6(Suppl 2):51S-209S.
5. Walsh MF, Flynn TJ. A 54-month evaluation of a popular very low calorie diet program. *J Fam Pract*. 1995;41(3):231-236.
6. [No authors listed] Position of the American Dietetic Association: weight management. *J Am Diet Assoc*. 1997;97(1):71-74.
7. Faires VM. *Thermodynamics*. New York, NY: Macmillan; 1967.
8. Jensen MD. Diet effects on fatty acid metabolism in lean and obese humans. *Am J Clin Nutr*. 1998;67(3 Suppl):531S-4S.
9. Agricultural Research Service. Fat intake continues to drop; veggies, fruits still low in the US diet. *Res News*. 1996.
10. Levine JA. Measurement of energy expenditure. *Public Health Nutr*. 2005;8(7A):1123-1132.
11. Facts About Thyroid Disease (2005). Available at http://www.aace.com/public/awareness/tam/2005/pdfs/thyroid_disease_fact_sheet.pdf. Accessed October 31, 2010.
12. American Diabetes Association—Diabetes Statistics (2007). Available at http://www.diabetes.org/diabetes-basics/diabetes-statistics/. Accessed October 31, 2010.
13. Dickerson RN, Roth-Yousey L. Medication effects on metabolic rate: a systematic review (part 1). *J Am Diet Assoc*. 2005;105:835-843.
14. Dickerson RN, Roth-Yousey L, Medication effects on metabolic rate: a systematic review (part 2). *J Am Diet Assoc*. 2005;105:1002-1009.
15. Mole PA. Impact of energy intake and exercise on resting metabolic rate. *Sports Med*. 1990;10(2):72-87.

16. Thompson J, Manore MM. Predicted and measured resting metabolic rate of male and female endurance athletes. *J Am Diet Assoc*. 1996;96(1):30-34.
17. Speakman JR, Westerterp KR. Associations between energy demands, physical activity, and body composition in adult humans between 18 and 96 y of age. *Am J Clin Nutr*. 2010;92(4):826-834.
18. Shils ME, Young VR. *Modern Nutrition in Health and Disease*. 7th ed. Philadelphia, PA: Lea & Febiger; 1988.
19. Rose WC, Haines WJ, Warner DT. The amino acid requirements of man. V. The role of lysine, arginine, and tryptophan. *J Biol Chem*. 1954;206:421-430.
20. Martineau A, Lecavalier L, Falardeau P, Chiasson, JL. Simultaneous determination of glucose turnover, alanine turnover, and gluconeogenesis in human using a double stable-isotope-labeled tracer infusion and gas chromatography-mass spectrometry analysis. *Anal Biochem*. 1985;151(2):495-503.
21. Berdanier CD. *Advanced Nutrition: Macronutrients*. Boca Raton, FL: CRC Press; 1995.
22. Block RJ, Mitchell HH. The correlation of the amino acid composition of proteins with their nutritive value. *Nutr Abstr Rev*. 1946;16:249-278.
23. Tarnopolsky MA, Atkinson SA, MacDougall JD, Chesley A, Phillip S, Schwarcz HP. Evaluation of protein requirements for trained strength athletes. *J Appl Physiol*. 1992;73(5):1986-1995.
24. Lemon PW, Tarnolpolsky MA, MacDougall JD, Atkinson SA. Protein requirements and muscle mass/strength changes during intensive training in novice bodybuilders. *J Appl Physiol*. 1992;73(2):767-775.
25. Keul J. The relationship between circulation and metabolism during exercise. *Med Sci Sports*. 1973;5:209-219.
26. Keul J, Doll E, Keppler D. *Energy Metabolism of Human Muscle*. Baltimore, MD: University Park Press; 1972.
27. Wahlberg JL, Leidy MK, Sturgill DJ, Hinkle DE, Ritchey SJ, Sebolt DR. Macronutrient content of a hypoenergy diet affects nitrogen retention and muscle function in weight lifters. *Int J Sports Med*. 1988;9(4):261-266.
28. Piatti PM, Monti F, Fermo I, et al. Hypocaloric high-protein diet improves glucose oxidation and spares lean body mass: comparison to hypocaloric high-carbohydrate diet. *Metabolism*. 1994;43(12):1481-1487.

29. Ruderman NB. Muscle amino acid metabolism and gluconeogenesis. *Annu Rev Med.* 1975;26:245-258.

30. Harper AE, Miller RH, Block KP. Branched-chain amino acid metabolism. *Annu Rev Nutr.* 1984;4:409-454.

31. Hood DA, Terjung RL. Amino acid metabolism during exercise and following endurance training. *Sports Med.* 1990;9(1):23-35.

32. Ahlborg G, Felig P, Hagenfeldt L, Hendler R, Wahren J. Substrate turnover during prolonged exercise in man. Splanchnic and leg metabolism of glucose, free fatty acids, and amino acids. *J Clin Invest.* 1974;53(4):1080-1090.

33. Lemon PW, Mullin JP. Effect of initial muscle glycogen levels on protein catabolism during exercise. *J Appl Physiol.* 1980;48(4):624-629.

34. White TP, Brooks GA. [U-14C]glucose, -alanine, and -leucine oxidation in rats at rest and two intensities of running. *Am J Physiol.* 1981;240(2):E155-165.

35. Knapik J, Meredith C, Jones B, Fielding R, Young V, Evans W. Leucine metabolism during fasting and exercise. *J Appl Physiol.* 1991;70(1):43-47.

36. Young VR. Metabolic and nutritional aspects of physical exercise. *Fed Proc.* 1985;44:341.

37. Allison JB, Bird JC. Elimination of nitrogen from the body. In: Munro HN, Allison JB, eds. *Mammalian Protein Metabolism*, Vol 1. New York, NY: Academic Press; 1964. 483-412.

38. Munro HN. Historical introduction: the origin and growth of our present concepts of protein metabolism. In: Munro HN, Allison JB, eds. *Mammalian Protein Metabolism*, Vol 1. New York, NY: Academic Press; 1964.

39. Waterlow JC, Garlick PJ, Millward DJ. *Protein Turnover in Mammalian Tissues and in the Whole Body.* New York, NY: North-Holland; 1978.

40. Kurzer MS, Calloway DH. Nitrate and nitrogen balances in men. *Am J Clin Nutr.* 1981;34(7):1305-1313.

41. Minghelli G, Schutz Y, Charbonnier A, Whitehead R, Jéquier E. Twenty-four-hour energy expenditure and basal metabolic rate measured in a whole-body indirect calorimeter in Gambian men. *Am J Clin Nutr.* 1990;51(4):563-570.

42. Spruce N. Plateaus and energy expenditure. Increased difficulty in attending fat or weight loss goals in healthy subjects. *J Natl Intramural Recreat Sports Assoc.* 1997;22(1):24-28.

43. Spiller GA, Jensen CD, Pattison TS, Chuck CS, Whittam JH, Scala J. Effect of protein dose on serum glucose and insulin response to sugars. *Am J Clin Nutr.* 1987;46(3):474-480.

44. Zawadzki KM, Yaspelkis BB 3rd, Ivy JL. Carbohydrate-protein complex increases the rate of muscle glycogen storage after exercise. *J Appl Physiol.* 1992;72(5):1854-1859.

45. Roy BD, Tarnopolsky MA. Influence of differing macronutrient intakes on muscle glycogen resynthesis after resistance exercise. *J Appl Physiol.* 1998;84(3):890-896.

46. Ziegenfuss TN, Landis J. Protein. In: Antonio J, Kalman D, Stout J, Greenwood M, Willoughby D, Haff G, eds. *Essentials of Sports Nutrition and Supplements.* Totowa NJ: Humana Press; 2008:251-266.

47. Anderson GH, Li ET, Glanville NT. Brain mechanisms and the quantitative and qualitative aspects of food intake. *Brain Res Bull.* 1984;12(2):167-173.

48. Gellebter AA. Effects of equicaloric loads of protein, fat and carbohydrate on food intake in the rat and man. *Physiol Behav.* 1979;22:267-273.

49. Van Zeggeren A, Li ET. Food intake and choice in lean and obese Zucker rats after intragastric carbohydrate preloads. *J Nutr.* 1990;120(3):309-316.

50. Li ET, Anderson GH. Meal composition influences subsequent food selection in the young rat. *Physiol Behav.* 1982;29(5):779-783.

51. Booth DA, Chase A, Campbell AT. Relative effectiveness of protein in the late stages of appetite suppression in man. *Physiol Behav.* 1970;5(11):1299-1302.

52. Barkeling B, Rössner S, Björvell H. Effects of a high-protein meal (meat) and a high-carbohydrate meal (vegetarian) on satiety measured by automated computerized monitoring of subsequent food intake, motivation to eat and food preferences. *Int J Obes.* 1990;14(9):743-751.

53. Wurtman RJ, Wurtman JJ. Carbohydrate craving, obesity and brain serotonin. *Appetite.* 1986;7(Suppl):99-103.

54. Drewnoski A, Oomura Y, Tarui S, Inoue S, Shmazu T, eds. *Progress in Obesity Research.* London: John Libbey; 1990.

55. Manore MM. Exercise and the Institute of Medicine recommendations for nutrition. *Curr Sports Med Rep.* 2005;4(4):193-198.

56. Rodriguez NR, DiMarco NM, Langley S; American Dietetic Association; Dietitians of Canada; American College of Sports Medicine. Position of the American Dietetic Association, Dietitians of Canada, and the American College of Sports Medicine: Nutrition and athletic performance. *J Am Diet Assoc.* 2009;109(3):509-527.

57. Lichtenstein AH, Kennedy E, Barrier P, et al. Dietary fat consumption and health. *Nutr Rev.* 1998;56(5 pt 2):S3-S19.

58. Hu FB, Stampfer MJ, Manson JE, et al. Dietary fat intake and the risk of coronary heart disease in women. *N Engl J Med.* 1997;337(21):1491-1499.

59. Kerstetter JE, Cas Dm, Mitnick ME, et al. Increased circulating concentrations of parathyroid hormone in healthy, young women consuming a protein restricted diet. *Am J Clin Nutr.* 1997;66:1188-1196.

60. Kerstetter JE, O'Brien KO, Insogna KI. Dietary protein affects intestinal calcium absorption. *Am J Clin Nutr.* 1998;68:859-865.

61. Kerstetter JE, Svastisalee CM, Caseria DM, Mitnick ME, Insogna KL. A threshold for low-protein-diet-induced elevations in parathyroid hormone. *Am J Clin Nutr.* 2000;72:168-173.

62. Manore M, Meyer N, Thompson J. *Sports Nutrition for Health and Performance.* 2nd ed. Champlaign, IL: Human Kinetics; 2009.

63. Smolin LA, Grosvenor MB. *Nutrition Science and Applications.* Orlando, FL: Saunders College Publishing; 1994.

64. Rolls BJ, Hill JO. *Carbohydrate and Weight Management.* Washington, DC: ILSI Press; 1998.

65. Jenkindrup AF, Jentjens R. Oxidation of carbohydrate feedings during prolonged exercise: current thoughts, guidelines and directions for future research. *Sports Med.* 2000;29(6):407-464.

66. Turcoatte LP, Hespel PJ, Graham TE, Richter EA. Impaired plasma FFA oxidation imposed by extreme CHO deficiency in contracting rat skeletal muscle. *J Appl Physiol.* 1994;77(2):517-525.

67. Sahlin K, Katz A, Broberg S. Tricarboxylic acid cycle intermediates in human muscle during prolonged exercise. *Am J Physiol.* 1990;259(5 Pt 1):C834-841.

68. Jenkins DJ, Vuksan V, Kendall CW, et al. Physiological effects of resistant starches on fecal bulk, short chain fatty acids, blood lipids and glycemic index. *J Am Coll Nutr.* 1998;17(6):609-616.

69. Lewis SJ, Heaton KW. Increasing butyrate concentration in the distal colon by accelerating intestinal transit. *Gut.* 1997;41(2):245-251.

70. Järvi AE, Karlström BE, Granfeldt YE, Björck IM, Vessby BO, Asp NG. The influence of food structure on postprandial metabolism in patients with non-insulin-dependent diabetes mellitus. *Am J Clin Nutr.* 1995;61(4):837-842.

71. Anderson JW, Smith BM, Gustafson NJ. Health benefits and practical aspects of high-fiber diets. *Am J Clin Nutr.* 1994;59(5 Suppl):1242S-1247S.

72. Wolk A, Manson JE, Stampfer MJ, et al. Long-term intake of dietary fiber and decreased risk of coronary heart disease among women. *JAMA.* 1999;281(21):1998-2004.

73. Ryan-Harshman M, Aldoori W. New dietary reference intakes for macronutrients and fibre. *Can Fam Physician.* 2006;52:177-179.

74. Aldoori WH, Giovanucci EL, Rockett HR, Sampson L, Rimm EB, Willett WC. A prospective study of dietary fiber types and symptomatic diverticular disease in men. *J Nutr.* 1998;128(4):714-719.

75. Rimm EB, Ascherio A, Giovanucci E, Spiegelman D, Stampfer MJ, Willett WC. Vegetable, fruit, and cereal fiber intake and risk of coronary heart disease among men. *JAMA.* 1996;275(6):447-451.

76. Anderson JW, Smith BM, Gustafson NJ. Health benefits and practical aspects of high-fiber diets. *Am J Clin Nutr.* 1994;59(5 Suppl):1242S-1247S.

77. Howe GR, Benito E, Castelleto R, et al. Dietary intake of fiber and decreased risk of cancers of the colon and rectum: evidence from the combined analysis of 13 case-control studies. *J Natl Cancer Inst.* 1992;84(24):1887-1896.

78. Fernstrom JD, Miller GD. *Appetite and Body Weight Regulation.* Boca Raton, FL: CRC Press; 1994.

79. Romijn JA, Coyle EF, Sidossis LS, et al. Regulation of endogenous fat and carbohydrate metabolism in relation to exercise intensity and duration. *Am J Physiol.* 1993;265(3 Pt 1):E380-391.

80. Berning JR, Steen SN. *Nutrition for Sport and Exercise.* Gaithersburg, MD: Aspen Publishers; 1998.

81. McArdle WD, Katch FI, Katch VL. *Sports and Exercise Nutrition.* 3rd ed. Baltimore MD: Lippincott Williams & Wilkins; 2008.

82. Phinney SD, Bistrian BR, Evans WJ, Gervino E, Blackburn GL. The human metabolic response to chronic ketosis without caloric restriction: preservation of submaximal exercise capability with reduced carbohydrate oxidation. *Metabolism.* 1983;32:769-776.

83. Lambert EV, Speechly DP, Dennis SC, Noakes TD. Enhanced endurance in trained cyclists during moderate intensity exercise following 2 weeks adaptation to a high-fat diet. *Eur J Appl Physiol Occup Physiol.* 1994;69(4):287-293.

84. Pendergast DR, Horvath PJ, Leddy JJ, Venkatraman JT. The role of dietary fat on performance, metabolism, and health. *Am J Sports Med.* 1996;24(6 Suppl):S53-58.

85. Fallowfield JL, Williams C. Carbohydrate intake and recovery from prolonged exercise. *Int J Sports Nutr.* 1993;3(2):150-164.

86. Simonsen JC, Sherman WM, Lamb DR, Dernbach AR, Doyle JA, Strauss R. Dietary carbohydrate, muscle glycogen, and power output during rowing training. *J Appl Physiol.* 1991;70(4):1500-1505.

87. Lambert EV, Hawley JA, Goedecke J, Noakes TD, Dennis SC. Nutritional strategies for promoting fat utilization and delaying the onset of fatigue during prolonged exercise. *J Sports Sci.* 1997;15(3):315-324.

88. Langfort J, Zarzeczny R, Pilis W, Nazar K, Kaciuba-Uscitko H. The effect of a low-carbohydrate diet on performance, hormonal and metabolic responses to a 30-s bout of supramaximal exercise. *Eur J Appl Physiol Occup Physiol.* 1997;76(2):128-133.

89. Balsom PD, Gaitanos GC, Söderlund K, Ekblom B. High-intensity exercise and muscle glycogen availability in humans. *Acta Physiol Scand.* 1999;165(4):337-345.

90. Helge JW, Richter EA, Kiens B. Interaction of training and diet on metabolism and endurance during exercise in man. *J Physiol (Lond).* 1996;492(Pt 1):293-306.

91. Sherman WM, Brodowicz G, Wright DA, Allen WK, Simonsen J, Dernbach A. Effects of 4 h preexercise carbohydrate feedings on cycling performance. *Med Sci Sports Exerc.* 1989;21:598-604.

92. Karlsson J, Saltin B. Diet, muscle glycogen, and endurance performance. *J Appl Physiol.* 1971;31:203-206.

93. Sherman WM, Costill DL, Fink WJ, Miller JM. The effect of exercise and diet manipulation on muscle glycogen and its subsequent use during performance. *Int J Sports Med.* 1981;2(2):114-118.

94. Coyle EF, Hagberg JM, Hurley BF, Martin WH, Ehsani AA, Holloszy JO. Carbohydrate feeding during prolonged strenuous exercise can delay fatigue. *J Appl Physiol.* 1983;55(1 Pt 1):230-235.

95. Coyle EF, Coggan AR, Hemmert WK, Ivy JL. Muscle glycogen utilization during prolonged strenuous exercise when fed carbohydrate. *J Appl Physiol.* 1986;61(1):165-172.

96. Wilber RL, Moffatt RJ. Influence of carbohydrate ingestion on blood glucose and performance in runners. *Int J Sports Nutr.* 1992;2(4):317-327.

97. Convertino VA, Armstrong LE, Coyle EF, et al. American College of Sports Medicine position stand: exercise and fluid replacement. *Med Sci Sports Exerc.* 1996;28:i-vii.

98. Below PR, Mora-Rodríguez R, González-Alonso J, Coyle EF. Fluid and carbohydrate ingestion independently improve performance during 1 h of intense exercise. *Med Sci Sports Exerc.* 1995;27(2):200-210.

99. Ivy JL, Lee MC, Broznick JT Jr, Reed MJ. Muscle glycogen storage after different amounts of carbohydrate ingestion. *J Appl Physiol.* 1988;65(5):2018-2023.

100. Liljeberg HG, Akerberg AK, Björck IM. Effect of the glycemic index and content of indigestible carbohydrates of cereal-based breakfast meals on glucose tolerance at lunch in healthy subjects. *Am J Clin Nutr.* 1999;69(4):647-655.

101. Raben A, Tagliabue A, Christensen NJ, Madsen J, Holst JJ, Astrup A. Resistant starch: the effect on postprandial glycemia, hormonal response, and satiety. *Am J Clin Nutr.* 1994;60(4):544-551.

102. Raben A, Christensen NJ, Madsen J, Holst JJ, Astrup A. Decreased postprandial thermogenesis and fat oxidation but increased fullness after a high-fiber meal compared with a low-fiber meal. *Am J Clin Nutr.* 1994;59(6):1386-1394.

103. Yang MU, Van Itallie TB. Composition of weight lost during short-term weight reduction. Metabolic responses of obese subjects to starvation and low-calorie ketogenic and nonketogenic diets. *J Clin Invest.* 1976;58(3):722-730.

104. Karlsson J, Saltin B. Lactate, ATP, and CP in working muscles during exhaustive exercise in man. *J Appl Physiol.* 1970;29(5):596-602.

105. Shick SM, Wing RR, Klem ML, McGuire MT, Hill JO, Seagle H. Persons successful at long-term weight loss and maintenance

continue to consume a low-energy, low-fat diet. *J Am Diet Assoc.* 1998;98(4):408-413.

106. McDowell MA, Briefel RR, Alaimo K, et al. Energy intakes of persons ages 2 months and over in the United States: Third National Health and Nutrition Examination Survey, Phase 1, 1988-91. *Adv Data.* 1994;24(255):1-24.

107. Ernst ND, Obarzanek E, Clark MB, Briefel RR, Brown CD, Donato K. Cardiovascular health risks related to overweight. *J Am Diet Assoc.* 1997;97(7 Suppl):S47-51.

108. US Department of Agriculture, Center for Nutrition Policy and Promotion. *Nutrient Content of the US Food Supply, 1909-94. Home Economics Research Report No. 53.* Washington, DC: US Department of Agriculture, Center for Nutrition Policy and Promotion; 1997.

109. US Department of Health and Human Services. *Physical Activity and Health: A Report of the Surgeon General.* Atlanta, GA: Centers for Disease Control and Prevention, 1996.

110. Lambert E, Bohlmann IMT, Cowling K. Physical activity for health: understanding the epidemiological evidence for risk benefits. *Int J Sports Med.* 2001;1:(5).

111. Flegal KM, Carroll MD, Kuczmarski RJ, Johnson CL. Overweight and obesity in the United States: prevalence and trends, 1960-1994. *Int J Obes Relat Metab Disord.* 1998;22(1):39-47.

112. Ogden CL, Carroll MD, McDowell MA, Flegal KM. *Obesity Among Adults in the United States—No Statistically Significant Change Since 2003-2004. NCHS Data Brief No 1.* Hyattsville, MD: National Center for Health Statistics; 2007.

113. Whitney EN, Rolfes SR. *Understanding Nutrition.* St. Paul, MN: West Publishing; 1996.

114. Groff JL, Gropper SS, Hunt SM. *Advanced Nutrition and Human Metabolism.* St. Paul, MN: West Publishing; 1995.

115. Simopoulos AP. Omega-3 fatty acids in health and disease and in growth and development. *Am J Clin Nutr.* 1991;54(3):438-463.

116. Simopoulos AP. Omega-3 fatty acids in the prevention-management of cardiovascular disease. *Can J Physiol Pharmacol.* 1997;75(3):234-239.

117. Lichtenstein AH, Ausman LM, Jalbert SM, Schaefer EJ. Effects of different forms of dietary hydrogenated fats on serum lipoprotein cholesterol levels [published correction appears in *N Engl J Med.* 1999;341(11):856]. *N Engl J Med.* 1999;340(25):1933-1940.

118. Tatò F. Trans-fatty acids in the diet: a coronary risk factor? *Eur J Med Res.* 1995;1(2):118-122.

119. Ascherio A, Willett WC. Health effects of trans fatty acids. *Am J Clin Nutr.* 1997;66(4 Suppl):1006S-1010S.

120. [NRC] National Research Council. *Recommended Dietary Allowances.* 10th ed. Washington, DC: National Academy Press; 1989.

121. Lissner L, Levitsky DA, Strupp BJ, Kalkwarf HJ, Roe DA. Dietary fat and the regulation of energy intake in human subjects. *Am J Clin Nutr.* 1987;46(6):886-892.

122. Lissner L, Heitmann BL. The dietary fat:carbohydrate ratio in relation to body weight. *Curr Opin Lipidol.* 1995;6(1):8-13.

123. Horton TJ, Drougas H, Reed GW, Peters JC, Hill JO. Fat and carbohydrate overfeeding in humans: different effects on energy storage. *Am J Clin Nutr.* 1995;62(1):19-29.

124. Leveille GA, Cloutier PF. Isocaloric diets: effects of dietary changes. *Am J Clin Nutr.* 1987;45(1 Suppl):158-163.

125. Stubbs RJ, Ritz P, Coward WA, Prentice AM. Covert manipulation of the ratio of dietary fat to carbohydrate and energy density: effect on food intake and energy balance in free-living men eating ad libitum. *Am J Clin Nutr.* 1995;62(2):330-337.

126. Jeukendrup AE, Saris WH, Schrauwen P, Brouns F, Wagenmakers AJ. Metabolic availability of medium-chain triglycerides coingested with carbohydrates during prolonged exercise. *J Appl Physiol.* 1995;79(3):756-762.

127. Van Zyl CG, Lambert EV, Hawley JA, Noakes TD, Dennis SC. Effects of medium-chain triglyceride ingestion on fuel metabolism and cycling performance. *J Appl Physiol.* 1996;80(6):2217-2225.

128. Misell LM, Lagomarcino ND, Schuster V, Kern M. Chronic medium-chain triacylglycerol consumption and endurance performance in trained runners. *J Sports Med Phys Fitness.* 2001;41(2):210-215.

129. Horowitz JF, Mora-Rodriguez R, Byerley LO, Coyle EF. Preexercise medium chain triglyceride ingestion does not alter muscle glycogen use during exercise. *J Appl Physiol.* 2000;88(1):219-225.

130. Goedecke JH, Clarke VR, Noakes TD, Lambert EV. The effects of medium-chain triacylglycerol and carbohydrate ingestion on ultra-endurance exercise performance. *Int J Sport Nutr. Exerc Metab.* 2005;15(1):15-27.

131. Shepherd PR, Kahn BB. Glucose transporters and insulin action—implications for insulin resistance and diabetes mellitus. *N Engl J Med.* 1999;341(4):248-257.

132. Buemann B, Tremblay A. Effects of exercise training on abdominal obesity and related metabolic complications. *Sports Med.* 1996;21(3):191-212.

133. Pandolfi C, Pellegrini L, Sbalzarini G, Mercantini F. Obesity and insulin resistance [in Italian]. *Minerva Med.* 1994;85(2):167-171.

134. Bloomgarden ZT. Insulin resistance: current concepts. *Clin Ther.* 1998;20(2):216-231.

135. Schraer CD, Risica PM, Ebbesson SO, Go OT, Howard BV, Mayer AM. Low fasting insulin levels in Eskimos compared to American Indians: are Eskimos less insulin resistant? *Int J Circumpolar Health.* 1999;58(4):272-280.

136. Beck-Nielsen H. General characteristics of the insulin resistance syndrome: prevalence and heritability. European Group for the Study of Insulin Resistance (EGIR). *Drugs.* 1999;58(Suppl 1):7-10.

137. Pi-Sunyer FX. Medical hazards of obesity. *Ann Intern Med.* 1993;119(7 Pt 2):655-660.

138. Grundy SM. Multifactorial causation of obesity: implications for prevention. *Am J Clin Nutr.* 1998;67(3 0Suppl):563S-569S.

139. Vaag A. On the pathophysiology of late onset non-insulin dependent diabetes mellitus. Current controversies and new insights. *Dan Med Bull.* 1999;46(3):197-234.

140. Parekh PI, Petro AE, Tiller JM, Feinglos MN, Surwit RS. Reversal of diet-induced obesity and diabetes in C57BL/6J mice. *Metabolism.* 1998;47(9):1089-1096.

141. Barnard RJ, Ugianskis EJ, Martin DA, Inkeles SB. Role of diet and exercise in the management of hyperinsulinemia and associated atherosclerotic risk factors. *Am J Cardiol.* 1992;69(5):440-444.

142. Wolinsky I, Hickson JF. *Nutrition in Exercise and Sport.* Boca Raton, FL: CRC Press; 1994.

143. Walsh RM, Noakes TD, Hawkey JA, Dennis SC. Impaired high-intensity cycling performance time at low levels of dehydration. *Int J Sports Med.* 1994;15(7):392-398.

144. Casa DJ, Clarkson PM, Roberts WO. American College of Sports Medicine roundtable on hydration and physical activity: consensus statements. *Curr Sports Med Rep.* 2005;4(3):115-127.

145. Cheuvront SN, Carter R III, Sawka MN. Fluid balance and endurance exercise performance. *Curr Sports Med Rep.* 2003;2(4):202-208.

146. Institute of Medicine. Water. In: *Dietary Reference Intakes for Water, Sodium, Chloride, Potassium and Sulfate*. Washington, DC: National Academy Press; 2005:73-185.

147. Dietary Guidelines for Guidelines for Americans 2005. US Department of Health and Human Services. US Department of Agriculture. Available at http://www.cnpp.usda.gov/Publications/DietaryGuidelines/2005/2005DGPolicyDocument.pdf. Accessed October 31, 2010.

148. Dansinger ML, Gleason JA, Griffith JL, Selker HP, Schaefer EJ. Comparison of Atkins, Ornish, Weight Watchers, and Zone diets for weight loss and heart disease risk reduction: a randomized trial. *JAMA.* 2005;293(1):43-53.

149. Foster D, Wyatt HR, Hill JO, et al. A randomized trial of a low carbohydrate diet for obesity. *N Engl J Med.* 2003;348(21) 2082-2090.

150. [No authors listed] Very low-calorie diets. National Task Force on the Prevention and Treatment of Obesity, National Institutes of Health. *JAMA.* 1993;270(8):967-974.

151. Heymsfield SB, van Mierlo CAJ, van der Knaap HCM, Heo M, Frier HI. Weight management using a meal replacement strategy: meta and pooling analysis from six studies. *Int J Obes Relat Metab Disord.* 2003;27:537-549.

Supplementation

OBJECTIVES

After studying this chapter, you will be able to:

✔ Define what dietary supplements are and describe the various classes and uses of them.

✔ Understand basic supplemental recommendations for optimizing health.

✔ Respond to questions about dietary supplements based on objective, scientific facts.

✔ Define the term *ergogenic* and common substances used to enhance performance.

Dietary Supplements

Introduction to Supplementation

During the first half of the twentieth century, the discovery that vitamins are essential components of food (along with tremendous growth in the understanding of human nutrient needs) set the foundation for the development of dietary supplements containing vitamins and minerals.

The traditional reason for use of a dietary supplement is to provide the body with nutrients that might not be supplied adequately by a person's typical diet. Around the middle of the twentieth century, the use of dietary supplements was primarily in the form of a "one-a-day" type of vitamin-mineral supplement. Although this continues to be the most commonly used type, the rapid growth of the dietary supplement industry has led to the development of a great variety of different types of supplements. Today, dietary supplements are much more than a low-dosage vitamin-mineral pill taken by a small percentage of the population. Contemporary dietary supplements often contain numerous chemical compounds other than nutrients, and people take dietary supplements for a wide variety of reasons other than meeting nutrient needs.

© iIolab/ShutterStock, Inc.

The popularity of dietary supplements has grown steadily in the United States, with sales in the supplement industry booming during the 1990s. Estimates put total sales at $3.3 billion for 1990 (1), growing to more than $100 billion in 2008 (2). Associated with this rapid growth, the Dietary Supplement Health and Education Act (DSHEA) was passed in 1994, providing a detailed legal definition of the term *dietary supplement*. These regulations for dietary supplements are separate from the regulations for foods and drugs (3).

What Are Dietary Supplements?

Dietary supplement A substance that completes or makes an addition to daily dietary intake.

The DSHEA defines **dietary supplements** as products (other than tobacco) intended to supplement the diet and meet at least one of the following criteria:

- Contains one or more of the following: vitamin; mineral; herb or other botanical; amino acid; dietary substance to supplement the diet by increasing the total dietary intake; concentrate, metabolite, constituent, or extract; or combination of any of the previously described ingredients.
- Intended for ingestion in a tablet, capsule, powder, softgel, gelcap, or liquid form.
- Labeled as a dietary supplement.
- Cannot be represented for use as a conventional food or as a sole item of a meal or diet.
- Cannot include an article that is approved as a drug or biologic.

Because the Food and Drug Administration (FDA) does not need to approve dietary supplements before being sold and instead the sole responsibility for determining the safety and effectiveness of a dietary supplement falls on the shoulders of the company that manufactures and markets it, almost anything that is not already classified as a drug can be put into a pill, capsule, or powder form and sold as a dietary supplement (4).

Rationale for the Use of Dietary Supplements

People take dietary supplements for a variety of reasons. Some take them to help prevent or treat a specific health problem. Others take dietary supplements in hopes of enhancing physical or mental performance, altering body composition, stimulating metabolism, controlling appetite, or slowing or reversing age-related changes in body

© Eky Studio/ShutterStock, Inc.

Did You Know?

Key Reasons for Taking Dietary Supplements
1. Low-energy weight-loss diet
2. Low-energy diet in elderly
3. Chronic disease prevention (e.g., calcium to prevent osteoporosis)
4. Special needs such as pregnancy and lactation
5. Extreme activity demands
6. Enhance recovery from exercise
7. Maintain normal immune function
8. Sport training
9. Before or after surgery
10. Therapeutic nutrition for specific health problems
11. Postbariatric surgery nutrition
12. Drug-induced increase in nutrient need (e.g., ibuprofen increases folate need)

structure and function. The use of dietary supplements that contain a broad spectrum of micronutrients (in low to moderate doses) can be especially beneficial for individuals consuming diets that do not meet their needs for all nutrients (5,6). Various studies have reported that people taking a multivitamin supplement experience a reduced risk of chronic disease development (6). However, comprehensive reviews on the overall safety and effectiveness of dietary supplements emphasizes the limited quantity and quality of scientific studies pertaining to the health consequences of multivitamin-mineral supplementation and the need for more studies (7).

Additionally, there are specific groups of individuals who may have greater need for dietary supplements. For example, older individuals often do not make proper adjustments in their diets when energy needs decline with age. Although calorie needs generally drop with age, the need for protein, vitamins, and minerals does not decline (8,9). Another group that can benefit from supplemented nutrients is women who are pregnant or breastfeeding. However, because of the potential for supplement toxicity or interactions with prescribed medications, it is extremely important for these groups to seek guidance on supplementation from qualified health professionals (10). Thus, whatever the goal for using a dietary supplement, the considerations for appropriate use are similar.

© Eky Studio/ShutterStock, Inc.

Did You Know?

Common Reasons Why Diets Do Not Contain Adequate Nutrients:

Inadequate food intake (especially diets <1,200 calories per day)
Disordered eating patterns

- Consuming mostly "junk" (nutrient-deficient) foods
- Avoidance of foods from specific food groups
- Eating only one major meal a day
- Irregular eating patterns (low-calorie diet one day, high-calorie the next)
- Eating too much or too little protein or carbohydrate
- Food phobias and "picky" eating
- Financial limitations affecting access to a variety of wholesome foods

SUMMARY

Vitamins (and many minerals) are essential components of food and are required in very small amounts by the body. The popularity of dietary supplements has increased dramatically in recent years. In 1994 the DSHEA was enacted by Congress, providing a detailed legal definition of the term *dietary supplement*. The U.S. FDA states that a dietary supplement is, basically, a labeled pill, capsule, tablet, or liquid intended to supplement the diet and contains one or more vitamins, minerals, botanicals, or amino acids. Almost anything not already classified as a drug can be sold as a dietary supplement. Taking low-to-moderate dose, broad-spectrum vitamin-mineral supplements is beneficial, especially for those whose diets do not meet all micronutrient requirements. There is evidence for a reduced risk of chronic diseases in people taking multivitamin supplements; however, this remains controversial and experts recommend additional research to clarify the relationships between supplements and diseases.

Supplementation Guidelines

General Guidelines for Responsible Use of Nutritional Dietary Supplements

Dietary supplements contain both natural and synthetic substances. Although dietary supplements are perceived to be safer than pharmaceutical drugs, that is not always the case as healthy people have died as a direct result of complications from taking dietary supplements. This section will give common guidelines for determining what quantity of a supplemental nutrient is likely to be adequate, safe, and beneficial and how much may be potentially excessive or detrimental to health.

Dietary Reference Intakes

In the United States, the Food and Nutrition Board (FNB) of the Institute of Medicine, National Academy of Sciences periodically reviews the current research on nutrient needs to provide authoritative, updated recommendations for nutrient intake. In 1997, the FNB released the first in a series of publications called "Dietary Reference Intakes" with the final volumes published in 2005 Table 18.1.

Dietary reference intake (DRI) values for nutrients provide good guidelines for what constitutes an adequate intake of a nutrient. For many nutrients, values also have been set for the amount considered to be excessive and potentially harmful. The DRIs are designed to estimate the nutrient needs of healthy people in various age groups and of both sexes. The values also are adjusted for the special needs of women during pregnancy and lactation.

Table 18.2 describes the DRI terminology used by the FNB. The DRIs most commonly used to evaluate or plan diets for individuals are the recommended dietary allowance (RDA), adequate intake (AI), and tolerable upper intake level (UL) values (described below) (17). The overall goal in designing a healthy diet is to provide nutrients at levels that represent a high probability of adequate intake (meeting RDA or AI levels) and also a low probability of excessive intake (not exceeding UL values).

TABLE 18.1 Dietary Reference Intake Publications	
Nutrients Reviewed	**Year of Publication**
Calcium, phosphorus, magnesium, vitamin D, and fluoride	1997[11]
Thiamin, riboflavin, niacin, vitamin B_6, folate, vitamin B_{12}, pantothenic acid, biotin, and choline	1998[12]
Vitamin C, vitamin E, selenium, and carotenoids	2000[13]
Vitamin A, vitamin K, arsenic, boron, chromium, copper, iodine, iron, manganese, molybdenum, nickel, silicon, vanadium, and zinc	2002[14]
Energy, carbohydrate, fiber, fat, fatty acids, cholesterol, protein, and amino acids	2005[15]
Water, potassium, sodium, chloride, and sulphate	2005[16]

Dietary Reference Intake Values and Guidelines

Table 18.3 summarizes the currently established adult DRI values for vitamins and minerals, including UL values and possible signs of excess intake of a nutrient. Except for vitamin E and magnesium, the UL values are set for total intake of each nutrient from food and supplements. The ULs for vitamin E and magnesium are set for levels of intake from supplements or pharmacologic sources only and do not include dietary intake.

TABLE 18.2 Dietary Reference Intake Terminology

Term	Definition
Estimated Average Requirement (EAR)	The average daily nutrient intake level that is estimated to meet the requirement of half the healthy individuals who are in a particular life stage and gender group.
Recommended Dietary Allowance (RDA)	The average daily nutrient intake level that is sufficient to meet the nutrient requirement of nearly all (97–98%) healthy individuals who are in a particular life stage and gender group.
Adequate Intake (AI)	A recommended average daily nutrient intake level, based on observed (or experimentally determined) approximations or estimates of nutrient intake that are assumed to be adequate for a group (or groups) of healthy people. This measure is used when RDA cannot be determined.
Tolerable Upper Intake Level (UL)	The highest average daily nutrient intake level likely to pose no risk of adverse health affects to almost all individuals in a particular life stage and gender group. As intake increases above the UL, the potential risk of adverse health effects increases.

TABLE 18.3 Comparison of Dietary Reference Intake Values (for Adult Men and Women) and Daily Values for Micronutrients with the Tolerable Upper Intake Levels, Safe Upper Levels, and Guidance Levels[a]

Nutrient	RDA/AI (Men/Women) ages 31–50	Daily Value (Food Labels)	UL	SUL or Guidance Level	Selected Potential Effects of Excess Intake
Vitamin A (µg)	900/700	1,500 (5,000 IU)	3,000	1,500[c] (5,000 IU)	Liver damage, bone and joint pain, dry skin, loss of hair, headache, vomiting
β-carotene (mg)				7 (11,655 IU)	Increased risk of lung cancer in smokers and those heavily exposed to asbestos

(Continued)

© ilolab/ShutterStock, Inc.

TABLE 18.3	(Continued)

© ilolab/ShutterStock, Inc.

Nutrient	RDA/AI (Men/ Women) ages 31–50	Daily Value (Food Labels)	UL	SUL or Guidance Level	Selected Potential Effects of Excess Intake
Vitamin D (μg)	5^b	10 (400 IU)	50	25 (1,000 IU)	Calcification of brain and arteries, increased blood calcium, loss of appetite, nausea
Vitamin E (mg)	15	20 (30 IU)	1,000	540 (800 IU)	Deficient blood clotting
Vitamin K (μg)	$120/90^b$	80	–	$1,000^c$	Red blood cell damage or anemia, liver damage
Thiamin (B_1) (mg)	1.2/1.1	1.5	–	100^c	Headache, nausea, irritability, insomnia, rapid pulse, weakness (7,000+ mg dose)
Riboflavin (B_2) (mg)	1.3/1.1	1.7	–	40^c	Generally considered harmless; yellow discoloration of urine
Niacin (mg)	16/14	20	35	500^c	Liver damage, flushing, nausea, gastrointestinal problems
Vitamin B_6 (mg)	1.3	2	100	10	Neurologic problems, numbness and pain in limbs
Vitamin B_{12} (μg)	2.4	6	–	$2,000^c$	No reports of toxicity from oral ingestion
Folic acid (μg)	400	400	1,000	$1,000^c$	Masks vitamin B_{12} deficiency (which can cause neurologic problems)
Pantothenic acid (mg)	5^b	10	–	200^c	Diarrhea and gastrointestinal disturbance (10,000+ mg/day)
Biotin (μg)	30^b	300	–	900^c	No reports of toxicity from oral ingestion
Vitamin C (mg)	90/75	60	2,000	$1,000^c$	Nausea, diarrhea, kidney stones
Boron (mg)			20	9.6	Adverse effects on male and female reproductive systems

Nutrient	RDA/AI (Men/ Women) ages 31–50	Daily Value (Food Labels)	UL	SUL or Guidance Level	Selected Potential Effects of Excess Intake
Calcium (mg)	$1,000^b$	1,000	2,500	$1,500^c$	Nausea, constipation, kidney stones
Chromium (μg)	35^b	120	–	$10,000^c$	Potential adverse effects on liver and kidneys; picolinate form possibly mutagenic
Cobalt (mg)				1.4^c	Cardiotoxic effects; not appropriate in a dietary supplement except as vitamin B_{12}
Copper (μg)	900	2,000	10,000	10,000	Gastrointestinal distress, liver damage
Fluoride (mg)	$4/3^b$		10		Bone, kidney, muscle, and nerve damage; supplement only with professional guidance
Germanium				$zero^c$	Kidney toxin; should not be in a dietary supplement
Iodine (μg)	150	150	1,100	500^c	Elevated thyroid hormone concentration
Iron (mg)	8/18	18	45	17^c	Gastrointestinal distress, increased risk of heart disease, oxidative stress
Magnesium (mg)	420/320	400	350^d	400^c	Diarrhea
Manganese (mg)	$2.3/1.8^b$	2	11	4^c	Neurotoxicity
Molybdenum	45	75	2,000	$zero^c$	Goutlike symptoms, joint pains, increased uric acid
Nickel (μg)				260^c	Increased sensitivity of skin reaction to nickel in jewelry
Phosphorus (mg)	700	1,000	4,000	250^c	Alteration of parathyroid hormone levels, reduced bone mineral density
Potassium (mg)				$3,700^c$	Gastrointestinal damage

(Continued)

TABLE 18.3 (Continued)					
Nutrient	RDA/AI (Men/ Women) ages 31–50	Daily Value (Food Labels)	UL	SUL or Guidance Level	Selected Potential Effects of Excess Intake
Selenium (μg)	55	70	400	450	Nausea, diarrhea, fatigue, hair and nail loss
Silicon (mg)				700	Low toxicity, possibility of kidney stones
Vanadium (mg)			1.8	zero	Gastrointestinal irritation; fatigue
Zinc (mg)	11/8	15	40	25	Impaired immune function, low HDL-cholesterol

aFood and Nutrition Board, Institute of Medicine (U.S.). Dietary Reference Intake Tables. Available at [http://www4.nationalacademies.org/IOM/IOMHome.nsf/Pages/Food+and+Nutrition+Board].
bIndicates adequate intake (AI).
cIndicates guidance levels, set by the Expert Group on Vitamins and Minerals of the Food Standards Agency, United Kingdom. These are intended to be levels of daily intake of nutrients in dietary supplements that potentially susceptible individuals could take daily on a lifelong basis without medical supervision in reasonable safety. When the evidence base was considered inadequate to set an SUL, guidance levels were set based on limited data. SULs and guidance levels tend to be conservative, and it is possible that for some vitamins and minerals, greater amounts could be consumed for short periods without risk to health. The values presented are for a 60-kg (132-lb) adult. Consult the full publication for values expressed per kilogram of body weight. This FSA publication, *Safe Upper Levels for Vitamins and Minerals*, is available at: [http://www.foodstandards.gov.uk/multimedia/pdfs/vitmin2003.pdf].
dThe UL for magnesium represents intake specifically from pharmacologic agents and dietary supplements in addition to dietary intake.
RDA, recommended dietary allowance; *UL*, tolerable upper intake level; *AI*, adequate intake; *SUL*, safe upper level.

Even essential nutrients are potentially toxic at some level of intake. For some nutrients, the level of intake that causes serious adverse effects is not presently known. For others, the adverse effects of excess have been documented. The effects of some nutrients can be extremely serious. Among the vitamin category of nutrients, excess vitamin A, D, and B$_6$ can produce serious adverse effects and are commonly available in dietary supplement form. Excess vitamin A, for example, can cause birth defects when a woman is taking too much at conception and during early pregnancy (14). Vitamin D excess can result in the calcification of blood vessels and eventually damage the function of the kidneys, heart, and lungs (11). Excessive intake of vitamin B$_6$ can cause permanent damage to sensory nerves (12).

Excess intake of mineral elements also can cause health problems. For example, excess (and inadequate) calcium intake can increase the risk of developing kidney stones. Excess intake of iron can interfere with the absorption of other minerals (such as zinc) and can cause gastrointestinal irritation (14).

It is important to remember that nutrient requirements and ULs are set for normal, healthy individuals. In some cases, a drug may increase or decrease the need for a nutrient. Anyone who is taking a medication may no longer fit into these DRI parameters. For example, large doses of anti-inflammatory drugs such as aspirin and ibuprofen may interfere with folic acid function and potentially increase folic acid requirements (12,18).

With respect to ULs, the nutrient levels that are perfectly safe for normal, healthy people can be life threatening for those with specific health problems. For example, supplementation with vitamins E and K can complicate conditions for people on anticoagulant therapy (or "blood thinners") (13,14). Consequently, the use of various drugs can contraindicate the use of specific nutrient supplements, as well as the consumption of some foods high in the specific nutrient. Therefore, people with serious health problems, and especially those taking drugs for health problems, should use dietary supplements only with guidance and monitoring by a physician, pharmacist, or other health professional knowledgeable in drug–nutrient interactions.

When no UL has been established for a nutrient, it does not mean that there is no potential for adverse effects from high intake. Rather, it may just mean that too little information is currently available to establish a UL value. Complete tables of the DRI values are available at the Web site for the USDA Food and Nutrition Information Center.

Another authoritative publication on upper limits for nutrient intake was produced by the Expert Group on Vitamins and Minerals of the Food Standards Agency in the United Kingdom. This publication, *Safe Upper Levels for Vitamins and Minerals*, provides "safe upper levels" (SUL) for eight nutrients and "guidance levels" for the 22 vitamins and minerals for which data were inadequate to set an SUL (19). These recommended upper levels of intake refer specifically to intake in the form of dietary supplements. The Expert Group on Vitamins and Minerals describes these terms as follows (19):

> The determination of SULs or Guidance Levels entails the determination of doses of vitamins and minerals that potentially susceptible individuals could take daily on a life-long basis, without medical supervision in reasonable safety. The setting of these levels provides a framework within which the consumer can make an informed decision about intake, having confidence that harm should not ensue. The levels so set will therefore tend to be conservative, and it is possible that for some vitamins and minerals larger amounts could be consumed for shorter periods without risk to health. However, there would be difficulties in deriving SULs for shorter term consumption because the available data are limited and relate to differing time periods. Although less susceptible individuals might be able to consume higher levels without risk to health, separate advice for susceptible individuals would be appropriate only if those individuals could recognize their own potential susceptibility.

Values for SULs and guidance levels are included in Table 18.3, for comparison with DRI values. It is interesting to note similarities and differences in the values set by the two different approaches. Guidance levels are based on very limited data and are not meant to be confused with, or used as, SULs. However, when no UL or SUL is available, guidance levels can provide a reasonable frame of reference.

Obviously, the bottom line is that it is preferable to consume nutrients within a range that is adequate to meet the body's needs. The optimal level of intake within this adequate range is not known. Whether optimal is closer to the RDA and AI or to the UL for a nutrient is unknown and likely differs for the various nutrients and also may differ from one individual person to another.

© ilolab/ShutterStock, Inc.

SUMMARY

Most dietary supplements contain potent natural chemicals that are generally considered safer than drugs. However, some precautions for appropriate use should still be taken, and guidelines should be followed. The most recent updated recommendations for nutrient intake are presented in a series of publications called "Dietary Reference Intakes."

DRI values are good guidelines for adequate, excessive, and potentially harmful intakes of a nutrient for normal, healthy individuals. The overall goal in designing a healthy diet is to provide nutrients that meet recommended daily allowance or adequate intake levels and also have a low probability of exceeding tolerable upper intake levels. Optimal intake may differ for the various nutrients and also may differ from one individual person to another.

Even essential nutrients and minerals are potentially toxic at some level of intake. Nutrient levels that are perfectly safe for normal, healthy people can be altered for those taking medication and even life threatening for those with specific health problems. These clients should use dietary supplements only with guidance and monitoring by a physician, pharmacist, or other health professional knowledgeable in drug–nutrient interactions.

Labels of Dietary Supplements

Units of Measure Used on Dietary Supplement Labels

Dietary supplement labels contain product information on "Supplement Facts" panels similar to the "Nutrition Facts" on food products **Figure 18.1**. Protein, carbohydrate, and fat are generally expressed in gram quantities, whereas vitamins, minerals,

---

FIGURE 18.1

Sample supplement facts panel used on a dietary supplement label.

Supplement Facts

Serving Size 1 Capsule

Amount per Capsule	% Daily Value
Calories 20	
Calories from fat 20	
Total Fat 2 g	3%*
Saturated Fat 0.5 g	3%*
Polyunsaturated Fat 1 g	†
Monounsaturated Fat 0.5 g	†
Vitamin A 4250 IU	85%
Vitamin D 425 IU	106%
Omega-3 fatty acids 0.5 g	†

* Percent Daily Values are based on a 2,000 calorie diet.
† Daily Value not established.

Ingredients: Cod liver oil, gelatin, water, and glycerin.

amino acids, and fatty acids are generally present and expressed in milligram (mg) or microgram (mcg or μg) quantities.

In addition to the nutrient amounts required on the supplement facts panel, dietary supplements must provide a "% Daily Value" for each nutrient listed. Daily values (DVs) were established specifically for food labeling and are intended to provide the consumer with a frame of reference that indicates how the amount of the nutrient present in a food or supplement compares with approximate levels of recommended intake. The DVs for vitamins and minerals are based on the 1968 RDAs for adults (using the higher of two recommended amounts, when there are differences between males and females). Thus, if a product indicates that the % DV for a nutrient is 50, it means that an adult will obtain about 50% of the amount commonly recommended on a daily basis for that nutrient.

The amounts and DVs for nutrients listed on a supplement facts panel are the amounts present in the serving size indicated at the top of the label. In Figure 18.1, the serving size is one capsule. However, some products may indicate more than one capsule, pill, tablet, and so forth as the serving size. Many components of supplements do not have DVs. When this is the case, there is an indication "Daily Value not established" at the bottom of the panel. Although the RDAs have been revised several times since 1968, the DVs have not changed since then. When DVs are used as a general ballpark guide, they still work reasonably well. However, some issues have evolved that will likely lead to a revision in the DVs to more closely match current nutritional recommendations. For example, the DV for iron is 18 mg/day, which was based on a menstruating woman's requirement. The current RDA for a man is 8 mg/day. Consequently, when a dietary supplement provides 100% of the DV for iron, it provides more than twice the RDA for a man.

The amounts of vitamins A, D, and E are expressed on supplement labels as international units (IUs). Table 18.4 compares the RDA values for these three nutrients expressed in microgram or milligram amounts to equivalent amounts expressed in IUs. This table also illustrates that the DVs that are used as reference amounts on food and supplement nutrition labels do not equal the most current RDA values for men and women. The DV for each of these three vitamins exceeds the current RDA for adult

| TABLE 18.4 | Comparison of RDA Adult Values for Vitamins A, D, and E with Tolerable Upper Intake Levels, Safe Upper Levels, and Daily Values Used for Food and Supplement Labels |

© ilolab/ShutterStock, Inc.

Vitamin	Men's RDA	Women's RDA	Adult UL/SUL	Label DV
Vitamin A (μg)	900	700	3,000/1,500	—
Vitamin A (IU)[a]	3,000	2,333	10,000/5,000	5,000
Vitamin D (μg)	5	5	50/25	—
Vitamin D (IU)	200	200	2,000/1,000	400
Vitamin E (μg)	15	15	1,000/540	—
Vitamin E (IU)[b]	22	22	1,490/800	30

[a]In the form of retinol (typically as retinyl palmitate).
[b]Based on natural vitamin E (D-α-tocopherol).
RDA, recommended dietary allowance; UL, tolerable upper intake level; SUL, safe upper level; DV, daily value.

males and females. Of particular interest, the DV for vitamin A is actually equal to the SUL value set by the Expert Committee on Vitamins and Minerals in the United Kingdom. Comparisons of other micronutrient DVs with current recommendations are shown in Table 18.4.

SUMMARY

Dietary supplement labels contain product information on "Supplement Facts" panels, expressed in quantities of mg or mcg or μg or IU. Also provided are "% Daily Value" for each nutrient listed. DVs for vitamins and minerals are based on the 1968 RDAs for adults, which still work reasonably well. However, some nutrients may not match current nutritional recommendations (such as vitamins A, D, and E, and iron).

Vitamin and Mineral Supplements

A variety of dietary supplements are used to enhance overall health or reduce the risk of various diseases. The most commonly used supplement is a multiple vitamin and mineral supplement (multi-vit/min) that is intended to compensate for nutrients that may be limited in a person's diet. The amounts of the various nutrients in a multi-vit/min that are reasonable and sensible depend on an individual's needs and their intake of nutrients from other sources. As a general rule of thumb, the safe level of most nutrients in a multi-vit/min should be around 100% of the DV. However, there are some notable exceptions to this general rule.

Vitamin A, if present in a supplement only as retinol (usually indicated as retinyl palmitate or vitamin A palmitate) rather than carotene, should be less than 100% of the DV. A high intake of retinol, but not β-carotene, is associated with increased incidence of hip fracture in older women (20). Also, as mentioned above, excess intake of retinol at conception and during early pregnancy increases the risk of birth defects (14).

Concerns also exist for including large doses of β-carotene in a dietary supplement (21). Two large intervention trials reported an increased incidence of lung cancer in smokers who were taking 20- to 30-mg/day supplements of β-carotene (22,23). However, a large study of 22,071 physicians reported no effect on cancer incidence or mortality in those taking 50 mg/day of β-carotene and found that supplementation in those with initially low blood levels of β-carotene helped reduce the incidence of prostate cancer (24). Still another large study conducted in China found that daily supplementation with 15 mg of β-carotene in combination with 50 μg of selenium and 30 mg of α-tocopherol was associated with a 13% reduction in cancer risk, mainly as a result of decreased incidence of gastric cancer (25). Consequently, supplementation with β-carotene remains controversial and appears to be most clearly contraindicated in smokers.

Calcium should be at low levels or absent in a multi-vit/min because taking 100% of the RDA, which is 1 g (1,000 mg) of elemental calcium, would make the supplement pill too large to swallow easily. Second, for best absorption, it is preferable to consume calcium with meals, spaced throughout the day, rather than to ingest 100% of daily needs at one time (26). Third, excess calcium consumed with other minerals can decrease the absorption of some important trace minerals (11).

Among the B vitamins, niacin, B$_6$, and folic acid have UL values. For niacin and folic acid, the adult ULs are only 2.2 and 2.5 times their respective RDA values. The UL for vitamin B$_6$ of 100 mg is 77 times the RDA. However, the FSA Expert Group on Vitamins and Minerals SUL value for daily consumption of supplemental vitamin B$_6$ is only 10 mg/day (19). At one tenth the UL value set by the U.S. Food and Nutrition Board, this value is based on the assumption that this SUL intake for supplemental B$_6$ is reasonably safe to consume over the lifetime of an adult (19).

Some B vitamins (B$_1$, B$_2$, B$_{12}$, pantothenic acid, and biotin) do not have UL values because of a lack of data on adverse effects (12). For these nutrients, the FSA Expert Group on Vitamins and Minerals established guidance levels that can at least provide a reasonable frame of reference (Table 18.2) (19).

Deficiencies of vitamins and minerals can impair the ability and desire to perform physical activity. In addition, many nutrient deficiencies can cause mental and emotional problems. Clearly, iron deficiency has been shown to affect both physical and mental function adversely (27,28). Also, a deficiency of some B vitamins can affect mental functions and emotional state. Perhaps the most common example of this is caused by vitamin B$_{12}$ deficiency, which is most commonly seen in the elderly and in those who avoid consuming animal foods (29,30). In the elderly, mental and emotional changes caused by vitamin B$_{12}$ deficiency are often mistaken for Alzheimer's disease and other dementias. The condition can be reversed if corrected early in the deficiency state. If not, nerve damage and dementia symptoms can be irreversible. However, correcting the deficiency will prevent further progression of the problems and potentially cause some reversal of symptoms. Because malabsorption is the usual cause of vitamin B$_{12}$ deficiency, the usual treatment is to receive monthly injections of the vitamin. However, some research indicates that high-dose oral supplementation in the range of 200 to 2,000 µg/day may be as effective as injections (31–33).

Selecting a multiple vitamin and mineral supplement with reasonable levels of each nutrient for an individual is not a simple task. It is not unusual to find multi-vit/mins with some nutrient levels that exceed the UL or SUL values. The information in Table 18.3 can provide some reasonable guidelines. Note that the upper level numbers (UL, SUL, and guidance level) for some nutrients are much closer to the RDA or AI than they are for others.

Table 18.5 compares the DV amounts (the reference values on food and dietary supplement labels) for four nutrients to current levels of recommended intake and upper limits. Because the recommended intakes for these nutrients are relatively close to common recommendations for upper limits, people are more likely to consume excessive amounts of these nutrients from supplements and fortified foods combined. Although the effects of vitamin D toxicity are known, vitamin D researchers are currently recommending that the recommended intake and the tolerable upper intake levels be substantially increased in the next revision of the Dietary Reference Intake values for the vitamin (34,35).

The amount of each nutrient in a supplement that is most appropriate for an individual depends on the amount of nutrients in his or her diet. Despite claims to the contrary, today's food supply is not devoid of nutrients. Certainly it is possible to select a diet composed mostly of overly refined foods that provide limited amounts of vitamins and minerals and plenty of calories. However, with the plethora of fortified foods (breakfast cereals, energy bars, protein powders, and just about everything with a calcium-fortified option), it is quite possible to consume excessive amounts of some nutrients even without taking dietary supplements. Consequently, decisions to use dietary supplements should be made in the context of a typical diet, with special attention to use of foods fortified with vitamins and minerals.

TABLE 18.5	Nutrients with the Greatest Potential for Excess Dosage in Dietary Supplements
Vitamin A	If a dietary supplement contains 100% of the Daily Value, it contains an amount of vitamin A that is more than twice the RDA for a woman, only half of the UL and equal to the Guidance Level.
Vitamin D	If a dietary supplement contains 100% of the Daily Value, it contains an amount of vitamin D that is twice the AI value. The UL is 5 times the DV, and the SUL is 2.5 times the DV. (Note: Vitamin D researchers are currently recommending that both the AI and UL values for vitamin D be increased to levels significantly greater than current recommendations.)
Iron	If a dietary supplement contains 100% of the Daily Value, it contains an amount of iron that is equal to the RDA for women, more than twice the RDA for men. The UL is only a little over twice the DV, and the Guidance Level is 1 milligram less than the DV.
Zinc	If a dietary supplement contains 100% of the Daily Value, it contains an amount of zinc that is almost twice the RDA for women. The UL is just a little over twice the DV, and the SUL is a little less than twice the DV.

Precaution Statements on Dietary Supplements Used for Specific Adaptation

1. Most people may benefit from the use of a multivitamin and mineral formula (in addition to a separate calcium supplement) to complement their best efforts to consume a proper diet.
2. Specific nutrient compounds, when ingested and manufactured properly, can allow the body to operate at full capacity, without disturbing its natural physiology.
3. The effects of dietary supplement use may vary among individuals based on dietary intake of nutrients and physiologic and psychologic individuality. Manufacturing methods and ingredients used to produce a supplement also may affect results.
4. The general population should not use dietary supplements for medicinal purposes, unless recommended by a qualified health professional. Such a practitioner will have experience in treating diseases and symptoms with both prescription drugs and natural compounds and will have performed the research to choose the safest and most effective therapy.

SUMMARY

The most commonly used supplement is a multi-vitamin that is intended to compensate for nutrients that may be limited in a person's diet. Deficiencies of vitamins and minerals can impair ability and desire to perform physical activity and also cause mental and emotional problems.

As a general rule of thumb, the safe level of most nutrients in a multi-vit/min should be around 100% of the DV. However, there are some exceptions, including:

◆ Vitamin A (present only as retinol) should be less than 100% of the DV.
◆ β-carotene is contraindicated in smokers.
◆ Calcium should be at low levels or absent in a multi-vit/min.

People are more likely to consume excessive amounts of the following nutrients from supplements and fortified foods combined:

◆ Vitamin A
◆ Vitamin D
◆ Iron
◆ Zinc

With the plethora of fortified foods available, it is quite possible to consume excessive amounts of some nutrients even without taking dietary supplements. Consequently, decisions to use dietary supplements should be made in the context of a typical diet, with special attention to the use of foods fortified with vitamins and minerals.

Ergogenic Aids

Introduction to Nonnutrient Ergogenic Aids

The term *ergogenic* literally means work generating. In popular use, the term ergogenic aid is something that enhances athletic performance. There are many ways that athletes and fitness enthusiasts attempt to boost their performance and training capacity. Some purported ergogenic aids make sense and some do not. It can be challenging for fitness professionals, athletes, trainers, and coaches to sort out which aids are potentially safe and effective and which are primarily unreasonable marketing hype based on pseudo-science. Dr. Ron Maughan, the prolific sport supplement researcher from the United Kingdom, states a reasonable axiom when considering ergogenic aids to improve performance: "If it works, it's probably banned. If it's not banned, it probably doesn't work."

This section provides an overview of popular substances that are promoted as potential ergogenic aids. A general understanding of popular ergogenic aids should exist to educate clients and provide *general* guidance in this area. It is likely that a fitness professional will be the first person approached with supplementation questions, so being confident about the nature of the relationship between ergogenic aids, fitness, and performance is essential. However, providing individual nutrition assessments, meal plans, or recommendations for sport supplements are best left to a Registered Dietician (RD). This means a qualified RD should be a valued partner for all fitness professionals. This becomes especially important if the client has health and medical concerns such as obesity, diabetes, heart disease, allergies, or hypertension.

Creatine Supplementation

For many sports, building muscle mass and strength are major goals. A wide variety of natural and synthetic substances have been tried (both legally and illegally) by athletes and fitness enthusiasts to assist the body's natural responses to strength training. A legal supplement common among strength athletes and bodybuilders is creatine.

Creatine is synthesized naturally in the human body from the amino acids methionine, glycine, and arginine. In resting skeletal muscle, about two thirds of the creatine exists in a phosphorylated form that can rapidly regenerate ATP (adenosine triphosphate) from ADP (adenosine diphosphate) to maintain high-intensity muscular efforts for up to about 10 seconds. Supplementation with creatine can increase muscle creatine levels and may enhance certain types of brief high-intensity efforts. When creatine supplementation is combined with a strength-training program, it has been shown to increase muscle mass, strength, and anaerobic performance (36). The typical dosing scheme begins with 5 to 7 days of supplementation at 20 g per day to rapidly increase muscle creatine. This is then followed by a maintenance phase of 2 to 5 g per day to sustain maximal muscle creatine levels. Creatine supplementation as part of a strength-training program typically causes an initial weight gain of 4 to 5 pounds that may be caused by the osmotic effect of creatine drawing water into muscles along with increased muscle protein synthesis (37).

The maintenance dose of creatine (2 to 5 g per day for maintenance) is apparently safe for normal healthy individuals for up to 5 years. However, possible effects of longer chronic use remain unknown. People with kidney problems should use creatine supplements only with medical guidance (38). Consuming creatine supplements in combination with carbohydrate can enhance muscle uptake of creatine and potentially increase muscle levels above that achieved without concurrent carbohydrate consumption (39). Creatine supplementation is under study for several therapeutic uses in various neuromuscular and neurodegenerative diseases, and it is now known that creatine plays an essential role in normal brain function (37).

Creatine supplementation is not banned by major sports governing bodies; however, the NCAA rules prohibit institutions from supplying creatine supplements directly to athletes. Creatine use is widespread in sports, and reasonable testing procedures for abnormal levels of this natural compound would be difficult to establish. It has been argued that creatine loading should be considered no different than carbohydrate loading because creatine is a substance found naturally in animal foods like red meat (40).

Stimulants (Caffeine)

Athletes and fitness enthusiasts have tried a wide variety of legal and illegal stimulants to obtain potential ergogenic benefits. These have ranged from herbal and synthetic sources of caffeine and ephedrine to controlled drugs such as amphetamine and cocaine. Because stimulants can affect both physical function and mental state, athletes involved in many different types of sports have attempted to get ergogenic benefits from the use of stimulants.

Many consider caffeine to be the most widely used drug in the world, oftentimes consumed in coffee, tea, cocoa, and other beverages with added caffeine. Foods such as chocolate and a wide variety of herbal supplements also provide caffeine. Caffeine acts as a stimulant that primarily affects the central nervous system, heart, and skeletal muscles.

Most carefully controlled studies have demonstrated ergogenic effects from caffeine, especially when tested on well-trained athletes performing endurance exercise (more than an hour) or high-intensity short-duration exercise lasting about 5 minutes. However, there does not appear to be an ergogenic effect on performance of sprint-type efforts lasting 90 seconds or less (41).

The most effective ergogenic response has been observed when the dosage of caffeine is about 3 to 6 mg per kg body weight and it is ingested about 1 hour before exercise. For a 70-kg person (~155 pounds), this dose is equivalent to 210 to 420 mg of caffeine. To put that into a coffee perspective, 16 ounces of black coffee likely ranges from about 200 to 350 mg of caffeine. The caffeine content of coffee can vary tremendously depending on the type of coffee, the amount used, and the brewing process. Caffeine doses greater than 6 mg per kg body weight generally show less performance benefit and have more risk of adverse effects (41).

Potential negative effects of caffeine can vary greatly from one person to another. Possible adverse effects range from the well-known insomnia and nervousness to lesser-known effects like nausea, rapid heart and breathing rates, convulsions, and increased urine production. Other symptoms that have been reported include headache, chest pain, and irregular heart rhythm (38).

Banned Stimulants

The World Anti-Doping Agency lists more than 50 different stimulants that are prohibited in sports competition. The list includes amphetamines and ephedrine, along with less commonly known drugs and substances with similar chemical structures or biologic effects (42). Many adverse side effects are common, including altered behavior (especially increased aggression), headache, disrupted heart function, overheating, and even death. Chronic use of these illegal stimulants can lead to addiction and the problems associated with withdrawal (43).

PROHORMONES

A variety of dietary supplements with hormone precursors have been used to promote building of strength and muscle mass. In general, research on these substances has demonstrated a lack of benefit and significant risk potential in young to middle-aged athletes. Dehydroepiandrosterone (DHEA) is produced naturally in the body and can serve as a precursor for androstenedione that, in turn, can be converted into testosterone or estrogens. There is some evidence that older individuals who have low levels of naturally produced DHEA can benefit from DHEA supplementation (44). However, high serum DHEA levels are associated with various health risks such as cancer (45). Consequently, it is recommended that supplementation with DHEA be conducted under medical supervision. Older athletes are the most likely to benefit from medical use of DHEA supplementation.

Androstenedione, a compound that the body can convert to testosterone or estrogens, has been used widely in an attempt to boost testosterone levels in men. Because androstenedione supplementation in men has been shown to boost estrogen levels more than testosterone levels (46), studies have been conducted with concurrent supplementation with natural compounds thought to inhibit the formation of estrogen from androstenedione to theoretically favor testosterone production. However, a combination of these inhibitors (Tribulis terrestris, chrysin, indole-3-carbinol, and saw palmetto) has failed to enhance testosterone production from androstenedione (47). Because of the apparent lack of potential benefit of these hormone precursors and blockers and the risks inherent in affecting natural hormone production, athletes and fitness enthusiasts should avoid the use of these products without careful medical supervision. Also, most of these substances are on the prohibited list of the World Anti-doping Code (42). Despite all the hype, androstenedione is unlikely to be ergogenic for any athlete in normal health and is clearly not worth its potential downside.

ANDROGENIC ANABOLIC STEROIDS

Androgenic anabolic steroids are drugs designed to mimic the effects of testosterone. These drugs have a long history of abuse by athletes, and their use is banned by all major athletic organizations. There is evidence that these drugs can promote the building of muscle mass, strength, and loss of body fat. However, these beneficial changes are accomplished at the risk of serious adverse health effects (48,49). Some of these undesirable health effects can persist even after drug withdrawal. Of particular concern is that the use of androgenic anabolic steroids by adolescents can cause early closure of the growth plates in bones and stunt the development of normal height. Refer to Table 18.6 for a summary of potential adverse effects of anabolic androgenic steroid use.

TABLE 18.6 **Partial Listing of Potential Adverse Side Effects of Androgenic-Anabolic Steroid Use**[a]

Men	Women[b]
Acne	General development of masculine traits
Increased body hair	Increased facial and body hair
Loss of head hair	Deepening of voice (more like a man's voice)
Gynecomastia (female-like breast and nipple enlargement)	Increased aggressiveness
Irritability	Increased appetite
Aggressive behavior	Acne
Increased or decreased sexual drive	Altered libido
Mood extremes (from well-being to depression)	Loss of head hair
Increased appetite	Alteration in pubic hair growth
Sleeplessness	Fluid retention
Fluid retention	Menstrual irregularities
Testicular shrinkage	Reduction of breast size
Decreased sperm production and infertility	Clitoris enlargement
Prostate gland enlargement	
Increased blood pressure	
Decreased HDL cholesterol	
Increased LDL cholesterol	
Stroke	
Impaired glucose tolerance	

[a]Adverse effects may vary because of individual differences and variation in the doses and types of steroids used.
[b]Availability of data about women is limited.
HDL, high-density lipoprotein; LDL, low-density lipoprotein.

Ethical and Legal Issues with Ergogenic Aids

When deciding to explore the use of a potential ergogenic aid, the athlete is presented with challenging decisions. The first question of most athletes is, Does it work? The answer to that question is not always simple and is generally heavily dependent on the type of physical activity or physical adaptation that the individual seeks to enhance, and the population the research is based on. In reality, the first question should be, Is it safe? The answer to this question is not always simple or obvious and must take into account many individual variables that may determine safety for a given individual. Not of least importance is the question, Is it legal or ethical? Again, the answer is not always simple. Even seemingly common herbal products can contain pharmaceutically active compounds that are banned and can result in a positive blood test for the banned substance. An international study that analyzed more than 600 nonhormonal nutritional supplements found that about 15% of the supplements contained undeclared anabolic androgenic steroids that could trigger a positive doping test. In some countries, 20% to 25% of the supplements were contaminated (50). Consequently, elite athletes who might qualify for a drug test must be especially careful in their choice of supplements. But all athletes need to be on notice as drug testing is moving beyond international and professional competitions and into scholastic arenas.

The temptation to use illegal performance-enhancing substances is great for many competitive athletes. The governing bodies of various sports are ethically bound to enforce controls on the use of banned substances. Unfortunately, the reputations of many great athletes have been sullied by illegal use of banned substances. For individual sports to maintain their reputations, their governing bodies carry the obligation to establish regulations for banned substance use and to enforce those regulations.

SUMMARY

Maximizing one's potential during high-level competition involves exploiting all available resources within known, healthful guidelines. There is no substitute for an appropriate training regimen and attitude, nor is there a magic pill that creates a world-class athlete out of anyone. However, when an athlete has obtained all he or she can from food intake, talent, training, and motivation, specific compounds used in proper dosages, forms, and schedules offer a safe and viable means of maximizing potential and enhancing results during training and competition. For example, when creatine supplementation is combined with a strength-training program, it has been shown to increase muscle mass, strength, and anaerobic performance. Keep in mind that individual results from the ingestion of similar specific compounds may vary because those results can be related to the physiologic and psychologic state of the competitive athletes who use them. However, banned substances and practices such as androgenic anabolic steroids should be avoided by all athletes and fitness enthusiasts. When deciding to explore the use of a potential ergogenic aid, the athlete or fitness enthusiast should ask three simple questions, Does it work? Is it safe? and Is it ethical and legal?

REFERENCES

1. Kurtzweil P. An FDA guide to dietary supplements. *FDA Consum.* 1998;32:28-35.

2. Nutrition Business Journal's 2009 Archived Annual U.S. Nutrition Industry Overview Web Seminar. Penton Media, 2009. Available at http://nutritionbusinessjournal.com/supplements/web-seminars/nutrition-industry-overview-webinar/.

3. U.S. 103rd Congress. Dietary Supplement Health and Education Act of 1994. Public Law 103-417. Available at http://www.fda.gov/opacom/laws/dshea.html.

4. U.S. Food and Drug Administration, Center for Food Safety and Applied Nutrition. Dietary Supplement Health and Education Act of 1994. December 1, 1995. Available at http://www.cfsan.fda.gov/~dms/dietsupp.html.

5. Fletcher RH, Fairfield KM. Vitamins for chronic disease prevention in adults: clinical applications. *JAMA.* 2002;287(23):3127-3129.

6. Fairfield KM, Fletcher RH. Vitamins for chronic disease prevention in adults: scientific review. *JAMA.* 2002;287(23):3116-3126.

7. Huang HY, Caballero B, Chang S, et al. Multivitamin/mineral supplements and prevention of chronic disease. *Evid Rep Technol Assess.* 2006;139:1-117.

8. Drewnowski A, Shultz JM. Impact of aging on eating behaviors, food choices, nutrition, and health status. *J Nutr Health Aging.* 2001;5(2):75-79.

9. Bidlack WR, Smith CH. Nutritional requirements of the aged. *Crit Rev Food Sci Nutr.* 1988;27(3):189-218.

10. Gunderson EP. Nutrition during pregnancy for the physically active woman. *Clin Obstet Gynecol.* 2003;46(2):390-402.

11. Food and Nutrition Board, Institute of Medicine. *Dietary Reference Intakes for Calcium, Phosphorus, Magnesium, Vitamin D, and Fluoride.* Washington, DC: National Academy Press; 1997.

12. Food and Nutrition Board, Institute of Medicine. *Dietary Reference Intakes for Thiamin, Riboflavin, Niacin, Vitamin B-6, Folate, Vitamin B-12, Pantothenic Acid, Biotin, and Choline.* Washington, DC: National Academy Press; 1998.

13. Food and Nutrition Board, Institute of Medicine. *Dietary Reference Intakes for Vitamin C, Vitamin E, Selenium, and Carotenoids.* Washington, DC: National Academy Press; 2000.

14. Food and Nutrition Board, Institute of Medicine. *Dietary Reference Intakes for Vitamin A, Vitamin K, Arsenic, Boron, Chromium, Copper, Iodine, Iron, Manganese, Molybdenum, Nickel, Silicon, Vanadium, and Zinc.* Washington, DC: National Academy Press; 2001.

15. Food and Nutrition Board, Institute of Medicine. *Dietary Reference Intakes for Energy, Carbohydrate, Fiber, Fat, Fatty Acids, Cholesterol, Protein, and Amino Acids.* Washington, DC: National Academy Press; 2005.

16. Food and Nutrition Board, Institute of Medicine. *Dietary Reference Intakes for Water, Potassium, Sodium, Chloride, and Sulfate.* Washington, DC: National Academy Press; 2005.

17. Food and Nutrition Board, Institute of Medicine. *Dietary Reference Intakes: Applications in Dietary Planning.* (prepublication copy/uncorrected proofs) Washington, DC: National Academy Press; 2003.

18. Baggott JE, Morgan SL, Ha T, Vaughn WH, Hine RJ. Inhibition of folate-dependent enzymes by non-steroidal anti-inflammatory drugs. *Biochem J.* 1992;282(Pt 1):197-202.

19. Expert Group on Vitamins and Minerals. Safe Upper Levels for Vitamins and Minerals. Food Standards Agency, United Kingdom, May 2003. Available at http://www.foodstandards.gov.uk/multimedia/pdfs/vitmin2003.pdf.

20. Feskanich D, Singh V, Willett WC, Colditz GA. Vitamin A intake and hip fractures among postmenopausal women. *JAMA.* 2002;287(1):47-54.

21. Albanes D, Heinonen OP, Taylor PR, et al. Alpha-tocopherol and beta-carotene supplements and lung cancer incidence in the Alpha-Tocopherol, Beta-Carotene Cancer Prevention Study: effects of baseline characteristics and study compliance. *J Natl Cancer Inst.* 1996;88:1560-1570.

22. Pryor WA, Stahl W, Rock CL. Beta carotene: from biochemistry to clinical trials. *Nutr Rev.* 2000;58(2 Pt 1):39-53.

23. Omen GS, Goodman G, Thornquist M, et al. The Beta-Carotene and Retinol Efficacy Trial (CARET) for chemoprevention of lung cancer in high risk populations: smokers and asbestos-exposed workers. *Cancer Res.* 1994;54:2038-2043.

24. Cook N, Lee IM, Manson J, et al. Effects of 12 years of beta-carotene supplementation on cancer incidence in the Physician's Health Study (PHS). *Am J Epidemiol.* 1999;149:270-279.

25. Blot WJ, Li JY, Taylor PR, et al. Nutritional intervention trials in Linxian, China: supplementation with specific vitamin/mineral combinations, cancer incidence, and disease specific mortality in the general population. *J Natl Cancer Inst.* 1993;85:1483-1492.

26. Heaney RP, Weaver CM, Fitzsimmons ML. Influence of calcium load on absorption fraction. *J Bone Miner Res.* 1990;5(11):1135-1138.

27. Benton D, Donohoe RT. The effects of nutrients on mood. *Public Health Nutr.* 1999;2(3A):403-409.

28. Risser WL, Lee EJ, Poindexter HB, et al. Iron deficiency in female athletes: its prevalence and impact on performance. *Med Sci Sports Exerc.* 1988;20(2):116-121.

29. Carmel R. Current concepts in cobalamin deficiency. *Annu Rev Med.* 2000;51:357-375.

30. Carmel R, Melnyk S, James SJ. Cobalamin deficiency with and without neurologic abnormalities: differences in homocysteine and methionine metabolism. *Blood.* 2003;101(8):3302-3308.

31. Andres E, Kaltenbach G, Noel E, et al. Efficacy of short-term oral cobalamin therapy for the treatment of cobalamin deficiencies related to food-cobalamin malabsorption: a study of 30 patients. *Clin Lab Haematol.* 2003;25(3):161-166.

32. Andres E, Perrin AE, Demangeat C, et al. The syndrome of food-cobalamin malabsorption revisited in a department of internal medicine. A monocentric cohort study of 80 patients. *Eur J Intern Med.* 2003;14(4):221-226.

33. Oh R, Brown DL. Vitamin B12 deficiency. *Am Fam Physician.* 2003;67(5):979-986.

34. Leidig-Bruckner G, Roth HJ, Bruckner T, Lorenz A, Raue F, Frank-Raue K. Are commonly recommended dosages for vitamin D supplementation too low? Vitamin D status and effects of supplementation on serum 25-hydroxyvitamin D levels: an observational study during clinical practice conditions. *Osteoporos Int.* 2010 Jun 17. [Epub ahead of print]

35. Hathcock JN, Shao A, Vieth R, Heaney R. Risk assessment for vitamin D. *Am J Clin Nutr.* 2007;85(1):6-18.

36. Branch JD. Effect of creatine supplementation on body composition and performance: a meta-analysis. *Int J Sport Nutr Exerc Metab.* 2003;13:198-226.

37. Brosnan JT, Brosnan ME. Creatine: endogenous metabolite, dietary, and therapeutic supplement. *Annu Rev Nutr.* 2007;27: 241-261.

38. Jellin JM, Gregory PJ, Batz F, et al. *Pharmacist's Letter/Prescriber's Letter Natural Medicines Comprehensive Database.* 5th ed. Stockton: Therapeutic Research Faculty; 2003.

39. Green AL, Simpson EJ, Littlewood JJ, et al. Carbohydrate ingestion augments creatine retention during creatine feeding in humans. *Acta Physiol Scand.* 1996;158:195-202.

40. Kreider RB. Creatine. In: Driskell JA, ed. *Sports Nutrition: Fats and Proteins.* Boca Raton, CRC Press; 2007:165-186.

41. Spriet LL. Caffeine and performance. *Int J Sport Nutr.* 1995;5 (Suppl):S84-99.

42. World Anti-Doping Agency. The World Anti-Doping Code: The 2008 Prohibited List. Available at http://www.wada-ama.org/rtecontent/document/2008_List_En.pdf. Accessed March 20, 2008.

43. Nuzzo NA, Waller DP. Drug abuse in athletes. In: Thomas JA, ed. *Drugs, Athletes, and Physical Performance.* New York: Plenum Publishing Corporation; 1988;141-167.

44. Villareal DT, Holloszy JO. DHEA enhances effects of weight training on muscle mass and strength in elderly women and men. *Am J Physiol Endocrinol Metab.* 2006;291:E1003-1008.

45. Johnson MD, Bebb RA, Sirrs SM. Uses of DHEA in aging and other disease states. *Ageing Res Rev.* 2002;1:29-41.

46. King DS, Sharp RL, Vukovich MD, et al. Effect of oral androstenedione on serum testosterone and adaptations to resistance training in young men: a randomized controlled trial. *JAMA.* 1999;281:2020-2028.

47. Brown GA, Vukovich M, King DS. Testosterone prohormone supplements. *Med Sci Sports Exerc.* 2006;38:1451-1461.

48. Bahrke MS, Yesalis CE. Abuse of anabolic androgenic steroids and related substances in sport and exercise. *Curr Opin Pharmacol.* 2004;4:614-620.

49. Hartgens F, Kuipers H. Effects of androgenic-anabolic steroids in athletes. *Sports Med.* 2004;34:513-54.

50. Geyer H, Parr MK, Mareck U, et al. Analysis of non-hormonal nutritional supplements for anabolic-androgenic steroids—results of an international study. *Int J Sports Med.* 2004;25:124-129.

SECTION 4

Client Interaction and Professional Development

Lifestyle Modification and Behavioral Coaching

After studying this chapter, you will be able to:

✔ Describe the characteristics of a positive client experience.

✔ Understand the stages of change model.

✔ Describe characteristics of what effective communication skills are.

✔ Describe the elements of effective SMART goal-setting techniques.

Introduction to Behavioral Coaching

Most American adults simply do not participate in enough regular exercise to improve and maintain their health and well-being. Despite the physiological and psychological benefits of exercise, including reduced anxiety, depression, and risk of cardiovascular disease, better weight control, and increased self-esteem, activity levels continue to decline (1). It is estimated that more than 75% of the American adult population does not partake, on a daily basis, in 30 minutes of low-to-moderate physical activity (2). If the benefits really do outweigh the barriers, and the current method of working with people is not working, how do successful personal trainers work differently with people to educate them about the advantages and disadvantages of exercise behavior and exercise adherence in a way that thoughtfully changes how people view exercise? This chapter explores some of the essential elements to help motivate clients and bring them closer to being able to exercise and to exercise adherence. Some of those essential elements include characteristics of a positive client experience, beginning the process of exercise, the initial session, the importance of effective communication skills, social influences on exercise, common barriers to exercise, strategies to enhance exercise adherence, and the psychological benefits of exercise.

Client Expectations of a Trainer

Personal trainers can have a significant influence on people; thus they have an obligation to design effective programs and give advice appropriate for individual clients. Their attitudes and behaviors and how they communicate greatly affect whether or not a person chooses to return for another personal training session. Personal trainers can train clients in positive ways that support the behavior change process, leading to increased adherence to exercise (3).

Personal trainers have 20 seconds to make a good first impression. That first impression includes:

- Making eye contact
- Introducing yourself by name and getting the client's name
- Smiling
- Shaking hands with the client
- Remembering the client's name and using it
- Using good body language

A new client will usually notice body language or facial expression before they hear anything. If a new client notices a personal trainer's poor body language or lack of congruency in body language and what they are saying in the first 20 seconds, it could significantly impact a personal trainer's relationship with a prospective new client permanently.

Besides attitudes, behaviors, and good communication, here are some other important qualities of a personal trainer (4):

- Personal trainers need to look professional: neat, clean, and well dressed.
- Personal trainers need to take time to build a relationship with new clients.
- Clients need to feel that the personal trainer is listening to them.
- Personal trainers need to maintain confidentiality and ensure the client's safety at all times.
- Personal trainers should be friendly, warm, interested, and compassionate.
- Personal trainers should collaborate with clients regarding their exercise routine.
- Personal trainers should model all exercises, explaining correct alignment and form.
- Personal trainers ask lots of good questions and perform comprehensive initial assessments.

Client Expectations of the Environment

It is important for personal trainers to consider what kind of environment they plan to work in. The environment in which personal trainers work is a reflection of who they are as a personal trainer and will determine the type of clientele they attract.

Some of the key predictors of exercise participation and adherence include:

- A large number of options for people to choose from
- A supportive, nurturing environment
- Convenient location
- Cost of membership and personal training

Besides the important key predictors of exercise participation and adherence, other supporting factors of a positive client experience include neat and clean facilities, detailed program information, an easy registration process, and friendly, organized support staff (4).

SUMMARY

Personal trainers can have a significant positive influence on people. Personal trainers should train clients in positive ways that support the behavior change process, leading to increased exercise adherence. Their attitudes and behaviors and how they communicate greatly affect whether or not a person chooses to return for another personal training session.

The recommended client expectations outlined above are not outside the realm of what is possible; they are factors we all come to expect from providers of goods and services. These recommendations along with a personal trainer's experiences will give them a good indication of the direction they need to go when working with various clients.

The Stages of Change

Unless people perceive there is a really good reason to change a health behavior, they probably will not do it. Change goes against human nature and what is familiar, stable, and routine. For most people change is scary and unpredictable. Most people strive to maintain the stability of what they know to be true about their lives. The behavior change process usually begins when there is a perceived problem or need for change.

One of the most widely used models of change with regard to exercise is the stages of change model **Figure 19.1**. Fitness professionals have found this model particularly helpful because of its useful applications when working with clients to change patterns of physical activity (5).

Most personal trainers will work with a client who has been exercising regularly for several years differently from the way they will work with a client who has never exercised before. Personal trainers need to tailor their actions and recommendations to a client's readiness to change.

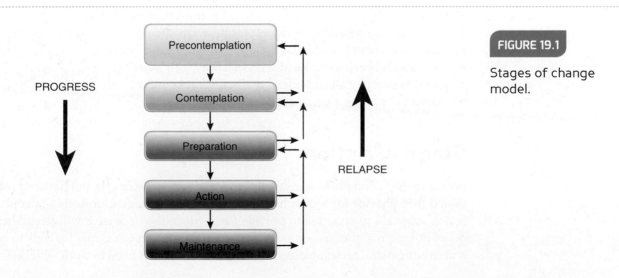

FIGURE 19.1

Stages of change model.

Stage 1: Precontemplation

Personal trainers will not usually see people in the precontemplation stage. People in this stage have no intention of changing. They do not exercise and do not intend to start in the next 6 months. The best strategy with precontemplators is education. Even though personal trainers cannot make anyone form the intention to become more active, they can suggest where they might get information to do so. Attractive, easy-to-read materials are helpful for precontemplators. If possible, personal trainers should make every effort to talk to precontemplators to find out what they think of exercise and try to dispel any myths they may have.

Stage 2: Contemplation

People in this stage do not exercise but are thinking about becoming more active in the next 6 months. Because contemplators are thinking about becoming more active, personal trainers can have a great deal of influence on what contemplators choose to do, whether or not they choose to exercise. Personal trainers need to be able to listen to what contemplators need and support them any way that they can. Contemplators are aware of some of the costs and benefits of exercise, but misconceptions may still be present.

The best strategy to use with contemplators is (still) education. Contemplators need information. Personal trainers need to find out what clients see as the pros and cons of exercise and suggest avenues of information for erroneous beliefs. It is important to discuss ways to deal with perceived cons of exercise. In this stage, personal trainers should help clients develop motivational programs that will lead to long-term adherence. Personal trainers can help contemplators move fairly quickly to the preparation stage of change.

Stage 3: Preparation

People in this stage do exercise (occasionally) but are planning to begin exercising regularly in the next month. They are believers in the health benefits of exercise. People in the preparation stage may have unrealistic expectations for the change they hope to achieve, which oftentimes leads to a high risk of disappointment and early dropout. The best strategies for working with people in the preparation stage include:

- Help clients at this stage clarify realistic goals and expectations.
- Help clients maintain their beliefs in the importance of exercise.
- Discuss programs that work best for different clients.
- Consider clients' schedules, preferences, and health concerns.
- Ask about previous successful experiences with exercise.
- Avoid exercise that could lead to discomfort or injury.
- Discuss building a social support network.

Stage 4: Action

People in the action phase are active. They have started to exercise, but have not yet maintained the behavior for 6 months. Some of the best strategies for keeping people in the action stage are to continue to provide them education because it will strengthen their belief in the pros of exercise. In this stage it is important to discuss barriers to exercise and to anticipate upcoming disruptions. Personal trainers need to work with their clients to develop action steps for overcoming any barriers or disruptions. Personal trainers should not be afraid to redesign exercise programs if time or intensity is a barrier.

Stage 5: Maintenance

People in the maintenance stage have maintained change for 6 months or more. Even though they have formed a change in their behavior in their exercise routine, they are still tempted to return to old habits of less exercise. There are good strategies to help clients maintain an exercise program. Personal trainers should suggest that clients have a maintenance check-in plan that includes reinforcing pros, discuss progress, and help them to change up their workout plan. Give suggestions tailored to personal preferences. People who have reached this stage sometimes go on to become instructors or trainers. Personal trainers can help enhance a person's motivation to exercise, provide social support, and help support exercise intentions (5).

Assessing a Client's Stage

Here are some questions to help guide you in assessing what stage a client may be in (5).

1. What experiences with physical activity have they had in the past?
2. What worked best to help them stick to an exercise program?
3. What worked the least? What contributed to their quitting an exercise program?
4. During the last 6 months, what kept them from exercising?
5. How did they keep up their exercise program when disruptions got in the way? Lack of time? Travel? Holidays?

If a client is in maintenance, questions 1 through 5 will give more information to help guide a personal trainer's work with that client.

If a personal trainer thinks a client is in the action stage, they might want to use questions 1, 2, 3, and 5; remember, in this stage clients struggle to find ways of dealing with exercise barriers.

If a personal trainer thinks a client is in the preparation stage, the discussion should be around questions 1, 2, and 3. Beyond the questions, suggest the client set realistic expectations and help him or her find social support.

If a personal trainer thinks a client is in the contemplation stage, then the job is to help him or her get ready for exercise. Questions 1, 2, 3, and 5 will help guide clients in that direction.

If a personal trainer believes a client is in the precontemplation stage, questions 1, 2, 3, and 5 may provide some useful information, but be prepared to ask other questions. For example, what keeps them from becoming active, or do they know that moderate-intensity exercise can be comfortable and still provide health benefits (5).

SUMMARY

Most fitness centers are designed for people in the action and maintenance stages. These people are psychologically prepared to sign up to take a class or to work with a personal trainer. People who are in the contemplative or preparation stages, however, are not psychologically prepared to sign up to take a class or to work with a personal trainer and usually find themselves floundering and quitting. Thus, the stages of change model suggests a variety of activities tailored to a wide range of people and should exert the greatest impact, particularly those in the contemplative and preparation stages (5). As a personal trainer this is important to realize and understand. What this means is that personal trainers need to have different approaches and conversations, be more collaborative in the process, and be more creative.

Understanding the behavior change process can help personal trainers meet their clients where they are, versus assuming that all clients have the same or similar exercise program needs. The stage of change model encourages a person-centered approach that will motivate clients and help them adhere to an exercise program that is likely to bring long-term success.

The Initial Session

Personal trainers have 20 seconds to make a good first impression. In those 20 seconds what is the first thing a client is going to see? Typically, before a client hears anything they tend to notice body language first. If a personal trainer's body language portrays a lack of welcoming, or a lack of friendliness and warmth, their 20-second impression is not going to be positive. Personal trainers need to develop a body language that portrays openness, friendliness, and a sense of warmth so clients feel comfortable.

If a personal trainer's initial 20-second impression is positive, it is important to continue moving in a positive direction. The initial session with clients does not consist of immediately giving them an exercise routine. The initial session is where the relationship begins. Building a relationship with clients initially is time spent getting to know who they are and what their needs and goals are. Personal trainers need to know that it is okay to let a client know that in the initial session they will spend at least 30 minutes just talking and getting to know them. It is in this session that personal trainers determine their client's readiness to exercise and decide what stage of change he or she is in. The initial conversation is when personal trainers start to engage, connect, and get to know their client. From this initial conversation with a client, a personal trainer can determine the direction that a client needs to go and how they need to go with him or her.

Besides determining clients' readiness to exercise, why is it important to spend time getting to know them? In the building period of any relationship there is testing, an uncertainty, and an opportunity for each person to get to know the other. It is usually in this trial period when both participants decide whether or not they want the relationship to continue. The relationship with clients goes through that same trial period. If clients determine in the trial period that they are not getting what they need, they will not come back. If clients determine in that trial period that they are getting what they need, they will continue to come back. If you want to ensure that clients come back, it is important to spend time getting to know them, getting to know their readiness for exercise, getting to know their goals, listening, showing support, and collaborating with them to design their exercise program.

In addition to assessing a client's stage, ask about other experiences with physical activity, and talk about what worked best to help a client stick to an exercise program and what worked the least. Some other initial conversation points to discuss are daily activities (e.g., gardening, housekeeping, and stair climbing), and the importance of physical activity in maintaining good health and preventing physical and emotional illness. Personal trainers should always tell clients why they think more physical activity is beneficial and why.

Discussing Health Concerns

Discussing health concerns is another important focus during the initial conversation, particularly with clients in the contemplation and preparation stages. Being able to have an intelligent conversation around the client's health concerns and how exercise can help can be motivating for a client to move toward exercise.

Health concerns are not only motivating for a client to exercise but they also provide the foundation for exercise prescription. Health concerns may be the reason a client has contacted you. Although the client may have filled out a health questionnaire or medical forms, it is important to have a verbal conversation around health concerns. Many clients may forget to write down important health information, especially if in a hurry. The conversation with clients about health concerns may include information about what health concerns they currently have, what health concerns they are concerned about potentially having, and health problems that run in their family. This conversation is also part of relationship building with your client. It allows personal trainers to connect with their client, hear their client's concerns, and show empathy for their client.

Exercise helps prevent, postpone, and treat many chronic health problems, and regular physical activity has been shown to reduce symptoms of many emotional health problems (6–8). Stress reduction is one of the primary reasons people stick to an exercise program. Ask clients about their stress levels and suggests that exercise might be beneficial.

Clarifying Fitness Goals

After personal trainers have established a good first impression and discussed health concerns, it is now important to talk with their clients about their fitness goals. It is important to understand what fitness improvements clients hope to achieve and to clarify what clients mean by feeling better, being stronger, improving appearance, and being fit. These kinds of phrases are used frequently but mean different things to different people. It is important to clarify with clients what they mean rather than trying to interpret what they mean. It is also important to have clients verbalize their goals, not only to clarify their goals for the personal trainer, but also to clarify their goals for themselves.

It is important for personal trainers to have an understanding of how to set goals and be able to work with their clients around setting goals. Clients often come up with unrealistic goals, and as a personal trainer it is important to be able to recognize what is unrealistic for a client. Unrealistic goals lead to demanding exercise programs that may be well beyond a client's ability, lifestyle, time limitations, or initial fitness level. This will often result in a client dropping out of an exercise program or possible injury.

Personal trainers should use experience and expertise when helping their client to set goals. These goals should be **S**pecific, **M**easurable, **A**ttainable, **R**ealistic, and **T**imely (known as SMART goals). Encourage clients to set goals that include physical skills, mental skills, and psychological benefits of exercise. Personal trainers should suggest that clients record their goals on paper and learn to refer to them frequently. Personal trainers should work with their clients to break down goals into small steps so their clients can accomplish them in a fairly short period of time. Accomplishing goals in a short period will help clients to feel successful (9).

There are two types of goals: process and product. It is most important to help a client focus on process goals. A client has more control over process goals then product goals, and if a client is focused on process goals then the outcome will be a result of that process. Tracking success in the process can be very motivating for a client. Something as simple as completing an exercise session represents the completion of a goal when the goal is participation (10).

It is important for personal trainers to determine when they will revisit with their clients to discuss their goals. Because every client is different, some clients progress more quickly than others, so it is important to discuss with each client when and how goals will be revisited and reevaluated. It is important to let clients know that everyone progresses differently and that is okay. It is also important to let clients know that it is okay to revise goals, add goals, or delete goals if necessary.

Reviewing Previous Exercise Experiences

To set up a well-rounded exercise plan it is important to understand a client's health concerns and fitness goals as well as to review previous exercise experiences. In discussing previous exercise experiences with a client, it is important to talk about not only the positive experiences but the negative experiences; what works and what does not work.

What worked? Personal trainers should have a conversation with their clients about what types of things have worked in the past and what factors may have helped them stick with an exercise program. Some clients may have to go back and have a discussion from when they were younger or when they were child. A client may not have current exercise history but asking a client to remember being physically active when he or she was a child can elicit positive memories and helps a client to remember that he or she has been successful.

Personal trainers are encouraged to talk with their clients about their positive experiences. Usually those positive experiences can be replicated into a new experience. If a client struggles to find something positive from past exercise experiences try asking the following questions:

- Did you ever feel good after working out?
- Did you ever notice having more energy during the day?
- Did you sleep better at night?
- Did you feel more relaxed?
- Were you able to think more clearly?

Some follow-up questions might be:

- Was exercise more successful at a certain time of the day?
- Was exercise more successful because of attending a class?
- Have you tried listening to music during exercise?
- Is it easier to stick to an exercise program when exercising with other people?
- What made past exercise experiences positive?
- What led to your quitting?

As personal trainers talk about previous exercise experiences with their clients there are usually a lot of reasons why a past exercise program did not work. Some of these reasons may be excuses, but others may be barriers that are difficult for a client to overcome. It is important for clients to have this information as an understanding of what factors could inhibit a new exercise program. By anticipating problems personal trainers can help their clients be more emotionally prepared to cope.

At this point in the conversation clients may mention several important factors that led to them dropping out of exercise: the exercise program was too difficult, they got injured, the exercise program took too much time, and life got too complicated. These are key indicators of factors that did not work for clients, and they are important for personal trainers to keep in mind when developing an exercise program for them. It is also important to take note of these things and check in with clients frequently about whether or not they are feeling any of these things. Personal trainers now know that if their clients are feeling any of these things, they are certain to drop out of their exercise program (3).

Finalizing the Program Design

By now personal trainers should have a really good sense of their client's health concerns, fitness goals, and past positive and negative exercise experiences. All of this information should give personal trainers a good sense of the direction that their client wants to go. It is at this point of the initial session with a client when the basics of an exercise plan are developed. Clients should be able to clearly see that a personal trainer has taken all of the information from their conversation to develop their program.

The rest of an initial session with a client should include gathering input from the client about what activities they want included in their exercise program. For example, if a client is interested in developing a strength program, it is important to take them through all training modalities: strength machines, free weights, balls, bands, medicine balls, and kettlebells. Once many of these training modalities have been covered, the conversation with the client can be continued about what he or she liked and did not like and the training program based on that information.

Lastly, the personal trainer can take the client through a detailed fitness assessment process to determine objective information such as body composition, cardiorespiratory fitness, and movement quality to further aid in program design. If the client agrees to a fitness assessment, personal trainers should perform these assessments where the client has some sense of privacy and out of the viewing eyes of other gym patrons. However, a fitness assessment may need to be performed on a following day (and can be used in conjunction with a first workout) if dealing with time constraints.

Help Clients Anticipate the Process

Probably one of the scariest parts of starting an exercise program for anyone new to exercise is having a sense of the first day on his or her own. Before the end of the first meeting, trainers should talk to their clients about the following: whether they are ready to begin, whether they have everything they need, whether they know where they are going, and whether they need more information.

If clients are new to a fitness facility, have a conversation with them about how to fit in. In this conversation it may be important to discuss the different kinds of members attending the facility. Clients will feel more comfortable knowing that there are other people who are similar to them. It is also important to discuss what clothing is appropriate to wear for exercise. Many people are not educated on appropriate workout clothing, and it is an important aspect of fitting in to a fitness facility. Having the knowledge that there are other people similar to them and understanding the appropriate workout clothing can help curb any social physique anxiety that clients may have.

Another important item to discuss with any new clients is the effect of other exercisers on their behavior. Other individuals in an exercise environment can influence another person's exercise behavior. Studies have shown that people increase their effort and performance when others are watching them, a principle called *social facilitation*. People want to create an impression that they are just as fit as the people exercising around them and may be reluctant to admit that a workout is more strenuous for them than for the person next to them. In self-reported studies, "people report lower ratings of perceived exertion (RPE) when they exercise next to a person who gives the impression that the exercise is very easy than when they are alone" (11). As a personal trainer, talk to clients about how they are affected by other people in the gym.

SUMMARY

In the initial session with a client there are several really important things to keep in mind. Communication is very important in the initial session and throughout working with a client. Listen carefully. Keep the conversation friendly and open and be as empathetic as possible. When talking about health concerns, educate about the dangers of a sedentary lifestyle and the specific health benefits associated with exercise. During any conversations about exercise goals, help clients identify goals that are realistic for them. Build self-confidence by helping clients identify areas of success but also discuss things that did not work, ensuring clients those factors will be considered when developing their exercise program. Allow clients to be involved in finalizing their exercise program and help them to anticipate what their first day will be like.

Importance of Effective Communication Skills

Effective communication is often the difference between success and failure for the relationship between a personal trainer and his or her client. It is important for personal trainers to understand the impact of verbal and nonverbal communication on their successes and failures. Moreover, effective communication skills are a learned behavior. Building the relationship with a client starts with the initial conversation; whether that is over the phone or in person. Regardless of the mode of communication, it is important to start building a positive relationship with new clients through proper communication skills.

Some skills to consider helping enhance communication with clients include the following (12):

* Explain important policies, procedures, and expectations so clients understand what is expected of them.
* Be sensitive to clients' feelings and connect emotionally to them (express empathy).
* Communicate consistently according to your personality and training style.
* Use a positive communication approach that includes encouragement, support, and positive reinforcement.
* Greet your client with a hello and a smile.

Nonverbal and Verbal Communication

In nonverbal communication what someone is thinking or feeling is reflected in his or her body language. Much nonverbal communication shows up in the face, such as a small movement in the lips or a change in the eyes. Other forms of nonverbal communication include physical appearance, posture, gestures, and body position. Humans are programmed to notice small nonverbal changes in other people. Many times the problem with nonverbal communication is how it is interpreted, although usually the impact of positive nonverbal communication is positive and the impact of negative nonverbal communication is negative. The negative effects of nonverbal communication generally will ensure that a client will not return (12).

Verbal messages must be clear to be received and interpreted correctly (12). For this to occur, messages need to be delivered at the right time and the right place. Not only the messages need to be delivered at the right time in the right place but the listener needs to clarify what he or she has heard from the speaker and the speaker needs to approve or reclarify with the listener.

Figure 19.2 illustrates a simple, four-step model of communication between a speaker and a listener. By examining this model in more detail, it is easy to see there is potential for error in virtually every step. First, it is not always clear what the speaker exactly wants to say. The speaker may choose words or phrases that are not completely accurate. The way a speaker communicates can vary in terms of tone, inflection, and enunciation. Moreover, what the listener actually hears may be all, some, or very little of what the speaker intended to communicate. The way a listener interprets the words that he or she heard may be very different than how the speaker interprets those same words. The result is miscommunication between the listener and speaker (13).

Active Listening

Active listening is more than having good communication skills. Active listening is about having an attitude and genuine interest in seeking a client's perspective and getting to know him or her. Active listening requires an individual to pay attention, avoid distractions, look the speaker in the eye, and provide feedback only when the speaker has finished.

Active listening in communication is not about convincing a client to do something, selling a program, or providing the right information. Active listening suggests that personal trainers seek to be respectful and genuinely care for clients, and that they desire to form partnerships or collaborative relationships with them. Instead of having the goal of communicating information, a personal trainer's goal should be to build a relationship with their client. This requires an attitude of honoring each client's perspective and a genuine interest in getting to know people. Arguably, it is more important to communicate understanding than to provide the right information.

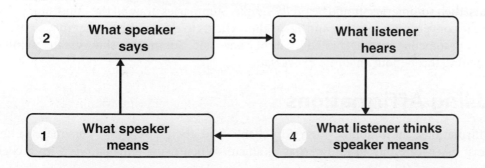

FIGURE 19.2

Verbal communication.

Fortunately, fairly simple communication strategies can be effective in helping clients feel supported, understood, and comfortable in forming a new relationship. These same simple communication strategies also minimize disagreements that may make the relationship with a client uncomfortable. By maximizing support and minimizing disagreements, personal trainers will help get people connected, and that connection is what leads to adherence to an exercise program.

Positive connections with clients give personal trainers the opportunity to be supportive of their client's pursuit of exercise. Lifestyle change seldom occurs all at once and without struggle. Gradual lifestyle change is often accompanied by a pattern of backsliding, stopping, and starting over. However, collaborative relationships with clients can and will provide the means to be supportive throughout the process.

Asking Questions

Closed-ended (directive) questions can be answered with one word. Although closed-ended questions can be important (for example, "What's your name,"), open-ended (nondirective) questions allow clients to give more information. Open-ended questions cannot be answered with a number, a place, or yes or no. They require clients to elaborate. Open-ended questions are very important for building collaborative relationships with a client because they invite discussion. They invite the client to express personal fears, barriers, failures, and successes. Open-ended questions are harder to ask than they seem. We do not typically use them in most of our daily conversations. Try listening to one of your typical conversations with a client. See how many closed questions you ask (13).

Reflecting

Reflections are conversational techniques that express the purported meaning of what was just heard (13). Reflections are rarely used in conversations but they are both subtle and powerful. They express caring and communicate understanding. Reflecting is an opportunity to make sure that what a client says is accurately understood, and it gives a client an opportunity to ensure they said what they thought or felt. Reflections are powerful because they show that active listening is occurring. If reflection is a new concept, reflections might seem like they come across as patronizing. It may seem like repeating every word a client says or going over information already covered is redundant, but it is not. As reflection becomes more fluent, the client naturally adds more information to what has been reflected. When done skillfully the conversation between a trainer and a client will flow, and all of the information will come from the client (14).

Summarizing

Summaries are a series of reflections. If a trainer has done a good job reflecting with clients, then summaries should be pretty simple. Summaries draw all the important points of the conversation together and again allow clients to clarify either what they have said or how someone has interpreted what they have said. Summaries show greater depth of listening throughout an entire conversation.

Using Affirmations

Affirmations show appreciation for clients and their strengths. Personal trainers must listen carefully to know what to affirm. When using affirmations with a client it is important to genuinely affirm something the client personally values. For example, affirming a client's workout clothes, sneakers, or heart rate monitor might seem appropriate, but generally, people will feel more validated by positive comments about their thoughts, plans, or skills. How are affirmations different from compliments? "Compliments typically have an evaluative judgment implicit within them" (15). Compliments usually begin with "I" statements. Changing "I" statements to "you" statements relocates the affirmation from an external advantage point to an internal client attribute. An affirmation communicates an appreciation of clients for who they are.

Asking Permission

Personal trainers oftentimes have the knowledge of what information is important and helpful for a client, but it is equally important to recognize as well that they do not always have the right information to share. Remember that clients are paying personal trainers to share information with them. However, before sharing information with a client it is important to ask permission to share that information. Asking permission to give advice softens the trainer's role as an authority figure, and supports a partnership in the decision-making process.

There are some basic ideas to keep in mind when communicating new information to a client. Some of those ideas are as follows (16):

- Imposing information on a client is likely to provoke resistance.
- Sometimes trainers may have information that they think will be beneficial for a client's success; however, it is important to ask permission, particularly if clients have not asked for the information.
- Provide information by using examples of work with other clients. For example, in my work with other clients this is what they found to be helpful.
- Give permission for clients to disagree with or disregard advice.
- Provide a menu of options.

 ## SUMMARY

A personal trainer's effectiveness depends on his or her ability to communicate with all types of people, clients, and colleagues. Personal trainers get paid to give good advice. And to a certain degree it seems that the more advice trainers provide, the more professional they are. Unfortunately, the need to give a lot of good advice has gotten in the way of being able to listen and the ability to get to know clients and what their needs are.

In recent years research has proven that what is more important than advice is how people engage and connect with clients. Engagement involves building a foundation with clients, listening and being able to understand their needs and wants and who they are overall as a person. Connecting with a client involves deepening all of the skills necessary for engagement including active listening, asking questions, reflecting, and affirming a client's beliefs.

Social Influences on Exercise

Social networks can strongly influence behavior and beliefs. People who are trying to change their exercise behavior and who have a strong social support fare better.

That social support can include family, friends, coworkers, personal trainers, and other people who provide encouragement, support, accountability, and companionship. Social support is one of the strongest predictors of exercise adherence.

During the first session with a new client, personal trainers should discuss the amount and type of social support the client may need or have. When talking about prior exercise successes, people may mention or attribute their past exercise successes to a workout buddy, a family member, or a friend. If a conversation does not go in this direction, some questions that might be asked include the following: Were other people involved in your past successes? Did family and friends help you stick to your exercise program? Who was the most important person that added to your exercise success? Inevitably exercise adherence and success can be partially attributed to social support.

Some clients may have a strong social support network whereas other clients may have a limited number of connections. For clients who have a strong social support network, have a conversation with them about how to use the social support they have available. For clients who have a limited social support network or no social support network, trainers should help clients find the social support they need to adhere to an exercise program. There are usually several opportunities within a fitness facility that will assist personal trainers in helping clients find areas of social support. One very simple way of helping a client find social support is to introduce them to other staff and members at the fitness facility. It is important for a client new to exercise to know people in their environment. Trainers can also design small-group training classes and encourage their existing clients to invite friends, coworkers, or family members. Lastly, provide informal orientation sessions for groups of new members, helping to connect them.

Although people with a strong social support fare better with exercise adherence, many people do enjoy exercising alone. Generally these people use exercise to get away from people, to spend some time alone, to think, or to destress and relax. It is important to respect their need for solitude and privacy. People who like to exercise alone may have strong social support at work or home that enables them to exercise regularly.

Helping clients to determine the kind and amount of social support they need to adhere to exercise is obtained in a conversation about past successful and unsuccessful exercise experiences. It is difficult for people to connect their successful exercise experiences to social support, just as it may be difficult for some clients to connect their unsuccessful exercise experiences to lack of social support. It is important to help clients make that connection (17).

What Are the Various Kinds of Support?

There are various kinds of support that help clients reach their health and fitness goals, and each of these support mechanisms has a significant impact on a client's successes or failures. Some of these support mechanisms include instrumental support, emotional support, informational support, and companionship support.

Instrumental Support

Instrumental support is the tangible and practical factors necessary to help a person adhere to exercise or achieve exercise goals. Some examples include transportation to a fitness facility, a babysitter, or a spotter for weightlifting at the gym. Components of instrumental support that are unsupported actually turn into barriers. It is practical to have a conversation with a client around these factors. People will not be able to adhere to an exercise program if there are tangible things that get in the way of them being able to exercise. For example, if a client does not have transportation, how is that client going to be able to get to the fitness facility every day?

Emotional Support

Emotional support is expressed through encouragement, caring, empathy, and concern. Praising a client for his or her efforts, encouraging a client to work harder, and sympathizing with a client when he or she complains about sore muscles are all examples of emotional support (18). Emotional support enhances self-esteem and reduces anxiety. Although emotional support goes a bit deeper, it can come in the form of an affirmation. As previously discussed, affirmations affirm intent and effort. Affirmations should be genuine and affirm something of value to clients.

Informational Support

Informational support is one of the main reasons that clients come to personal trainers in the first place. This type of support includes the directions, advice, or suggestions given to clients about how to exercise and the feedback regarding their progress. As discussed in the communication section, how trainers provide this type of information is also important. Informational support can come from formal sources such as personal trainers, group exercise instructors, or other health and fitness professionals or it can come from informal sources such as family and friends who share their own exercise experiences.

Companionship Support

Companionship support is probably the most familiar type of support. As discussed in the first few paragraphs of this section, similar to social support, companionship support includes the availability of family, friends, and coworkers with whom clients can exercise. Companionship during exercise produces positive feelings and may distract people from negative exercise-related feelings such as fatigue, pain, and boredom. Companionship also provides a sense of camaraderie and accountability.

Group Influences on Exercise

There are various persons whose influence may either help or hinder clients' abilities to reach their fitness and wellness goals. Some of these influences include spouses, parents, exercise leaders, and peers participating in a fitness group.

Family

The positive effects of a supportive spouse or partner on exercise behavior have been consistently demonstrated in published research. For example, healthy married adults who joined a fitness program with their spouse had significantly better attendance and were less likely to drop out of the program than married people who joined without their spouse (18).

There can be several downsides to family support. When family members pressure or make loved ones feel guilty about exercise, that person may actually respond by exercising less. This is known as *behavioral reactants*. People generally do not like to be controlled by others and on feeling pressured and controlled to exercise will do the opposite. Family members may also provide a sense of negative support. Negative support of exercise may include overprotectiveness. Family members may be overprotective of people with chronic disease or disability, and parents may be overprotective of their children's participation in physical activities that are perceived to have a high risk of injury. Other forms of negative support may include family members providing a sense of guilt because exercise is taking away from family time and family obligations.

Parental

Parental support at a young age is important for a developing child. It is important for a child to grow up understanding the importance of exercise and the negative impact of inactivity. Children need parents who model healthy and appropriate physical activity. It provides a sense of routine and familiarity for children that can last a lifetime. Besides being important for parents to model healthy and appropriate physical activity, it is important for children to be exposed to a variety of physical activities and for parents to empower their children with the ability to be able to choose the appropriate physical activities for themselves.

Exercise Leader

An exercise leader plays a role similar to that of a personal trainer. A big part of this job is engaging, connecting, and getting to know the members in the class. Group exercise instructors should introduce themselves, ask and remember members' names, acknowledge new class participants and ensure they are properly set up for class, introduce new class participants to veteran class members, talk to members about their goals and expectations, and check in with members after class. Compassionate exercise leaders generally have a positive social influence on exercisers and may contribute to increases in their self-confidence, enjoyment, and motivation to exercise (18).

Group exercise participants who experienced a socially supportive leadership style reported the following:

◆ greater self-efficacy
◆ more energy and enthusiasm
◆ less social physique anxiety
◆ more enjoyment of the class and the ability to try new things
◆ greater confidence

These results indicate that a socially supportive group exercise instructor can have positive effects on participants in a single exercise class. Because group exercise instructors are seen as reliable sources of health and fitness, many exercisers look at them as role models. As role models it is important that group exercise instructors use their influence to promote healthy and balanced attitudes and behaviors toward exercise. For example, instructors who exercise even when they are ill or exercise excessively may not be sending the appropriate message.

The Exercise Group

A sense of cohesion in a group exercise setting is related to whether or not an individual adheres to an exercise program. Some principles shown to increase group cohesiveness include the following: having a group distinctiveness, giving group members responsibilities for particular tasks, establishing group norms, providing opportunities to make sacrifices for the group, and increasing social interactions before, during, and after class.

Size

Research has suggested that the instructor's role is clearest in the largest and the smallest classes. In large classes participants expect there to be a group-oriented approach to teaching whereby the instructor addresses and reinforces the group as a whole. In a small class participants expect and usually receive a more individually oriented approach to teaching whereby the instructor addresses and reinforces individual members of the group. In a medium-sized group exercise class, research has shown that it may be unclear whether a group- or individual-oriented approach is best. The research goes on to say that there may be discrepancies between what participants expect and what approach is used by the instructor. Instructors may also be unsure about which approach is best in a medium-size class and use both styles inconsistently. Such inconsistency could contribute to dissatisfaction with the class and the instructor (18).

Composition

There is some evidence to suggest that the characteristics of the people in a group exercise class can affect the exercise experience of everyone in the group. Some of these characteristics that affect an individual's experience include sex, assimilation, and enthusiasm. The gender makeup of a group exercise class is one group composition factor that can affect an exerciser's experience. Women often report feeling uncomfortable in an environment that is made up of primarily men. In response, some health clubs have decided to offer classes for women only. Feeling similar to other group members in a group exercise setting can affect comfort level and motivation. People would prefer to exercise in an environment with people who are of similar body type and similar ability. Feeling less competent in a group exercise setting can diminish an exerciser's self-confidence and motivation. Personal trainers should keep this in mind, if they are planning on leading small groups or boot camps.

In a study with group exercise participants who were enthusiastic, encouraging of one another, and socially interactive, most participants reported greater enjoyment and stronger intentions to join an exercise group. Some first-time exercisers reported concerns about embarrassing themselves and being evaluated by other members in the group. For this group, encouragement and attention from other group members elicited feelings of self-consciousness and anxiety. For people who are new to exercise it may be important to help them focus on mastering the exercise skills before introducing them to an enthusiastic group (18).

SUMMARY

Personal trainers should encourage clients to consider their social support needs. It is critical that individuals consider whether or not they require support in exercise settings and what kind of support they need. Some people may need companionship support, whereas other people need instrumental support. Once an individual's support needs have been identified, personal trainers can help an exerciser identify where to get that support.

Other important social influences on exercise include the exercise instructor and the group exercise class. It is important for the group exercise instructor to develop a positive, socially supportive leadership style and for the class to create a cohesive group environment to help create a more comfortable group exercise experience that may prevent exercisers from quitting. Knowing this information will help you have these conversations with your clients and allow you to gain insight into what environments may be best for a variety of people.

Common Barriers to Exercise

Sticking to a regular exercise schedule is not easy, especially for somebody new to exercise. There are plenty of potential barriers and obstacles for an individual to overcome, such as a busy schedule, a poor social support network, and low self-confidence. However, there are practical strategies for overcoming common barriers to fitness.

Time

The most frequent reason given for not exercising is lack of time (19). Usually a closer look at an exerciser's schedule reveals that what people perceive as a lack of time is not in reality. One technique that exercise psychologists use with clients is a time journal. A time journal allows clients to keep track of what they do during the day for 3 or 4 days to gain a general sense of how the exerciser uses his or her time. In most cases the problem lies in how the exerciser prioritizes the day. For example, in many cases free time is used to watch television, to surf the Web, or to send e-mails. Being able to bring awareness to how much time an exerciser spends participating in these types of activities is important and can shed light on where to cut back to make time for physical activity (19,20).

Unrealistic Goals

When done properly goal setting is designed to help increase motivation, to build self-esteem, and for an exerciser to see and feel successful. Unrealistic goals, on the other hand, lower motivation, decrease self-esteem, and do not provide the exerciser a sense of success. It is not uncommon for someone to try and make up for missing weeks or years of exercise by engaging in unrealistic and intense exercise programs that lead to unnecessary injury.

It is important for personal trainers to help their clients define what is realistic. It is very difficult for people who are newer to exercise to understand what is realistic and what is not realistic. After weeks, months, or years, something has triggered your client to start exercising but that does not mean that he or she had any sense of how to start, what to do, or what is necessary to sustain exercise for a lifetime of health. In fact, many people in this position start off way too fast with far too many unrealistic goals. For example, a goal to lose a large amount of weight in a relatively short time is unrealistic and unhealthy. It is your responsibility to talk to your client about setting up a plan for losing weight in a realistic and healthy way (4).

Lack of Social Support

Social support is probably the most important type of social influence on exercise. Social support is the perceived physical and emotional comfort that a person receives from others (18). There is evidence to support the motivational and adherence value in exercisers having social support (21). There are various types of social support: instrumental, emotional, informational, and companionship. Personal trainers need to define what type and amount of social support their clients need to exercise that will help support their current exercise program and their adherence to exercise.

Social Physique Anxiety

Social physique anxiety is a concern with body image. In an exercise setting this includes a sense of difference in body type and attire preferences. Exercisers who experience social physique anxiety overemphasize the difference between their body type and the body types of others when in a fitness facility. Their perception is that they are more overweight and more out of shape than most others and then less able (capable) to participate in exercise. Similarly problematic for people who experience social physique anxiety are situations in which fitness facilities design exercise programs for people of similar body types. People in this situation do not feel comfortable being singled out.

Studies done on women in a group exercise setting and the clothes they wore revealed that women with higher social physique anxiety stood further away from the instructor and wore less revealing clothing. For these women, standing at the back of a group exercise class and wearing long, baggy exercise attire are strategies that they might use to ward off other people seeing and evaluating their bodies. Social physique anxiety is a real problem for many people, particularly those who are new to exercise. As a personal trainer you should try to work with your client to normalize their body type. One suggestion is introducing your client to people of similar body types who have become comfortable in a similar exercise environment (22).

For a client who is dealing with social physique anxiety it is vital to talk to your client about appropriate attire for an exercise environment and where to buy that clothing. A client new to exercise may not know what attire is appropriate for exercise nor will they know where to buy the appropriate attire.

Convenience

Access to facilities, classes, personal trainers, and instructors may be limited based on physical location or lack of adequate financial resources. Sometimes convenience of the physical location of a fitness facility is based on an individual's perception rather than the actual proximity of the facility. Examine all options available to clients, and if exercising at home will help some clients, come up with a program that is affordable and easy to do at home outside of an exercise facility (23).

SUMMARY

There are many barriers to exercise. Some of those barriers to exercise include time, unrealistic goals, lack of social support, social physique anxiety, and convenience of exercising. Some of these barriers are real and some are perceived. For clients to adhere to exercise they need to know their barriers, understand how those barriers affect their exercise, and have a plan to overcome them. Talk to clients about what gets in the way of their being able to exercise and help them find ways of dealing with those things that get in the way.

Strategies to Enhance Exercise Adherence

Starting and continuing an exercise program can be a challenging yet rewarding experience. Yet many individuals who attempt a new exercise regimen drop out within the first 6 months, fail to adopt a healthy, physically active lifestyle, and may require additional support mechanisms (24). Personal trainers should become aware of behavioral and cognitive factors that can improve exercise adherence and lasting lifestyle changes for their clients.

Behavioral Strategies

Behavioral strategies aim to change a client's behaviors and actions to improve exercise adherence and maintain a physically active lifestyle. Behavioral strategies include self-management, goal setting, and self-monitoring.

Self-Management

Self-management refers to individuals managing their own behaviors, thoughts, and emotions. Self-management skills improve an individual's ability to look at his or her behaviors, thoughts, and emotions and to change whatever is not working, for example, coping with and adapting to lifestyle changes such as those associated with beginning or returning to an exercise program.

Self-management of behaviors might include setting up an initial exercise program that is realistic and easy to follow. Managing individual behaviors, thoughts, and feelings incorporates looking at how individuals see life and the way they talk to themselves. For example, when people feel stressed they figure out the source of the stress and take action to deal with it.

Effective self-management skills maximize self-control energy, channeling it into the most important areas. Self-management skills increase the likelihood that desired changes in behavior will occur. These skills help clients change their environments in ways that support their exercise program adherence and help clients cope with difficulties that might otherwise short-circuit plans to exercise regularly (17).

Self-management skills are rarely taught, and it is generally not until clients have had an experience in which they need self-management training that they look for help. For example, some clients have the ability to talk themselves into exercising even when they do not want to while others struggle to exercise when they do not feel like doing it. The following are a few helpful self-management skills for improving exercise adherence.

Goal Setting

Goal setting is a process that involves assessing one's current level of fitness or performance; creating a specific, measurable, realistic, and challenging goal for one's future level of fitness or performance; and detailing the actions to be taken to achieve that goal (25).

Initial goal-setting sessions with new clients should be focused on coming up with long-term goals first. Clients' long-term goals should be based on their personal values, for example; who do they want to be and what is important to them. If clients' goals are an extension of their values, then they will have passion and inspiration and remain focused. Using the following questions may help clients determine their long-term goals (26).

- What do I want to accomplish in 6 months?
- What do I want to accomplish in the next year?
- What do I want to accomplish in the next 5 years?
- What is my dream accomplishment?

The next part of creating a goal-setting plan with a client is to create achievable short-term goals from the long-term goals already established. Long-term goals are made up of many short-term goals. Short-term goals not only provide a focused path, but also provide motivation and confidence when the client sees the benefit of achieving each short-term goal. Short-term goals help to focus the client's attention on the now. One key to setting short-term goals is to help clients narrow down goals to the ones that are the most important so that they do not get overwhelmed.

A client's short-term goals should not only include physical skills but also include mental skills. For example, your client lists motivation as a goal. Your client states that he or she is at a 2 in motivation but feels he or she should be at a 9. You now know that it is important for you to work with your client to set goals around becoming more motivated.

Effective goal setting stems from the acronym SMART. As mentioned earlier, SMART refers to specific, measurable, attainable, realistic, and timely. SMART goals use the following principles:

- **Specific**
  - » A specific goal is one that is clearly defined in such a way that anyone could understand what the intended outcome is. Goals should contain a detailed description of what is to be accomplished; when a client wants to accomplish it by; and the action(s) that will be taken to accomplish it.
- **Measurable**
  - » Goals need to be quantifiable. Establish a way to assess the progress toward each goal. If a goal cannot be measured, a client cannot manage it. For example, "I want to look better" is not measurable, but "to reduce body fat by 5% in 12 weeks" is measurable.
- **Attainable**
  - » Attainable goals are the right mix of goals that are challenging, but not extreme. Goals that are too easily accomplished do not stretch a client or make him or her grow as a person because they are not challenging enough.
- **Realistic**
  - » To be realistic, a goal must represent an objective toward which an individual is both *willing* and *able* to work. A goal is probably realistic if the individual truly believes that it can be accomplished. Additional ways to know whether a goal is realistic is to determine whether a client has accomplished anything similar in the past or to ask what conditions would have to exist to accomplish this goal.
- **Timely**
  - » A goal should always have a specific date of completion. The date should be realistic, but not too distant in the future. For example, set goals that can be achieved tomorrow *and* in 3 months.

The last piece of a personal trainer's goal-setting plan should include developing an action plan for how a client will reach his or her goals. This can be done by developing an action plan that clearly spells out how to achieve each short-term goal. To develop an action plan, a few action-oriented questions must be answered (26):

◆ What is my objective (goal)?
◆ What is the target date to complete my goal?
◆ What resources are needed to accomplish my goal (money, time, equipment, people)?
◆ What do I need to accomplish on a daily basis to reach my goal?
◆ What is the current status of my goal?
◆ What are some possible difficulties I may have to overcome to reach my objective?

Part of the goal-setting process is regularly reviewing a client's goals and the difficulties that he or she may have in reaching his or her goals. A client's priorities and circumstances may change, and it is important to be able to adjust goals when circumstances change.

There are many benefits to setting goals. The following is a list of some of the benefits:

◆ Goals direct attention to important elements of the skill being performed
◆ Learning what is within your client's control
◆ Empowerment
◆ Satisfaction
◆ Self-confidence
◆ Increased focus
◆ Increased motivation

Some common problems with goal setting include the following (26–29):

◆ Failure to convince exercisers of the importance
◆ Setting only outcome-oriented goals
◆ Failure to set SMART goals
◆ Setting too many goals
◆ Not knowing which goals are the priority
◆ Failure to adjust goals
◆ Lack of support

Self-Monitoring

Self-monitoring is usually done in the form of a daily written record of the behavior that a client is trying to change. Clients who are new to exercise may choose to keep an exercise log. An exercise log can have a variety of forms: journal, calendar, or a workout card. It is important for a client to find an effective, individual method of self-monitoring. A trainer may suggest that clients include not only time, exercises, calories expended, and perceived heart rate but also how much sleep they are getting, the kind of food they are eating, and how they are feeling emotionally. The following are benefits of self-monitoring (25):

◆ This log gives clients the opportunity to look at progress over time.
◆ Being able to see progress builds self-confidence and self-esteem, which leads to exercise adherence.

◆ The exercise log can be used as a form of accountability. In that sense if clients know you are going to ask them to show their exercise log each week, it can help keep them motivated.

◆ Self-monitoring encourages clients to be honest about their activity, which encourages them to stick to an exercise program.

◆ Logging a workout serves as a reward.

◆ Self-monitoring helps clients identify challenging situations and barriers to exercise.

Cognitive Strategies

Cognitive strategies aim to change a client's thoughts and attitudes toward exercise and physical activity. Cognitive strategies include positive self-talk, psyching up, and imagery.

Positive Self-Talk

For someone new to exercise there is a high degree of negativity and negative thoughts around exercise. Some of those thoughts include I can't do this, it's too hard, it takes too much time, and it's too painful. Helping your client to develop positive self-talk is essential. Here is how you can help coach an exerciser from a negative state to a more positive state:

◆ Help your clients become aware of their negative thought process by making a list of any negative thoughts they might have around exercise.

◆ Next, help your clients come up with a list of positive thoughts they might use with regard to exercise. For example, I can do it, I feel good, I can keep going, and I will stick with it.

◆ Train your clients to notice negative thoughts, stop those negative thoughts, and translate those negative thoughts into something positive from the list of positive thoughts you generated.

Another alternative is to generate a list of positive, motivating key words that your clients can use as an awareness tool and in place of negative thoughts to keep them motivated (30). For example, fast, energetic, go, focus, and get it.

Psyching Up

For someone new to exercise it is difficult to be motivated and get psyched up to exercise. For this reason it is valuable to give your clients the knowledge and skills to be able to develop the necessary positive energy to exercise. We want new exercisers to feel excited, positive, engaged, and energetic before exercise. These feelings will promote a desire for your client to work out.

The dialogue about getting psyched up to exercise should include any techniques your clients currently might use to get psyched up for other situations in their lives. It is important to use outside examples of how your clients get psyched up for work, shopping, or other projects. Using that information with regard to exercise can help make the transition much smoother.

Personal trainers need to help clients come up with a list of things that will help get them psyched up for exercise. Some examples include positive thoughts, keywords, imagery, specific food, and music. Because not all things work in all situations, on all days, or during different times, part of that fine tuning may include figuring out what does work in different situations, on different days, and during different times. Work with clients to fine-tune what will work in different situations.

The ability to continue having conversations with clients around whether or not they are psyched up to exercise, what is working and what is not working, is important in ensuring they will adhere to an exercise program. This is something that trainers will have to continue to revisit with their clients because it may continue to change.

Imagery

Imagery is a form of stimulation. It is similar to a real experience in that it includes all the senses, but it occurs in the mind. In everyday life we dream during the day and at night. In those dreams we conjure up all kinds of images, including how we will deliver certain types of information, what we will have for dinner, and how we will handle certain types of situations.

Exercise imagery is the process created to produce internalized experiences to support or enhance exercise participation. Whatever you can imagine pertaining to performance and participation might foster positive behavior change and goal attainment. Clients can imagine themselves approaching their activities with greater confidence. They can visualize performing with greater relaxation and muscular control. They can rehearse their performances with positive feelings and outcomes. They can manage pain and discomfort. They can create images of highly focused actions. And they can imagine positive outcomes that motivate their continuing motivation (31).

There are some things to think about when developing a piece of imagery with a client. Has the client had a similar past positive experience? If not, what other experiences can be used to help develop the client's imagery? If a client has a similar past positive experience, use that experience as the basis to create a piece of imagery. It is always best to draw from a client's own past experiences. It gives clients a sense of control and feelings associated with overcoming and being successful at whatever it is that they are currently struggling with. Work with clients to write down as much information as they can remember about that past positive experience: thoughts, feelings, sounds, tastes, smells, and sights. The more vivid the image, the more real it will feel. For example, if a client is struggling to get to the gym but in the past has found successful ways to overcome that barrier, use that information. Make sure to include the entire experience. Include as many thoughts, feelings, sounds, tastes, smells, and sights as you can. An entire piece of imagery may last for 10, 15, or even 20 minutes.

If a client does not have a past positive experience, you can work with your client to develop one by using television shows, videos, or role models. In developing this type of imagery, get a sense of how this has impacted a client and his or her rationale for using this information.

Once a trainer has worked with a client to develop a positive, successful piece of imagery, it is time to figure out the best times to use it. A client can use imagery at any time but particularly during a time when he or she may not be feeling motivated or positive about exercising. Many clients find it appropriate to record (CD, phone, or iPod) their piece of imagery and listen to it in the car or before going to bed.

Exercise imagery The process created to produce internalized experiences to support or enhance exercise participation.

SUMMARY

There are numerous techniques for helping clients enhance their exercise adherence. The most important aspect of helping clients enhance exercise adherence is to help them find the most appropriate technique for them. There are behavioral strategies, which include goal setting and self-monitoring, and there are several cognitive strategies, such as positive self-talk, helping a client to get psyched up for exercise, and visualization. These strategies can be used alone or in combination with each other.

Psychological Benefits of Exercise

The psychological benefits of exercise are well documented (6–8). Some of the proposed psychological benefits of exercise include promoting a positive mood, reducing stress, improving sleep, and reducing depression and anxiety.

Promotes Positive Mood

Many times people who exercise report feeling good after a workout. Feeling good means different things for different people, but it mainly signifies a positive mood encompassing feelings of satisfaction. Clients will often feel energized after exercise, which leads to a more positive outlook on life. Exercise also promotes feelings of relaxation and stress reduction, alertness, and improved ability to concentrate and focus, all leading to a positive mood.

Reduces Stress

Stress is the outcome of challenging situations in our lives. There are physical symptoms such as headaches and stomachaches, and there are emotional symptoms including frustration, pressure, and uncertainty. Exercise has been shown to be effective at reducing stress and can lead to immediate and long-term results (3). Many people report feeling less angry and irritable as a result of regular exercise. This is important because anger is most strongly associated with harmful health effects such as hypertension and heart disease.

For people who exercise as a way of dealing with stress it is a good idea to exercise during the time of day that is most beneficial. An early-morning workout might prepare someone for the day's stressors. A midday workout might provide a break in the day's stress and allow people to feel less angry and irritable throughout the rest of the day. A workout later in the day or early evening can provide a client with a method for decreasing the tensions and worries of the day and an opportunity to refresh before going home and going to sleep.

Improves Sleep

Many people report having better sleep when they exercise regularly. Typical improvements include falling asleep more quickly, longer periods of deep sleep, and feeling more refreshed in the morning (3,32). Because exercise has a positive impact on stress, anxiety, and depression, all of which interfere with sleep, exercise helps improve sleep

© ilolab/ShutterStock, Inc.

and reduce emotional health problems. Outdoor exercise is beneficial because it also provides light therapy, adding extra sleep benefits. There are many important qualities inherent in a good night's sleep, including:

- resistance to stress-related illnesses and immune function
- start the day feeling invigorated and refreshed
- reduced feelings of stress and an improved mood
- allows you to experience all the effects of regular exercise

Reduces Depression and Anxiety

According to research, regular exercise is associated with reductions in anxiety and depression (3,33). Anxiety refers to feelings of worry, self-doubt, fear, and uncertainty. Trait anxiety is a stable personality trait. If this person is new to exercise and exhibits high trait anxiety, his or her anxiety around exercise will start off high. If this person is new to exercise and exhibits low trait anxiety, his or her anxiety around exercise will start off low. State anxiety is situational, temporary feelings of anxiety. For example, rapid heart rate, sweaty palms, and butterflies in the stomach before a marathon are all examples of state anxiety. This translates into some people experiencing anxiety in certain situations but not all. If this person is new to exercise and exhibits high trait anxiety, his or her anxiety around exercise will start off high and may continue to increase. If this person is new to exercise and exhibits low trait anxiety, his or her anxiety around exercise will start off low but will more than likely increase because of the environment.

About one in four Americans suffers from clinical depression. It is well known for its symptoms of negative mood and feelings of hopelessness, which for many people become so severe they interfere with daily life. Exercise appears to be associated with improved mood in people who have depression. Research has shown that regular exercise has the greatest impact on depression and is comparable in effectiveness to psychotherapy and medication for mild to moderate depression.

SUMMARY

In an exercise program the primary goal of practitioners is to get sedentary or irregularly active individuals to adopt a regular exercise program and keep individuals who are in maintenance active (34). Some of the first steps in that process are for practitioners to have a basic understanding of what is important to clients, learning to communicate with clients, understanding the stages of change, knowing the benefits of exercise adoption and adherence, and being familiar with clients' barriers to exercise adoption and adherence to lend support and guidance in motivating clients to regular exercise. Hopefully you have come away from reading this chapter with the following insights:

- Not everyone approaches exercise in the same way.
- Exercise is no longer (only) concerned with providing someone a strength and cardio program.
- The most beneficial exercise program is developed with and for an individual based on who they are and what they need, physically and psychologically.
- Exercise is no longer contained in a prescription but is in relation to building a strong relationship through good communication.

The consensus on guidelines to help support the adoption and adherence to an exercise program includes interventions that are applied based on the personal and environmental characteristics and barriers of an individual (34). However, it is always important that health and fitness professionals make exercise enjoyable, provide social support, and offer participants a wide range of activities to choose from.

REFERENCES

1. Centers for Disease Control and Prevention. Prevalence of self-reported physically active adults—United States, 2007. *MMWR Morb Mortal Wkly Rep.* 2008;57(48):1297-1300. Available at http://www.cdc.gov/mmwr/preview/mmwrhtml/mm5748a1.htm. Accessed October 25, 2010.
2. Lambert VE, Bohlmann IMT, Cowling K. Physical activity for health: understanding the epidemiological evidence for risk benefits. *Int J Sports Med.* 2001;1:1-15.
3. Brehm B. *Successful Fitness Motivation Strategies.* Champaign, IL: Human Kinetics; 2004:91-111.
4. Anshel MH. *Applied Exercise Psychology: A Practitioners Guide.* New York, NY: Springer Publishing; 2006:53-66.
5. Brehm B. *Successful Fitness Motivation Strategies.* Champaign, IL: Human Kinetics; 2004:21-40.
6. Knubben K, Reischies FM, Adli M, Schlattmann P, Bauer M, Dimeo F. A randomised, controlled study on the effects of a short-term endurance training programme in patients with major depression. *Br J Sports Med.* 2007;41(1):29-33.
7. Dimeo F, Bauer M, Varahram I, Proest G, Halter U. Benefits from aerobic exercise in patients with major depression: a pilot study. *Br J Sports Med.* 2001;35(2):114-117.
8. Scully D, Kremer J, Meade MM, Graham R, Dudgeon K. Physical exercise and psychological well being: a critical review. *Br J Sports Med.* 1998;32:111-120.
9. Brehm B. *Successful Fitness Motivation Strategies.* Champaign, IL: Human Kinetics; 2004:41-61.
10. Annesi JJ. *Enhancing Exercise Motivation: A Guide to Increasing Fitness Center Member Retention.* Los Angeles, CA: Fitness Management Magazine; 1996.
11. Lox LL, Martin Ginis KA, Petruzzella SJ. *The Psychology of Exercise Integrating Theory and Practice.* Scottsdale, AZ: Holcomb Publishing; 2006:133.
12. Weinberg RS, Gould D. *Foundations of Sport and Exercise Psychology.* Champaign, IL: Human Kinetics; 2007:232.
13. *YMCA Activate America Listen First: Learn and Implement Workbook.* Chicago, IL: YMCA of the USA; 2007: 1-15.
14. Fuller C, Taylor P. *A Toolkit of Motivational Skills Encouraging and Supporting Change in Individuals.* Hoboken, NJ: John Wiley & Sons; 2008.
15. Rosengren DB. *Building Motivational Interviewing Skills: A Practitioner Workbook.* New York, NY: Guilford Press; 2009:62.
16. Rosengren DB. *Building Motivational Interviewing Skills: A Practitioner Workbook.* New York, NY: Guilford Press; 2009:58-87.
17. Brehm B. *Successful Fitness Motivation Strategies.* Champaign, IL: Human Kinetics; 2004:63-75.
18. Lox LL, Martin Ginis KA, Petruzzella SJ. *The Psychology of Exercise: Integrating Theory and Practice.* Scottsdale, AZ: Holcomb Publishing; 2006:101-138.
19. Strazdins L, Broom DH, Banwell C, McDonald T, Skeat H. Time limits? Reflecting and responding to time barriers for healthy, active living. *Health Promot Int.* 2010 Oct 15. [Epub ahead of print]
20. Van Duyn MA, McCrae T, Wingrove BK, et al. Adapting evidence-based strategies to increase physical activity among African Americans, Hispanics, Hmong, and Native Hawaiians: a social marketing approach. *Prev Chronic Dis.* 2007;4(4):A102.
21. King AC. Clinical and community interventions to promote and support physical activity participation. In: Dishman RK, ed. *Advances in Exercise Adherence.* Champaign, IL: Human Kinetics; 1994:183-212.
22. Bowden RG, Rust DM, Dunsmore S, Briggs J. Changes in social physique anxiety during 16-week physical activity courses. *Psychol Rep.* 2005;96(3 Pt 1):690-692.
23. Anshel MH, Seipel SJ. Self-monitoring and selected measures of aerobic and strength fitness and short-term exercise attendance. *J Sport Behav.* 2009; June. http://findarticles.com/p/articles/mi_hb6401/is_2_32/ai_n31872073/. Accessed December 14, 2010.
24. Mcauley E, Courneya KS, Rudolph DL, Lox CL. Enhancing exercise adherence in middle-aged males and females. *Prev Med.* 1994;23(4):498-506.
25. Lox LL, Martin Ginis KA, Petruzzella SJ. *The Psychology of Exercise: Integrating Theory and Practice.* Scottsdale, AZ: Holcomb Publishing; 2006:139-174.
26. Effective Time Management. Available at http://www.effective-time-management-strategies.com/fitness-goal-setting.html. Accessed November 1, 2010.
27. Williams J. *Applied Sport Psychology Personal Growth to Peak Performance.* Mountain View, CA: Mayfield Publishing Company; 1998.
28. Gavin J. *Exercise and Sports Psychology.* Champaign, IL: Human Kinetics; 2005:44-45.
29. Weinberg RS, Gould D. *Foundations of Sport and Exercise Psychology.* Champaign, IL: Human Kinetics; 2007.
30. McAuley E, Talbot HM, Martinez S. Manipulating self-efficacy in the exercise environment in women: influences on affective responses. *Health Psychol.* 1999;18(3):288-294.
31. Gavin J. *Exercise and Sports Psychology.* Champaign, IL: Human Kinetics; 2005:46.
32. Reid KJ, Baron KG, Lu B, Naylor E, Wolfe L, Zee PC. Aerobic exercise improves self-reported sleep and quality of life in older adults with insomnia. *Sleep Med.* 2010;11(9):934-940.
33. Salmon P. Effects of physical exercise on anxiety, depression, and sensitivity to stress: a unifying theory. *Clin Psychol Rev.* 2001;21(1):33-61.
34. Buckworth J, Dishman, RK. *Exercise Psychology.* Champaign, IL: Human Kinetics; 2002.

© Vlas2000/ShutterStock, Inc.

© Eky Studio/ShutterStock, Inc.

© Ilolab/ShutterStock, Inc.

Developing a Successful Personal Training Business

After studying this chapter, you will be able to:

✔ Describe the qualities and characteristics of uncompromising customer service.

✔ Describe strategies for finding an ideal workplace.

✔ Understand the process for writing a resume.

✔ Understand the four Ps of marketing.

✔ Understand basic membership sales techniques, including strategies for solicitation of new sales and how to close sales.

The Business of Personal Training

Although generating revenue in excess of expenses, i.e., "making a profit," is the assumed goal of any business, profit alone is not the only or even "sole" purpose of the business itself. The main purpose of creating and running a successful business is to create and keep a loyal customer base or following. Successful businesses are very interested in who their customers are, for example, where do they live, where they come from, what are their likes and dislikes, and what can they do to attract new customers to their business and more importantly, what can the business do to keep customers returning. Running a *successful* personal training business, whether as an independent business owner, as an independent contractor, or an employee in a health club setting, is no different than running a successful Fortune 500 business; the motto is always "the customer always comes first!"

When profit alone is the primary focus of any business, the source of that profit (nearly always the customer or consumer) at some point will get neglected. Once a business loses sight of what is creating revenue, the revenue will begin to drop if not disappear altogether and threaten the future of the business. Conversely, organizations (and individuals) that possess a fanatical customer focus reinvent themselves continually to provide an ever-growing level of value to their customers. Long-term profit generation is largely the result of creating and keeping customers. Most successful business have clearly defined mission and vision statements that define exactly what the business is about and what their goals are; many of them mention "customer service."

Good customer service is all the things that businesses do to attract and keep customers happy that go beyond the day-to-day activities of simply running the business. These activities are intended to increase customer satisfaction. For personal trainers, good customer service starts the second you approach a new prospective client (remember they are sizing you up as well). The ultimate goal of good customer service is to always strive to meet, and when possible exceed, the expectations of your customers. Satisfied and delighted customers are customers who are happy and content, share your name with their friends, and are proud and excited to be your client, and more importantly, customer service is instrumental in the long-term success of any business.

This chapter provides the personal trainer with the initial steps to take to enter into the personal training profession; basic marketing strategies; and a progressive, customer-focused process for creating a distinctive level of value and developing a highly successful client base. By mastering the OPT™ model, completing NASM's CPT certification, and applying the tools and solutions learned with clients, you will be able to create or greatly increase your personal level of success.

Starting Out

Most personal trainers are passionate about fitness and living a healthy lifestyle. They enjoy learning about new exercises, nutrition requirements, and gym equipment. They believe in this lifestyle so much they've decided to make it their profession. However, there is much more to personal training than nutrition and exercise. Personal training requires skills in sales, marketing, and finance. Whether a personal trainer plans to work independently or at a local health club, successfully running a personal training business is no different than starting any other business; it takes time, determination, preparation, and a well thought-out and detailed plan. As discussed in chapter 6 (Fitness Assessment), personal trainers must perform detailed and comprehensive fitness assessments to design individualized exercise programs based on their client's goals, needs, and abilities. Similarly, to have a successful, customer-focused, and profitable career, personal trainers should perform detailed financial assessments and develop strategic business and marketing plans to meet their needs. The first step in this process is education.

The Importance of Education

Earning a certification from a recognized and accredited organization should be an aspiring fitness trainer's first goal. Education is vital in teaching individuals the entire scope of practice of personal training, including how to properly assess and instruct their clients through safe and effective workouts. The International Health Racquet & Sportsclub Association (IHRSA) recommends earning a certification from an organization that has either received accreditation or is in the process of receiving accreditation of their programs from an accrediting body such as the National Commission for Certifying Agencies (NCCA) (1). In addition to earning a certification, higher education—such as a college degree in an exercise science related field (e.g., exercise science, exercise physiology, kinesiology, biomechanics, or physical education)—will help enhance marketability, experience, and knowledge regarding health, wellness, and exercise prescription. Currently there are no government regulations that require personal trainers to earn a certification or college degree; however, most gyms and health clubs enforce certification as a minimum requirement. Gyms and health clubs more often are taking IHRSA's advice, which requires that individuals earn a certification that has earned third-party accreditation. Unaccredited certifications are becoming a thing of the past, and the fitness community is demanding more education from today's fitness professionals.

Memory Jogger

Scope of Practice

Personal trainers are health and fitness professionals who perform individualized assessments and design safe, effective, and individualized exercise and conditioning programs that are scientifically valid and based on clinical evidence for clients who have no medical or special needs. They provide guidance to help clients achieve their personal health, fitness, and performance goals via the implementation of exercise programs, nutritional recommendations, and suggestions for lifestyle modification. They hold a current emergency cardiac care (cardiopulmonary resuscitation) certification and respond appropriately during emergency situations. Certified Personal Trainers do not diagnose and/or treat areas of pain or disease, and they refer clients to other health care professionals/practitioners when appropriate. They abide by NASM's Code of Professional Conduct at all times.

Where to Work?

Once the certification process is complete, it is time to search for employment. There are a number of facilities that allow a gradual development of the skills necessary to become a successful fitness professional. It is important to facilitate the skills learned during the certification course in a pleasant atmosphere where one can make modifications in presentation skills, rapport building, and acquire observational skills. Some example facilities include:

◆ YMCA
◆ Jewish Community Centers (JCC)
◆ Local Town Recreation & Park Services
◆ Women-only facilities
◆ Commercial fitness clubs

Most new professionals become successful when the intangible skills (i.e., building rapport, maintaining basic people skills, and coaching) are developed early on in a career. Many facilities provide the necessary hands-on training needed to help solidify these skills and ensure long-term success.

Once the basic characteristics in the fitness professional are harnessed, a more lucrative position in the fitness field is often desired. Although most individuals enter the fitness field with a passion to help others reach healthy goals, a lucrative tenure is usually a foundation for long-term achievement. A profitable career will help make a profession more enjoyable because it provides financial stability and personal growth. Often a personal trainer will be required to sell his or her services to receive monetary rewards (i.e., profit, bonus, or higher salary).

Commercial Fitness Facilities

Commercial fitness facilities usually rely on revenue growth and member retention for survival. Personal training and other fitness services are sometimes known as "profit centers" because they add to the base revenue generator. Typically, the base revenue generator for most clubs is memberships. In this setting, the personal trainer will be expected to regularly sell personal training services to club attendants. Most staff professionals will have weekly, monthly, or quarterly sales quotas. In most commercial fitness facilities, pay rates are structured on a leveled system that meets the needs of the club and helps develop the selling techniques of the fitness professional. For example, personal trainers with multiple fitness-related certifications, numerous years of service, or high client retention will often earn a higher base salary or bonus incentive.

Not all facilities are the same. Some facilities may require no selling on the part of the personal trainer and only require exercise instruction. These facilities usually have membership advisors that sell fitness services at the point of the club membership sale. However, personal trainers should not solely rely on the sales staff but rather be proactive in attaining clientele (discussed later in this chapter).

Some commercial fitness clubs also provide in-house training in advanced exercise techniques, nutrition, youth training, senior training, and salesmanship. Some clubs also invest in the latest cardiovascular, strength, balance, and flexibility equipment. This is advantageous because it allows personal trainers to work with the latest equipment and learn updated fitness and conditioning concepts. Ultimately, the more information a personal trainer acquires regarding exercise equipment and exercise techniques, the more marketable they become for professional growth. Coincidently, the more rehearsed and educated a personal trainer becomes with advanced information and tools, the more confidence is developed. One cannot suggest that this is only gained at the commercial fitness club because every facility is different. Most facilities, both nonprofit and for-profit, are dependent on budget management and areas of expertise.

Independent Contractors

An independent contractor can be a person, business, or corporation that provides goods or services to another entity under terms specified in a contract or within a verbal agreement. Unlike an employee, an independent contractor does not work regularly for an employer but works as and when required. These individuals do not receive the benefits of full-time employees, such as health insurance or retirement packages (e.g., a 401K), but rather work on a contract basis. As an independent contractor, a personal trainer typically pays a fee to a gym or health club in return for the ability to train clients at that facility. Personal trainers can be very successful as independent contractors because they learn the necessary business skills to help them advance into private practice and network with local businesses. Although independent contractors are not employed by the club, they still represent the business and service the club provides. Being an independent contractor allows a fitness professional to learn how to budget his or her time, market himself or herself within a club, and improve organizational skills. This setting can be a stepping stone to a fitness professional owning a facility or studio.

In-Home Personal Training

Some personal trainers also elect to work with clientele in their homes. This option requires the fitness professional to travel and use portable equipment. Clients receive services in the convenience of their own homes, and the fitness professional gains notoriety in the community, which allows for networking opportunities and referrals. Some advantages to this position are no overhead costs for a physical building (e.g., rent, utilities) and autonomy to develop one's own business model. There are some disadvantages that present themselves when traveling between client locations. The fitness professional must equip his or her vehicle with obtuse equipment (stability balls, BOSU® ball, weights, etc.), which increases gasoline expenditure depending on the travel distance. They also must plan ahead to set up the equipment in the client's home, which may make sessions spill over into the next hour. These travel and set-up periods can lengthen visits and cost the professional opportunities to work with additional clients. Most personal trainers succeed in building a clientele within a certain mile-radius in their community and only transport certain pieces of equipment. Other options include setting up affiliations with manufacturers that allow clients to purchase exercise equipment for the home through the fitness professional. These means prove advantageous for the fitness professional because they cut costs and set-up times drastically.

Owning a Facility

Many fitness professionals dream of being their own boss. Although the dream can be wished by anyone in any occupation, there is still an enormous amount of work that goes into building a business around one's own model. Owning a facility or studio can be an advantageous endeavor simply because the demand for service can be appealing to the fitness professional and the bottom line. Marketing and networking is done at the discretion of the fitness professional and the target population is usually what the fitness professional specializes in working with. However, owning a facility also involves overhead costs, hiring and firing staff, community networking, facility ordinances, taxes, insurance, and preserving a continuous stream of clientele for business. Most fitness professionals that elect to set up their own business are experienced and understand the nuances to enter the business world and be successful. Table 20.1 outlines the advantages and disadvantages of various employment opportunities.

Resume Writing for the Fitness Professional

In conjunction with researching potential employment opportunities, aspiring personal trainers need to write a first-rate resume. Personal trainers that want to get noticed in a sea of applicants for that "most desired" training position need a well-structured resume. A resume is a selling tool that outlines a fitness professional's education, skills, and experience so employers can see at a glance how the trainer might contribute to their company. *A resume does its job successfully if it does not exclude one from consideration.* In many cases, it may take less than 30 seconds for employers to decide if a resume ends up in the "consider" pile or the "reject" pile.

The most effective resumes clearly focus on a specific job title (e.g., Personal Trainer, Group Exercise Instructor, General Manager) and address the employer's

TABLE 20.1	Employment Advantages and Disadvantages	
	Advantages	**Disadvantages**
Commercial Fitness Clubs	• Salesmanship provides business learning opportunity • Provide in-house training in various areas (nutrition, sports training, business, etc) • Pay rates structured on client retention with incentives and fitness professional's level of education • Updated equipment and exercise protocols	• Selling may impose challenge with monthly & quarterly quotas • Pay rates may begin at a lower level to motivate sales • Club dictates marketing and business practices
Independent Contractors	• Professional may control schedule • In control of marketing and business practices • No overhead costs for building or ordinances	• Not employed by club, therefore no benefits (medical, vacation, 401K, etc) • Business and marketing not totally supported by club • Club may take percentage of session fees
Owning a Facility	• Appeal to personalized clientele • Can be financially rewarding if proper business model is used • Networking & marketing tailored to target population	• Responsible for overhead costs, local ordinances, taxes, hiring and firing staff, community networking, & client retention

stated requirements for the position. Knowing about the duties and skills required for a specific position helps aspiring applicants organize and tailor their resume around these points to get noticed and be successful.

Tips for Writing an Effective Resume

◆ An "objective" is a statement that expresses an employment goal in one or two short phrases. Aspiring personal trainers should emphasize what they can offer rather than what they are seeking. *Example:* "I am a reliable fitness professional eager to make a positive difference" versus "I am seeking a position as a training professional in your organization." The latter is implied when you submit a resume.)

◆ List all college degrees, fitness certifications, advanced specializations, and completed continuing education courses.

◆ New college graduates should list their education before their work experience, especially if they have limited work history. Fitness professionals with no or little college experience should list their work experience first. Listing the most attractive features near the beginning of a resume will help give a good first impression to potential employers.

- Aspiring personal trainers should list all work experience that has taught important, relevant, and applicable skills such as sales, customer service, leadership, and multitasking, even if the work experience was not in the fitness industry.
- List references on a separate sheet of paper. It's much better to use space on a resume for important skills, experience, and education. You may note "references provided upon request" at the bottom of your resume.
- Avoid listing family members as references. Former managers, supervisors, mentors, and college professors make excellent references.
- Avoid spelling and grammar errors.
- Ask a mentor, teacher, or friend to review your resume.
- Use clean, high-quality, white, 8½- × 11-inch paper and a plain, easy to read font.
- After dropping off resumes with potential employers, aspiring personal trainers should follow up with a "thank you" phone call or email. A proper follow-up will leave a lasting impression with the hiring managers.

Interviewing

It is a good idea that fitness professionals who are seeking employment practice their interviewing skills before their first interview with a hiring manager. By asking a friend or relative to play the part of the interviewer, aspiring fitness professionals can rehearse their answers, which may decrease anxiety and help give a good first impression. Answers during an interview should be concise, eloquent, and personable.

An interview is a fitness professional's chance to shine. Before the interview begins, it is equally important to shake the interviewer's hand, smile, and make eye contact when introduced. While conversing it is important for an individual to talk about their good qualities. For example, if one has limited experience working as a fitness trainer, he or she should discuss previous jobs and how they relate to personal training, such as experiences in customer service and sales. Personal training can relate to many fields and most health clubs are willing to hire new trainers as long as they show potential and an eagerness to learn.

 SUMMARY

Personal training requires skills in sales, marketing, and finance. Whether a fitness professional plans to work independently or at a local health club, successfully running a personal training business is no different than running any other business. It takes time, determination, preparation, and a well thought out and detailed plan.

The first step to becoming a certified personal trainer is education. Education is vital in teaching the fitness professional how to properly assess and instruct their clients through safe and effective workouts. The IHRSA recommends earning a certification from an organization that has either received accreditation or is in the process of receiving accreditation of their programs.

Once the certification process is complete, it is time to search for employment. There are a number of facilities and avenues available to aspiring personal trainers, including the YMCA, JCC, recreation and park services, women-only facilities, commercial facilities, independent contracting, and ownership.

Personal trainers who want to get noticed in a sea of applicants for that "most desired" training position need a well-structured resume. A resume is a selling tool that outlines a fitness professional's education, skills, and experience so employers can see at a glance how they might contribute to their company. The most effective resumes are clearly focused on a specific job title and address the employer's stated requirements for the position.

Lastly, it is a good idea for fitness professionals who are seeking employment to practice their interviewing skills before an actual interview. Answers during an interview should be concise, eloquent, and personable.

Marketing 101

Many personal trainers mistakenly identify marketing as simply advertising a product or service. Though advertising is an element of marketing, it is not the only or the most important part. Merriam Webster's dictionary defines marketing as "the process or techniques of promoting, selling, and distributing a product or service" (2). Although this definition is rather simplistic, it begins to demonstrate how marketing encompasses many elements above and beyond creating signage and other forms of advertisements.

Marketing is the process of promoting a product or service (such as personal training) by communicating the features and benefits to potential customers. Effective marketing requires identifying the customer's needs, developing the appropriate products or services to satisfy those needs, and promoting services and solutions in a cost-effective manner. The ultimate goal of marketing is to understand the wants and needs of consumers so well that selling becomes nonessential because the product or service sells itself.

Whether working in a commercial facility, as an independent contractor, or as a business owner, personal trainers must develop a comprehensive marketing plan to achieve a full book of business. This requires a detailed understanding of potential clients' wants, needs, demographics, and socioeconomic statuses. For example, if a personal trainer is working in a health club that mostly caters to working parents and young adults, he or she should provide services to accommodate these individuals' goals and work or school schedules, such as early morning and evening classes. Conversely, if a personal trainer works mostly with stay-at-home parents and retirees, this personal trainer can create incentive packages for training during afternoon hours when clubs are typically less crowded.

The Marketing Mix (The Four Ps of Marketing)

To have a successful marketing plan, fitness professionals must have an understanding of the marketing mix, also known as the four Ps of marketing. The marketing mix refers to activities that a personal trainer can control to produce the response he or she wants from a target market. The four Ps of marketing include:

- **Product:** The specific product or service offered to customers.
- **Price:** The amount charged for a product or service, including volume discounts, seasonal pricing, and bundle packages.
- **Place (distribution):** Channels a product or service will go through to reach the customer.
- **Promotion**: The communication of information about a product or service with the goal of generating a positive customer response. Some marketing communication strategies include advertising, sales, social media, and public relations.

Product

As is the case with any other business, it is important to identify the specific product that is being delivered to the customer. Most services provided by a personal trainer are sold by the hour or by the session, which leads some to believe that it is time with the client that is being sold. In other scenarios, it might be assumed that the product is the education that the client receives from working with the trainer. This type of education may come in the form of how to use equipment properly, how to eat correctly, or how to lose weight. Others may venture to say that the motivation to exercise is the product being sold.

The fitness professional may provide all of the previously mentioned services; however, ultimately, the product delivered to the customer is the result that is trying to be achieved. If a client wants to lose weight, he or she may opt to get involved in personal training to "have the motivation to go to the gym" or "learn how to exercise properly"; however, these are paths that lead to the end result of weight loss. It is important for a personal trainer always to keep in mind that the obligation lies in the result rather than the path. Remembering this will allow you to never lose sight of your purpose and need for this position. It is when the fitness professional assumes the service they are providing is a path rather than a result that professional productivity declines and the impact of the business is lost.

Developing a Niche or Specialty

Having a specialty or a niche is a great way to help personal trainers stand out and provide a unique product in a competitive market. Earning additional certifications, advanced specializations, or a higher educational degree may enable fitness professionals to offer their services to a select group of clients. For example, fitness professionals may choose to become specialists in weight management, corrective exercise, sport-specific conditioning, or even working with a certain sex or age group. Targeting a specific category with many potential clients and very few other trainers can position the fitness professional to dominate their specific niche and greatly improve their earning potential.

Price

Personal training pay rates vary across the country and depend on many factors including the socioeconomic status of clientele; the type of training offered (boot camps, small-group training, personal training); volume discounts; and the education and experience level of the fitness professional. Moreover, personal training in populated and affluent areas is generally more expensive than in rural areas. Before determining a set price, fitness professionals should research the demographics and socioeconomic status of potential clients in their area. Equally important is research into competitor's prices. Based on this information, fitness professionals can begin to find an *appropriate* price for their services. Keep in mind that there is no such thing as the "perfect price"; inevitably, a small percentage of clients will be unable to afford your services.

Place

Place refers to where and how a product or service is distributed and sold. In the case of personal training, most think of a gym or health club; however, new trends in the industry are emerging that will allow personal trainers to offer their services through a variety of distribution channels, including:

- Online and phone coaching
- Youth sports groups and after school programs
- Boot-camps held at local parks, schools, or beaches
- Corporate wellness programs
- Sport training centers
- Senior centers

Promotion

Promoting personal training services involves communicating important information to potential clients with the goal of generating a positive customer response. Some marketing communication strategies include traditional advertising (e.g., print advertisements, posters, and brochures); promotional sales; sponsorships; and community service. Additionally, web-based communications such as a professional website; online advertising (banner ads); and social media (e.g., Facebook, Twitter, and LinkedIn) are extremely useful and engaging mediums by which personal trainers can advertise their services. Online marketing can be a successful form of advertising that will help personal trainers maximize their return on investment. Moreover, the unique features of social media enable personal trainers to advertise and interact with potential clients in real time.

Promotions can be categorized into two separate entities: push or pull. Advertising *pulls* a consumer towards a fitness professional by making the consumer aware of his or her services. An incentive, such as seasonal or bulk discounts, *pushes* a personal trainer's services by encouraging potential clients to purchase in volume.

SUMMARY

Many personal trainers mistakenly identify marketing as simply advertising a product or service. Although advertising is an element of marketing, it is not the only nor the most important part. Effective marketing requires identifying the customer's needs, developing the appropriate products or services to satisfy those needs, and promoting services and solutions in a cost-effective manner.

To have a successful marketing plan, fitness professionals must have an understanding of the marketing mix, also known as the "four Ps of marketing." The marketing mix refers to activities that a personal trainer can control to produce the response he or she wants from a target market. The four Ps of marketing include:

- **Product:** The specific product or service offered to customers.
- **Price:** The amount charged for a product or service including volume discounts, seasonal pricing, and bundle packages.
- **Place (distribution):** Channels a product or service will go through to reach the customer.
- **Promotion:** The communication of information about a product or service with the goal of generating a positive customer response. Some marketing communication strategies include advertising, sales, social media, and public relations.

Providing Uncompromising Customer Service

Success in the fitness industry does not end with successful attainment of a personal training position and a basic understanding of marketing. Success depends, to a great degree, on reputation. Those known for excellence and distinction in their profession gain a competitive advantage over everyone else working in the same position. It is essential to have a strong commitment to excellence, knowledge, and professionalism to be thought of with high regard. The best personal trainers operate with the utmost level of integrity and refuse to settle for anything less than their personal best.

To develop a reputation as an excellent personal trainer, one must first develop a reputation for uncompromising customer service. *Uncompromising customer service* means being unwavering in providing an experience and level of assistance that is rarely, if ever, experienced anywhere else. Develop an obsession for becoming artistic in your approach to helping people. The most successful personal trainers never settle for average, never stop trying to improve themselves or their business, never settle for second best, and are always looking ahead.

An important business strategy to remember is that most if not all buying decisions are based on emotion. Clients have many choices regarding where to exercise, and who to exercise with. Thus, how a client goes about choosing a personal trainer is based on how they *feel* (often first impressions) about a given facility and the personal trainers that work there. This feeling is often based on the level of customer service received and that client's perception of the value offered. Those who adapt to uncompromising customer service as the minimal acceptable standard of professionalism will give clients positive feelings. It is clear that relationships are the most powerful competitive advantage in a service profession.

Guidelines for Uncompromising Customer Service

In everyday business, there is always a tendency to get caught up in tasks and details, which sometimes results in overlooking the bigger picture, in this case the customer. Successful personal trainers never think of any of their clients as an interruption of work; instead they are the entire reason their business exists in the first place!

Keys to developing an uncompromising customer service philosophy include the following:

1. Take every opportunity to meet and get to know all potential clientele. Each and every time you walk into the club or onto the workout floor is an opportunity to create a professional relationship with a potential new client and, eventually, make a sale.
2. Remember to represent a positive image and high level of professionalism every minute of the day.
3. Never give the impression that any question is inconvenient, unnecessary, or unintelligent.
4. Express ideas well through verbal communication, vocal tonality, and body language, which all work together to convey a message.
5. Obsess on opportunities to create moments that strengthen professional relationships.
6. Do not merely receive complaints, but take ownership of them.

Successful personal trainers routinely ask themselves the following question: *If my entire future were based on the way this one client evaluated his experience with me right now, would I change anything?* They may also ask, *Did I exceed this client's expectations?* If the answer to either of these questions is "no," committed fitness professionals would continue to look for ways to improve themselves. NASM's education, application, integrity, solutions, and tools are the foundation for creating "yes" answers to these questions and providing optimal performance and results for clients.

SUMMARY

The primary purpose of a business is to create and keep customers. A customer-focused process, using the keys to uncompromising customer service, will create a distinctive level of value and develop success in finding, building, and retaining clients. Establish a reputation for excellence and distinction as a fitness professional, then develop a reputation for uncompromising customer service. Leave each club member with a positive impression.

A client's buying decisions are based on how he or she feels about a certain facility and its fitness professionals. These feelings are influenced by the level of customer service received and perception of value offered. As such, clients are never an interruption of work, but rather the entire purpose behind it. Each client's experience should be treated as if it affects the entire career of the fitness professional, because it does.

Know Who Your Customers Are

Fitness clientele may seek out the services of a personal trainer for a variety of reasons, including the desire to improve their appearance, sports performance, or general health and to increase their physical capacity in activities of daily living. Whatever the reason(s) clients seek out personal trainers, the ultimate motivation is the desire to improve their quality of life.

Advanced technology is not synonymous with better health although that is a widely held assumption. If anything, because advances in technology have replaced so many aspects of everyday movement, in reality it is associated more so with poor health than anything else. Decreases in physical activity are directly associated with greater risk and rates of obesity, diabetes, heart disease, and musculoskeletal dysfunction, as well as numerous other chronic diseases (3–8). It is obvious that the need for professional, personalized physical training is increasing. Personal fitness training may once have been viewed as a luxury, but it is moving toward becoming a necessity. In the very near future, health care may play a pivotal role in the success and growth of the fitness industry. NASM's certified personal trainers will be qualified to deliver the OPT system and tools, producing remarkable results for clients.

In today's sedentary culture, who is a potential client? Everybody! It is difficult to imagine anyone who does not have a desire to look and feel better, perform at a higher level, be healthier and more confident, enjoy a better quality of life, and reduce chronic pain.

Approaching Potential Clients

Far too often, young, inexperienced, or sometimes even experienced, personal trainers never reach their full career potential because they do not know how to sell themselves. They confuse selling their services as selling in the traditional sense (such as selling cars or stereo equipment), when in fact it is not really selling at all. Instead of viewing sales in a negative sense, personal trainers learning to attract new clients should think of sales as self-promotion. All they are really doing is confirming to others what they already know, which is that they are the "*best of the best.*"

The first step in learning to self-promote yourself is to not be afraid to approach potential new clients, especially if you have never met them before. Stand up straight, walk up to them with poise and confidence, and without even saying a word convey to them that you are the best personal trainer around and that if they want results, they need to be with you! Remember that personal trainers can change the life of a client, which is an awesome responsibility.

Openly provide that uncompromising customer service by doing any of the following:

- Say "hello" to every member while working out or while working a shift.
- Make eye contact, smile, and be personable to every member.
- Offer members a towel or some water.
- Roam the floor, clean up equipment, and make sure that the workout floor is impeccable and represents the highest standard of appearance.
- Do not hide behind the fitness desk, a computer, or a magazine.
- At the very least, simply introduce yourself by name and ask members for their names as well.
- Let members know that you are there to enrich the club experience, by attending to *any* need. Then just do it!
- First interactions with new members should be professional, pleasant, and most important, nonthreatening.
- Once you have made an initial contact with a new member, now you are in a better position to offer valuable assistance. If a member is performing an exercise incorrectly, tell him or her about a positive benefit of that exercise. Then, offer to help that person "maximize the exercise." State that you have just attended a seminar or read a book (which should always be true) that offers an alternative to what he or she is already doing. If the member says "No, thanks," leave him or her alone. However, if he or she says "Yes," provide specific help with the exercise and articulate the benefit that the member will receive related directly to his or her goal. Continue to offer him or her assistance throughout the workout.

There are also ways that have been shown to be immediately off-putting to members. Potential clients are very unreceptive to any approach that may challenge their belief systems or judgments regarding an exercise or competencies. Avoid any of the following opening lines:

- May I make a suggestion?
- Can I recommend a better way of doing that?
- Can I show you a different technique?
- Let me show you the right way.
- Can I help you with that?
- What's your goal for that exercise?

Creating Value

The increased need for personal training does not guarantee the success of all fitness professionals. Just because people have a need or a desire does not mean that they will take action. In the clients' minds, the value of the service must outweigh the cost. *Cost* refers to the price of the services as well as the time, effort, and commitment involved in training.

In addition, individuals may have reservations created by the potential for failure. It is the fitness professional's personal responsibility to create and display the value of their services.

To be successful at attracting and keeping clients, personal trainers must be familiar with the NASM–BOC Code of Professional Conduct and they must use the systematic approach presented throughout this text.

In addition to adhering to the NASM–BOC Code of Professional Conduct, NASM personal trainers shall:

♦ Excel at using NASM's integrated fitness assessments (including subjective and objective information) and various movement observations to accurately assess the needs and goals of the individual.

♦ Have the ability to design an OPT training program and correctly fill out an OPT template.

♦ Explain to clients how each component of the exercise program focuses on their personal goals and needs.

♦ Be able to demonstrate exercises and implement individually tailored exercise programs for a wide range of clients.

♦ Demonstrate to clients how the OPT system offers them the greatest benefits possible.

Clients need to believe in the personal trainer they choose to work with and trust that he or she will help them achieve their personal health and wellness goals and objectives. It is important to remember that the OPT system is a map to success and a systematic approach that ensures results.

© Eky Studio/ShutterStock, Inc.

Did You Know?

NASM–BOC Code of Professional Conduct

In following and adhering to the NASM–BOC Code of Professional Conduct, NASM personal trainers shall:

1. Maintain their competencies through continuing education
2. Adhere to safe and ethical training practices (e.g., OSHA)
3. Adhere to strict facility maintenance (e.g., equipment, safety, layout, disinfection)
4. Understand scope of practice with respect to special considerations for training diverse clientele (e.g., age, sex, cultural background, and ability)
5. Clearly understand the role and professional limitations of a personal trainer (e.g., referral to registered dieticians, allied healthcare professionals)
6. Adhere to professionalism and ethical business practices
   a. Liability insurance
   b. Record keeping
   c. Medical clearance
   d. Physical appearance and attire
   e. Timeliness
   f. Sexual harassment awareness
   g. Client confidentiality (e.g., HIPAA)

For a complete transcript of the NASM Code of Professional Conduct, log onto www.nasm.org

SUMMARY

Clients use the services of personal trainers for a variety of reasons, but all with the motivation to improve quality of life. In today's sedentary culture, everyone can be considered a potential client. There are countless people who desire to look and feel better, be healthier and more confident, perform better, enjoy a higher quality of life, and reduce chronic pain. Personal training is moving toward becoming a necessity, and health care may soon play a pivotal role in the success and growth of the industry.

However, simply because someone has a desire to do so does not mean that person will take action. The value of personal training services must outweigh their price, time, effort, and commitment. It is the fitness professional's personal responsibility to create and display that value.

Personal trainers need to be proactive when approaching prospective new clients. Avoid making members feel uncomfortable by saying things such as, *"Can I recommend a better way of doing that?"* Instead, do things such as:

- Roam the floor and say "Hello" to every member, while offering towels and water and making sure that everything is clean and safe.
- Introduce yourself and ask members for their names, letting them know that you can help them with any of their needs.
- Avoid overeducating new clients. However, if a member is performing an exercise incorrectly, find out what it is about the exercise that is important to him or her. Then, offer to help that person "maximize the exercise." Use movement and postural observations for screening and the OPT model to customize the exercise and other recommendations. Continue to offer the potential client assistance throughout the workout.

To secure a client, the fitness professional must use the OPT system as a map to success and use its systematic approach, which ensures results by:

- Using NASM's integrated fitness assessment and movement observations to accurately assess and design exercise programs based on the needs and goals of the individual.
- Designing OPT training programs and correctly filling out an OPT template.
- Explaining to clients how the OPT system offers the highest benefit and how each program component focuses on personal goals and needs.
- Explaining first, then demonstrating exercises to new clients.

Sales Techniques

It is probable that a high level of customer service will, in turn, increase sales of personal training. To the personal trainer, that means sales to clients. However, there are many negative connotations regarding sales. Many personal trainers are reluctant to ask for a sale because they associate selling with either rejection or doing something that is ethically wrong.

It is not through manipulation but concern and professionalism that sales are created. There are numerous benefits related to performance, health, self-esteem, and quality of life that can be gained through the fitness professional's services, using the OPT solutions and tools. The fact is that until a potential client makes a purchase, he or she cannot benefit from these services. The sale is the first essential step to helping a client to achieve results.

Ten Steps to Success

Developing a list of good clientele depends on how well personal trainers learn to self-promote themselves while out on the floor. Personal trainers should not make the mistake of relying on sales consultants to schedule all potential client orientations, because it is a philosophy that is dependent on the productivity of someone else and causes personal trainers to give up control of how many presentations they are able to make each week.

Set up a plan based on a desired annual income goal. Use the following 10 steps and corresponding questions to direct the design of that plan.

Step 1: What is the Desired Annual Income?

An annual income goal is the achievable desired sum total of monthly earnings over 12 months. After clearly identifying a desired annual income, move on to step 2.

Example: Based on her expenses and lifestyle, Christy would like to earn $40,000 annually as a fitness professional.

Step 2: How Much Must Be Earned per Week to Achieve the Annual Goal?

Divide the desired annual income by 50 to figure out what will need to be earned on a weekly basis. (Instead of dividing by the 52 weeks in a year, use the number 50 to allow for 2 weeks of vacation, sick time, jury duty, and so on.)

Example: Christy divides $40,000 by 50, which equals $800. She knows that she will need to earn $800 each week to hit her goal.

Step 3: To Earn the Weekly Goal, How Many Sessions Need to Be Performed?

To earn the weekly amount, how many clients or sessions are needed each week? To establish this number, take the weekly goal and divide it by the amount earned per session.

Example: Christy divides $800 by $25 per hour. Now, Christy knows that she will need to perform 32 sessions per week to hit her goal.

Also, take the current average number of paid sessions performed weekly and divide it by the number of clients currently signed up.

Example: Christy currently performs 20 sessions per week and has 11 regular clients. She divides and gets a number of 1.82. So, Christy divides her goal of 32 sessions by 1.82 and can now estimate that she needs at least 18 clients to hit her income goals.

Step 4: What Is the Closing Percentage?

Personal trainers need to figure out their closing percentage. This number is determined by the total number of people helped on the floor compared with how many of them purchased training packages.

> *Example: Christy looks back at her contact log and ascertains that she has spoken to 60 members in the last 30 days. Of those 60 members, she managed to sign up 5 of them as clients. When she divides 5 by 60, she sees that her closing rate is 8%.*

Step 5: In What Timeframe Will New Clients Be Acquired?

Unrealistic timeframes will likely lead to frustration and disappointment. However, if a timeframe is set too far in the future, it will not create the sense of urgency necessary to maximize performance.

> *Example: Since she now has 11 clients and needs to have at least 18 to hit her goals, Christy decides that she wants to gain at least 7 more clients. She decides to set a time frame of 3 weeks to gain 7 new clients.*

Step 6: How Many Potential Clients Need to Be Interacted with Overall to Gain Clients within the Timeframe?

Take the desired number of new clients and divide that number by the closing percentage.

> *Example: Christy wants 7 new clients and her closing rate is 8%. She divides 7 by 8% and comes up with 87.5. Christy must have excellent contact with at least 88 members during the next 3 weeks to come close to her goal of 7 new clients.*

Break down the number of members that need to be interacted with overall into weekly increments to make the process more manageable.

> *Example: Christy needs to contact at least 88 members during the next 3 weeks. She divides 88 by 3 and realizes that she has to contact about 30 members each week.*

Step 7: How Many Potential Clients Need to Be Contacted Each Day?

Further break down the number of members that need to be interacted with on a weekly basis into daily increments to create concrete goals for each workday.

> *Example: Christy is aiming to contact 30 members each week. She works 5 days per week. So, she divides 30 by 5 and discovers that she only needs to talk to 6 members each day. This is a much more manageable number than she originally thought.*

Step 8: How Many Potential Clients Need to Be Contacted Each Hour of the Day?

Once more, break down the number of members that need to be contacted on a daily basis into hourly increments to form easy, solid plans for each hour on the floor.

Example: Now that she knows she only needs to approach 6 members each day, Christy divides that number by her actual floor time. She generally conducts four 1-hour sessions each day during her 8-hour shift. She also takes a half-hour lunch and usually conducts one half-hour orientation. That leaves her with 3 hours on the floor to contact her goal of 6 members. Christy now knows that after dividing 6 by 3, she must talk to a member every 30 minutes to achieve her goals.

For each contact in that hour, provide measurable, personalized assistance that is related to the goal of the person being approached. These contacts, even if they do not develop into sales, add to a valuable future prospect base.

Step 9: Ask Each Member Spoken to for His or Her Contact Information

The NASM-certified personal trainer possesses core competencies of individualized assessment, OPT program design, and exercise selection. These personal trainers automatically have the capacity to provide a personalized, results-oriented experience for any member they make a connection with.

If a good level of rapport has been built with a member, do not be afraid to ask him or her for their contact information. Offer to develop a few exercises to help him or her achieve the goals discussed. Contact the member and arrange a time to assist them in implementing the new exercises during his or her next visit to the club.

Step 10: Follow Up

It should be clear by now that every exercise is an assessment. Regardless of the exercise that a member was doing on the floor, write down what you saw according to the five kinetic chain checkpoints in general movement and postural observations. Write and keep detailed notes on each member. Within 24 hours, mail the member a handwritten thank-you card for the time they spent with you in the club. This is classy and considerate, causing members to remember you.

Give the card 2 to 3 days to arrive, and then call the member 1 week from initial contact. During the call, work toward the following goals:

◆ Make sure the member got the card.
◆ Thank him or her personally for his or her time.
◆ Let the member know that you have thought about his or her goals and would like to go over some exercises that will be helpful.
◆ Be clear that it will only take about 10 minutes the next time he or she is in the club.
◆ Determine the next time he or she is coming to the club.
◆ Schedule an informal appointment during his or her next visit.

When you see the member again, be sure to:

◆ Implement a couple of the exercises on the floor and explain how they relate to the member's goal.
◆ Offer the member a more thorough assessment, an individualized program design, and a single training session to maximize the results he or she is currently seeing.
◆ Directly ask the member to sign up for a package of sessions.

Asking for the Sale

Most sales are lost because they are not asked for. Failure to close a sale comes down to one or more of the following four reasons:

1. There was not enough value built into the sale.
2. An insufficient level of rapport makes the potential client hesitant to go ahead.
3. The health and fitness professional did not affirmatively ask for the sale.
4. The potential client legitimately does not have the ability to pay.

The first three can be directly controlled. Many personal trainers are able to offer high value and have outstanding personalities, but do not ask for the sale because they fear rejection.

After following the above 10 steps and then directly asking for the sale, 9 of 10 members will say no. That may seem incredibly discouraging. However, even with a 10% closing ratio, thousands of personal trainers in the industry have been able to develop a steady clientele. If the personal trainer has established rapport, had empathy for why the client's goals are important to him or her, conducted a thorough assessment, and made the right program recommendations, then rejection is considerably less likely. For example:

> **Personal Trainer:** Sarah, we have outlined what is most important to you and developed the OPT program to get you there. Let's go through the OPT template and I'll explain all the parts to you. Ask me any questions that come up. Once you feel like you understand it, let's get started today.

When a potential client says yes to a product, program, or personal training package, go through the following steps:

1. Finish the sales transaction.
2. Schedule the client's first appointment within 48 hours.
3. Send the client a thank-you card within 24 hours.
4. Call to confirm before the first appointment.
5. Go over the client's goals again and briefly reiterate how he or she will achieve those goals.
6. Congratulate the client and acknowledge him or her for taking the first step in achieving his or her goals.

If a potential client declines to take the appointment or purchase services:

- Remain professional and helpful.
- Thank the potential client for participating in the session.
- Make sure to have the potential client's contact information.
- Ask to call him or her in a couple of weeks to check on program status.
- Send a thank-you card immediately.
- Schedule a follow-up call in 14 days in a daily planner.
- Every 30 days, send information that pertains to the potential client's goals (such as pertinent points from article clippings, trade journals, fitness Web sites, and so forth).
- Make sure to follow through on all of the above tasks.
- Keep a record of all points of contact.

Successful personal trainers keep in consistent contact. They understand that a "no" today is not a "no" indefinitely. They realize that contacts equal opportunity and that the more contacts they make, the more opportunity they will have to change lives. Finally, these individuals know that the greater the number of people who consider them "expert" resources, the larger their referral base will be.

SUMMARY

Personal trainers must work the floor and greet members to develop rapport, build relationships, and eventually close sales. Use the 10-step plan to work toward an overall goal:

1. Choose a desired annual income.
2. Determine how much must be earned per week to achieve the annual goal.
3. Figure out how many sessions need to be performed to earn the weekly goal (and how many clients are needed for those sessions).
4. Calculate closing percentage.
5. Decide in what timeframe new clients will be acquired.
6. Determine the number of potential clients that need to be interacted with overall to gain clients within the timeframe. Figure out a weekly contact rate based on that number.
7. Break down the weekly contact rate into daily increments.
8. Further break down the daily contact rate into the number of hourly contacts.
9. Ask each contact for his or her contact information.
10. Follow up with a thank-you card and a call, and schedule an informal appointment during the member's next visit.

Most sales are lost because they are not asked for. The sale is the first essential step to helping a client benefit from the personal trainer services. Rejection is much less likely when the fitness professional has established rapport, built a relationship, had empathy for why the client's goals are important to him or her, conducted a thorough assessment, and made the right OPT program recommendations. Whether a potential client says "yes" or "no" to a product, it is important to remain professional and helpful, get the potential client's contact information, send out a thank-you card immediately, call to check in, stay in contact, make sure to follow through, and finally, keep a record of all points of contact. A "no" today is not a "no" indefinitely. Having a large base of people who consider a fitness professional an "expert" resource will surely increase his or her referral base. More contacts create more opportunities.

REFERENCES

1. The International Health, Racquet & Sportsclub Association. Available at: http://www.ihrsa.org/home/2010/1/14/accreditation-announcement-to-ihrsa-members.html. Accessed January 24, 2010.
2. Merriam-Webster's Dictionary. Available at: http://www.merriam-webster.com/dictionary/marketing. Accessed January 24, 2010.
3. Haskell WL, Lee IM, Pate RR, et al. American College of Sports Medicine, American Heart Association. Physical Activity and Public Health: Updated Recommendation for Adults from the American College of Sports Medicine and the American Heart Association; *Med Sci Sports Exerc.* 2007; Aug;39(8):1423-1434.
4. Pedersen BK, Saltin B. Evidence for prescribing exercise as therapy in chronic disease. *Scand J Med Sci Sports.* 2006;16 (Suppl 1):3-63.
5. Sherman SE, Agostino RBD, Silbershatz H, Kannel WB. Comparison of past versus recent physical activity in the prevention of premature death and coronary artery disease. *Am Heart J.* 1999;138:900-907.
6. Centers for Disease Control and Prevention. Prevalence of physical activity, including lifestyle activities among adults—United States, 2000–2001. *MMWR Morb Mortal Wkly Rep.* 2003;52(32):764-769.
7. Zack MM, Moriarty DG, Stroup DF, Ford ES, Mokdad AH. Worsening trends in adult health-related quality of life and self-rated health—United States, 1993–2001. *Public Health Rep.* 2004;119(5):493-505.
8. Harkness EF, Macfarlane GJ, Silman AJ, McBeth J. Is musculoskeletal pain more common now than 40 years ago? Two population-based cross-sectional studies. *Rheumatology (Oxford).* 2005;44(7):890-895.

© Eky Studio/ShutterStock, Inc.

© ilolab/ShutterStock, Inc.

Exercise Library

© ilolab/ShutterStock, Inc.

Flexibility

Self-Myofascial Release

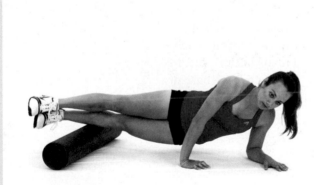

Peroneals

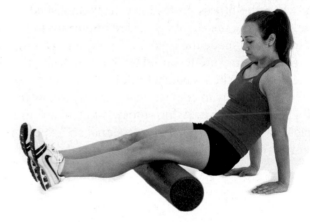

Hamstrings

Flexibility *continued*

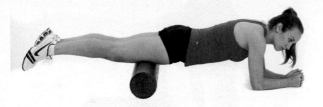

Quadriceps

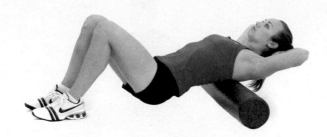

Thoracic spine

Static Stretching

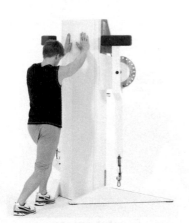

Soleus

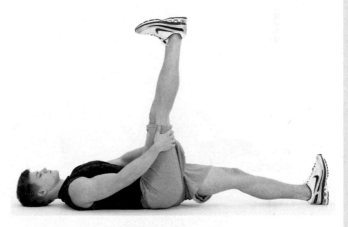

90/90 hamstring

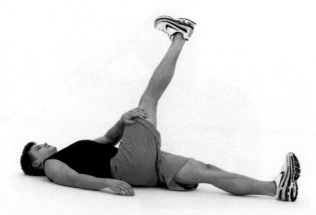

Supine biceps femoris

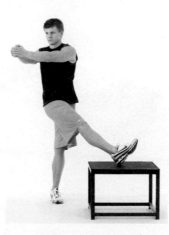

Standing biceps femoris

Flexibility *continued*

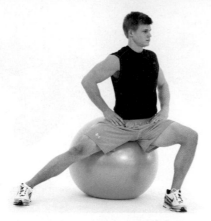

Seated ball adductor

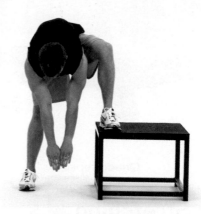

Adductor magnus

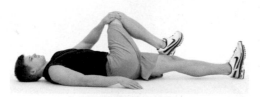

Supine piriformis

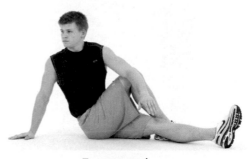

Erector spinae

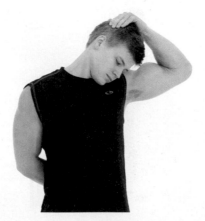

Levator scapulae

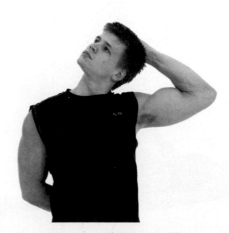

Sternocleidomastoid

Flexibility *continued*

Active-Isolated Stretching

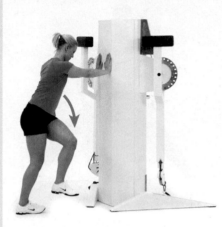 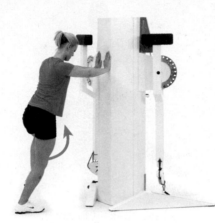 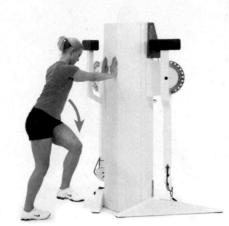

Soleus (supination/pronation)

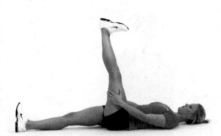 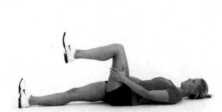 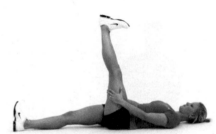

90/90 hamstring

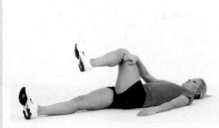 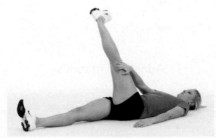 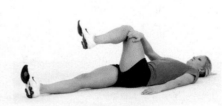

Supine biceps femoris

Flexibility *continued*

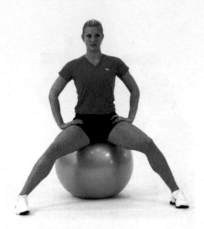 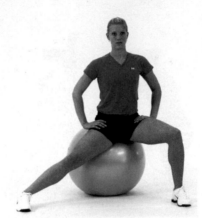 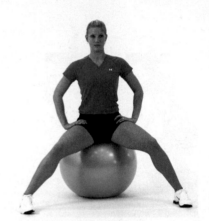

Seated ball adductor

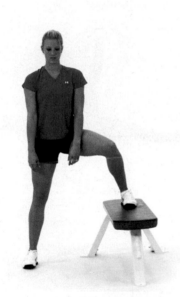 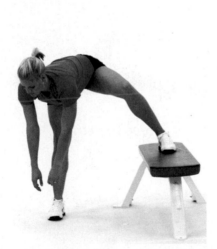 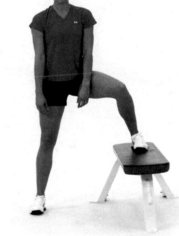

Adductor magnus

Flexibility *continued*

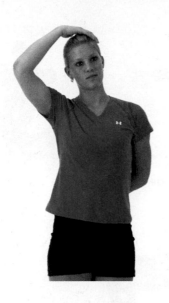
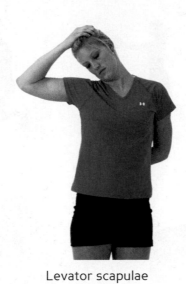
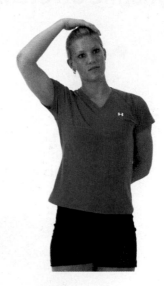

Levator scapulae

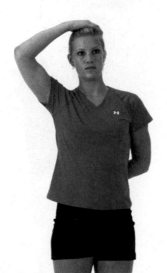
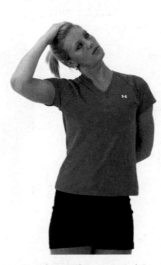
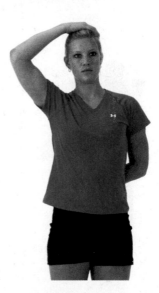

Sternocleidomastoid

© ilolab/ShutterStock, Inc.

Flexibility *continued*

Dynamic Stretching

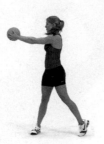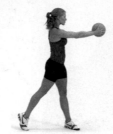

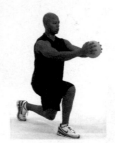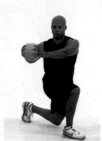

Medicine ball rotation

Lunge with rotation

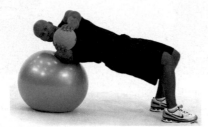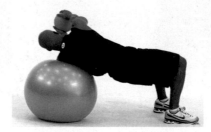

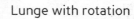

Russian twist

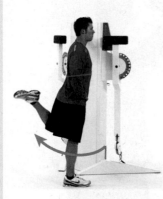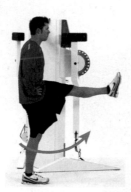

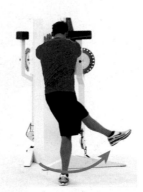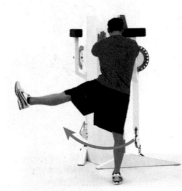

Leg swings: front to back

Leg swings: side to side

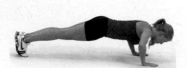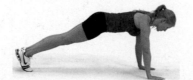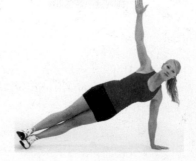

Push-up with rotation

Core

Core-Stabilization

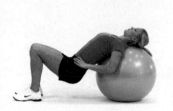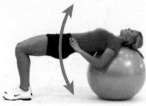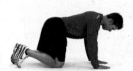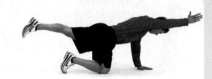

Ball bridge   Quadruped opposite arm/leg raise

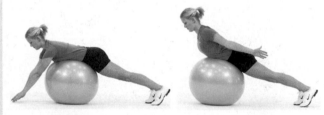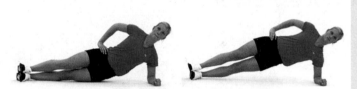

Ball cobra   Side iso-abs (side plank)

Core-Strength

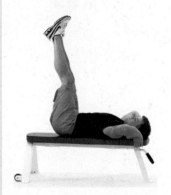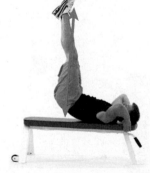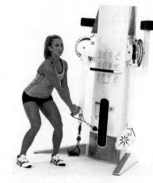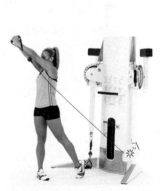

Knee-up   Cable lift

Core *continued*

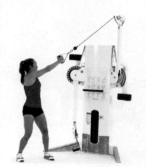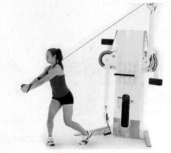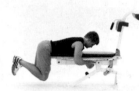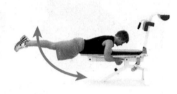

Cable chop

Reverse hypers

Core-Power

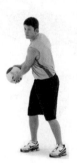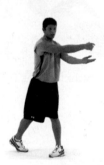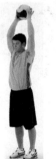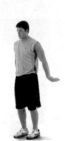

Side medicine ball oblique throw

Soccer throw

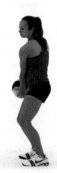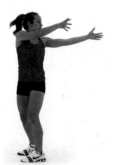

Medicine ball back extension throw

Balance

Balance-Stabilization

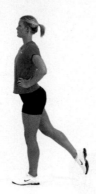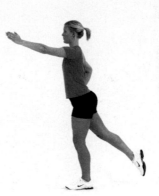

Single-leg arm and leg motion

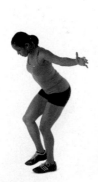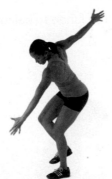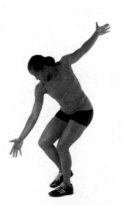

Single-leg windmill

Balance-Strength

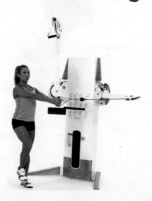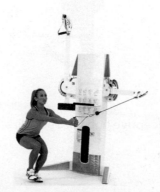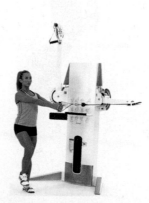

Single-leg squat with cable assistance

Balance *continued*

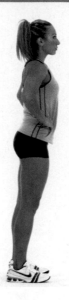
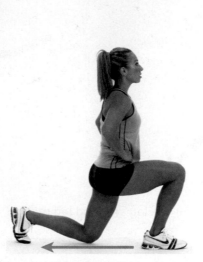
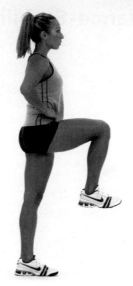

Reverse lunge to balance

Balance-Power

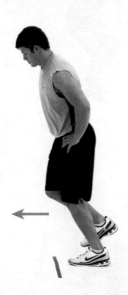
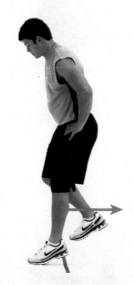
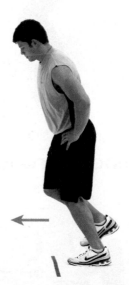

Single-leg proprioceptive hop with stabilization: sagittal plane

Balance *continued*

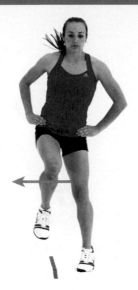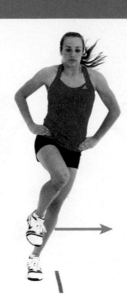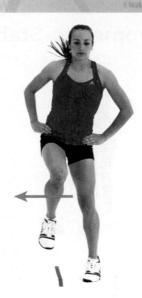

Single-leg proprioceptive hop with stabilization: frontal plane

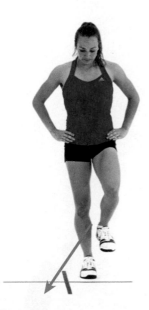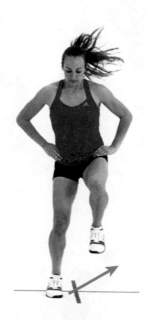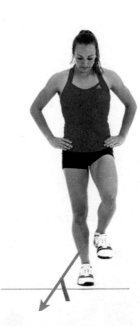

Single-leg proprioceptive hop with stabilization: transverse plane

© ilolab/ShutterStock, Inc.

Plyometric

Plyometric-Stabilization

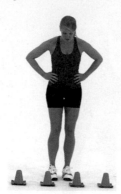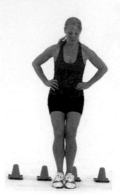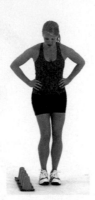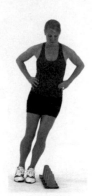

Cone jumps with stabilization: sagittal plane   Cone jumps with stabilization: frontal plane

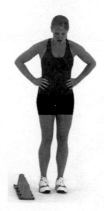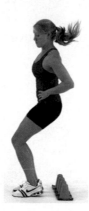

Cone jumps with stabilization: transverse plane

Plyometric-Strength

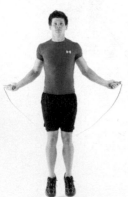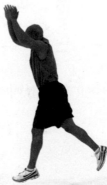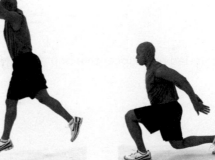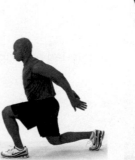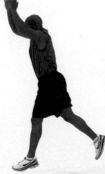

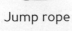
Jump rope   Lunge jumps

Plyometric *continued*

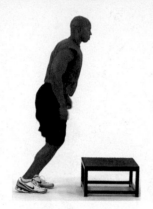
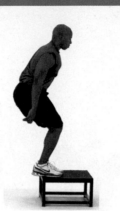
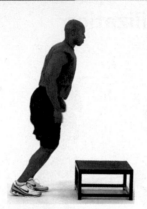
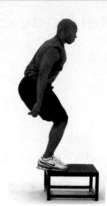

Repeat box jumps

Plyometric-Power

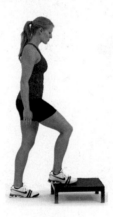
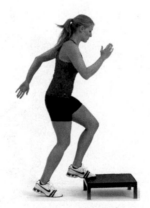
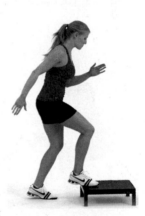

Box run steps: sagittal plane

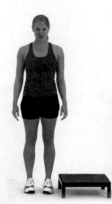
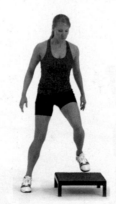
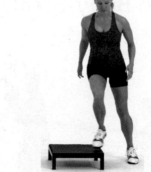

Box run steps: frontal plane

Resistance

Total Body-Stabilization

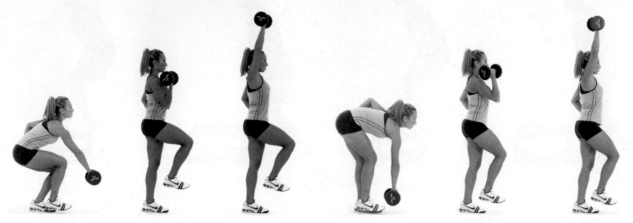

Single-leg squat touchdown, curl, to overhead press   Single-leg Romanian deadlift, curl, to overhead press

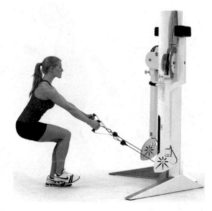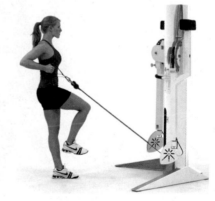

Single-leg squat to row

Total Body-Strength

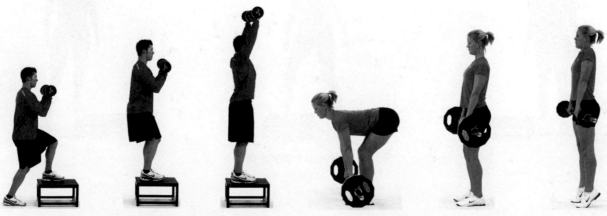

Step-up to overhead press: sagittal plane   Romanian deadlift, shrug to calf raise

Resistance *continued*

Total Body-Power

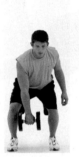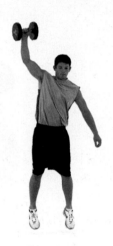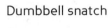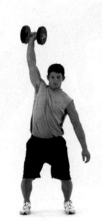

Dumbbell snatch

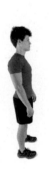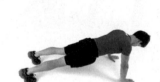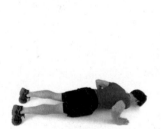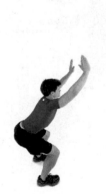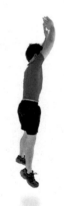

Squat thrust (burpies)

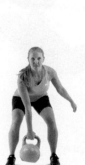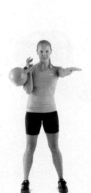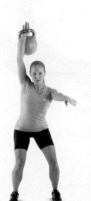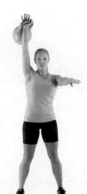

KB hang clean and jerk

Resistance *continued*

Chest-Stabilization

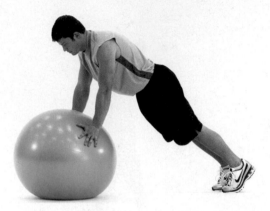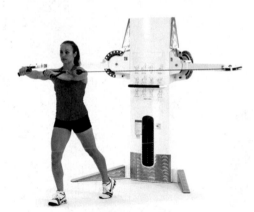

Ball push-up: hands on ball

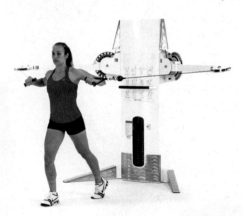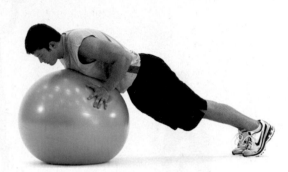

Standing cable chest press

Chest-Strength

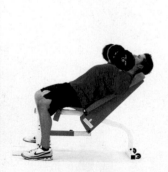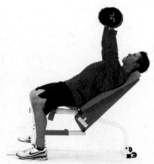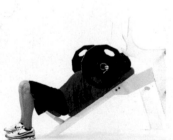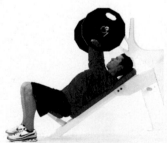

Incline dumbbell chest press   Incline barbell bench press

Resistance *continued*

Chest-Power

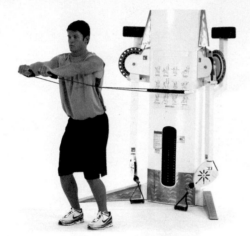
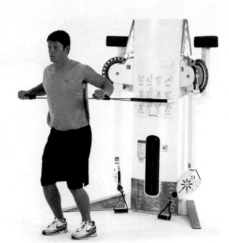

Speed tubing chest press

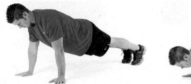
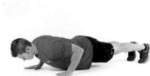
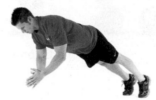
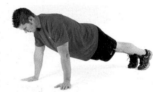

Plyometric push-up

Back-Stabilization

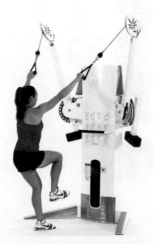
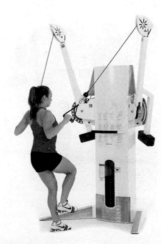

Single-leg pulldown

Resistance *continued*

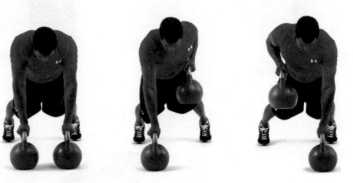

Ball cobra

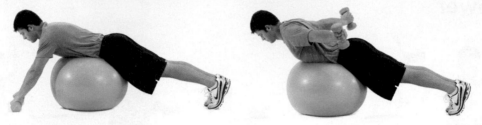

KB renegade row

Back-Strength

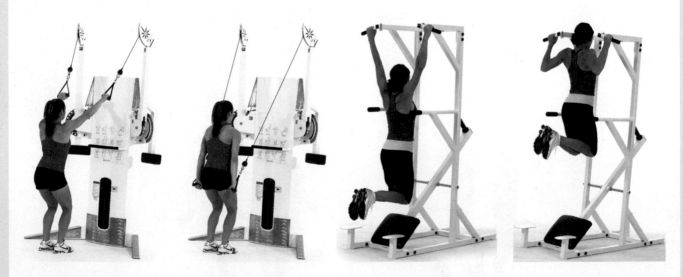

Straight-arm pulldown   Pull-up

Resistance *continued*

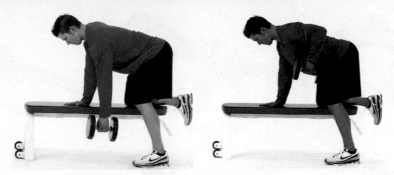

Supported dumbbell row

Back-Power

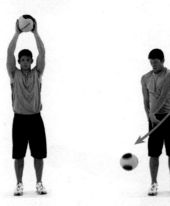

Woodchop throw

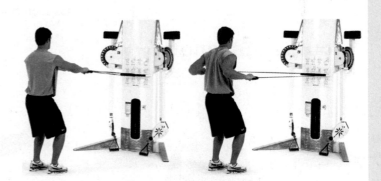

Speed tubing row

Shoulder-Stabilization

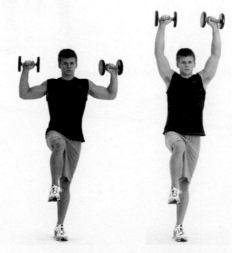

Single-leg overhead press

Resistance *continued*

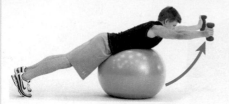 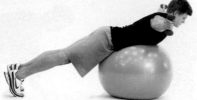 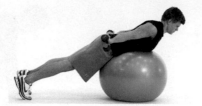

Ball combo I

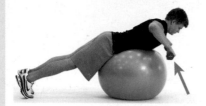 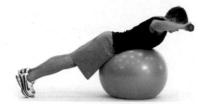 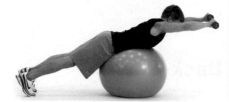

Ball combo II

Shoulder-Strength

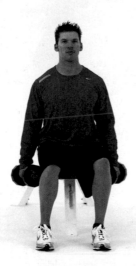 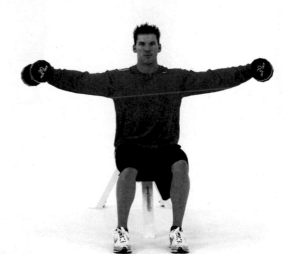

Seated dumbbell lateral raise

Resistance *continued*

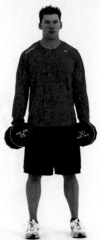
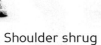

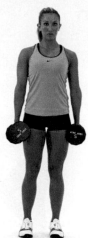

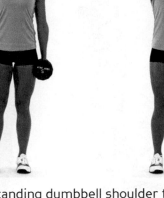

Shoulder shrug

Standing dumbbell shoulder flexion

Shoulder-Power

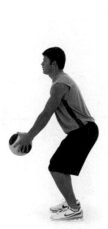
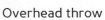

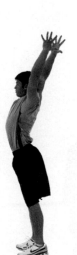

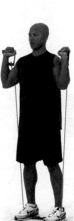

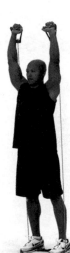

Overhead throw

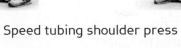

Speed tubing shoulder press

Resistance *continued*

Biceps-Stabilization

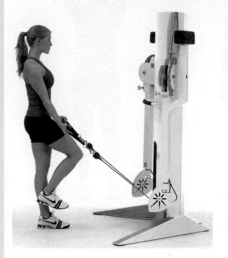
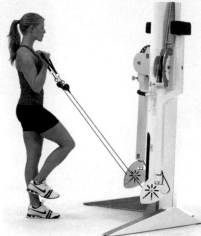
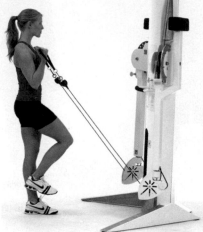

Single-leg cable curl

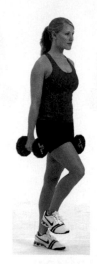
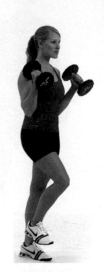

Single-leg hammer curl

Biceps-Strength

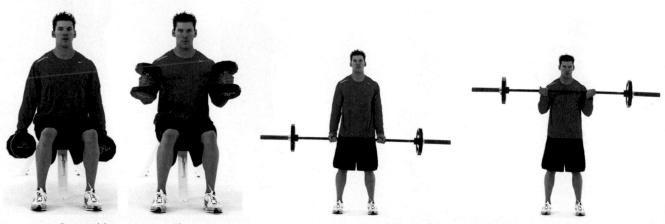

Seated hammer curl   Standing barbell curl

Resistance *continued*

Triceps-Stabilization

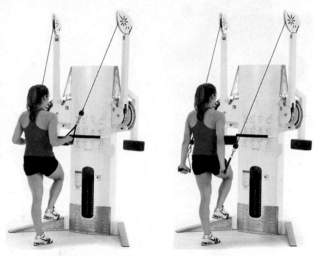

Single-leg cable pressdown

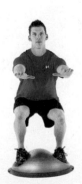

Narrow grip push-up

Triceps-Strength

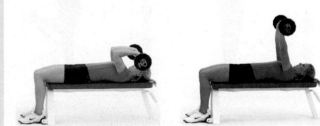

Supine bench barbell triceps extension

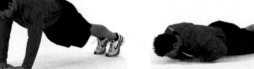

Narrow grip bench press

Legs-Stabilization

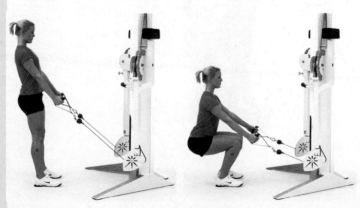

Cable squat

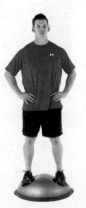

BOSU ball squat

Resistance *continued*

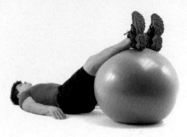
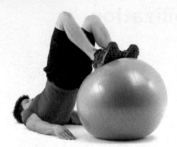

Ball hamstring curl

Leg-Strength

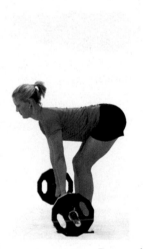
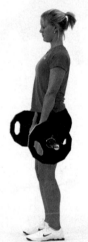
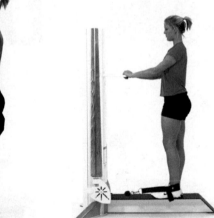
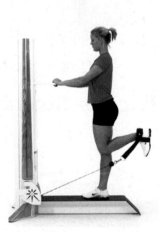

Romanian deadlift

Cable hamstring curl

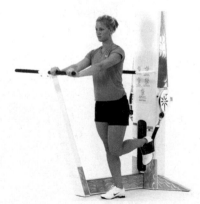
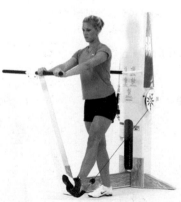

Cable leg extension

Resistance *continued*

Leg-Power

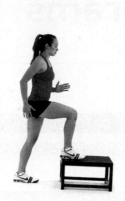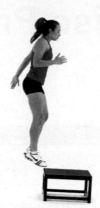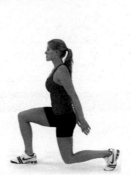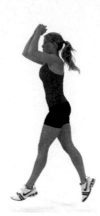

Power step-up   Lunge jumps

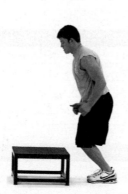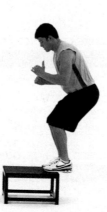

Box jumps

© Eky Studio/ShutterStock, Inc.

© ilolab/ShutterStock, Inc.

OPT Exercise Programs

Professional's Name: Brian Sutton

NASM
NATIONAL ACADEMY OF SPORTS MEDICINE

CLIENT'S NAME: JOHN SMITH   **DATE: 6/01/13**

GOAL: FAT LOSS   **PHASE: 1 STABILIZATION ENDURANCE**

WARM-UP

Exercise	Sets	Duration	Coaching Tip
SMR: Calves, IT-Band, Lats	1	30 s.	Hold each tender area for 30 sec
Static Stretch: Calves, Hip Flexors, Lats	1	30 s.	Hold each stretch for 30 sec
Treadmill	1	5–10 min	Brisk walk to slow jog

CORE / BALANCE / PLYOMETRIC

Exercise	Sets	Reps	Tempo	Rest	Coaching Tip
Floor Bridge	2	15	Slow	0	Circuit
Floor Prone Cobra	2	15	Slow	0	
Single-Leg Balance Reach: Frontal Plane	2	8	Slow	0	8 reaches each leg
Squat Jump w/Stabilization	2	5	Slow	90 s.	Hold landing 3–5 sec

SPEED, AGILITY, QUICKNESS

Exercise	Sets	Reps	Rest	Coaching Tip
Optional				
Optional				

RESISTANCE

Exercise		Sets	Reps	Tempo	Rest	Coaching Tip
Total Body	Ball Squat Curl to Press	2	15	Slow	0	Vertical loading
Chest	Ball Dumbbell Chest Press	2	15	Slow	0	
Back	Standing Cable Row	2	15	Slow	0	
Shoulders	Single-Leg Dumbbell Scaption	2	15	Slow	0	
Biceps	*Optional*					
Triceps	*Optional*					
Legs	Step-Up to Balance	2	15	Slow	60 s.	

COOL-DOWN

Exercise	Sets	Duration	Coaching Tip
Treadmill (*Optional*)	1	5–10 min	Brisk walk; gradually reduce speed
SMR: Calves, IT-Band, Lats	1	30 s.	Hold each tender area for 30 sec
Static Stretch: Calves, Hip Flexors, Lats	1	30 s.	Hold each stretch for 30 sec

Coaching Tips:

National Academy of Sports Medicine

Professional's Name: Brian Sutton

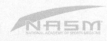

CLIENT'S NAME: JOHN SMITH   DATE: 7/01/13

GOAL: FAT LOSS   PHASE: 2 STRENGTH ENDURANCE

WARM-UP

Exercise	Sets	Duration	Coaching Tip
SMR: Calves, IT-Band, Lats	1	30 s.	Hold each tender area for 30 sec
Active Stretch: Calves, Hip Flexors, Lats	1	10 reps	Hold each stretch for 1–2 sec
Treadmill	1	5–10 min	

CORE / BALANCE / PLYOMETRIC

Exercise	Sets	Reps	Tempo	Rest	Coaching Tip
Ball Crunch	2	10	Medium	0	Circuit
Back Extension	2	10	Medium	0	
Single-Leg Squat	2	10	Medium	0	
Squat Jump	2	10	Medium	60 s.	

SPEED, AGILITY, QUICKNESS

Exercise	Sets	Reps	Rest	Coaching Tip
Optional				
Optional				

RESISTANCE

Exercise		Sets	Reps	Tempo	Rest	Coaching Tip
Total Body	Optional					
Chest	Bench Press		12	Medium	0	Vertical loading
	Push-Up	2	12	Slow	0	
Back	Lat Pulldown		12	Medium	0	
	Ball Dumbbell Row	2	12	Slow	0	
Shoulders	Shoulder Press Machine		12	Medium	0	
	Single-Leg Scaption	2	12	Slow	0	
Biceps	Optional					
Triceps	Optional					
Legs	Leg Press		12	Medium	0	
	Step-Up to Balance	2	12	Slow	60 s.	

COOL-DOWN

Exercise	Sets	Duration	Coaching Tip
Treadmill (Optional)	1	5–10 min	Brisk walk; gradually reduce speed
SMR: Calves, IT-Band, Lats	1	30 s.	Hold each tender area for 30 sec
Static Stretch: Calves, Hip Flexors, Lats	1	30 s.	Hold each stretch for 30 sec

Coaching Tips: Resistance exercises for each body part will be performed as supersets.

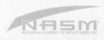

Professional's Name: Brian Sutton

CLIENT'S NAME: JOHN SMITH   DATE: 6/01/13

GOAL: LEAN BODY MASS GAIN   PHASE: 1 STABILIZATION ENDURANCE

WARM-UP

Exercise	Sets	Duration	Coaching Tip
SMR: Calves, IT-Band, Lats	1	30 s.	Hold each tender area for 30 sec
Static Stretch: Calves, Hip Flexors, Lats	1	30 s.	Hold each stretch for 30 sec
Treadmill	1	5–10 min	Brisk walk to slow jog

CORE / BALANCE / PLYOMETRIC

Exercise	Sets	Reps	Tempo	Rest	Coaching Tip
Prone Iso-Abs	2	n/a	Slow	0	Hold for desired time
Floor Bridge	2	15	Slow	0	
Single-Leg Balance Reach: Frontal Plane	2	8	Slow	60 s	8 reaches each leg

SPEED, AGILITY, QUICKNESS

Exercise	Sets	Reps	Rest	Coaching Tip
Optional				
Optional				

RESISTANCE

Exercise		Sets	Reps	Tempo	Rest	Coaching Tip
Total Body	Optional					
Chest	Ball Dumbbell Chest Press	2	15	Slow	0	Vertical loading
Back	Standing Cable Row	2	15	Slow	0	
Shoulders	Single-Leg Scaption	2	15	Slow	0	
Biceps	Single-Leg Barbell Curl	2	15	Slow	0	
Triceps	Supine Ball DB Triceps Extensions	2	15	Slow	0	
Legs	Ball Squat	2	15	Slow	90 s.	

COOL-DOWN

Exercise	Sets	Duration	Coaching Tip
Treadmill (Optional)	1	5–10 min	Brisk walk; gradually reduce speed
SMR: Calves, IT-Band, Lats	1	30 s.	Hold each tender area for 30 sec
Static Stretch: Calves, Hip Flexors, Lats	1	30 s.	Hold each stretch for 30 sec

Coaching Tips:

Professional's Name: Brian Sutton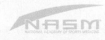

CLIENT'S NAME: JOHN SMITH   DATE: 7/01/13

GOAL: LEAN BODY MASS GAIN   PHASE: 2 STRENGTH ENDURANCE

WARM-UP

Exercise	Sets	Duration	Coaching Tip
SMR: Calves, IT-Band, Lats	1	30 s.	Hold each tender area for 30 sec
Active Stretch: Calves, Hip Flexors, Lats	1	10 reps	Hold each stretch for 1–2 sec
Treadmill	1	5–10 min	Brisk walk to slow jog

CORE / BALANCE / PLYOMETRIC

Exercise	Sets	Reps	Tempo	Rest	Coaching Tip
Ball Crunch	2	12	Medium	0	Circuit
Back Extension	2	12	Medium	0	
Single-Leg Squat	2	12	Medium	0	
Squat Jump	2	8	Medium	60 s.	

SPEED, AGILITY, QUICKNESS

Exercise	Sets	Reps	Rest	Coaching Tip
Optional				
Optional				

RESISTANCE

Exercise		Sets	Reps	Tempo	Rest	Coaching Tip
Total Body	Optional					
Chest	Flat Dumbbell Chest Press		10	Medium	0	
	Ball Dumbbell Chest Press	2	10	Slow	60 s.	Superset
Back	Seated Cable Row		10	Medium	0	
	Ball Dumbbell Row	2	10	Slow	60 s.	Superset
Shoulders	Standing Dumbbell Shoulder Press		10	Medium	0	
	Single-Leg Scaption	2	10	Slow	60 s.	Superset
Biceps	Biceps Curl Machine		10	Medium	0	
	Single-Leg Dumbbell Curl	2	10	Slow	60 s.	Superset
Triceps	Cable Pushdown		10	Medium	0	
	Prone Ball DB Triceps Extensions	2	10	Slow	60 s.	Superset
Legs	Leg Press		10	Medium	0	
	Ball Squat	2	10	Slow	60 s.	Superset

COOL-DOWN

Exercise	Sets	Duration	Coaching Tip
Treadmill (Optional)	1	5–10 min	Brisk walk; gradually reduce speed
SMR: Calves, IT-Band, Lats	1	30 s.	Hold each tender area for 30 sec
Static Stretch: Calves, Hip Flexors, Lats	1	30 s.	Hold each stretch for 30 sec

Coaching Tips: Resistance program can be split into 2, 3, or 4-day workout routine. Ex. 3-day routine: Day 1 (chest/back) Day 2 (legs) Day 3 (shoulder/biceps/triceps)

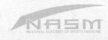

Professional's Name: Brian Sutton

CLIENT'S NAME: JOHN SMITH   DATE: 8/01/13

GOAL: LEAN BODY MASS (BACK, BICEPS, LEGS)   PHASE: 3 HYPERTROPHY

WARM-UP

Exercise	Sets	Duration	Coaching Tip
SMR: Calves, IT-Band, Lats	1	30 s.	Hold each tender area for 30 sec
Active Stretch: Calves, Hip Flexors, Lats	1	10 reps	Hold each stretch 1–2 sec
Treadmill	1	5–10 min	Brisk walk to slow jog

CORE / BALANCE / PLYOMETRIC

Exercise	Sets	Reps	Tempo	Rest	Coaching Tip
Reverse Crunch	2	12	Medium	0	
Cable Rotations	2	12	Medium	60 s	

SPEED, AGILITY, QUICKNESS

Exercise	Sets	Reps	Rest	Coaching Tip
Optional				
Optional				

RESISTANCE

Exercise		Sets	Reps	Tempo	Rest	Coaching Tip
Total Body						
Chest						
Back	Lat Pulldown	3	8	Medium	60 s	Horizontal Loading
	Seated Cable Row	3	8	Medium	60 s.	
Shoulders						
Biceps	Seated Dumbbell Curls	3	8	Medium	60 s	
	Seated Hammer Curls	3	8	Medium	60 s.	
Triceps						
Legs	Barbell Squat	3	8	Medium	60 s	
	Romanian Deadlift	3	8	Medium	60 s.	

COOL-DOWN

Exercise	Sets	Duration	Coaching Tip
Treadmill (Optional)	1	5–10 min	Brisk walk; gradually reduce speed
SMR: Calves, IT-Band, Lats	1	30 s.	Hold each tender area for 30 sec
Static Stretch: Calves, Hip Flexors, Lats	1	30 s.	Hold each stretch for 30 sec

Coaching Tips: Extra stretching for the back, biceps, and legs may be necessary during the cool-down.

Professional's Name: Brian Sutton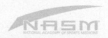

CLIENT'S NAME: JOHN SMITH	DATE: 8/03/13

GOAL: LEAN BODY MASS (CHEST, SHOULDERS TRICEPS)	PHASE: 3 HYPERTROPHY

WARM-UP

Exercise	Sets	Duration	Coaching Tip
SMR: Calves, IT-Band, Lats	1	30 s.	Hold each tender area for 30 sec
Active Stretch: Calves, Hip Flexors, Lats	1	10 reps	Hold each stretch 1–2 sec
Treadmill	1	5–10 min	Brisk walk to slow jog

CORE / BALANCE / PLYOMETRIC

Exercise	Sets	Reps	Tempo	Rest	Coaching Tip
Ball Crunch	2	12	Medium	0	Circuit
Back Extension	2	12	Medium	60 s	

SPEED, AGILITY, QUICKNESS

Exercise	Sets	Reps	Rest	Coaching Tip
Optional				
Optional				

RESISTANCE

Exercise		Sets	Reps	Tempo	Rest	Coaching Tip
Total Body						
Chest	Barbell Bench Press	3	8	Medium	60 s.	Horizontal Loading
	Incline Dumbbell Chest Press	3	8	Medium	60 s.	
Back						
Shoulders	Seated Dumbbell Shoulder Press	3	8	Medium	60 s.	
	Seated Dumbbell Lateral Raise	3	8	Medium	60 s.	
Biceps						
Triceps	Cable Pressdown	3	8	Medium	60 s.	
	Supine Bench Barbell Triceps Extensions	3	8	Medium	60 s.	
Legs						

COOL-DOWN

Exercise	Sets	Duration	Coaching Tip
Treadmill (*Optional*)	1	5–10 min	Brisk walk; gradually reduce speed
SMR: Calves, IT-Band, Lats	1	30 s.	Hold each tender area for 30 sec
Static Stretch: Calves, Hip Flexors, Lats	1	30 s.	Hold each stretch for 30 sec

Coaching Tips: Extra stretching for the chest, shoulders, and triceps may be necessary during the cool-down.

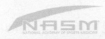

© Iiolab/ShutterStock, Inc.

Professional's Name: Brian Sutton

CLIENT'S NAME: JOHN SMITH   **DATE:** 9/03/13

GOAL: LEAN BODY MASS (BACK, BICEPS, LEGS)   **PHASE: 4 MAX STRENGTH**

WARM-UP

Exercise	Sets	Duration	Coaching Tip
SMR: Calves, IT-Band, Lats	1	30 s.	Hold each tender area for 30 sec
Active Stretch: Calves, Hip Flexors, Lats	1	10 reps	Hold each stretch for 1–2 sec
Treadmill	1	5–10 min	Brisk walk to slow jog

CORE / BALANCE / PLYOMETRIC

Exercise	Sets	Reps	Tempo	Rest	Coaching Tip
Ball Crunches	2	8	Medium	0	Circuit
Reverse Crunch	2	8	Medium	60 s.	

SPEED, AGILITY, QUICKNESS

Exercise	Sets	Reps	Rest	Coaching Tip
Optional				
Optional				

RESISTANCE

Exercise		Sets	Reps	Tempo	Rest	Coaching Tip
Total Body						
Chest						
Back	Seated Rows	5	5	Explosive	3 min	Horizontal Loading
	Lat Pulldown	5	5	Explosive	3 min	
Shoulders						
Biceps	Standing Barbell Curls	5	5	Explosive	3 min	
Triceps						
Legs	Barbell Squat	5	5	Explosive	3 min	
	Russian Deadlifts	5	5	Explosive	3 min	
	Standing Calf Raise	5	5	Explosive	3 min	

COOL-DOWN

Exercise	Sets	Duration	Coaching Tip
Treadmill (*Optional*)	1	5–10 min	Brisk walk; gradually reduce speed
SMR: Calves, IT-Band, Lats	1	30 s.	Hold each tender area for 30 sec
Static Stretch: Calves, Hip Flexors, Lats	1	30 s.	Hold each stretch for 30 sec

Coaching Tips: Extra stretching for the back, biceps, and legs may be necessary during the cool-down.

National Academy of Sports Medicine

Professional's Name: Brian Sutton

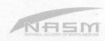

CLIENT'S NAME: JOHN SMITH   DATE: 9/01/13

GOAL: LEAN BODY MASS   PHASE: 4 MAX STRENGTH
(CHEST, SHOULDERS, TRICEPS)

WARM-UP

Exercise	Sets	Duration	Coaching Tip
SMR: Calves, IT-Band, Lats	1	30 s.	Hold each tender area for 30 sec
Active Stretch: Calves, Hip Flexors, Lats	1	10 reps	Hold each stretch for 1–2 sec
Treadmill	1	5–10 min	Brisk walk to slow jog

CORE / BALANCE / PLYOMETRIC

Exercise	Sets	Reps	Tempo	Rest	Coaching Tip
Cable Rotations	2	8	Medium	0	Circuit
Back Extension	2	8	Medium	60 s.	

SPEED, AGILITY, QUICKNESS

Exercise	Sets	Reps	Rest	Coaching Tip
Optional				
Optional				

RESISTANCE

Exercise		Sets	Reps	Tempo	Rest	Coaching Tip
Total Body						
Chest	Bench Press	5	5	Explosive	3 min	Horizontal Loading
	Incline Bench Press	5	5	Explosive	3 min	
Back						
Shoulders	Barbell Military Press	5	5	Explosive	3 min	
Biceps						
Triceps	Cable Pressdown	5	5	Explosive	3 min	
Legs						

COOL-DOWN

Exercise	Sets	Duration	Coaching Tip
Treadmill (*Optional*)	1	5–10 min	Brisk walk; gradually reduce speed
SMR: Calves, IT-Band, Lats	1	30 s.	Hold each tender area for 30 sec
Static Stretch: Calves, Hip Flexors, Lats	1	30 s.	Hold each stretch for 30 sec

Coaching Tips: Extra stretching for the chest, shoulders, and triceps may be necessary during the cool-down.

Professional's Name: Brian Sutton

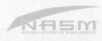

CLIENT'S NAME: JOHN SMITH   DATE: 6/01/13

GOAL: GENERAL PERFORMANCE   PHASE: 1 STABILIZATION ENDURANCE

WARM-UP

Exercise	Sets	Duration	Coaching Tip
SMR: Calves, IT-Band, Lats	1	30 s.	Hold each tender area for 30 sec
Static Stretch: Calves, Hip Flexors, Lats	1	30 s.	Hold each stretch for 30 sec
Treadmill	1	5–10 min	Brisk walk to slow jog

CORE / BALANCE / PLYOMETRIC

Exercise	Sets	Reps	Tempo	Rest	Coaching Tip
Prone Iso-Ab	2	n/a	Slow	0	Hold for desired time
Floor Bridge	2	15	Slow	0	
Single-Leg Throw and Catch	2	8	Slow	0	8 throws each side
Box Jump-Up w/ Stabilization	2	5	Slow	60 s.	Hold landing 3–5 sec

SPEED, AGILITY, QUICKNESS

Exercise	Sets	Reps	Rest	Coaching Tip
Speed Ladder: 1-ins, 2-ins, side shuffle	2	n/a	60 s.	
Box Drill	2	n/a	60 s.	

RESISTANCE

Exercise		Sets	Reps	Tempo	Rest	Coaching Tip
Total Body	Ball Squat Curl to Press	2	15	Slow	0	Vertical loading
Chest	Ball Dumbbell Chest Press	2	15	Slow	0	
Back	Single-Leg Cable Row	2	15	Slow	0	
Shoulders	Single-Leg Dumbbell Scaption	2	15	Slow	0	
Biceps	*Optional*					
Triceps	*Optional*					
Legs	Step-Up to Balance	2	15	Slow	90 s.	

COOL-DOWN

Exercise	Sets	Duration	Coaching Tip
Treadmill (*Optional*)	1	5–10 min	Brisk walk; gradually reduce speed
SMR: Calves, IT-Band, Lats	1	30 s.	Hold each tender area for 30 sec
Static Stretch: Calves, Hip Flexors, Lats	1	30 s.	Hold each stretch for 30 sec

Coaching Tips:

Professional's Name: Brian Sutton

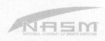

CLIENT'S NAME: JOHN SMITH   DATE: 7/01/13

GOAL: GENERAL PERFORMANCE   PHASE: 2 STRENGTH ENDURANCE

WARM-UP

Exercise	Sets	Duration	Coaching Tip
SMR: Calves, IT-Band, Lats	1	30 s.	Hold each tender area for 30 sec
Active Stretch: Calves, Hip Flexors, Lats	1	10 reps	Hold each stretch for 1–2 sec
Dynamic Stretch: Prisoner Squat, Tube Walking, Push-Up with Rotation	1	10 reps	Dynamic stretching will replace general cardio warm-up

CORE / BALANCE / PLYOMETRIC

Exercise	Sets	Reps	Tempo	Rest	Coaching Tip
Ball Crunch	2	10	Medium	0	Circuit
Single-Leg Romanian Deadlift	2	10	Medium	0	
Squat Jump	2	10	Medium	60 s.	

SPEED, AGILITY, QUICKNESS

Exercise	Sets	Reps	Rest	Coaching Tip
Speed Ladder: 1-ins, 2-ins, ali shuffle, side shuffle, zig-zag, in-in-out-out	2	n/a	60 s.	
T-Drill	2	n/a	60 s.	

RESISTANCE

Exercise		Sets	Reps	Tempo	Rest	Coaching Tip
Total Body	Optional					
Chest	Bench Press		10	Medium	0	Vertical loading
	Push-Up	2	10	Slow	60 s.	
Back	Lat Pulldown		10	Medium	0	
	Ball Dumbbell Row	2	10	Slow	60 s.	
Shoulders	Seated Dumbbell Shoulder Press		10	Medium	0	
	Single-Leg Scaption	2	10	Slow	60 s.	
Biceps	Optional					
Triceps	Optional					
Legs	Leg Press		10	Medium	0	
	Step-Up to Balance	2	10	Slow	60 s.	

COOL-DOWN

Exercise	Sets	Duration	Coaching Tip
Treadmill (Optional)	1	5–10 min	Brisk walk; gradually reduce speed
SMR: Calves, IT-Band, Lats	1	30 s.	Hold each tender area for 30 sec
Static Stretch: Calves, Hip Flexors, Lats	1	30 s.	Hold each stretch for 30 sec

Coaching Tips: Resistance exercises for each body part will be performed as supersets.

Professional's Name: Brian Sutton

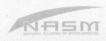

CLIENT'S NAME: JOHN SMITH	DATE: 8/01/13

GOAL: GENERAL PERFORMANCE	PHASE: 5 POWER

WARM-UP

Exercise	Sets	Duration	Coaching Tip
SMR: Calves, IT-Band, Lats	1	30 s.	Hold each tender area for 30 sec
Dynamic Stretch: Tube Walking, Multiplanar Lunges, Med Ball Lift and Chop	1	10 reps	

CORE / BALANCE / PLYOMETRIC

Exercise	Sets	Reps	Tempo	Rest	Coaching Tip
Ball Med Ball Pullover Throw	2	12	Fast	0	Circuit
Rotation Chest Pass	2	12	Fast	0	
Multiplanar Single-Leg Hop w/ Stabilization	2	10	Medium	60 s.	

SPEED, AGILITY, QUICKNESS

Exercise	Sets	Reps	Rest	Coaching Tip
Speed Ladder: 1-ins, 2-ins, side shuffle, Ali shuffle, zig-zag, in-in-out-out	2	n/a	60 s.	
5–10–5 Drill	2	n/a	60 s.	

RESISTANCE

Exercise		Sets	Reps	Tempo	Rest	Coaching Tip
Total Body	*Optional*					
Chest	Bench Press Plyometric Push-Up	3	5 10	Explosive	0 2 min	Superset
Back	Lat Pulldown Soccer Throw	3	5 10	Explosive	0 2 min	Superset
Shoulders	Seated Dumbbell Shoulder Press Overhead Medicine Ball Throw	3	5 10	Explosive	0 2 min	Superset
Biceps	*Optional*					
Triceps	*Optional*					
Legs	Barbell Squat Tuck Jump	3	5 10	Explosive	0 2 min	Superset

COOL-DOWN

Exercise	Sets	Duration	Coaching Tip
Treadmill (*Optional*)	1	5–10 min	Brisk walk; gradually reduce speed
SMR: Calves, IT-Band, Lats	1	30 s.	Hold each tender area for 30 sec
Static Stretch: Calves, Hip Flexors, Lats	1	30 s.	Hold each stretch for 30 sec

Coaching Tips: Perform resistance exercises for each body part as a superset in a vertically loaded fashion.

National Academy of Sports Medicine

Professional's Name: Brian Sutton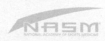

CLIENT'S NAME: JOHN SMITH   DATE: 6/01/13

GOAL: SUSPENSION (TRX) PROGRAM   PHASE: 1 STABILIZATION ENDURANCE

WARM-UP

Exercise	Sets	Duration	Coaching Tip
SMR: Calves, IT-Band, Lats	1	30 s.	Hold each tender area for 30 sec
Static Stretch: Calves, Hip Flexors, Lats	1	30 s.	Hold each stretch for 30 sec
Treadmill	1	5–10 min	Brisk walk to slow jog

CORE / BALANCE / PLYOMETRIC

Exercise	Sets	Reps	Tempo	Rest	Coaching Tip
Floor Bridge	2	15	Slow	0	Circuit
Floor Prone Cobra	2	15	Slow	0	
Single-Leg Balance Reach: Frontal Plane	2	8	Slow	0	8 reaches each leg
Squat Jump w/ Stabilization	2	5	Slow	60 s.	Hold landing 3–5 sec

SPEED, AGILITY, QUICKNESS

Exercise	Sets	Reps	Rest	Coaching Tip
Optional				
Optional				

RESISTANCE

Exercise		Sets	Reps	Tempo	Rest	Coaching Tip
Total Body	Optional					
Chest	TRX Chest Press: offset stance	2	15	Slow	0	Vertical loading
Back	TRX Low Row: offset stance	2	15	Slow	0	
Shoulders	TRX Y Deltoid Fly	2	15	Slow	0	
Biceps	TRX High Biceps Curl	2	15	Slow	0	
Triceps	TRX Triceps Press	2	15	Slow	0	
Legs	TRX Squat	2	15	Slow	90 s.	

COOL-DOWN

Exercise	Sets	Duration	Coaching Tip
Treadmill (Optional)	1	5–10 min	Brisk walk; gradually reduce speed
SMR: Calves, IT-Band, Lats	1	30 s.	Hold each tender area for 30 sec
Static Stretch: Calves, Hip Flexors, Lats	1	30 s.	Hold each stretch for 30 sec

Coaching Tips: This program focuses on stabilization endurance training. It includes a mix of TRX suspension bodyweight exercises and traditional exercises.

Professional's Name: Brian Sutton

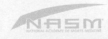

CLIENT'S NAME: JOHN SMITH	DATE: 7/01/13

GOAL: SUSPENSION (TRX) PROGRAM	PHASE: 2 STRENGTH ENDURANCE

WARM-UP

Exercise	Sets	Duration	Coaching Tip
SMR: Calves, IT-Band, Lats	1	30 s.	Hold each tender area for 30 sec
Active Stretch: Calves, Hip Flexors, Lats	1	10 reps	Hold each stretch for 1–2 sec
Treadmill	1	5–10 min	

CORE / BALANCE / PLYOMETRIC

Exercise	Sets	Reps	Tempo	Rest	Coaching Tip
Ball Crunch	2	10	Medium	0	Circuit
Single-Leg Squat	2	10	Medium	0	
Squat Jump	2	10	Medium	60 s.	

SPEED, AGILITY, QUICKNESS

Exercise	Sets	Reps	Rest	Coaching Tip
Optional				
Optional				

RESISTANCE

Exercise		Sets	Reps	Tempo	Rest	Coaching Tip
Total Body	Optional					
Chest	Bench Press		12	Medium	0	Vertical loading
	TRX Chest Press: Single-Leg	2	12	Slow	60 s.	
Back	Lat Pulldown		12	Medium	0	
	TRX Back Row	2	12	Slow	60 s.	
Shoulders	Shoulder Press Machine		12	Medium	0	
	TRX T Deltoid Fly	2	12	Slow	60 s.	
Biceps	Optional					
Triceps	Optional					
Legs	Leg Press		12	Medium	0	
	TRX Hip Press	2	12	Slow	60 s.	

COOL-DOWN

Exercise	Sets	Duration	Coaching Tip
Treadmill (Optional)	1	5–10 min	Brisk walk; gradually reduce speed
SMR: Calves, IT-Band, Lats	1	30 s.	Hold each tender area for 30 sec
Static Stretch: Calves, Hip Flexors, Lats	1	30 s.	Hold each stretch for 30 sec

Coaching Tips: This program focuses on strength endurance training. It includes a mix of TRX suspension bodyweight exercises and traditional exercises. Resistance exercises for each body part will be performed as supersets.

Professional's Name: Brian Sutton

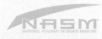

CLIENT'S NAME: JOHN SMITH   DATE: 6/01/13

GOAL: VIBRATION (POWER PLATE)   PHASE: 1 STABILIZATION ENDURANCE

WARM-UP

Exercise	Sets	Duration	Coaching Tip
SMR: Calves, IT-Band, Lats	1	30 s.	Hold each tender area for 30 sec
Static Stretch: Calves, Hip Flexors, Lats	1	30 s.	Hold each stretch for 30 sec
Treadmill	1	5–10 min	Brisk walk to slow jog

CORE / BALANCE / PLYOMETRIC

Exercise	Sets	Time/Reps	Hz/Tempo	Amplitude	Rest	Coaching Tip
Prone Iso-Ab (plank)	2	30 s.	30 Hz	Low	0 s.	Circuit
Ball Bridge	2	12 reps	Slow	n/a	0 s.	
Multiplanar Single-Leg Balance Reach	2	30 s.	30 Hz	Low	60 s.	15 sec each leg

SPEED, AGILITY, QUICKNESS

Exercise	Sets	Reps	Rest	Coaching Tip
Optional				
Optional				

RESISTANCE

Exercise		Sets	Time/Reps	Hz/Tempo	Amplitude	Rest	Coaching Tip
Total Body	Ball Squat, Curl, to Press	2	15 reps	Slow	n/a	0 s.	
Chest	Push-Up	2	30 s.	30 Hz	Low	0 s.	Hands on the plate and feet on a step
Back	Standing Cable Row	2	15 reps	Slow	n/a	0 s.	
Shoulders	Single-Leg DB Scaption	2	15 reps	Slow	n/a	0 s.	
Biceps	Optional						
Triceps	Optional						
Legs	Step-Up to Balance: Sagittal Plane	2	30 s.	30 Hz	Low	90 s.	

COOL-DOWN

Exercise	Sets	Duration	Hz	Amplitude	Coaching Tip
Treadmill (Optional)	1	5–10 min	n/a	n/a	Brisk walk
Massage: Calves, IT-Band, Lats	1	60 s.	35 Hz	High	
Static Stretch: Calves, Hip Flexors, Lats	1	30 s.	30 Hz	Low	

Coaching Tips: This program focuses on stabilization endurance training. It includes a mix of Power Plate exercises and traditional exercises. Perform all resistance exercises in a vertically loaded (circuit) fashion.

Professional's Name: Brian Sutton

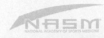

CLIENT'S NAME: JOHN SMITH	DATE: 7/01/13

GOAL: VIBRATION (POWER PLATE)	PHASE: 2 STRENGTH ENDURANCE

WARM-UP

Exercise	Sets	Duration	Coaching Tip
SMR: Calves, IT-Band, Lats	1	30 s.	Hold each tender area for 30 sec
Active Stretch: Calves, Hip Flexors, Lats	1	10 reps	Hold each stretch for 1–2 sec
Treadmill	1	5–10 min	Brisk walk to slow jog

CORE / BALANCE / PLYOMETRIC

Exercise	Sets	Time/Reps	Hz/Tempo	Amplitude	Rest	Coaching Tip
Ball Crunch	2	12 reps	Medium	n/a	0 s.	Circuit
Single-Leg Squat	2	45 s.	35 Hz	Low	0 s.	45 sec each leg
Squat Jump	2	10 reps	Medium	n/a	60 s.	

SPEED, AGILITY, QUICKNESS

Exercise	Sets	Reps	Rest	Coaching Tip
Optional				
Optional				

RESISTANCE

Exercise		Sets	Time/Reps	Hz/Tempo	Amplitude	Rest	Coaching Tip
Total Body	Optional						
Chest	Bench Press		12 reps	Medium	n/a	0 s.	
	Push-Up	2	12 reps	40 Hz	Low	30 s.	Hands on plate
Back	Iso Row (off machine)		30 s.	40 Hz	Low	0 s.	Use straps
	Single-Leg Cable Row	2	12 reps	Medium	n/a	30 s.	
Shoulders	DB Shoulder Press		12 reps	Medium	n/a	0 s.	
	DB Scaption on Plate	2	30 s.	30 Hz	Low	30 s.	
Biceps	Optional						
Triceps	Optional						
Legs	Iso Deadlift		30 s.	40 Hz	Low	0 s.	Use straps
	Single-Leg RDL	2	12 reps	Slow	n/a	30 s.	

DB = dumbbell, RDL = Romanian Deadlift

COOL-DOWN

Exercise	Sets	Duration	Hz	Amplitude	Coaching Tip
Treadmill (Optional)	1	5–10 min	n/a	n/a	Brisk walk
Massage: Calves, IT-Band, Lats	1	60 s.	35 Hz	High	
Static Stretch: Calves, Hip Flexors, Lats	1	30 s.	30 Hz	Low	

Coaching Tips: This program focuses on strength endurance training. It includes a mix of Power Plate exercises and traditional exercises. Resistance exercises for each body part will be performed as supersets.

Professional's Name: Brian Sutton

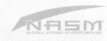

CLIENT'S NAME: JOHN SMITH

DATE: 8/01/13

GOAL: VIBRATION (POWER PLATE)

PHASE: 3 HYPERTROPHY

WARM-UP

Exercise	Sets	Duration	Coaching Tip
SMR: Calves, IT-Band, Lats	1	30 s.	Hold each tender area for 30 sec
Active Stretch: Calves, Hip Flexors, Lats	1	10 reps	Hold each stretch for 1–2 sec
Treadmill	1	5–10 min	Brisk walk to slow jog

CORE / BALANCE / PLYOMETRIC

Exercise	Sets	Time/Reps	Hz/Tempo	Amplitude	Rest	Coaching Tip
Reverse Crunch	2	10 reps	Medium	n/a	0 s.	Circuit
Cable Rotations	2	10 reps	Medium	n/a	0 s.	
Single-Leg Romanian Deadlift	2	45 s.	35 Hz	Low	60 s	45 sec each leg

SPEED, AGILITY, QUICKNESS

Exercise	Sets	Reps	Rest	Coaching Tip
Optional				
Optional				

RESISTANCE

Exercise		Sets	Time/Reps	Hz/Tempo	Amplitude	Rest	Coaching Tip
Total Body	Optional						
Chest	Bench Press	3	8 reps	Medium	n/a	30 s.	
Back	Lat Pulldown	3	8 reps	Medium	n/a	30 s.	
Shoulders	Lateral Raise	3	45 s.	30 Hz	High	30 s.	Use straps
Biceps	Biceps Curl	3	45 s.	30 Hz	High	30 s.	Use straps
Triceps	Triceps Kickback	3	45 s.	30 Hz	High	30 s.	Use straps
Legs	Dumbbell Lunge: Sagittal Plane	3	8 reps	Medium	n/a	30 s.	

COOL-DOWN

Exercise	Sets	Duration	Hz	Amplitude	Coaching Tip
Treadmill (Optional)	1	5–10 min	n/a	n/a	Brisk walk
Massage: Calves, IT-Band, Lats	1	60 s.	35 Hz	High	
Static Stretch: Calves, Hip Flexors, Lats	1	30 s.	30 Hz	Low	

Coaching Tips: This program focuses on hypertrophy training. It includes a mix of Power Plate exercises and traditional exercises.

Professional's Name: Brian Sutton

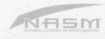

CLIENT'S NAME: JOHN SMITH   DATE: 9/01/13

GOAL: VIBRATION (POWER PLATE)   PHASE: 5 POWER

WARM-UP

Exercise	Sets	Duration	Coaching Tip
SMR: Calves, IT-Band, Lats	1	30 s.	Hold each tender area for 30 sec
Dynamic Stretch: Prisoner Squats, Tube Walking: Side to Side, Push-Up w/ Rotation	1	10 reps	

CORE / BALANCE / PLYOMETRIC

Exercise	Sets	Reps	Tempo	Rest	Coaching Tip
Ball MB Pullover Throw	2	12	Explosive	0	
Single-Leg Hop with Stabilization	2	10	Medium	60 s.	10 each leg

SPEED, AGILITY, QUICKNESS

Exercise	Sets	Reps	Rest	Coaching Tip
Optional				
Optional				

RESISTANCE

	Exercise	Sets	Reps/Time	Hz/Tempo	Amplitude	Rest	Coaching Tip
Total Body	*Optional*						
Chest	Bench Press Plyomeytric Push-Up	3	5 reps 45 s.	Explosive 30 Hz	n/a Low	0 2 min	
Back	Lat Pulldown MB Soccer Throw	3	5 reps 45 s.	Explosive 30 Hz	n/a High	0 2 min	Stand on machine
Shoulders	Seated Shoulder Press MB Front Oblique Throw	3	5 reps 45 s.	Explosive 30 Hz	n/a High	0 2 min	Stand on machine
Biceps	*Optional*						
Triceps	*Optional*		5 reps				
Legs	Deadlift Tuck Jumps	3	5 reps 10 reps	Explosive Explosive	n/a n/a	0 2 min	

COOL-DOWN

Exercise	Sets	Duration	Hz	Amplitude	Coaching Tip
Treadmill (*Optional*)	1	5–10 min	n/a	n/a	Brisk walk
Massage: Calves, IT-Band, Lats	1	60 s.	35 Hz	High	
Static Stretch: Calves, Hip Flexors, Lats	1	30 s.	30 Hz	Low	

Coaching Tips: This program focuses on power training. It includes a mix of Power Plate exercises and traditional exercises. Perform resistance exercises for each body part as a superset.

Professional's Name: Brian Sutton

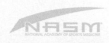

CLIENT'S NAME: JOHN SMITH   DATE: 6/01/13

GOAL: KETTLEBELL PROGRAM   PHASE: 1 STABILIZATION ENDURANCE

WARM-UP

Exercise	Sets	Duration	Coaching Tip
SMR: Calves, IT-Band, Lats	1	30 s.	Hold each tender area for 30 sec
Static Stretch: Calves, Hip Flexors, Lats	1	30 s.	Hold each stretch for 30 sec
Treadmill	1	5–10 min	Brisk walk to slow jog

CORE / BALANCE / PLYOMETRIC

Exercise	Sets	Reps	Tempo	Rest	Coaching Tip
Floor Bridge	1	15	Slow	0	Circuit
Prone Iso-Ab (plank)	1	n/a	n/a	0	Hold for desired time
Single-Leg Balance Reach: Frontal Plane	1	8	Slow	0	8 reaches each leg
Squat Jump w/ Stabilization	1	5	Slow	60 s.	Hold landing 3–5 sec

SPEED, AGILITY, QUICKNESS

Exercise	Sets	Reps	Rest	Coaching Tip
Optional				
Optional				

RESISTANCE

Exercise		Sets	Reps	Tempo	Rest	Coaching Tip
Total Body	KB Swing: 2-arm	2	12	Medium	30 s.	KB swings can't be performed with slow tempo
Chest	Push-Up: Hands on top of KB	2	15	Slow	30 s.	
Back	KB Renegade Row	2	15	Slow	30 s.	
Shoulders	KB Single-Leg Overhead Press: 1-arm	2	15	Slow	30 s.	
Biceps	Optional	2	15	Slow	30 s.	
Triceps	Optional	2	15	Slow	30 s.	
Legs	KB Single-Leg Squat Touchdown	2	15	Slow	30 s.	

COOL-DOWN

Exercise	Sets	Duration	Coaching Tip
Treadmill (Optional)	1	5–10 min	Brisk walk; gradually reduce speed
SMR: Calves, IT-Band, Lats	1	30 s.	Hold each tender area for 30 sec
Static Stretch: Calves, Hip Flexors, Lats	1	30 s.	Hold each stretch for 30 sec

Coaching Tips: KB swings are performed in smooth arc up and away from body, with arms straight. Allow KB to follow same path on the way up and down, absorbing it at the bottom. Keep back and hips in a neutral position and be sure to power through the swing with your glutes, core, and legs.

Professional's Name: Brian Sutton

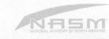

CLIENT'S NAME: JOHN SMITH	DATE: 7/01/13
GOAL: KETTLEBELL PROGRAM	PHASE: 2 STRENGTH ENDURANCE

WARM-UP

Exercise	Sets	Duration	Coaching Tip
SMR: Calves, IT-Band, Lats	1	30 s.	Hold each tender area for 30 sec
Active Stretch: Calves, Hip Flexors, Lats	1	10 reps	Hold each stretch for 1–2 sec
Treadmill	1	5–10 min	

CORE / BALANCE / PLYOMETRIC

Exercise	Sets	Reps	Tempo	Rest	Coaching Tip
Ball Crunch	2	10	Medium	0	Circuit
Back Extension	2	10	Medium	0	
KB Single-Leg Romanian Deadlift	2	10	Medium	0	
Squat Jump	2	10	Medium	60 s.	

SPEED, AGILITY, QUICKNESS

Exercise	Sets	Reps	Rest	Coaching Tip
Optional				
Optional				

RESISTANCE

Exercise		Sets	Reps	Tempo	Rest	Coaching Tip
Total Body	Optional					Vertical Loading
Chest	Bench Press		10	Medium	0	
	KB Press on Floor: Alternate arms	2	12	Slow	60 s.	
Back	Cable Row		10	Medium	0	
	KB Renegade Row	2	12	Slow	60 s.	
Shoulders	Shoulder Press Machine		10	Medium	0	
	KB Single-Leg Overhead Press	2	12	Slow	60 s.	
Biceps	Optional					
Triceps	Optional					
Legs	Leg Press		10	Medium	0	
	KB Single-Leg Squat Touchdown	2	12	Slow	60 s.	

COOL-DOWN

Exercise	Sets	Duration	Coaching Tip
Treadmill (Optional)	1	5–10 min	Brisk walk; gradually reduce speed
SMR: Calves, IT-Band, Lats	1	30 s.	Hold each tender area for 30 sec
Static Stretch: Calves, Hip Flexors, Lats	1	30 s.	Hold each stretch for 30 sec

Coaching Tips: Superset each body part during resistance training in a vertically loaded fashion.

National Academy of Sports Medicine

Professional's Name: Brian Sutton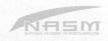

CLIENT'S NAME: JOHN SMITH   DATE: 8/01/13

GOAL: KETTLEBELL PROGRAM   PHASE: 5 POWER

WARM-UP

Exercise	Sets	Duration	Coaching Tip
SMR: Calves, IT-Band, Lats	1	30 s.	Hold each tender area for 30 sec
Dynamic Stretch: Tube Walking, Multiplanar Lunges, Med Ball Lift and Chop	1	10 reps	

CORE / BALANCE / PLYOMETRIC

Exercise	Sets	Reps	Tempo	Rest	Coaching Tip
Ball Med Ball Pullover Throw	2	12	Explosive	0	Circuit
Multiplanar Single-Leg Hop w/ Stabilization	2	10	Medium	60 s.	

SPEED, AGILITY, QUICKNESS

Exercise	Sets	Reps	Rest	Coaching Tip
Optional				
Optional				

RESISTANCE

Exercise		Sets	Reps	Tempo	Rest	Coaching Tip
Total Body	Optional					
Chest	Barbell Bench Press	3	5		0	
	MB Chest Pass		10	Explosive	2 min	Superset
Back	KB Row: 1-arm	3	5		0	
	Soccer Throw		10	Explosive	2 min	Superset
Shoulders	Standing KB Overhead Press	3	5		0	
	MB Front Oblique Throw		10	Explosive	2 min	Superset
Biceps	Optional					
Triceps	Optional					
Legs	KB Lunge: Sagittal Plane	3	5		0	
	Squat Jump		10	Explosive	2 min	Superset

COOL-DOWN

Exercise	Sets	Duration	Coaching Tip
Treadmill (Optional)	1	5–10 min	Brisk walk; gradually reduce speed
SMR: Calves, IT-Band, Lats	1	30 s.	Hold each tender area for 30 sec
Static Stretch: Calves, Hip Flexors, Lats	1	30 s.	Hold each stretch for 30 sec

Coaching Tips: This program focuses on power training. It includes a mix of kettlebell exercises and traditional exercises. Perform resistance exercises for each body part as a superset.

One Repetition Maximum Conversion

Pounds	10 reps	9 reps	8 reps	7 reps	6 reps	5 reps	4 reps	3 reps	2 reps
5	7	6	6	6	6	6	6	5	5
10	13	13	13	12	12	11	11	11	11
15	20	19	19	18	18	17	17	16	16
20	27	26	25	24	24	23	22	22	21
25	33	32	31	30	29	29	28	27	26
30	40	39	38	36	35	34	33	32	32
35	47	45	44	42	41	40	39	38	37
40	53	52	50	48	47	46	44	43	42
45	60	58	56	55	53	51	50	49	47
50	67	65	63	61	59	57	56	54	53
55	73	71	69	67	65	63	61	59	58
60	80	77	75	73	71	69	67	65	63
65	87	84	81	79	76	74	72	70	68
70	93	90	88	85	82	80	78	76	74
75	100	97	94	91	88	86	83	81	79
80	107	103	100	97	94	91	89	86	84
85	113	110	106	103	100	97	94	92	89
90	120	116	113	109	106	103	100	97	95
95	127	123	119	115	112	109	106	103	100
100	133	129	125	121	118	114	111	108	105

Pounds	10 reps	9 reps	8 reps	7 reps	6 reps	5 reps	4 reps	3 reps	2 reps
105	140	135	131	127	124	120	117	114	111
110	147	142	138	133	129	126	122	119	116
115	153	148	144	139	135	131	128	124	121
120	160	155	150	145	141	137	133	130	126
125	167	161	156	152	147	143	139	135	132
130	173	168	163	158	153	149	144	141	137
135	180	174	169	164	159	154	150	146	142
140	187	181	175	170	165	160	156	151	147
145	193	187	181	176	171	166	161	157	153
150	200	194	188	182	176	171	167	162	158
155	207	200	194	188	182	177	172	168	163
160	213	206	200	194	188	183	178	173	168
165	220	213	206	200	194	189	183	178	174
170	227	219	213	206	200	194	189	184	179
175	233	226	219	212	206	200	194	189	184
180	240	232	225	218	212	206	200	195	189
185	247	239	231	224	218	211	206	200	195
190	253	245	238	230	224	217	211	205	200
195	260	252	244	236	229	223	217	211	205
200	267	258	250	242	235	229	222	216	211
205	273	265	256	248	241	234	228	222	216
210	280	271	263	255	247	240	233	227	221
215	287	277	269	261	253	246	239	232	226
220	293	284	275	267	259	251	244	238	232
225	300	290	281	273	265	257	250	243	237
230	307	297	288	279	271	263	256	249	242
235	313	303	294	285	276	269	261	254	247
240	320	310	300	291	282	274	267	259	253
245	327	316	306	297	288	280	272	265	258
250	333	323	313	303	294	286	278	270	263

(Continued)

Pounds	10 reps	9 reps	8 reps	7 reps	6 reps	5 reps	4 reps	3 reps	2 reps
255	340	329	319	309	300	291	283	276	268
260	347	335	325	315	306	297	289	281	274
265	353	342	331	321	312	303	294	286	279
270	360	348	338	327	318	309	300	292	284
275	367	355	344	333	324	314	306	297	289
280	373	361	350	339	329	320	311	303	295
285	380	368	356	345	335	326	317	308	300
290	387	374	363	352	341	331	322	314	305
295	393	381	369	358	347	337	328	319	311
300	400	387	375	364	353	343	333	324	316
305	407	394	381	370	359	349	339	330	321
310	413	400	388	376	365	354	344	335	326
315	420	406	394	382	371	360	350	341	332
320	427	413	400	388	376	366	356	346	337
325	433	419	406	394	382	371	361	351	342
330	440	426	413	400	388	377	367	357	347
335	447	432	419	406	394	383	372	362	353
340	453	439	425	412	400	389	378	368	358
345	460	445	431	418	406	394	383	373	363
350	467	452	438	424	412	400	389	378	368
355	473	458	444	430	418	406	394	384	374
360	480	465	450	436	424	411	400	389	379
365	487	471	456	442	429	417	406	395	384
370	493	477	463	448	435	423	411	400	389
375	500	484	469	455	441	429	417	405	395
380	507	490	475	461	447	434	422	411	400
385	513	497	481	467	453	440	428	416	405
390	520	503	488	473	459	446	433	422	411
395	527	510	494	479	465	451	439	427	416
400	533	516	500	485	471	457	444	432	421
405	540	523	506	491	476	463	450	438	426

Pounds	10 reps	9 reps	8 reps	7 reps	6 reps	5 reps	4 reps	3 reps	2 reps
410	547	529	513	497	482	469	456	443	432
415	553	535	519	503	488	474	461	449	437
420	560	542	525	509	494	480	467	454	442
425	567	548	531	515	500	486	472	459	447
430	573	555	538	521	506	491	478	465	453
435	580	561	544	527	512	497	483	470	458
440	587	568	550	533	518	503	489	476	463
445	593	574	556	539	524	509	494	481	468
450	600	581	563	545	529	514	500	486	474
455	607	587	569	552	535	520	506	492	479
460	613	594	575	558	541	526	511	497	484
465	620	600	581	564	547	531	517	503	489
470	627	606	588	570	553	537	522	508	495
475	633	613	594	576	559	543	528	514	500
480	640	619	600	582	565	549	533	519	505
485	647	626	606	588	571	554	539	524	511
490	653	632	613	594	576	560	544	530	516
495	660	639	619	600	582	566	550	535	521
500	667	645	625	606	588	571	556	541	526
505	673	652	631	612	594	577	561	546	532
510	680	658	638	618	600	583	567	551	537
515	687	665	644	624	606	589	572	557	542
520	693	671	650	630	612	594	578	562	547
525	700	677	656	636	618	600	583	568	553
530	707	684	663	642	624	606	589	573	558
535	713	690	669	648	629	611	594	578	563
540	720	697	675	655	635	617	600	584	568
545	727	703	681	661	641	623	606	589	574
550	733	710	688	667	647	629	611	595	579
555	740	716	694	673	653	634	617	600	584

(Continued)

Pounds	10 reps	9 reps	8 reps	7 reps	6 reps	5 reps	4 reps	3 reps	2 reps
560	747	723	700	679	659	640	622	605	589
565	753	729	706	685	665	646	628	611	595
570	760	735	713	691	671	651	633	616	600
575	767	742	719	697	676	657	639	622	605
580	773	748	725	703	682	663	644	627	611
585	780	755	731	709	688	669	650	632	616
590	787	761	738	715	694	674	656	638	621
595	793	768	744	721	700	680	661	643	626
600	800	774	750	727	706	686	667	649	632
605	807	781	756	733	712	691	672	654	637
610	813	787	763	739	718	697	678	659	642
615	820	794	769	745	724	703	683	665	647
620	827	800	775	752	729	709	689	670	653
625	833	806	781	758	735	714	694	676	658
630	840	813	788	764	741	720	700	681	663
635	847	819	794	770	747	726	706	686	668
640	853	826	800	776	753	731	711	692	674
645	860	832	806	782	759	737	717	697	679
650	867	839	813	788	765	743	722	703	684
655	873	845	819	794	771	749	728	708	689
660	880	852	825	800	776	754	733	714	695
665	887	858	831	806	782	760	739	719	700
670	893	865	838	812	788	766	744	724	705
675	900	871	844	818	794	771	750	730	711
680	907	877	850	824	800	777	756	735	716
685	913	884	856	830	806	783	761	741	721
690	920	890	863	836	812	789	767	746	726
695	927	897	869	842	818	794	772	751	732
700	933	903	875	848	824	800	778	757	737
705	940	910	881	855	829	806	783	762	742
710	947	916	888	861	835	811	789	768	747

Pounds	10 reps	9 reps	8 reps	7 reps	6 reps	5 reps	4 reps	3 reps	2 reps
715	953	923	894	867	841	817	794	773	753
720	960	929	900	873	847	823	800	778	758
725	967	935	906	879	853	829	806	784	763
730	973	942	913	885	859	834	811	789	768
735	980	948	919	891	865	840	817	795	774
740	987	955	925	897	871	846	822	800	779
745	993	961	931	903	876	851	828	805	784
750	1000	968	938	909	882	857	833	811	789
755	1007	974	944	915	888	863	839	816	795
760	1013	981	950	921	894	869	844	822	800
765	1020	987	956	927	900	874	850	827	805
770	1027	994	963	933	906	880	856	832	811
775	1033	1000	969	939	912	886	861	838	816
780	1040	1006	975	945	918	891	867	843	821
785	1047	1013	981	952	924	897	872	849	826
790	1053	1019	988	958	929	903	878	854	832
795	1060	1026	994	964	935	909	883	859	837
800	1067	1032	1000	970	941	914	889	865	842
805	1073	1039	1006	976	947	920	894	870	847
810	1080	1045	1013	982	953	926	900	876	853
815	1087	1052	1019	988	959	931	906	881	858
820	1093	1058	1025	994	965	937	911	886	863
825	1100	1065	1031	1000	971	943	917	892	868
830	1107	1071	1038	1006	976	949	922	897	874
835	1113	1077	1044	1012	982	954	928	903	879
840	1120	1084	1050	1018	988	960	933	908	884
845	1127	1090	1056	1024	994	966	939	914	889
850	1133	1097	1063	1030	1000	971	944	919	895
855	1140	1103	1069	1036	1006	977	950	924	900
900	1200	1161	1125	1091	1059	1029	1000	973	947

(Continued)

Pounds	10 reps	9 reps	8 reps	7 reps	6 reps	5 reps	4 reps	3 reps	2 reps
905	1207	1168	1131	1097	1065	1034	1006	978	953
910	1213	1174	1138	1103	1071	1040	1011	984	958
915	1220	1181	1144	1109	1076	1046	1017	989	963
920	1227	1187	1150	1115	1082	1051	1022	995	968
925	1233	1194	1156	1121	1088	1057	1028	1000	974
930	1240	1200	1163	1127	1094	1063	1033	1005	979
935	1247	1206	1169	1133	1100	1069	1039	1011	984
940	1253	1213	1175	1139	1106	1074	1044	1016	989
945	1260	1219	1181	1145	1112	1080	1050	1022	995
950	1267	1226	1188	1152	1118	1086	1056	1027	1000
955	1273	1232	1194	1158	1124	1091	1061	1032	1005
960	1280	1239	1200	1164	1129	1097	1067	1038	1011
965	1287	1245	1206	1170	1135	1103	1072	1043	1016
970	1293	1252	1213	1176	1141	1109	1078	1049	1021
975	1300	1258	1219	1182	1147	1114	1083	1054	1026
980	1307	1265	1225	1188	1153	1120	1089	1059	1032
985	1313	1271	1231	1194	1159	1126	1094	1065	1037
990	1320	1277	1238	1200	1165	1131	1100	1070	1042
995	1327	1284	1244	1206	1171	1137	1106	1076	1047
1000	1333	1290	1250	1212	1176	1143	1111	1081	1053

Muscular System

The traditional perception of muscles is that they work concentrically and predominantly in one plane of motion. However, to more effectively understand motion it is imperative to view muscles functioning in all planes of motion and through the entire muscle action spectrum. The following section describes the isolated (concentric) and integrated (isometric, eccentric) actions of the major muscles of the human movement system.

The following section describes each muscles' origin, insertion, and function. The origin and insertion refer to the anatomic locations of where a muscle attaches (usually a bone). The origin refers to the proximal attachment site that remains relatively fixed during contraction. The insertion refers to the muscle's distal attachment site to a moveable bone.

Lower Leg Musculature

Anterior Tibialis

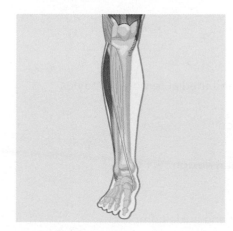

Origin
- Lateral condyle and proximal two thirds of the lateral surface of the tibia

Insertion
- Medial and plantar aspects of the medial cuneiform and the base of the first metatarsal

Isolated Function
- Concentrically accelerates dorsiflexion and inversion

Integrated Function
- Eccentrically decelerates plantarflexion and eversion
- Isometrically stabilizes the arch of the foot

Posterior Tibialis

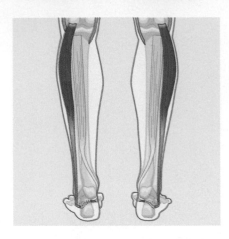

Origin
- Proximal two thirds of posterior surface of the tibia and fibula

Insertion
- Every tarsal bone (naviular, cuneiform, cuboid) but the talus plus the bases of the second through the fourth metatarsal bones. The main insertion is on the navicular tuberosity and the medial cuneiform bone

Isolated Function
- Concentrically accelerates plantarflexion and inversion of the foot

Integrated Function
- Eccentrically decelerates dorsiflexion and eversion of the foot
- Isometrically stabilizes the arch of the foot

Soleus

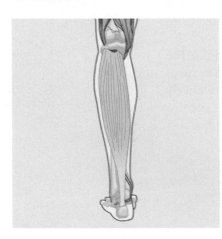

Origin
- Posterior surface of the fibular head and proximal one third of its shaft and from the posterior side of the tibia

Insertion
- Calcaneus via the Achilles tendon

Isolated Function
- Concentrically accelerates plantarflexion

Integrated Function
- Decelerates ankle dorsiflexion
- Isometrically stabilizes the foot and ankle complex

Gastrocnemius

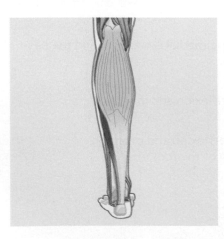

Origin
- Posterior aspect of the lateral and medial femoral condyles

Insertion
- Calcaneus via the Achilles tendon

Isolated Function
- Concentrically accelerates plantarflexion

Integrated Function
- Decelerates ankle dorsiflexion
- Isometrically stabilizes the foot and ankle complex

Peroneus Longus

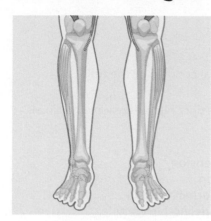

Origin
- Lateral condyle of tibia, head, and proximal two thirds of the lateral surface of the fibula

Insertion
- Lateral surface of the medial cuneiform and lateral side of the base of the first metatarsal

Isolated Function
- Concentrically plantarflexes and everts the foot

Integrated Function
- Decelerates ankle dorsiflexion
- Isometrically stabilizes the foot and ankle complex

Hamstring Complex

Biceps Femoris—Long Head

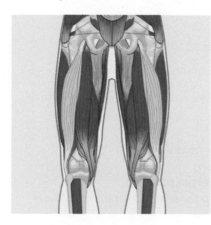

Origin
- Ischial tuberosity of the pelvis, part of the sacrotuberous ligament

Insertion
- Head of the fibula

Isolated Function
- Concentrically accelerates knee flexion and hip extension
- Tibial external rotation

Integrated Function
- Eccentrically decelerates knee extension
- Eccentrically decelerates hip flexion
- Eccentrically decelerates tibial internal rotation at mid-stance of the gait cycle
- Isometrically stabilizes the lumbo-pelvic-hip complex and knee

Biceps Femoris—Short Head

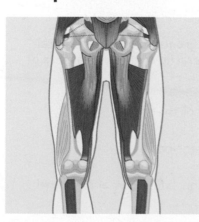

Origin
- Lower one third of the posterior aspect of the femur

Insertion
- Head of the fibula

Isolated Function
- Concentrically accelerates knee flexion and tibial external rotation

Integrated Function
- Eccentrically decelerates knee extension
- Eccentrically decelerates tibial internal rotation
- Isometrically stabilizes the knee

Semimembranosus

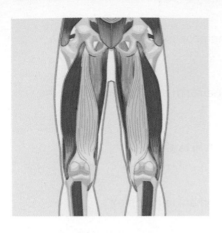

Origin
• Ischial tuberosity of the pelvis

Insertion
• Posterior aspect of the medial tibial condyle of the tibia

Isolated Function
• Concentrically accelerates knee flexion, hip extension, and tibial internal rotation

Integrated Function
• Eccentrically decelerates knee extension
• Eccentrically decelerates hip flexion
• Eccentrically decelerates tibial external rotation
• Isometrically stabilizes the lumbo-pelvic-hip complex and knee

Semitendinosus

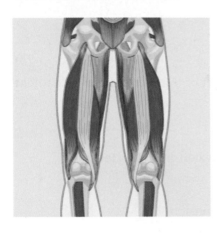

Origin
• Ischial tuberosity of the pelvis and part of the sacrotuberous ligament

Insertion
• Proximal aspect of the medial tibial condyle of the tibia (pes anserine)

Isolated Function
• Concentrically accelerates knee flexion, hip extension, and tibial internal rotation

Integrated Function
• Eccentrically decelerates knee extension
• Eccentrically decelerates hip flexion
• Eccentrically decelerates tibial external rotation
• Isometrically stabilizes the lumbo-pelvic-hip complex and knee

Quadriceps

Vastus Lateralis

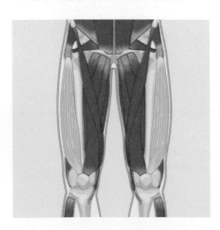

Origin
• Anterior and inferior border of the greater trochanter, lateral region of the gluteal tuberosity, lateral lip of the linea aspera of the femur

Insertion
• Base of patella and tibial tuberosity of the tibia

Isolated Function
• Concentrically accelerates knee extension

Integrated Function
• Eccentrically decelerates knee flexion, adduction, and internal rotation
• Isometrically stabilizes the knee

Vastus Medialis

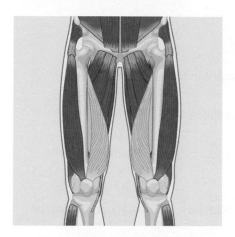

Origin
- Lower region of intertrochanteric line, medial lip of linea aspera, proximal medial supracondylar line of the femur

Insertion
- Base of patella, tibial tuberosity of the tibia

Isolated Function
- Concentrically accelerates knee extension

Integrated Function
- Eccentrically decelerates knee flexion, adduction, and internal rotation
- Isometrically stabilizes the knee

Vastus Intermedius

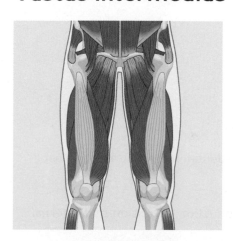

Origin
- Anterior-lateral regions of the upper two thirds of the femur

Insertion
- Base of patella, tibial tuberosity of the tibia

Isolated Function
- Concentrically accelerates knee extension

Integrated Function
- Eccentrically decelerates knee flexion, adduction, and internal rotation
- Isometrically stabilizes the knee

Rectus Femoris

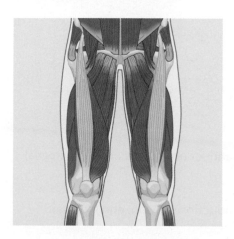

Origin
- Anterior-inferior iliac spine of the pelvis

Insertion
- Base of patella, tibial tuberosity of the tibia

Isolated Function
- Concentrically accelerates knee extension and hip flexion

Integrated Function
- Eccentrically decelerates knee flexion, adduction, and internal rotation
- Decelerates hip extension
- Isometrically stabilizes the lumbo-pelvic-hip complex and knee

Hip Musculature

Adductor Longus

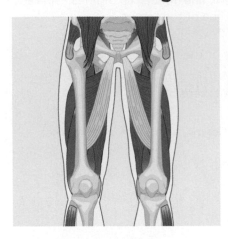

Origin
- Anterior surface of the inferior pubic ramus of the pelvis

Insertion
- Proximal one third of the linea aspera of the femur

Isolated Function
- Concentrically accelerates hip adduction, flexion, and internal rotation

Integrated Function
- Eccentrically decelerates hip abduction, extension, and external rotation
- Isometrically stabilizes the lumbo-pelvic-hip complex

Adductor Magnus—Anterior Fibers

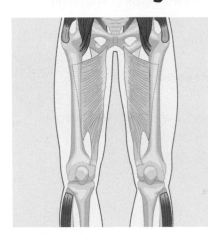

Origin
- Ischial ramus of the pelvis

Insertion
- Linea aspera of the femur

Isolated Function
- Concentrically accelerates hip adduction, flexion, and internal rotation

Integrated Function
- Eccentrically decelerates hip abduction, extension, and external rotation
- Dynamically stabilizes the lumbo-pelvic-hip complex

Adductor Magnus—Posterior Fibers

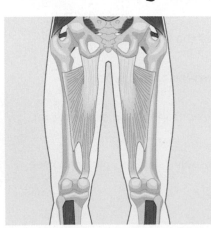

Origin
- Ischial tuberosity of the pelvis

Insertion
- Adductor tubercle on femur

Isolated Function
- Concentrically accelerates hip adduction, extension, and external rotation

Integrated Function
- Eccentrically decelerates hip abduction, flexion, and internal rotation
- Isometrically stabilizes the lumbo-pelvic-hip complex

Adductor Brevis

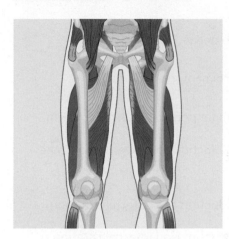

Origin
- Anterior surface of the inferior pubic ramus of the pelvis

Insertion
- Proximal one third of the linea aspera of the femur

Isolated Function
- Concentrically accelerates hip adduction, flexion, and internal rotation

Integrated Function
- Eccentrically decelerates hip abduction, extension, and external rotation
- Isometrically stabilizes the lumbo-pelvic-hip complex

Gracilis

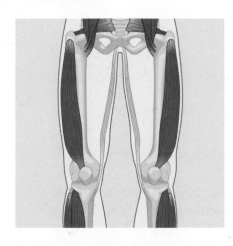

Origin
- Anterior aspect of lower body of pubis

Insertion
- Proximal medial surface of the tibia (pes anserine)

Isolated Function
- Concentrically accelerates hip adduction, flexion, and internal rotation
- Assists in tibial internal rotation

Integrated Function
- Eccentrically decelerates hip abduction, extension, and external rotation
- Isometrically stabilizes the lumbo-pelvic-hip complex and knee

Pectineus

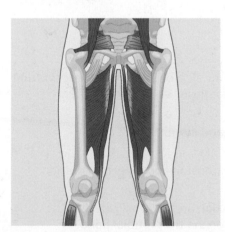

Origin
- Pectineal line on the superior pubic ramus of the pelvis

Insertion
- Pectineal line on the posterior surface of the upper femur

Isolated Function
- Concentrically accelerates hip adduction, flexion, and internal rotation

Integrated Function
- Eccentrically decelerates hip abduction, extension, and external rotation
- Isometrically stabilizes the lumbo-pelvic-hip complex

Gluteus Medius

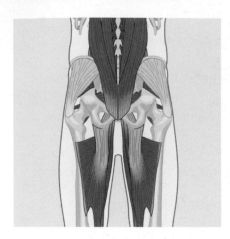

Origin
- Outer surface of the ilium of the pelvis

Insertion
- Lateral surface of the greater trochanter on the femur

Isolated Function
- Concentrically accelerates hip abduction and internal rotation (anterior fibers)
- Concentrically accelerates hip abduction and external rotation (posterior fibers)

Integrated Function
- Eccentrically decelerates hip adduction and external rotation (anterior fibers)
- Eccentrically decelerates hip adduction and internal rotation (posterior fibers)
- Isometrically stabilizes the lumbo-pelvic-hip complex

Gluteus Minimus

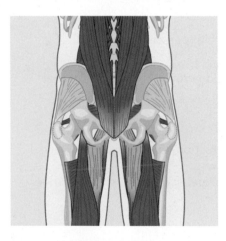

Origin
- Ilium of the pelvis between the anterior and inferior gluteal line

Insertion
- Greater trochanter of the femur

Isolated Function
- Concentrically accelerates hip abduction and internal rotation

Integrated Function
- Eccentrically decelerates hip adduction and external rotation
- Isometrically stabilizes the lumbo-pelvic-hip complex

Gluteus Maximus

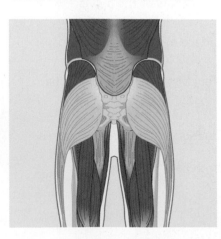

Origin
- Outer ilium of the pelvis, posterior side of sacrum and coccyx, and part of the sacrotuberous and posterior sacroiliac ligament

Insertion
- Gluteal tuberosity of the femur and iliotibial tract

Isolated Function
- Concentrically accelerates hip extension and external rotation

Integrated Function
- Eccentrically decelerates hip flexion and internal rotation
- Decelerates tibial internal rotation via the iliotibial band
- Isometrically stabilizes the lumbo-pelvic-hip complex

Tensor Fascia Latae (Including the Iliotibial Band)

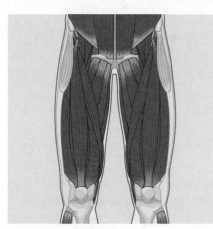

Origin
- Outer surface of the iliac crest just posterior to the anterior-superior iliac spine of the pelvis

Insertion
- Proximal one third of the iliotibial band

Isolated Function
- Concentrically accelerates hip flexion, abduction, and internal rotation

Integrated Function
- Eccentrically decelerates hip extension, adduction, and external rotation
- Isometrically stabilizes the lumbo-pelvic-hip complex

Psoas

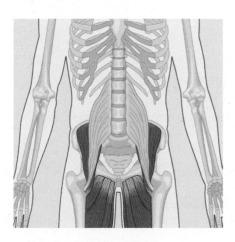

Origin
- Transverse processes and lateral bodies of the last thoracic and all lumbar vertebrae including intervetebral disks

Insertion
- Lesser trochanter of the femur

Isolated Function
- Concentrically accelerates hip flexion and external rotation
- Concentrically extends and rotates lumbar spine

Integrated Function
- Eccentrically decelerates hip internal rotation
- Eccentrically decelerates hip extension
- Isometrically stabilizes the lumbo-pelvic-hip complex

Iliacus

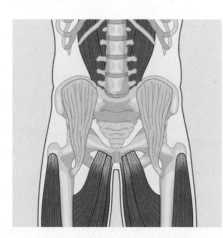

Origin
- Superior two thirds of iliac fossa, inner lip of the iliac crest

Insertion
- Lesser trochanter of femur

Isolated Function
- Concentrically accelerates hip flexion and external rotation

Integrated Function
- Eccentrically decelerates hip extension and internal rotation
- Isometrically stabilizes the lumbo-pelvic-hip complex

Sartorius

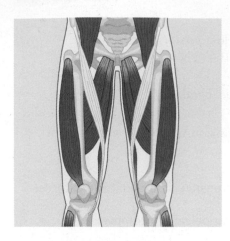

Origin
- Anterior-superior iliac spine of the pelvis

Insertion
- Proximal medial surface of the tibia

Isolated Function
- Concentrically accelerates hip flexion, external rotation, and abduction
- Concentrically accelerates knee flexion and internal rotation

Integrated Function
- Eccentrically decelerates hip extension and internal rotation
- Eccentrically decelerates knee extension and external rotation
- Isometrically stabilizes the lumbo-pelvic-hip complex and knee

Piriformis

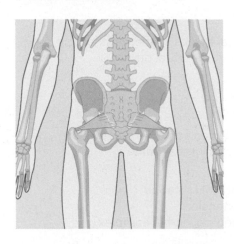

Origin
- Anterior side of the sacrum

Insertion
- The greater trochanter of the femur

Isolated Function
- Concentrically accelerates hip external rotation, abduction, and extension

Integrated Function
- Eccentrically decelerates hip internal rotation, adduction, and flexion
- Isometrically stabilizes the hip and sacroiliac joints

Abdominal Musculature

Rectus Abdominis

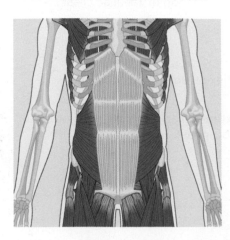

Origin
- Pubic symphysis of the pelvis

Insertion
- Ribs 5–7
- Xiphoid process of the sternum

Isolated Function
- Concentrically accelerates spinal flexion, lateral flexion, and rotation

Integrated Function
- Eccentrically decelerates spinal extension, lateral flexion, and rotation
- Isometrically stabilizes the lumbo-pelvic-hip complex

External Oblique

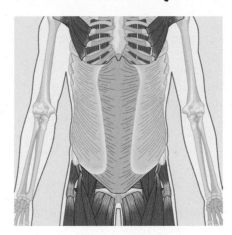

Origin
- External surface of ribs 4–12

Insertion
- Anterior iliac crest of the pelvis, linea alba, and contralateral rectus sheaths

Isolated Function
- Concentrically accelerates spinal flexion, lateral flexion, and contralateral rotation

Integrated Function
- Eccentrically decelerates spinal extension, lateral flexion, and rotation
- Isometrically stabilizes the lumbo-pelvic-hip complex

Internal Oblique

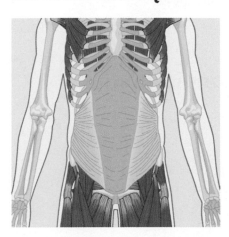

Origin
- Anterior two thirds of the iliac crest of the pelvis and thoracolumbar fascia

Insertion
- Ribs 9–12, linea alba, and contralateral rectus sheaths

Isolated Function
- Concentrically accelerates spinal flexion, lateral flexion, and ipsilateral rotation

Integrated Function
- Eccentrically decelerates spinal extension, rotation, and lateral flexion
- Isometrically stabilizes the lumbo-pelvic-hip complex

Transverse Abdominis

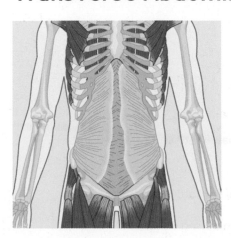

Origin
- Ribs 7–12, anterior two thirds of the iliac crest of the pelvis, and thoracolumbar fascia

Insertion
- Lineae alba and contralateral rectus sheaths

Isolated Function
- Increases intra-abdominal pressure
- Supports the abdominal viscera

Integrated Function
- Isometrically stabilizes the lumbo-pelvic-hip complex

Diaphragm

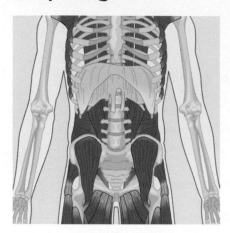

Origin
- Costal part: inner surfaces of the cartilages and adjacent bony regions of ribs 6–12
- Sternal part: posterior side of the xiphoid process
- Crural (lumbar) part: (1) two aponeurotic arches covering the external surfaces of the quadratus lumborum and psoas major; (2) right and left crus, originating from the bodies of L1–L3 and their intervertebral disks

Insertion
- Central tendon

Isolated Function
- Concentrically pulls the central tendon inferiorly, increasing the volume in the thoracic cavity

Integrated Function
- Stabilizes the lumbo-pelvic-hip complex

Back Musculature

Superficial Erector Spinae: Iliocostalis, Longissimus, and Spinalis

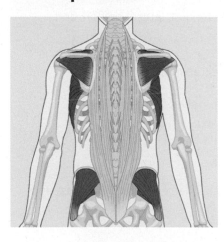

Division in the Group
- Lumborum (lumbar)
- Thoracis (thoracic)
- Cervicis (cervical)

Common Origin
- Iliac crest of the pelvis
- Sacrum
- Spinous and transverse process of T11–L5

Insertion
Iliocostalis
- Lumborum: Inferior border of ribs 7–12
- Thoracis: Superior border of ribs 1–6
- Cervicis: Transverse process of C4–C6

Longissimus
- Thoracis: Transverse process T1–T12; ribs 2–12
- Cervicis: Transverse process of C6–C2
- Capitis: Mastoid process of the skull

Spinalis
- Thoracis: Spinous process of T7–T4
- Cervicis: Spinous process of C3–C2
- Capitis: Between the superior and inferior nuchal lines on occipital bone of the skull

Isolated Function
- Concentrically accelerates spinal extension, rotation, and lateral flexion

Integrated Function
- Eccentrically decelerates spinal flexion, rotation, and lateral flexion
- Dynamically stabilizes the spine during functional movements

Quadratus Lumborum

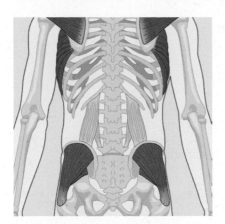

Origin
- Iliac crest of the pelvis

Insertion
- 12th rib
- Transverse process L2–L5

Isolated Function
- Spinal lateral flexion

Integrated Function
- Eccentrically decelerates contralateral lateral spinal flexion
- Isometrically stabilizes the lumbo-pelvic-hip complex

Multifidus

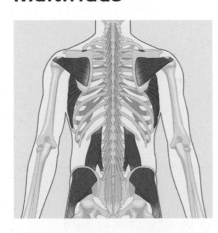

Origin
- Posterior aspect of the sacrum
- Processes of the lumbar, thoracic, and cervical spine

Insertion
- Spinous processes one to four segments above the origin

Isolated Function
- Concentrically accelerates spinal extension and contralateral rotation

Integrated Function
- Eccentrically decelerates spinal flexion and rotation
- Isometrically stabilizes the spine

Latissimus Dorsi

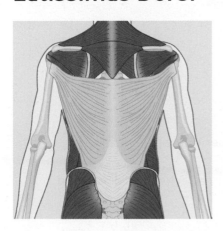

Origin
- Spinous processes of T7–T12
- Iliac crest of the pelvis
- Thoracolumbar fascia
- Ribs 9–12

Insertion
- Inferior angle of the scapula
- Intertubercular groove of the humerus

Isolated Function
- Concentrically accelerates shoulder extension, adduction, and internal rotation

Integrated Function
- Eccentrically decelerates shoulder flexion, abduction, and external rotation
- Eccentrically decelerates spinal flexion
- Isometrically stabilizes the lumbo-pelvic-hip complex and shoulder

Shoulder Musculature

Serratus Anterior

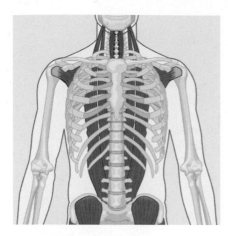

Origin
- Ribs 4–12

Insertion
- Medial border of the scapula

Isolated Function
- Concentrically accelerates scapular protraction

Integrated Function
- Eccentrically decelerates dynamic scapular retraction
- Isometrically stabilizes the scapula

Rhomboid Major

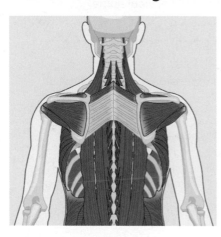

Origin
- Spinous processes C7–T5

Insertion
- Medial border of the scapula

Isolated Function
- Concentrically produces scapular retraction and downward rotation

Integrated Function
- Eccentrically decelerates scapular protraction and upward rotation
- Isometrically stabilizes the scapula

Rhomboid Minor

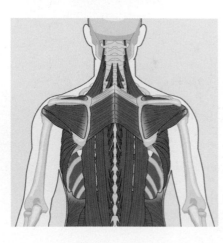

Origin
- Spinous processes C7–T1

Insertion
- Medial border of the scapula superior to spine

Isolated Function
- Concentrically produces scapular retraction and downward rotation

Integrated Function
- Eccentrically decelerates scapular protraction and upward rotation
- Isometrically stabilizes the scapula

Lower Trapezius

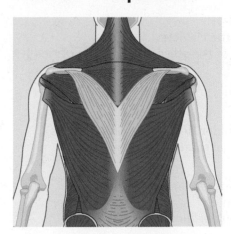

Origin
- Spinous processes of T6–T12

Insertion
- Spine of the scapula

Isolated Function
- Concentrically accelerates scapular depression

Integrated Function
- Eccentrically decelerates scapular elevation
- Isometrically stabilizes the scapula

Middle Trapezius

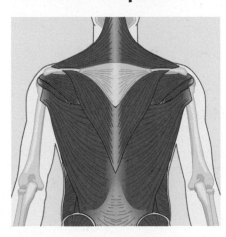

Origin
- Spinous processes of T1–T5

Insertion
- Acromion process of the scapula
- Superior aspect of the spine of the scapula

Isolated Function
- Concentrically accelerates scapular retraction

Integrated Function
- Eccentrically decelerates scapular elevation
- Isometrically stabilizes the scapula

Upper Trapezius

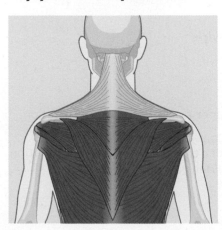

Origin
- External occipital protuberance of the skull
- Spinous process of C7

Insertion
- Lateral third of the clavicle
- Acromion process of the scapula

Isolated Function
- Concentrically accelerates cervical extension, lateral flexion, and rotation
- Concentrically accelerates scapular elevation

Integrated Function
- Eccentrically decelerates cervical flexion, lateral flexion, and rotation
- Eccentrically decelerates scapular depression
- Isometrically stabilizes the cervical spine and scapula

Pectoralis Major

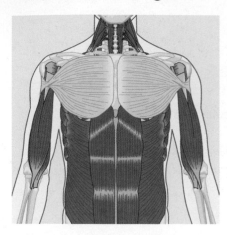

Origin
- Clavicular: Anterior surface of the clavicle
- Sternocostal: Anterior surface of the sternum, cartilage of ribs 1–7

Insertion
- Greater tubercle of the humerus

Isolated Function
- Concentrically accelerates shoulder flexion (clavicular fibers), horizontal adduction, and internal rotation

Integrated Function
- Eccentrically decelerates shoulder extension, horizontal abduction, and external rotation
- Isometrically stabilizes the shoulder girdle

Pectoralis Minor

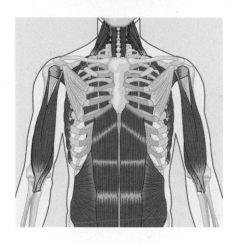

Origin
- Ribs 3–5

Insertion
- Coracoid process of the scapula

Isolated Function
- Concentrically protracts the scapula

Integrated Function
- Eccentrically decelerates scapular retraction
- Isometrically stabilizes the shoulder girdle

Anterior Deltoid

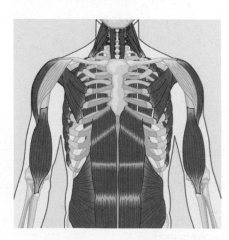

Origin
- Anterior: Lateral third of the clavicle

Insertion
- Deltoid tuberosity of the humerus

Isolated Function
- Concentrically accelerates shoulder flexion and internal rotation

Integrated Function
- Eccentrically decelerates shoulder extension and external rotation
- Isometrically stabilizes the shoulder girdle

Medial Deltoid

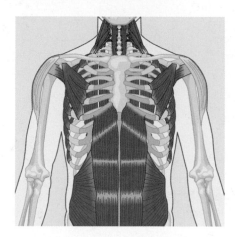

Origin
- Acromion process of the scapula

Insertion
- Deltoid tuberosity of the humerus

Isolated Function
- Concentrically accelerates shoulder abduction

Integrated Function
- Eccentrically decelerates shoulder adduction
- Isometrically stabilizes the shoulder girdle

Posterior Deltoid

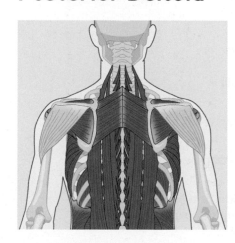

Origin
- Posterior: Spine of the scapula

Insertion
- Deltoid tuberosity of the humerus

Isolated Function
- Concentrically accelerates shoulder extension and external rotation

Integrated Function
- Eccentrically decelerates shoulder flexion and internal rotation
- Isometrically stabilizes the shoulder girdle

Teres Major

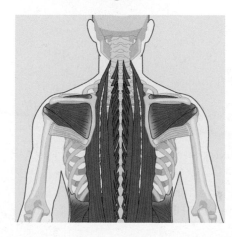

Origin
- Inferior angle of the scapula

Insertion
- Lesser tubercle of the humerus

Isolated Function
- Concentrically accelerates shoulder internal rotation, adduction, and extension

Integrated Function
- Eccentrically decelerates shoulder external rotation, abduction, and flexion
- Isometrically stabilizes the shoulder girdle

Rotator Cuff

Teres Minor

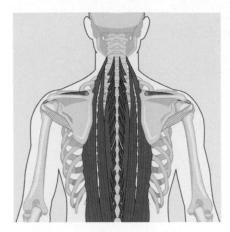

Origin
• Lateral border of the scapula

Insertion
• Greater tubercle of the humerus

Isolated Function
• Concentrically accelerates shoulder external rotation

Integrated Function
• Eccentrically decelerates shoulder internal rotation
• Isometrically stabilizes the shoulder girdle

Infraspinatus

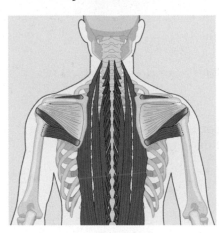

Origin
• Infraspinous fossa of the scapula

Insertion
• Middle facet of the greater tubercle of the humerus

Isolated Function
• Concentrically accelerates shoulder external rotation

Integrated Function
• Eccentrically decelerates shoulder internal rotation
• Isometrically stabilizes the shoulder girdle

Subscapularis

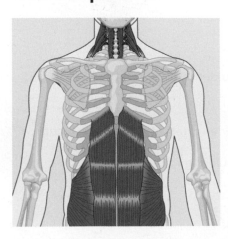

Origin
• Subscapular fossa of the scapula

Insertion
• Lesser tubercle of the humerus

Isolated Function
• Concentrically accelerates shoulder internal rotation

Integrated Function
• Eccentrically decelerates shoulder external rotation
• Isometrically stabilizes the shoulder girdle

Supraspinatus

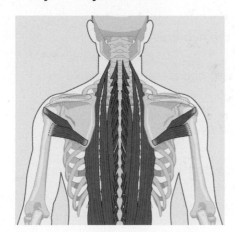

Origin
- Supraspinous fossa of the scapula

Insertion
- Superior facet of the greater tubercle of the humerus

Isolated Function
- Concentrically accelerates abduction of the arm

Integrated Function
- Eccentrically decelerates adduction of the arm
- Isometrically stabilizes the shoulder girdle

Arm Musculature

Biceps Brachii

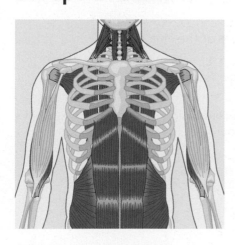

Origin
- Short head: Coracoid process of the scapula
- Long head: Tubercle above glenoid cavity on the humerus

Insertion
- Radial tuberosity of the radius

Isolated Function
- Concentrically accelerates elbow flexion, supination of the radioulnar joint, and shoulder flexion

Integrated Function
- Eccentrically decelerates elbow extension, pronation of the radioulnar joint, and shoulder extension
- Isometrically stabilizes the elbow and shoulder girdle

Triceps Brachii

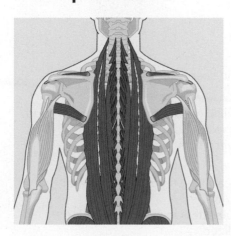

Origin
- Long head: Infraglenoid tubercle of the scapula
- Short head: Posterior humerus
- Medial head: Posterior humerus

Insertion
- Olecranon process of the ulna

Isolated Function
- Concentrically accelerates elbow extension and shoulder extension

Integrated Function
- Eccentrically decelerates elbow flexion and shoulder flexion
- Isometrically stabilizes the elbow and shoulder girdle

Brachioradialis

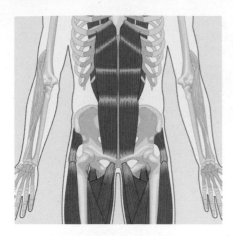

Origin
- Lateral supracondylar ridge of the humerus

Insertion
- Lateral surface of distal radius, immediately above styloid process

Isolated Function
- Concentrically accelerates elbow flexion

Integrated Function
- Eccentrically decelerates elbow extension
- Isometrically stabilizes the elbow

Brachialis

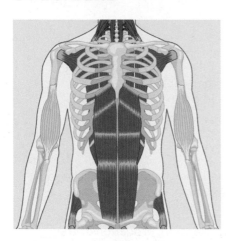

Origin
- Lower 1/2 of the anterior surface of the humerus

Insertion
- Tuberosity and coronoid process of the ulna

Isolated Function
- Concentrically accelerates elbow flexion

Integrated Function
- Eccentrically decelerates elbow extension
- Isometrically stabilizes the elbow

Neck Musculature

Levator Scapulae

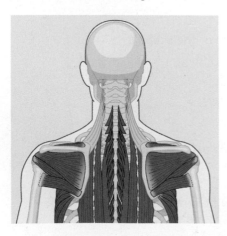

Origin
- Transverse processes of C1–C4

Insertion
- Superior vertebral border of the scapulae

Isolated Function
- Concentrically accelerates cervical extension, lateral flexion, and ipsilateral rotation when the scapulae is anchored
- Assists in elevation and downward rotation of the scapulae

Integrated Function
- Eccentrically decelerates cervical flexion and contralateral cervical rotation and lateral flexion
- Eccentrically decelerates scapular depression and upward rotation when the neck is stabilized
- Stabilizes the cervical spine and scapulae

Sternocleidomastoid

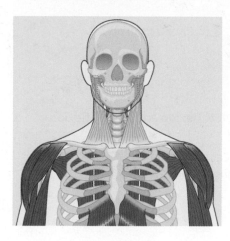

Origin
- Sternal head: Top of manubrium of the sternum
- Clavicular head: Medial one third of the clavicle

Insertion
- Mastoid process, lateral superior nuchal line of the occiput of the skull

Isolated Function
- Concentrically accelerates cervical flexion, rotation, and lateral flexion

Integrated Function
- Eccentrically decelerates cervical extension, rotation, and lateral flexion
- Isometrically stabilizes the cervical spine and acromioclavicular joint

Scalenes

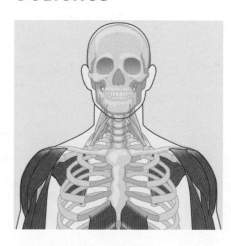

Origin
- Transverse processes of C3–C7

Insertion
- First and second ribs

Isolated Function
- Concentrically accelerates cervical flexion, rotation, and lateral flexion
- Assists rib elevation during inhalation

Integrated Function
- Eccentrically decelerates cervical extension, rotation, and lateral flexion
- Isometrically stabilizes the cervical spine

Longus Coli

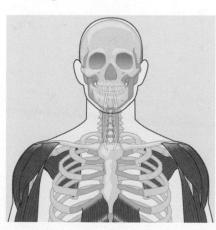

Origin
- Anterior portion of T1–T3

Insertion
- Anterior and lateral C1

Isolated Function
- Concentrically accelerates cervical flexion, lateral flexion, and ipsilateral rotation

Integrated Function
- Eccentrically decelerates cervical extension, lateral flexion, and contralateral rotation
- Isometrically stabilizes the cervical spine

Longus Capitis

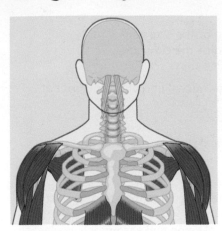

Origin
- Transverse processes of C3–C6

Insertion
- Inferior occipital bone

Isolated Function
- Concentrically accelerates cervical flexion and lateral flexion

Integrated Function
- Eccentrically decelerates cervical extension
- Isometrically stabilizes the cervical spine

Exam Prep Material

Fitness Assessment Considerations

Maximal Heart Rate Method for Prescribing Exercise Intensity

Traditionally the formula 220-age has been used to determine Heart Rate Max (HRmax). Updated research has shown that this formula has little scientific merit for use in exercise physiology and related fields. It is for this reason that the regression formula of $208 - (0.7 \times age)$ has been adopted. This equation is very simple to use, and can be easily implemented as a general starting point for measuring cardiorespiratory training intensity. The fitness professional should keep in mind that this, or any other simple formula, is not a definitive HRmax value.

Quick Check
What is the protocol for taking a client's pulse?

Assessment Adjustments for the Pregnant Population

In the 2nd and 3rd trimesters:

◆ Power and speed assessments should be avoided.
◆ Push-up assessments should be modified to be performed on the knees.
◆ The single-leg squat assessment should be modified to a single-leg balance.
◆ ROM for the OHS should be decreased.

Quick Check
What are normal Heart Rate and Blood Pressure measurements?

Assessment Adjustments for the Obese Population

Adjustment Considerations for Obese Populations:

◆ The Rockport walk test is a preferred cardiorespiratory assessment for this population.
◆ A single-leg balance should be considered in replacement of the single-leg squat.
◆ Modified push-ups on a bench or from the knees should be considered for push-up tests.

Assessment Adjustments for Common Injuries

Clients with low back pain:

◆ Watch for anterior or posterior rotation of the pelvis during the overhead squat, pushing, and pulling assessments, as this may indicate core weakness.
◆ The push-up position may be too difficult due to the demands on the core, in which case it may be more appropriate for clients to perform this assessment on their knees or with their hands on a bench.

Clients with a history of shoulder injuries:

◆ Watch for the arms falling forward during the overhead squat and/or the shoulders elevating and the head migrating forward during pushing and pulling assessments.
◆ Placing individuals in positions in which a large amount of stress is being placed on the shoulder complex may be eliminated or adjusted to decrease stress to the area.

Additional Considerations for Foot, Ankle, and Knee Compensations

Compensations seen in the overhead and single-leg squat assessments can determine if other assessments should or should not be performed. For example, an athlete whose knee excessively adducts during the single-leg squat assessment should probably not do a shark skill test, because not only will the client's performance be hindered, it may increase the risk of injury due to the dynamic nature of the assessment. Another option may be to perform the shark skill test using two legs versus one if the assessment is key to the client's programming and demands of his or her sport. In this case, the fitness professional would note on the assessment form that it was modified in order to meet the client's needs.

Additional Considerations for Lumbo-Pelvic-Hip Complex Compensations

Gravity is a constant downward directed force that can have a great impact on the demands of the core, particularly in the prone position. The force of gravity can be manipulated to lessen the demands on the core by decreasing the body's lever length in relation to gravity. This can be done by putting an individual in a more inclined position (e.g., hands on a bench with feet on the floor) or bringing the pivot point closer to the center of gravity (e.g., performing prone assessments with knees on the floor).

Performance Assessments

The following are additional performance assessments for the fitness professional to apply to clients seeking performance enhancement.

Vertical Jump Test

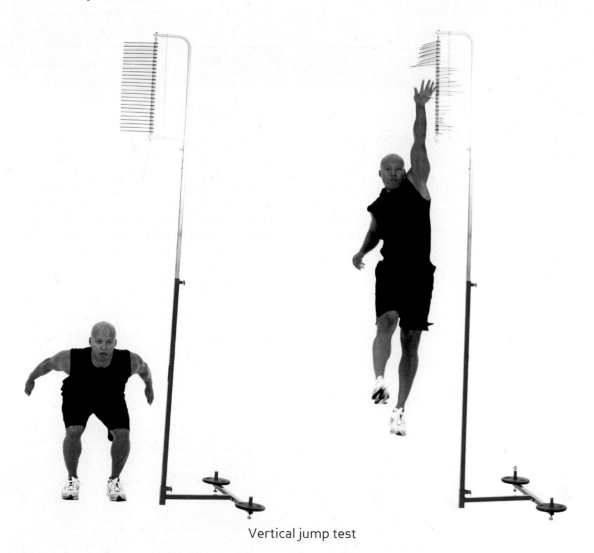

Vertical jump test

Purpose	The purpose of the vertical jump test is to assess lower extremity power.
Position	The client stands with their side next to a wall and reaches up with the hand closest to the wall. Keeping the feet flat on the ground, the point of the fingertips is marked or recorded. This is called the *standing reach height*.
Movement	1. The client then stands away from the wall, and leaps vertically (without stepping) as high as possible, using both arms and legs to assist in projecting the body upwards, and touches the wall. 2. Mark the location where the client touched. 3. The difference in distance between the standing reach height and the jump height is the score. The best of three attempts is recorded. 4. When reassessing, the individual's jump height should be higher.

40-yard Dash

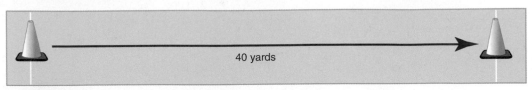

40-yard dash

Quick Check
What is body composition
testing and what
are common testing
protocols?

Purpose	The purpose of the 40-yard dash is to assess acceleration and speed. This assessment is best performed on a track or field of at least 60 yards. The professional should also have a stopwatch and set up cones 40 yards apart.
Position	The client starts from a comfortable, stationary, three-point-stance position with the front foot behind the starting line. This starting position should be held for 3 seconds prior to starting.
Movement	1. When ready, the client sprints to the end cone. 2. Begin timing at the client's first movement and stop timing the moment the client's chest crosses the end cone. 3. Typically, two trials are allowed, with the best time recorded. 4. When reassessing, the individual's time should be less.

Pro Shuttle Test

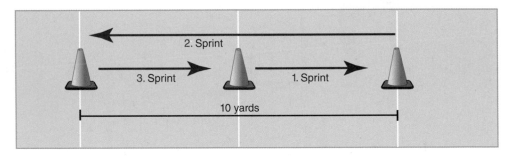

Pro shuttle test

Quick Check
When should you take
someone's circumference
measurements?

Purpose	The purpose of the pro shuttle test is to assess speed, explosion, body control, and the ability to change direction (agility). The fitness professional will need a stopwatch and three cones. The assessment should be performed on a flat, nonslip surface.
Position	Three marker cones are placed along a line 5 yards apart. The client stands at the middle cone.
Movement	1. On the signal "Go" the client turns and runs 5 yards to the right side and touches the line with the right hand. 2. Client then runs 10 yards to the left and touches the other line with the left hand. 3. Finally, the client turns and finishes by running back through the start/finish line (the middle cone). 4. The best time seen in three trials is recorded. 5. When reassessed, the time should be lower.

LEFT Test

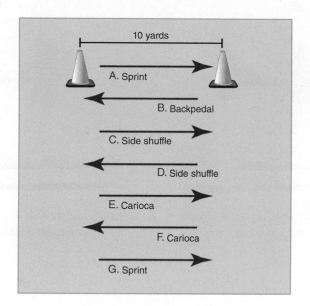

LEFT test

Quick Check
What are muscle actions, joint motions, planes of motion, Davis's law, and the sliding filament theory?

Purpose	The purpose of the LEFT test is to assess agility, acceleration, deceleration, and neuromuscular control. The fitness professional will need a stopwatch and two marker cones. The assessment should be performed on a flat, nonslip surface.
Position	Two marker cones are placed 10 yards apart.
Movement	1. On the signal "Go," the client sprints from cone 1 to cone 2, backpedals back to cone 1, side shuffles to cone 2 then to cone 1, Carioca's to cone 2 then to cone 1, and finishes with a sprint to cone 2. 2. The time is recorded. 3. When reassessed, the time should be lower.

Gait Assessment

Purpose	Assessment of dynamic posture during ambulation.
Position	Walk at a comfortable pace at a 0-degree incline on a treadmill.
Movement	1. From an anterior view, observe the feet and knees. The feet should remain straight, with the knees in line with the toes. From a lateral view, observe the low back, shoulders, and head. The low back should maintain a neutral lordotic curve. The shoulders and head should also be in neutral alignment. From a posterior view, observe the feet and lumbo-pelvic-hip complex (LPHC). The feet should remain straight and the LPHC should remain level. The time is recorded. 2. Feet: Do the feet flatten and/or turn out? 3. Knees: Do the knees move inward? 4. LPHC: Does the low back arch? 5. Shoulders and head: Do the shoulders round? Does the head migrate forward? 6. Feet: Do the feet flatten and/or turn out? 7. LPHC: Is there excessive pelvic rotation? Do the hips hike?

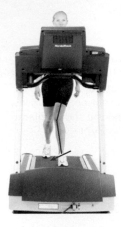
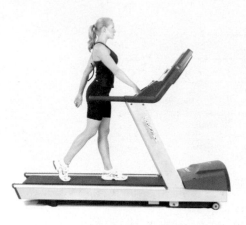
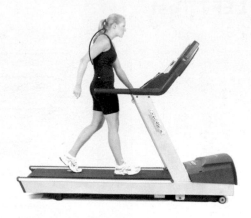

Gait treadmill walking assessment compensations: Feet flatten/knees move inward.

Gait treadmill walking assessment compensations: Low back arches.

Gait treadmill walking assessment compensations: Shoulders round.

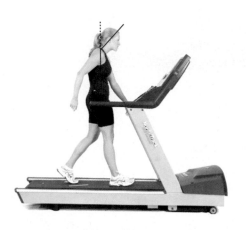
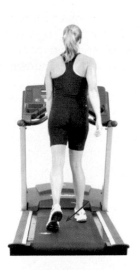
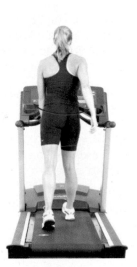
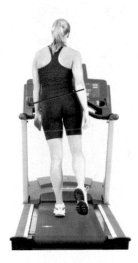

Gait treadmill walking assessment compensations: Head forward.

Gait treadmill walking assessment compensations: Feet flatten and/or turn out.

Gait treadmill walking assessment compensations: Pelvic rotation.

Gait treadmill walking assessment compensations: Hip hikes.

Quick Check
What is synergistic dominance?

Cardio Considerations for Client's Feet Turn Out Compensation

The following are suggested cardio activities for clients with turned out feet:

- *Treadmill*: Clients can use the treadmill *after* doing flexibility, and if the speed is a level at which they can focus on keeping the five kinetic chain checkpoints aligned.

			© ilolab/ShutterStock, Inc.
TABLE E.1	**Kinetic Chain Compensations for the Gait Assessment**		
Checkpoint	**Compensation**	**Probable Overactive Muscles**	**Probable Underactive Muscles**
Feet	Flatten	Peroneal complex Lat. Gastrocnemius Biceps femoris (short head) TFL	Anterior tibialis Posterior tibialis Med. Gastrocnemius Gluteus medius
	Turn out	Soleus Lat. Gastrocnemius Biceps femoris (short head) Tensor fascia lata (TFL)	Med. Gastrocnemius Med. Hamstring Gluteus medius/maximus Gracilis Sartorius Popliteus
Knees	Move inward (Valgus)	Adductor complex Biceps femoris (short head) TFL Lat. Gastrocnemius Vastus lateralis	Med. Hamstring Med. Gastrocnemius Gluteus medius/maximus Vastus medialis oblique Anterior tibialis Posterior tibialis
LPHC	Low back arches	Hip flexor complex Erector spinae Latissimus dorsi	Gluteus maximus Intrinsic core stabilizers Hamstrings
	Excessive rotation	External obliques Adductor complex Hamstrings	Gluteus medius/maximus Intrinsic core stabilizers
	Hip hike	Quadratus lumborum (opposite side) TFL/Gluteus minimus (same side)	Adductor complex (same side) Gluteus medius (same side)
Shoulders	Rounded	Pectorals Latissimus dorsi	Middle and lower trapezius Rotator cuff
Head	Forward	Upper trapezius Levator scapulae Sternocliedomastoid	Deep cervical flexors

- *Elliptical trainer*: When the client is on the elliptical, the foot can be positioned straight and the pad will help maintain it.
- *Rowing machine*: The foot is in a position that does not require as much control.
- *Versa climber*: The versa climber uses a foot pad that can assist in maintaining a neutral foot position.

Quick Check
What is reciprocal
inhibition?

Cardio Considerations for Clients with Arms Falling Forward or Rounded Posture

The following are some exercises in which it is challenging to maintain good upper body posture:

◆ *Stationary bike/cycling*: Cycling with upright posture is better for clients with upper body compensations.
◆ *Stair climber*: Standing upright is better for the upper body and puts the weight back on the legs where it should be.
◆ *Treadmill*: Ensure that the clients avoid holding the treadmill rails, which pulls the upper body forward into the compensation.
◆ *Anything with a television*: If the TV is positioned too high, the individual may have to put the head into excessive extension, leading to the head protruding forward.

Working with Post-Cardiac Rehabilitation Clients

Cardiac rehabilitation is a four-phase process, separate from the OPT Model, that is important for those who have experienced a heart attack, heart valve repair, artery bypass surgery, angioplasty, or those who suffer from chronic chest pain.

Phase One of Cardiac Rehab	Cardiac rehabilitation conducted at a medical facility that generally involves 36 outpatient visits over 12 weeks, which include directly supervised exercise and lifestyle modification education.
Phase Two of Cardiac Rehab	Prescribed by a physician if continued improvement under direct supervision is needed. May last up to another 12 weeks and is also conducted in a cardiac rehabilitation setting.
Phases Three–Four of Cardiac Rehab	Self-paced programs that involve exercise direction and motivation to sustain lifestyle changes and healthy behaviors. These phases may be conducted outside of a medical facility but require interaction between the physician and the fitness professional to ensure safety.

Concepts for Program Design

Progressive Resistance Exercise

Quick Check
How do assessments
apply to program design?

The principle of progressive resistance exercise shows that resistance training programs should start with light loads and increase as strength adaptations are achieved.

Applying Undulating Periodization to the OPT Model

Two ways that the OPT model can be used in an undulating, nonlinear fashion are:

◆ Using weekly cycles composed of various phases of the OPT model.
◆ Using weekly cycles composed of one phase of the OPT model, but with intensities and volume varied throughout the week.

Core Considerations

The following should be considered with regard to core exercises:

♦ *The Floor Bridge*: To activate the correct muscles the client should move the feet to hip width and keep them straight to avoid activating the adductors.
♦ *Prone Iso-Abs*: A common hand and arm position during the prone iso-abs is to bring the hands together, internally rotating at the shoulders. The arms should run parallel to each other when performing the prone iso-abs exercise.

Balance Considerations

The following should be considered with regard to single-leg balance exercise:

♦ *Monitor feet turn out*: The foot will turn out with the increased challenge of balance training in an attempt to increase the base of support.
♦ *Monitor anterior pelvic tilt*: Single-leg balance is an exercise that can be incredibly demanding on the muscles around the hips and spine. Therefore, it is not unusual to see a client demonstrate compensations around the hips during this exercise. During single-leg stance the gluteal muscles need to work with the abdominal muscles to keep the hips and the stance leg in proper position.

Resistance Training Considerations

The following should be considered with regard to resistance training:

♦ *Monitor feet turn out*: During the staggered stance, it is very common for the rear leg to turn out, exacerbating the compensation of the feet turning out. The rear leg should be straight, and if necessary the client can get the rear leg into a triple-extended position.
♦ *Monitor anterior pelvic tilt*: If the hip flexors are restricting this motion, then the front of the hips will likely be pulled down, exacerbating the compensation.
♦ *Monitor arms falling forward*: Performing many repetitions of lat pull-downs, pull-ups, or heavy chest exercises may make the compensation worse. If the client moves into an anterior pelvic tilt, overhead movements should be avoided until proper extensibility has been restored to the lats and pectorals.

Client Homework

Homework should include exercises that engage the clients and help them progress toward their goals. Several different factors should be considered when convincing clients to complete homework:

♦ *Client attitudes toward homework*. Try to avoid the negative connotation that often comes with the word "homework." It is important to get clients to realize that repetition enables them to progress more quickly.
♦ *Client goals*. Many clients pursuing a weight loss goal suffer from a lack of motivation or even anxiety toward exercise. Some will be motivated to go the gym and perform an hour-long workout session without the trainer, whereas others may prefer to perform flexibility and light cardio, such as a walk in the neighborhood.
♦ *Task difficulty*. To encourage completion, training should begin with simple tasks, and fitness professionals should periodically assess the client's readiness to take on more complex exercises.

Quick Check
What are the acute variables for all phases of and modes of training in the OPT Model?

Quick Check
What are the acute variables, goals and rationale for cardio stage training?

Quick Check
What are the program design modifications for special populations?

Trainer Templates and Record Keeping

In order to keep track of each client's progress, it is important to keep records of each session. This record keeping will be an asset to the client now and in the future. For the fitness professional, this is the foundation of a good business. Informative records do not ensure success, but success without them is unlikely.

A training template should track five items:

- Phase of training.
- Exercise selection.
- Intensity.
- Volume.
- *Outcome.*

Movement and Muscle Balance

Muscle imbalances can in large part be attributed to the client's lifestyle and daily activity pattern. There is no amount of foam-rolling, stretching, or strengthening that can correct poor daily habits. This is often seen when the client is not progressing after 1 month of proper training. If the overhead squat assessment is not getting better, either the program design needs to be considered or the daily patterns that occur outside of the gym need to be addressed by the fitness professional.

Fitness professionals should teach their clients how to move when performing basic tasks throughout their day. The client learning how to move properly when not in the gym may be the most important factor when considering muscle imbalances. This will require the fitness professional to provide the client with movement-specific homework.

Exercise Selection—Common Exercises

10 Exercises Effective in Most Individuals

Quick Check
How do you progress, regress, and classify exercises within the OPT Model?

Supine bridge	Engages the gluteal muscles, which should be very powerful muscles.
Prone iso-abs	Teaches the muscles that are designed to stabilize the spine to engage.
Scaption	Safe shoulder exercise that uses the entire shoulder girdle in the most functional plane of motion.
Single-leg balance reach	This is the recommended beginning exercise for most clients once the client is able to coordinate the muscular activity.
Squat jump to stabilization	Can be used with any movement compensation as long as the client can safely perform it.
Back row	Rowing motions will teach scapular retraction and depression as well as strengthen muscles that are often weak.
Squat to row	Uses two of the largest muscle groups in the body, the back and the gluteals, as well as all of the muscles around the core.
Squat	The squat requires work from many very large muscles, and adequate range of motion in some very important joints.

Lunge	Think of the lunge as a squat with a different footprint, requiring many of the same muscles and range of motion.
Deadlift	The deadlift becomes very important for clients who do not have the range of motion to squat but still need to work their gluteal muscles.

Quick Check
What is triple extension and when is it used?

Exercises to Avoid

Compensations and Exercises to Avoid Until Specific Movement Compensations Are Corrected

Feet Turning Out	• *Calf raises*: The feet typically turn out because the calves are shortened and overactive.
Knees Caving In	• *Adductor machine*: The knees cave in because the adductors are already overactive. • *Abductor machine*: The abductor machine may appear to be indicated with the knees caving in. • *Leg extension*: Leg extension machines focus on the quadriceps muscle group. Therefore, to isolate the quads with that movement compensation could potentially make it worse.
Anterior Pelvic Tilt	• *Leg press*: The leg press is a quad-dominant machine and does not allow the gluteal muscles to work to their full potential. • *Adductor machine*: Some of the adductors also serve as hip flexors (pectineus and adductor brevis). Isolating the adductors will potentially make the compensation worse. • *Leg raises*: The hip flexors are overactive in an anterior pelvic tilt. Strengthening the hip flexors with this exercise may exacerbate the movement dysfunction. • *Leg extension*: Leg extension is designed to isolate the quadriceps. Therefore, isolating the quadriceps is not recommended in the presence of an anterior pelvic tilt. • *Leg curl*: This exercise may be performed incorrectly due to the inflexibility of the quadriceps and hip flexors, the weakness of the hamstrings, and overactivity of the low back muscles; all indicated by anterior pelvic tilt.
Arms Falling Forward	• *Lat pull-down*: Muscles that control the scapula in upward rotation should be worked on before performing lat strengthening work. • *Chest press machine*: The chest press machine, however, is often used with a significant amount of weight. This will increase the strength of the prime movers without teaching proper stabilization. • *Shoulder press*: The shoulder press is not harmful, but if the lats are inflexible then clients will likely arch their low back in order to successfully execute the shoulder press.

Quick Check
How do you safely and effectively spot, cue, and modify various exercises?

Quick Check
What is the flexibility continuum and how does it apply to the OPT Model?

Hydration Concepts

Quick Check
What are the nutritional guidelines including macronutrient percentages and how many grams of each equals one calorie?

TABLE E.2	Recommended Water Intake
Gender or Exercise Status	**Recommended Intake**
Women	2.7 L (91 oz.) per day
Men	3.7 L (125 oz.) per day
2 hours pre-exercise	14–20 oz.
15 minutes pre-exercise	16 oz., if tolerated
During exercise	4–8 oz. every 15–20 minutes or 16–32 ounces every hour
Postexercise	50 ounces for every kilogram (2.2 pounds) of body weight lost

Data from: *Dietary Reference Intakes*, Institute of Medicine, 2004

TABLE E.3 Water Balance from Intake and Output

Water Intake		Water Output	
Source	*Intake*	*Source*	*Loss*
Food	600–800 mL	Urine	900–1,200 mL
Beverages	1,000 mL	Mild sweating	400 mL
Metabolic water (from digestion)	200–300 mL	Lungs	300 mL
		Feces	200 mL
Total	**1,800–2,100 mL**	**Total**	**1,800–2,100 mL**

Hewlings & Medeiros, 2011

Quick Check
When should you ingest each macronutrient for maximum performance benefit?

TABLE E.4 Signs of Dehydration

Dry mouth	Headache	Rapid heartbeat
Sleepiness or tiredness	Constipation	Rapid breathing
Thirst	Dizziness	Fever
Decreased urine output	Sunken eyes	Delirium
Dry skin	Low blood pressure	Unconsciousness

TABLE E.5	Guidelines for Fluid Replacement and Exercise

© ilolab/ShutterStock, Inc.

Before Exercise

Ensure high fluid intake for several days before competition (urine should be pale in color).

Consume 14–20 ounces (1.75–2.5 cups) of fluid 2 hours before exercise.

Consume 16 ounces about 15 minutes before exercise, if tolerated.

Consume water or sports drinks rather than soda or juice.

Fluid absorption is accelerated with a 6% carbohydrate drink (any popular sports drink).

Cold water or fluid is more rapidly absorbed.

During Exercise

Drink 4–8 ounces (0.5–1.0 cup) every 15–20 minutes or 16–32 ounces of fluid every hour.

If the weather is very hot, more fluid may be required.

Consuming fluids with 500–700 grams of sodium per 33 ounces of water enhances fluid replacement.

Drink sports drinks containing 6–8% glucose for exercise lasting longer than 60 minutes.

Sodas, teas, and juices are not ideal, and may result in the reverse of the desired effect.

Drinking plain water without electrolytes can also be a problem.

Take electrolyte pills with water and/or eat food if sports drinks are not favorable.

After Exercise

Consume 50 ounces of fluid for every kilogram (2.2 pounds) of body weight lost.

For exercise longer than 1 hour in duration, consuming a drink containing sodium and glucose will promote rapid rehydration.

Data from American College of Sports Medicine. (2009). ACSM position stand: Exercise and fluid replacement. *Medicine and Science in Sports and Exercise*, *39*(2), 377–390.

Fitness Technologies and Trends

Mobile Applications

Advantages of including the use of a mobile app into a personal training service include:

- Provides guidance to clients while they are traveling or even through remote personal training.
- Organizes and tracks exercise order (with visual demonstrations of exercise technique), sets, reps, and even rest periods can be prescribed through an app, allowing the client to complete workouts on their own while on vacation, traveling for business, or away from the gym.
- Professionals can use these apps to monitor workload, whether the workout is performed in person or remote.
- Facilitates encouragement and motivation from the professional and surrounding community by using social networks.
- Nutritional apps can also provide valuable information and assistance on client's habits throughout the day/week.

Quick Check
How do you apply common anatomy directional terms (medial, proximal, superior, inferior, etc.)?

Quick Check
What nutritional guidelines should be given to clients to help them lose weight?

© Ifolab/ShutterStock, Inc.

Activity Trackers

Quick Check
What are the differences between the Golgi Tendon Organs and Muscle Spindles?

These apps or devices can track movement and provide information regarding physical activity patterns. By monitoring physical activity throughout the day among their clients, fitness professionals can help guide people toward greater activity and facilitate faster results. Some activity trackers allow for the monitoring of heart rate, which can be valuable data for a fitness professional. Lower heart rate during work and rest signifies a more efficient and fit cardiorespiratory system. Sleep patterns can be tracked by some activity trackers, enabling for the evaluation of quality of sleep along with alterations in training plans as needed. Fitness professionals should explain to clients how various mobile apps will be utilized and why their use is beneficial.

Social Media

Fitness professionals should consider the different audiences that each outlet can help them access and utilize each in strategic ways. Each social media outlet is a powerful method of inexpensive promotion of personal training services and offers a unique opportunity for the fitness professional to position himself/herself. Social media is instrumental in helping develop relationships between professionals and their clients.

The primary goals of utilizing social media to further personal training business are:

- Connect with current and potential clients outside of the gym
- Establish a position of expertise and leadership
- Share information about services, events, and training opportunities

Additional goals of utilizing social media to further personal training business are:

- Encourage and motivate clients
- Provide educational messages
- Show relevancy in the industry
- Establish credibility

The following are examples of educational posts that can help the professional gain credibility:

Quick Check
What is the structure of the heart and how does blood flow through it?

- Short videos discussing exercise techniques for various modalities
- Blog posts discussing a recent research article
- Suggestions for creative ways of overcoming barriers to fitness
- Recommendations of training strategies for specific populations such as weight loss or older adults
- Examples of training plans for a variety of clients
- Philosophical statements that describe the fitness professional's approach to program design along with examples of how programs are altered based on individual needs
- Fitness tip of the day

Emerging Technologies

Determining what fitness trends are simply fads and what technologies will develop and thrive is helpful to planning ahead in the fitness industry. Unfortunately, it may be difficult to really know what consumers will gravitate towards in coming years.

Wearable technology appears to be an area that will continue to see the greatest interest and development in fitness technology (Vogel, 2015; Suciu, 2013). Devices that can be synched to smart phones to track and display exercise habits in real time may be an area of rapid growth as well as the development of new apps and greater physiological variables being monitored by each device. The development of fitness apps is projected to continue, especially now that app developers are becoming more accessible to fitness professionals.

Quick Check
What are SMART Goals?

Behavior Change Strategies for Client Results

Self-Confidence

Self-confidence can lead to greater exercise adherence, which, in turn, results in more confidence, which leads to increased exercise. Therefore, fitness professionals should try to build their clients' confidence so they can initiate and maintain a commitment to exercise.

Sources of Self-Confidence	
Performance Accomplishments	This is the strongest source of self-confidence. It focuses on personal task improvement and success, rather than on comparisons with others.
Modeling	Watching other, similar individuals successfully perform the desired task can increase a person's confidence in his or her ability to complete the task, too.
Verbal Persuasion	Being persuaded by someone else (e.g., fitness professional, coach, friend) that he or she can perform the task successfully.
Imagery	When people imagine themselves performing a task, it increases their confidence that they will actually be able to perform it.

Motivational Interviewing

Motivational interviewing has been defined as a collaborative person-centered form of guiding to elicit and strengthen motivation for change. The foundation of this technique is an empathetic, person-centered style, emphasizing evoking and strengthening the client's own motivation for healthy change.

Motivational interviewing involves knowledge and skills in four areas (Rollnick, Miller, and Butler, 2007):

- Expressing empathy
- Helping the client realize the gap between values and problematic behavior (developing discrepancy)
- Respecting the client's resistance as being normal
- Supporting the client's self-efficacy

Quick Check
What are the different stages of the Transtheoretical Model and how do you identify them?

Quick Check
What is the purpose of
active listening?

The spirit of motivational interviewing can be captured in the following fitness-related principles (Breckon, 2002):

- It is the client's task, not the fitness professional's, to articulate the client's ambivalence (exercise vs. not exercising).
- Motivation to change is elicited from the client.
- Readiness to change is not a client trait, but rather a fluctuating product of interpersonal interaction (the fitness professional might be assuming a greater readiness for change than is the case).

Autonomy-Supportive Coaching

The autonomy-supportive style of coaching focuses on creating an environment that emphasizes self-improvement, rather than beating others (i.e., direct competition).

Fitness professionals can support their clients' autonomy by:

- Providing choices within limits
- Offering rationales for activity structures
- Recognizing clients' feelings and perspectives
- Creating opportunities for clients to demonstrate initiative
- Avoiding overt control and criticism
- Providing informational feedback
- Limiting clients' ego involvement throughout their program (i.e., focus on self-improvement instead of comparing to others)

Behavior Modification Approaches

By effectively applying these tools, the client will be better equipped to make the modifications for long-term behavior change. The following approaches and techniques were shown to be successful in behavior modification (Dishman and Buckworth,1997).

Prompting:

- A prompt is a cue that initiates a behavior.
- Prompts can be verbal, physical, or symbolic.
- A verbal prompt can be a slogan or phrase that encourages the client.
- A physical prompt might be helping someone get over a "sticking point" in an activity.
- A symbolic prompt generally reminds a person to begin or continue a behavior, such as leaving out one's workout gear the night before to promote physical activity.
- The goal is to increase cues for the desired behavior and decrease cues for competing behaviors.

Quick Check
What is the Scope of
Practice of a fitness
professional and how
does it apply to nutrition,
behavior change, and
diagnosing?

Contracting:

- Written statements that outline specific behaviors and establish consequences for fulfillment (or lack thereof) are known as contracts.
- Contracts typically specify expectations, responsibilities, and contingencies for behavioral change.
- The purpose of contracts is to help the client take action, establishing criteria for meeting goals, and providing a means for clarifying consequences (Kanfer and Gaelick, 1986).
- Contracts increase the individual's public commitment and foster a sense of self-control.

Charting Attendance and Participation:

- Public reporting strategy
- A performance or attendance graph usually represents data in a form that is easily understood by everyone involved.
- The visual representation of progress by a chart is extremely helpful because a client can note even small changes in behavior and performance.
- This public information allows fitness professionals and the clients to offer praise and encouragement for the client on the chart.

Providing Feedback on Progress:

- Capitalizing on individuals' inherent interest to reach certain outcomes provides periodic, positive feedback on the progress that has been made.
- Feedback is provided with specific information on performing the behavior in question.

Cognitive-Behavioral Approach

This approach focuses on ways to help someone solve current issues. Ultimately, the focus will rely upon addressing thoughts and behaviors that are detrimental to the growth of the individual.

Association and Dissociation:

- Involves thoughts, which will eventually affect behavior.
- Association occurs when the focus is on internal body feedback (e.g., how their muscles feel or their breathing feels).
- Dissociation occurs when the focus is on the external environment (e.g., noticing how pretty the scenery is or listening to music while exercising).

Social Support:

- Refers to an individual's favorable attitude toward another person's involvement in an exercise program.

Intrinsic Approach:

- Emphasizes the internal enjoyment and fun of exercise, and making it something to look forward to—not just as a means to an external goal such as weight loss (Kimiecik, 2002).
- Professionals should help clients find activities they enjoy.

Record Keeping

Keeping accurate records is an important part of a fitness professional's job both for business purposes and for designing and implementing workouts. Details matter in running a successful long-lasting business.

Fitness professionals often see several clients in a row, which makes it all the more important to write down an outline for the workout in each person's file. With all the other responsibilities of the job, it can be tough to leave everything to memory. Having a chart/folder to refer to, and making notes during or soon after the session, makes for better and more efficient fitness professionals. It is important that fitness professionals record not only clients' objective workout results, but also what was discussed during the workout:

- How did they feel?
- What are their goals for the week or month?
- Do they have any new aches and pains?

Quick Check
What is the Code of Conduct and professional responsibility of an NASM Certified Personal Trainer?

Quick Check
How many CEUs does an NASM trainer need every year?

Quick Check
What are some good referral sources for a personal trainer?

Fitness professionals should keep two types of records. The first type is concerned with clients' progress. Clients come in with different abilities, needs, and goals; these should be individualized and tracked on a daily, weekly, or monthly basis, depending on what is most germane to the client. The other type of records that professionals should keep is concerned with the business aspect of the job.

The specific items recorded will vary based on the job responsibilities, but the following are some typical records that are kept on a daily, weekly, monthly, or yearly basis:

- Number of days worked
- Average income (per hour)
- Number of days off
- Client hours cancelled/rescheduled
- Percentage of cancellations that were paid
- Mileage driven (to in-home clients)
- Average number of sessions
- Average time spent in the gym not getting paid

Exam Taking Best Practices and Preparation

Study Approach

A multitude of tactics can be used to study the content you have learned in your CPT course to prepare for the credentialing exam. Use the study approach that maximizes your ability to retain and recall the information you learned. However, regardless of the study approach, it is important to prepare for the CPT exam in a kinesthetic way. This will allow you to have the same memory recall while taking the CPT exam.

Example of Kinesthetic Learning:
Performing an isolated contraction would give you firsthand experience on how a problematic muscle feels. So, if you are stuck on a question that tests the concept of a problematic muscle, you may practice the movement of the muscle to refresh your memory.

Mental Preparation Checklist

- Don't try to learn everything the night before the exam. Structure your schedule to allow for ample time to study and review the CPT material.
- Get 8 hours of sleep before the exam. It is essential to get enough rest to be able to focus during the exam.
- Eat before the exam. Ensuring you have sufficient energy to sit through the exam is vital for your ability to focus.

Taking the Exam Best Practices

- Focus on the test in front of you.
- If you don't know an answer, mark it and move on. Spending time on a question you don't know will do little good.
- Don't worry if others finish before you. Finishing first or last has nothing to do with your score. Make good use of the time allotted to you.
- All questions are multiple choice, providing you four answer choices with 4 choices.
- The CPT exam questions are focused on the objective criteria rather than the subjective criteria.

Glossary

A

A-Band The region of the sarcomere where myosin filaments are predominantly seen with minor overlap of the actin filaments.

Abduction A movement in the frontal plane away from the midline of the body.

Acceleration When a muscle exerts more force than is being placed on it, the muscle will shorten; also known as a concentric contraction or force production.

Acidosis The accumulation of excessive hydrogen that causes increased acidity of the blood and muscle.

Actin One of the two major myofilaments, actin is the "thin" filament that acts along with myosin to produce muscular contraction.

Action Potential Nerve impulse that allows neurons to transmit information.

Active Flexibility The ability of agonists and synergists to move a limb through the full range of motion while their functional antagonist is being stretched.

Active-Isolated Stretch The process of using agonists and synergists to dynamically move the joint into a range of motion.

Acute Variables Important components that specify how each exercise is to be performed.

Adaptive Capable of changing for a specific use.

Adduction Movement in the frontal plane back toward the midline of the body.

Adenosine Diphosphate (ADP) A high-energy compound occurring in all cells from which adenosine triphosphate (ATP) is formed.

Adenosine Triphosphate (ATP) Energy storage and transfer unit within the cells of the body.

Adequate Intake (AI) A recommended average daily nutrient intake level, based on observed (or experimentally determined) approximations or estimates of nutrient intake that are assumed to be adequate for a group (or groups) of healthy people; this measure is used when an RDA cannot be determined.

Advanced Stage The second stage of the dynamic pattern perspective theory when learners gain the ability to alter and manipulate the movements more efficiently to adapt to environmental changes.

Aerobic Activities requiring oxygen.

Afferent Neurons (Also known as sensory neurons) They gather incoming sensory information from the environment and deliver it to the central nervous system.

Agility The ability to accelerate, decelerate, stabilize, and change direction quickly while maintaining proper posture.

Agonist Muscles that are the primary movers in a joint motion; also known as prime movers.

Alarm Reaction The first stage of the General Adaptation Syndrome (GAS), the initial reaction to a stressor.

Altered Reciprocal Inhibition The concept of muscle inhibition, caused by a tight agonist, which inhibits its functional antagonist.

Amortization Phase   The electromechanical delay a muscle experiences in the transition from eccentric (reducing force and storing energy) to concentric (producing force) muscle action.

Anaerobic   Activities that do not require oxygen.

Anaerobic Threshold   The point during high-intensity activity when the body can no longer meet its demand for oxygen and anaerobic metabolism predominates; also called lactate threshold.

Anatomic Locations   Refers to terms that describe locations on the body.

Anatomic Position   The position with the body erect with the arms at the sides and the palms forward. The anatomic position is of importance in anatomy because it is the position of reference for anatomic nomenclature. Anatomic terms such as anterior and posterior, medial and lateral, and abduction and adduction apply to the body when it is in the anatomic position.

Annual Plan   Generalized training plan that spans 1 year to show when the client will progress between phases.

Antagonist   Muscles that act in direct opposition to agonists (prime movers).

Anterior (or Ventral)   On the front of the body.

Aortic Semilunar Valve   Controls blood flow from the left ventricle to the aorta going to the entire body.

Appendicular Skeleton   Portion of the skeletal system that includes the upper and lower extremities.

Arteries   Vessels that transport blood away from the heart.

Arterioles   Small terminal branches of an artery, which end in capillaries.

Arteriosclerosis   A general term that refers to hardening (and loss of elasticity) of arteries.

Arthritis   Chronic inflammation of the joints.

Arthrokinematics   1. Joint motion. 2. The motions of joints in the body.

Arthrokinetic Dysfunction   1. A biomechanical and neuromuscular dysfunction in which forces at the joint are altered, resulting in abnormal joint movement and proprioception. 2. Altered forces at the joint that result in abnormal muscular activity and impaired neuromuscular communication at the joint.

Arthrokinetic Inhibition   The neuromuscular phenomenon that occurs when a joint dysfunction inhibits the muscles that surround the joint.

Articular (Hyaline) Cartilage   Cartilage that covers the articular surfaces of bones.

Articulation   Junctions of bones, muscles, and connective tissue at which movement occurs; also known as a joint.

Assessment   A process of determining the importance, size, or value of something.

Association Stage   Fitt's second stage in which learners become more consistent with their movement with practice.

Atherosclerosis   1. Clogging, narrowing, and hardening of the body's large arteries and medium-sized blood vessels. Atherosclerosis can lead to stroke, heart attack, eye problems, and kidney problems. 2. Buildup of fatty plaques in arteries that leads to narrowing and reduced blood flow.

Atmospheric Pressure   Everyday pressure in the air.

Atrioventricular (AV) Node   A small mass of specialized cardiac muscle fibers, located in the wall of the right atrium of the heart, that receives heartbeat impulses from the sinoatrial node and directs them to the walls of the ventricles.

Atrioventricular Valves   Allow for proper blood flow from the atria to the ventricles.

Atrium   The superior chamber of the heart that receives blood from the veins and forces it into the ventricles.

Augmented Feedback   Information provided by some external source such as a fitness professional, videotape, or a heart rate monitor.

Autogenic Inhibition   The process by which neural impulses that sense tension are greater than the impulses that cause muscles to contract, providing an inhibitory effect to the muscle spindles.

Autonomous Stage   Fitt's third stage of motor learning in which the learner has refined the skill to a level of automation.

Axial Skeleton   Portion of the skeletal system that consists of the skull, rib cage, and vertebral column.

Axon   A cylindric projection from the cell body that transmits nervous impulses to other neurons or effector sites.

B

Backside Mechanics   Proper alignment of the rear leg and pelvis during sprinting, which includes ankle plantar flexion, knee extension, hip extension, and neutral pelvis.

Balance   **1.** The ability to sustain or return the body's center of mass or line of gravity over its base of support. **2.** When the body is in equilibrium and stationary, meaning no linear orangular movement.

Ball-and-Socket Joint   Most-mobile joints that allow motion in all three planes. Examples would include the shoulder and hip.

Basal Ganglia   A portion of the lower brain that is instrumental in the initiation and control of repetitive voluntary movements such as walking and running.

Beta-oxidation (β-oxidation)   The breakdown of triglycerides into smaller subunits called free fatty acids (FFAs) to convert FFAs into acyl-CoA molecules, which then are available to enter the Krebs cycle and ultimately lead to the production of additional ATP.

Bicuspid (Mitral) Valve   Two cusps control the blood flow from the left atrium to the left ventricle.

Bioenergetic Continuum   Three main pathways used by the kinetic chain to produce ATP.

Bioenergetics   The study of energy in the human body.

Biomechanics   **1.** A study that uses principles of physics to quantitatively study how forces interact within a living body. **2.** The science concerned with the internal and external forces acting on the human body and the effects produced by these forces.

Bipenniform Muscle Fibers   Muscle fibers that are arranged with short, oblique fibers that extend from both sides of a long tendon. An example would be the rectus femoris.

Blood   Fluid that circulates in the heart, arteries, capillaries, and veins, carries nutrients and oxygen to all parts of the body, and also rids the body of waste products.

Blood Lipids   Also known as cholesterol and triglycerides, blood lipids are carried in the blood stream by protein molecules known as high-density lipoproteins (HDL) and low-density lipoproteins(LDL).

Blood Vessels   Network of hollow tubes that circulates blood throughout the body.

Bones   Provide a resting ground for muscles and protection of vital organs.

Bracing   Occurs when you have contracted both the abdominal, lower back, and buttock muscles at the same time.

Brainstem   The link between the sensory and motor nerves coming from the brain to the body and vice versa.

C

calorie   The amount of heat energy required to raise the temperature of 1 g of water 1°C.

Calorie   A unit of expression of energy equal to 1000 cal. The amount of heat energy required to raise the temperature of kilogram or lit of water 1°C.

Cancer   Any of various types of malignant neoplasms, most of which invade surrounding tissues, may metastasize to several sites, and are likely to recur after attempted removal and to cause death of the patient unless adequately treated.

Capillaries   The smallest blood vessels, and the site of exchange of chemicals and water between the blood and the tissues.

Carbohydrates   1. Organic compounds of carbon, hydrogen, and oxygen, which include starches, cellulose, and sugars, and are an important source of energy. All carbohydrates are eventually broken down in the body to glucose, a simple sugar. 2. Neutral compounds of carbon, hydrogen, and oxygen (such as sugars, starches, and celluloses).

Cardiac Muscle   Heart muscle.

Cardiac Output (Q̇)   Heart rate × stroke volume, the overall performance of the heart.

Cardiorespiratory Fitness   The ability of the circulatory and respiratory systems to supply oxygen rich blood to skeletal muscles during sustained physical activity.

Cardiorespiratory System   A system of the body composed of the cardiovascular and respiratory systems.

Cardiorespiratory Training   Any physical activity that involves and places stress on the cardiorespiratory system.

Cardiovascular Control Center (CVC)   Directs impulses that will either increase or decrease cardiac output and peripheral resistance based on feedback from all structures involved.

Cardiovascular System   A system of the body composed of the heart, blood, and blood vessels.

Cell Body   The portion of the neuron that contains the nucleus, lysosomes, mitochondria, and a Golgi complex.

Central Controller   Controls heart rate, left ventricular contractility, and arterial blood pressure by manipulating the sympathetic and parasympathetic nervous systems.

Central Nervous System   The portion of the nervous system that consists of the brain and spinal cord.

Cerebellum   A portion of the lower brain that compares sensory information from the body and the external environment with motor information from the cerebral cortex to ensure smooth coordinated movement.

Cerebral Cortex   A portion of the central nervous system that consists of the frontal lobe, parietal lobe, occipital lobe, and temporal lobe.

Cervical Spine   The area of the spine containing the seven vertebrae that compose the neck.

Chain   A system that is linked together or connected.

Chemoreceptors   Sensory receptors that respond to chemical interaction (smell and taste).

Chronic Obstructive Lung Disease   The condition of altered airflow through the lungs, generally caused by airway obstruction as a result of mucus production.

Circuit Training System   This consists of a series of exercises that an individual performs on after another with minimal rest.

Co-contraction   Muscles contract together in a force-couple.

Cognitive Stage   Fitt's first stage of motor learning that describes how the learner spends much of the time thinking about what they are about to perform.

Collagen   A protein that is found in connective tissue that provides tensile strength. Collagen, unlike elastin, is not very elastic.

Compound-Sets   Involve the performance of two exercises for antagonistic muscles. For example, a set of bench presses followed by cable rows (chest/back).

Concentric Muscle Action   When a muscle is exerting force greater than the resistive force, resulting in shortening of the muscle.

Conduction Passageway   Consists of all the structures that air travels through before entering the respiratory passageway.

Condyles   Projections protruding from the bone to which muscles, tendons, and ligaments can attach; also known as a process, epicondyle, tubercle, and trochanter.

Condyloid Joint   A joint where the condyle of one bone fits into the elliptical cavity of another bone to form the joint. An example would include the knee joint.

Contralateral   Positioned on the opposite side of the body.

Controlled Instability   Training environment that is as unstable as can safely be controlled by an individual.

Core   1. The center of the body and the beginning point for movement. 2. The structures that make up the lumbo-pelvic-hip complex (LPHC), including the lumbar spine, the pelvic girdle, abdomen, and the hip joint.

Core Strength   The ability of the lumbo-pelvic-hip complex musculature to control an individual's constantly changing center of gravity.

Coronal Plane   An imaginary plane that bisects the body to create front and back halves; also known as the frontal plane.

Corrective Flexibility   Designed to improve muscle imbalances and altered arthrokinematics.

Creatine Phosphate   A high-energy phosphate molecule that is stored in cells and can be used to resynthesize ATP immediately.

Cumulative Injury Cycle   A cycle whereby an injury will induce inflammation, muscle spasm, adhesions, altered neuromuscular control, and muscle imbalances.

D

Davis's Law   States that soft tissue models along the line of stress.

Decelerate   When the muscle is exerting less force than is being placed on it, the muscle lengthens; also known as an eccentric muscle action or force reduction.

Deconditioned   A state of lost physical fitness, which may include muscle imbalances, decreased flexibility, and a lack of core and joint stability.

Dendrites   A portion of the neuron that is responsible for gathering information from other structures.

Depressions   Flattened or indented portions of bone, which can be muscle attachment sites.

Delayed-Onset Muscle Soreness   Pain or discomfort often felt 24 to 72 hours after intense exercise or unaccustomed physical activity.

Diabetes Mellitus   Chronic metabolic disorder caused by insulin deficiency, which impairs carbohydrate usage and enhances usage of fats and proteins.

Diaphysis   The shaft portion of a long bone.

Dietary Supplement   A substance that completes or makes an addition to daily dietary intake.

Diffusion   The process of getting oxygen from the environment to the tissues of the body.

Distal   Positioned farthest from the center of the body, or point of reference.

Dorsal   Refers to a position on the back or toward the back of the body.

Dorsiflexion   When applied to the ankle, the ability to bend at the ankle, moving the front of the foot upward.

Dynamic Balance   The ability to move and change directions under various conditions without falling.

Drawing-In Maneuver   **1.** Activation of the transverse abdominis, multifidus, pelvic floor muscles, and diaphragm to provide core stabilization. **2.** A maneuver used to recruit the local core stabilizers by drawing the navel in toward the spine.

Dynamic Functional Flexibility   Multiplanar soft tissue extensibility with optimal neuromuscular efficiency throughout the full range of motion.

Dynamic Joint Stabilization   The ability of the stabilizing muscles of a joint to produce optimum stabilization during functional, multiplanar movements.

Dynamic Pattern Perspective (DPP)   The theory that suggests that movement patterns are produced as a result of the combined interactions among many systems (nervous, muscular, skeletal, mechanical, environmental, past experiences, and so forth).

Dynamic Range of Motion   The combination of flexibility and the nervous system's ability to control this range of motion efficiently.

Dynamic Stabilization   When a muscle is exerting force equal to the force being placed on it. Also known as an isometric contraction.

Dynamic Stretching   **1.** Uses the force production of a muscle and the body's momentum to take a joint through the full available range of motion. **2.** The active extension of a muscle, using force production and momentum, to move the joint through the full available range of motion.

E

Eccentric Muscle Action   An eccentric muscle action occurs when a muscle develops tension while lengthening.

Effectors   Any structure innervated by the nervous system including organs, glands, muscle tissue, connective tissue, blood vessels, bone marrow, and so forth.

Efferent Neurons   Neurons that transmit nerve impulses from the brain or spinal cord to the effector sites such as muscles or glands; also known as motor neurons.

Elastin   A protein that is found in connective tissue that has elastic properties.

Empathy   Action of awareness, understanding, and sensitivity of the thoughts, emotions, and experience of another without personally having gone through the same.

Endocrine System   The system of glands in the human body that is responsible for producing hormones.

Endomysium   The deepest layer of connective tissue that surrounds individual muscle fibers.

Endurance Strength   The ability to produce and maintain force for prolonged periods.

Energy   The capacity to do work.

Energy-Utilizing   When energy is gathered from an energy-yielding source by some storage unit (ATP) and then transferred to a site that can use this energy.

Enjoyment   The amount of pleasure derived from performing a physical activity.

Epicondyle   Projections protruding from the bone to which muscles, tendons, and ligaments can attach; also known as a condyle, process, tubercle, and trochanter.

Epimysium   A layer of connective tissue that is underneath the fascia and surrounds the muscle.

Epiphyseal Plates   The region of long bone connecting the diaphysis to the epiphysis. It is a layer of subdividing cartilaginous cells in which growth in length of the diaphysis occurs.

Epiphysis   The end of long bones, which is mainly composed of cancellous bone, and house much of the red marrow involved in red blood cell production. They are also one of the primary sites for bone growth.

Equilibrium   A condition of balance between opposed forces, influences, or actions.

Erythrocytes   Red blood cells.

Estimated Average Requirement (EAR)   The average daily nutrient intake level that is estimated to meet the requirement of half the healthy individuals who are in a particular life stage and gender group.

Eversion   A movement in which the inferior calcaneus moves laterally.

Excess Postexercise Oxygen Consumption (EPOC)   The state in which the body's metabolism is elevated after exercise.

Excitation-Contraction Coupling   The process of neural stimulation creating a muscle contraction.

Exercise Imagery   Is the process created to produce internalized experiences to support or enhance exercise participation.

Exercise Metabolism   The examination of bioenergetics as it relates to the unique physiologic changes and demands placed on the body during exercise.

Exercise Order   Refers to the order in which the exercises are performed during a workout.

Exercise Selection   The process of choosing appropriate exercises for a client's program.

Exhaustion   The third stage of the General Adaptation Syndrome (GAS), when prolonged stress or stress that is intolerable produces exhaustion or distress to the system.

Expert Stage   The third stage of the dynamic pattern perspective model in which the learner now focuses on recognizing and coordinating their joint motions in the most efficient manner.

Expiration   The process of actively or passively relaxing the inspiratory muscles to move air out of the body.

Explosive Strength   The ability to develop a sharp rise in force production once a movement pattern has been initiated.

Extensibility   Capability to be elongated or stretched.

Extension   A straightening movement in which the relative angle between two adjacent segments increases.

External Feedback   Information provided by some external source, such as a health and fitness professional, videotape, mirror, or heart rate monitor, to supplement the internal environment.

External Rotation   Rotation of a joint away from the middle of the body.

F

Fan-Shaped Muscle   A muscular fiber arrangement that has muscle fibers span out from a narrow attachment at one end to a broad attachment at the other end. An example would be the pectoralis major.

Fascia   The outermost layer of connective tissue that surrounds the muscle.

Fascicle   A grouping of muscle fibers that house myofibrils.

Fast Twitch Fibers   Muscle fibers that can also be characterized by the term type IIA and IIB. These fibers contain fewer capillaries, mitochondria, and myoglobin. These fibers fatigue faster than type I fibers.

Fat   One of the three main classes of foods and a source of energy in the body. Fats help the body use some vitamins and keep the skin healthy. They also serve as energy stores for the body. In food, there are two types of fats, saturated and unsaturated.

Feedback   **1.** The utilization of sensory information and sensorimotor integration to aid the kinetic chain in the development of permanent neural representations of motor patterns. **2.** The use of sensory information and sensorimotor integration to help the human movement system in motor learning.

Flat Bones   A classification of bone that is involved in protection and provides attachment sites for muscles. Examples include the sternum and scapulae.

Flexibility   The normal extensibility of all soft tissues that allows the full range of motion of a joint.

Flexibility Training   Physical training of the body that integrates various stretches in all three planes of motion to produce the maximum extensibility of tissues.

Flexion   A bending movement in which the relative angle between two adjacent segments decreases.

Force   An influence applied by one object to another, which results in an acceleration or deceleration of the second object.

Force-Couple   Muscle groups moving together to produce movement around a joint.

Force-Velocity Curve   The ability of muscles to produce force with increasing velocity.

Formed Elements   Refers to the cellular component of blood that includes erythrocytes, leukocytes, and thrombocytes.

Fossa   A depression or indented portion of bone, which could be a muscle attachment site; also known as a depression.

Frequency   The number of training sessions in a given timeframe.

Frontal Lobe   A portion of the cerebral cortex that contains structures necessary for the planning and control of voluntary movement.

Frontal Plane   An imaginary bisector that divides the body into front and back halves.

Frontside Mechanics   Proper alignment of the lead leg and pelvis during sprinting, which includes ankle dorsiflexion, knee flexion, hip flexion, and neutral pelvis.

Fructose   Known as fruit sugar; a member of the simple sugars carbohydrate group found in fruits, honey and syrups, and certain vegetables.

Functional Efficiency   The ability of the nervous and muscular systems to move in the most efficient manner while placing the least amount of stress on the kinetic chain.

Functional Flexibility   Integrated, multiplanar, soft tissue extensibility with optimum neuromuscular control through the full range of motion.

Functional Strength   The ability of the neuromuscular system to perform dynamic eccentric, isometric, and concentric contractions efficiently in a multiplanar environment.

Fusiform   A muscular fiber arrangement that has a full muscle belly that tapers off at both ends. An example would include the biceps brachii.

G

General Adaptation Syndrome (GAS)   **1.** A syndrome in which the kinetic chain responds and adapts to imposed demands. **2.** A term used to describe how the body responds and adapts to stress.

Generalized Motor Program (GMP)   A motor program for a distinct category of movements or actions, such as overhand throwing, kicking, or running.

General Warm-Up   **1.** Consists of movements that do not necessarily have any movement specificity to the actual activity to be performed. **2.** Low-intensity exercise consisting of movements that do not necessarily relate to the more intense exercise that is to follow.

Gliding Joint   A nonaxial joint that moves back and forth or side to side. Examples would include the carpals of the hand and the facet joints.

Gluconeogenesis   The formation of glucose from noncarbohydrate sources, such as amino acids.

Glucose   A simple sugar manufactured by the body from carbohydrates, fat, and to a lesser extent protein, which serves as the body's main source of fuel.

Glycemic Index   A ranking of carbohydrate-containing foods based on the food's effect on blood sugar compared with a standard reference food's effect.

Glycogen   The complex carbohydrate molecule used to store carbohydrates in the liver and muscle cells. When carbohydrate energy is needed, glycogen is converted into glucose for use by the muscle cells.

Golgi Tendon Organs   Receptors sensitive to change in tension of the muscle and the rate of that change.

Goniometric Assessment   Technique measuring angular measurement and joint range of motion.

Gravity   The attraction between earth and the objects on earth.

Ground Reaction Force (GRF)   The equal and opposite force that is exerted back onto the body with every step that is taken.

H

Heart   A hollow muscular organ that pumps a circulation of blood through the body by means of rhythmic contraction.

Heart Rate (HR)   The rate at which the heart pumps.

Hemoglobin   Oxygen-carrying component of red blood cells and also gives blood its red color.

Hierarchical Theories   Theories that propose all planning and implementation of movement result from one or more higher brain centers.

Hinge Joint   A uniaxial joint that allows movement in one plane of motion. Examples would include the elbow and ankle.

Hobbies   Activities that a client may partake in regularly, but which may not necessarily be athletic in nature.

Homeostasis   The ability or tendency of an organism or a cell to maintain internal equilibrium by adjusting its physiologic processes.

Horizontal Abduction   Movement of the arm or thigh in the transverse plane from an anterior position to a lateral position.

Horizontal Adduction   Movement of the arm or thigh in the transverse plane from a lateral position to an anterior position.

Horizontal Loading   Performing all sets of an exercise or body part before moving on to the next exercise or body part.

Human Movement Science   The study of functional anatomy, functional biomechanics, motion learning, and motor control.

Human Movement System   The combination and interrelation of the nervous, muscular, and skeletal systems.

Hypercholesterolemia   Chronic high levels of cholesterol in the bloodstream.

Hyperglycemia   Abnormally high blood sugar.

Hyperlipidemia   Elevated levels of blood fats (e.g., triglycerides, cholesterol).

Hyperextension   Extension of a joint beyond the normal limit or range of motion.

Hypertension   Consistently elevated arterial blood pressure, which, if sustained at a high enough level, is likely to induce cardiovascular or end-organ damage.

Hypertrophy   Enlargement of skeletal muscle fibers in response to overcoming force from high volumes of tension.

H-Zone   The area of the sarcomere where only myosin filaments are present.

I

I-Band   The area of the sarcomere where only actin filaments are present.

Inferior   Positioned below a point of reference.

Insertion   The part of a muscle by which it is attached to the part to be moved—compare with origin.

Inspiration   The process of actively contracting the inspiratory muscles to move air into the body.

Insulin   A protein hormone released by the pancreas that helps glucose move out of the blood and into the cells in the body, where the glucose can be used as energy and nourishment.

Integrated Cardiorespiratory Training   Cardiorespiratory training programs that systematically progress clients through various stages to achieve optimal levels of physiologic, physical, and performance adaptations by placing stress on the cardio-respiratory system.

Integrated Fitness Profile   A systematic problem-solving method that provides the fitness professional with a basis for making educated decisions about exercise and acute variable selection.

Integrated Flexibility Training   A multifaceted approach integrating various flexibility techniques to achieve optimum soft tissue extensibility in all planes of motion.

Integrated Performance Paradigm   To move with efficiency, forces must be dampened (eccentrically), stabilized (isometrically), and then accelerated (concentrically).

Integrated Training   A concept that incorporates all forms of training in an integrated fashion as part of a progressive system. These forms of training include flexibility training; cardiorespiratory training; core training; balance training; plyometric (reactive) training; speed, agility, and quickness training; and resistance training.

Integrative (Function of Nervous System)   The ability of the nervous system to analyze and interpret sensory information to allow for proper decision making, which produces the appropriate response.

Intensity   The level of demand that a given activity places on the body.

Intermittent Claudication   The manifestation of the symptoms caused by peripheral arterial disease.

Internal Feedback   The process whereby sensory information is used by the body to reactively monitor movement and the environment.

Internal Rotation   Rotation of a joint toward the middle of the body.

Interneurons   Transmit nerve impulses from one neuron to another.

Intermuscular Coordination   The ability of the neuromuscular system to allow all muscles to work together with proper activation and timing between them.

Intramuscular Coordination   The ability of the neuromuscular system to allow optimal levels of motor unit recruitment and synchronization within a muscle.

Intrapulmonary Pressure   Pressure within the thoracic cavity.

Inversion   A movement in which the inferior calcaneus moves medially.

Ipsilateral   Positioned on the same side of the body.

Irregular Bones   A classification of bone that has its own unique shape and function, which does not fit the characteristics of the other categories. Examples include the vertebrae and pelvic bones.

Isokinetic Muscle Action   When a muscle shortens at a constant speed over the full range of motion.

Isometric Muscle Action   When a muscle is exerting force equal to the force being placed on it leading to no visible change in the muscle length.

J

Joints   Junctions of bones, muscles, and connective tissue at which movement occurs; also known as an articulation.

Joint Motion   Movement in a plane occurs about an axis running perpendicular to the plane.

Joint Receptors   Receptors surrounding a joint that respond to pressure, acceleration, and deceleration of the joint.

Joint Stiffness   Resistance to unwanted movement.

K

Kilocalorie   A unit of expression of energy equal to 1000 calories. The amount of heat energy required to raise the temperature of kilogram or liter of water 1°Celsius.

Kinetic   Force.

Kinetic Chain   The combination and interrelation of the nervous, muscular, and skeletal systems.

Knowledge of Performance (KP)   A method of feedback that provides information about the quality of the movement pattern performed.

Knowledge of Results (KR)   A method of feedback after the completion of a movement to inform the client about the outcome of their performance.

Kyphosis   Exaggerated outward curvature of the thoracic region of the spinal column resulting in a rounded upper back.

L

Lactic Acid   An acid produced by glucose-burning cells when these cells have an insufficient supply of oxygen.

Lateral   Positioned toward the outside of the body.

Lateral Flexion   The bending of the spine (cervical, thoracic, or lumbar) from side to side.

Law of Acceleration   Acceleration of an object is directly proportional to the size of the force causing it, in the same direction as the force, and inversely proportional to the size of the object.

Law of Action-Reaction   Every force produced by one object onto another produces an opposite force of equal magnitude.

Law of Gravitation   Two bodies have an attraction to each other that is directly proportional to their masses and inversely proportional to the square of their distance from each other.

Law of Thermodynamics   Weight reduction can only take place when there is more energy burned than consumed.

Length-Tension Relationship   The resting length of a muscle and the tension the muscle can produce at this resting length.

Leukocytes   White blood cells.

Ligament   Primary connective tissue that connects bones together and provides stability, input to the nervous system, guidance, and the limitation of improper joint movement.

Limit Strength   The maximum force a muscle can produce in a single contraction.

Lipids   A group of compounds that includes triglycerides (fats and oils), phospholipids, and sterols.

Long Bones   A characteristic of bone that has a long cylindric body with irregular or widened bony ends. Examples include the clavicle and humerus.

Longitudinal Muscle Fiber   A muscle fiber arrangement in which its fibers run parallel to the line of pull. An example would include the sartorius.

Lower-Brain   The portion of the brain that includes the brainstem, the basal ganglia, and the cerebellum.

Lower-Extremity Postural Distortion   An individual who has increased lumbar lordosis and an anterior pelvic tilt.

Lumbar Spine   The portion of the spine, commonly referred to as the small of the back. The lumbar portion of the spine is located between the thorax (chest) and the pelvis.

Lumbo-Pelvic-Hip Complex   Involves the anatomic structures of the lumbar and thoracic spines, the pelvic girdle, and the hip joint.

Lumbo-Pelvic-Hip Postural Distortion   Altered joint mechanics in an individual that lead to increased lumbar extension and decreased hip extension.

M

Maximal Oxygen Consumption ($\dot{V}O_{2max}$)   The highest rate of oxygen transport and utilization achieved at maximal physical exertion.

Maximal Strength   The maximum force an individual's muscle can produce in a single voluntary effort, regardless of the rate of force production.

Mechanical Specificity   **1.** The specific muscular exercises using different weights and movements that are performed to increase strength or endurance in certain body parts. **2.** Refers to the weight and movements placed on the body.

Mechanoreceptors   Sensory receptors responsible for sensing distortion in body tissues.

Medial   Positioned near the middle of the body.

Mediastinum   The space in the chest between the lungs that contains all the internal organs of the chest except the lungs.

Medullar Cavity   The central cavity of bone shafts where marrow is stored.

Metabolic Specificity   **1.** The specific muscular exercises using different levels of energy that are performed to increase endurance, strength, or power. **2.** Refers to the energy demand placed on the body.

Metabolism   All of the chemical reactions that occur in the body to maintain itself. Metabolism is the process in which nutrients are acquired, transported, used, and disposed of by the body.

Mitochondria   The mitochondria are the principal energy source of the cell. Mitochondria convert nutrients into energy as well as doing many other specialized tasks.

M-Line   The portion of the sarcomere where the myosin filaments connect with very thin filaments called titin and create an anchor for the structures of the sarcomere.

Mode   Type of exercise performed.

Momentum   The product of the size of the object (mass) and its velocity (speed with which it is moving).

Monthly Plan   Generalized training plan that spans one month and shows which phases will be required each day of each week.

Motor Behavior   **1.** The manner in which the nervous, skeletal, and muscular systems interact to produce an observable mechanical response to the incoming sensory information from the internal and external environments. **2.** Motor response to internal and external environmental stimuli.

Motor Control   **1.** The involved structures and mechanisms that the nervous system uses to gather sensory information and integrate it with previous experiences to produce a motor response. **2.** How the central nervous system integrates internal and external sensory information with previous experiences to produce a motor response.

Motor Development   The change in motor skill behavior over time throughout the lifespan.

Motor (Function of Nervous System)   The neuromuscular response to the sensory information.

Motor Learning   The integration of motor control processes with practice and experience that lead to relatively permanent changes in the capacity to produced skilled movements.

Motor (Efferent) Neurons   Transmit nerve impulses from the brain and spinal cord to effector sites.

Motor Unit   A motor neuron and all of the muscle fibers it innervates.

Multipenniform   Muscles that have multiple tendons with obliquely running muscle fibers.

Multiple-Set System   The system consists of performing multiple sets of the same exercise.

Multisensory Condition   Training environment that provides heightened stimulation to proprioceptors and mechanoreceptors.

Muscle Action Spectrum   The range of muscle actions that include concentric, eccentric, and isometric actions.

Muscle Fiber Arrangement   Refers to the manner in which the fibers are situated in relation to the tendon.

Muscle Fiber Recruitment   Refers to the recruitment pattern of muscle fiber or motor units in response to creating force for a specific movement.

Muscle Hypertrophy   **1.** Characterized by the increase in the cross-sectional area of individual muscle fibers and believed to result from an increase in the myofibril proteins. **2.** Enlargement of skeletal muscle fibers in response to overcoming force from high volumes of tension.

Muscle Imbalance   Alteration of muscle length surrounding a joint.

Muscle Spindles   Receptors sensitive to change in length of the muscle and the rate of that change.

Muscle Synergies   Groups of muscles that are recruited by the central nervous system to provide movement.

Muscular Endurance   **1.** A muscle's ability to contract for an extended period. **2.** The ability to produce and maintain force production over prolonged periods of time.

Muscular System   Series of muscles that moves the skeleton.

Myofibrils   A portion of muscle that contains myofilaments.

Myofilaments   The contractile components of muscle, actin, and myosin.

Myosin   One of the two major myofilaments known as the thick filament that works with actin to produce muscular contraction.

N

Nervous System   A conglomeration of billions of cells specifically designed to provide a communication network within the human body.

Neural Activation   The contraction of a muscle generated by neural stimulation.

Neural Adaptation   An adaptation to strength training in which muscles are under the direct command of the nervous system.

Neuromuscular Efficiency   **1.** The ability of the neuromuscular system to enable all muscles to efficiently work together in all planes of motion. **2.** The ability of the neuromuscular system to allow agonists, antagonists, and stabilizers to work synergistically to produce, reduce, and dynamically stabilize the entire kinetic chain in all three planes of motion.

Neuromuscular Junction   The point at which the neuron meets the muscle to allow the action potential to continue its impulse.

Neuromuscular Specificity   **1.** The specific muscular exercises using different speeds and styles that are performed to increase neuromuscular efficiency. **2.** Refers to the speed of contraction and exercise selection.

Neuron   The functional unit of the nervous system.

Neurotransmitters   Chemical messengers that cross the neuromuscular junction (synapse) to transmit electrical impulses from the nerve to the muscle.

Neutralizer   Muscles that counteract the unwanted action of other muscles.

Nociceptors   Sensory receptors that respond to pain.

Nonsynovial Joints   Joints that do not have a joint cavity, connective tissue, or cartilage.

Novice Stage   The first stage of the dynamic pattern perspective model in which the learner simplifies movements by minimizing the specific timing of joint motions, which tends to result in movement that is rigid and jerky.

Nutrition   The process by which a living organism assimilates food and uses it for growth and repair of tissues.

O

Obesity   **1.** The condition of being considerably overweight, and refers to a person with a body mass index of 30 or greater, or who is at least 30 pounds over the recommended weight for their height. **2.** The condition of subcutaneous fat exceeding the amount of lean body mass.

Occipital Lobe   A portion of the cerebral cortex that deals with vision.

Optimal Strength   The ideal level of strength that an individual needs to perform functional activities.

Optimum Performance Training™ (OPT™)   A systematic, integrated, and functional training program that simultaneously improves an individual's biomotor abilities and builds high levels of functional strength, neuromuscular efficiency, and dynamic flexibility.

Origin   The more fixed, central, or larger attachment of a muscle—compare with insertion.

Osteoarthritis   Arthritis in which cartilage becomes soft, frayed, or thins out, as a result of trauma or other conditions.

Osteoblasts   A type of cell that is responsible for bone formation.

Osteoclasts   A type of bone cell that removes bone tissue.

Osteopenia   A decrease in the calcification or density of bone as well as reduced bone mass.

Osteoporosis   Condition in which there is a decrease in bone mass and density as well as an increase in the space between bones, resulting in porosity and fragility.

Overtraining   Excessive frequency, volume, or intensity of training, resulting in fatigue (which is also caused by a lack of proper rest and recovery).

Overweight   Refers to a person with a body mass index of 25 to 29, or, who is between 25 to30 pounds over the recommended weight for their height.

Oxygen Uptake   The usage of oxygen by the body.

Oxygen Uptake Reserve (V̇o2R)   The difference between resting and maximal or peak oxygen consumption.

P

Parietal Lobe   A portion of the cerebral cortex that is involved with sensory information.

Pattern Overload   **1.** Repetitive physical activity that moves through the same patterns of motion, placing the same stresses on the body over time. **2.** Consistently repeating the same pattern of motion, which may place abnormal stresses on the body.

Perception   The integrating of sensory information with past experiences or memories.

Perimysium   The connective tissue that surrounds fascicles.

Periodization   Division of a training program into smaller, progressive stages.

Periosteum   A dense membrane composed of fibrous connective tissue that closely wraps(invests) all bone, except that of the articulating surfaces in joints, which are covered by a synovial membrane.

Peripheral Arterial Disease   A condition characterized by narrowing of the major arteries that are responsible for supplying blood to the lower extremities.

Peripheral Heart Action System (PHA)   A variation of circuit training in which the client performs four to six exercises in a row, rests for 30 to 45 seconds, then moves to the next sequence of different exercise and continues the pattern.

Peripheral Nervous System   Cranial and spinal nerves that spread throughout the body.

Peripheral Vascular Disease   A group of diseases in which blood vessels become restricted or blocked, typically as a result of atherosclerosis.

Phases of Training   Smaller divisions of training progressions that fall within the three building blocks of training.

Photoreceptors   Sensory receptors that respond to light (vision).

Physical Activity Readiness Questionnaire (PAR-Q)   A questionnaire that has been designed to help qualify a person for low-to-moderate-to-high activity levels.

Pivot Joint   Allows movement in predominately the transverse plane; examples would include the alantoaxial joint at the base of the skull and between the radi-oulnar joint.

Plane of Motion   Refers to the plane (sagittal, frontal, or transverse) in which the exercise is performed.

Plantarflexion   Ankle motion such that the toes are pointed toward the ground.

Plasma   Aqueous liquidlike component of blood.

Plyometric (Reactive) Training   Exercises that generate quick, powerful movements involving an explosive concentric muscle contraction preceded by an eccentric muscle action.

Posterior (Dorsal)   On the back of the body.

Posterior Pelvic Tilt   A movement in which the pelvis rotates backward.

Postural Distortion Patterns   Predictable patterns of muscle imbalances.

Postural Equilibrium   The ability to efficiently maintain balance throughout the body segments.

Posture   Position and bearing of the body for alignment and function of the kinetic chain.

Power   Ability of the neuromuscular system to produce the greatest force in the shortest time.

Pregnancy   The condition of a female who contains an unborn child within the body.

Preprogrammed   Activation of muscles in healthy people that occurs automatically and independently of other muscles before movement.

Prime Mover   The muscle that acts as the initial and main source of motive power.

Principle of Individualism   Refers to the uniqueness of a program to the client for whom it is designed.

Principle of Overload   Implies that there must be a training stimulus provided that exceeds the current capabilities of the kinetic chain to elicit the optimal physical, physiologic, and performance adaptations.

Principle of Progression   Refers to the intentional manner in which a program is designed to progress according to the physiologic capabilities of the kinetic chain and the goals of the client.

Principle of Specificity *or* **Specific Adaptation to Imposed Demands (SAID Principle)**   Principle that states the body will adapt to the specific demands that are placed on it.

Processes   Projections protruding from the bone where muscles, tendons, and ligaments can attach.

Program Design   A purposeful system or plan put together to help an individual achieve a specific goal.

Pronation   A triplanar movement that is associated with force reduction.

Proprioception   The cumulative sensory input to the central nervous system from all mechanoreceptors that sense body position and limb movements.

Proprioceptively Enriched Environment   An unstable (yet controllable) physical situation in which exercises are performed that causes the body to use its internal balance and stabilization mechanisms.

Protein   Amino acids linked by peptide bonds, which consist of carbon, hydrogen, nitrogen, oxygen, and usually sulfur, and that have several essential biologic compounds.

Proximal   Positioned nearest the center of the body or point of reference.

Pulmonary Arteries   Deoxygenated blood is pumped from the right ventricle to the lungs through these arteries.

Pulmonary Capillaries   Surround the alveolar sacs. As oxygen fills the sacs it diffuses across the capillary membranes and into the bloodstream.

Pulmonary Semilunar Valve   Controls blood flow from the right ventricle to the pulmonary arteries going to the lungs.

Pyramid System   Involves a triangle or step approach that either progress up in weight with each set or decreases weight with each set.

Pyruvate   A byproduct of anaerobic glycolysis.

Q

Quadrilateral Muscle Fiber An arrangement of muscle fibers that is usually flat and four-sided. An example would include the rhomboid.

Quickness The ability to react and change body position with maximal rate of force production, in all planes of motion and from all body positions, during functional activities.

R

Range of Motion Refers to the range that the body or bodily segments move during an exercise.

Rapport Aspect of a relationship characterized by similarity, agreement, or congruity.

Rate Coding Muscular force can be amplified by increasing the rate of incoming impulses from the motor neuron after all prospective motor units have been activated.

Rate of Force Production Ability of muscles to exert maximal force output in a minimal amount of time.

Reactive Strength The ability of the neuromuscular system to switch from an eccentric contraction to a concentric contraction quickly and efficiently.

Reactive Training Exercises that use quick, powerful movements involving an eccentric contraction immediately followed by an explosive concentric contraction.

Reciprocal Inhibition The simultaneous contraction of one muscle and the relaxation of its antagonist to allow movement to take place.

Recommended Dietary Allowance (RDA) The average daily nutrient intake level that is sufficient to meet the nutrient requirement of nearly all (97 to 98%) healthy individuals who are in a particular life stage and gender group.

Recreation A client's physical activities outside of their work environment.

Relative Flexibility The tendency of the body to seek the path of least resistance during functional movement patterns.

Relative Strength The maximum force that an individual can generate per unit of body weight, regardless of the time of force development.

Remodeling The process of resorption and formation of bone.

Repetition One complete movement of a single exercise.

Repetition Tempo The speed with which each repetition is performed.

Resistance Development The second stage of the General Adaptation Syndrome (GAS), when the body increases its functional capacity to adapt to the stressor.

Respiratory Passageway Collects the channelled air coming from the conducting passageway.

Respiratory Pump Is composed of skeletal structures (bones) and soft tissues (muscles) that work together to allow proper respiratory mechanics to occur and help pump blood back to the heart during inspiration.

Respiratory System A system of organs (the lungs and respiratory passageways) that collects oxygen from the external environment and transports it to the bloodstream.

Rest Interval The time taken to recuperate between sets.

Restrictive Lung Disease The condition of a fibrous lung tissue, which results in a decreased ability to expand the lungs.

Rheumatoid Arthritis   Arthritis primarily affecting connective tissues, in which there is a thickening of articular soft tissue, and extension of synovial tissue over articular cartilages that have become eroded.

Roll   The joint motion that depicts the rolling of one joint surface on another. Examples would include that of the femoral condyles over the tibial condyles during a squat.

Root Cause Analysis   A method of asking questions on a step-by-step basis to discover the initial cause of a fault.

Rotary Motion   Movement of the bones around the joints.

S

Saddle Joint   One bone is shaped as a saddle, the other bone is shaped as the rider; the only example is in the carpometacarpal joint in the thumb.

Sagittal Plane   An imaginary bisector that divides the body into left and right halves.

Sarcolemma   A plasma membrane that surrounds muscle fibers.

Sarcomere   The functional unit of muscle that produces muscular contraction and consists of repeating sections of actin and myosin.

Sarcoplasm   Cell components that contain glycogen, fats, minerals, and oxygen that are contained within the sarcolemma.

Scapular Depression   Downward (inferior) motion of the scapula.

Scapular Elevation   Upward (superior) motion of the scapula.

Scapular Protraction   Abduction of scapula; shoulder blades move away from the midline.

Scapular Retraction   Adduction of scapula; shoulder blades move toward the midline.

Self-Myofascial Release   Another form of flexibility that focuses on the fascial system in the body.

Self-Organization   This theory, which is based on the dynamic pattern perspective, provides the body with the ability to overcome changes that are placed on it.

Semilunar Valves   Allow for proper blood flow from the ventricles to the aorta and pulmonary arteries.

Sensation   The process whereby sensory information is received by the receptor and transferred either to the spinal cord for reflexive motor behavior or to higher cortical areas for processing.

Sensorimotor Integration   **1.** The ability of the nervous system to gather and interpret sensory information to anticipate, select, and execute the proper motor response. **2.** The cooperation of the nervous and muscular system in gathering and interpreting information and executing movement.

Sensors   Provide feedback from the effectors to the central controller and cardiovascular control system. They include baroreceptors, chemoreceptors, and muscle afferents.

Sensory Feedback   The process whereby sensory information is used to reactively monitor movement and the environment.

Sensory (Function of Nervous System)   The ability of the nervous system to sense changes in either the internal or external environment.

Set   A group of consecutive repetitions.

Sensory (Afferent) Neurons   Transmit nerve impulses from effector sites (such as muscles and organs) via receptors to the brain and spinal cord.

Short Bones   A classification of bone that appears cubical in shape. Examples include the carpals and tarsals.

Single-Set System   The individual performs one set of each exercise, usually 8 to 12 repetitions at a slow, controlled tempo.

Sinoatrial (SA) Node   A specialized area of cardiac tissue, located in the right atrium of the heart, which initiates the electrical impulses that determine the heart rate; often termed the pacemaker for the heart.

Skeletal System   The body's framework, composed of bones and joints.

Skin-Fold Caliper   An instrument with two adjustable legs to measure thickness of a skin fold.

Slide   The joint motion that depicts the sliding of a joint surface across another. Examples would include the tibial condyles moving across the femoral condyles during a knee extension.

Sliding Filament Theory   The proposed process by which the contraction of the filaments within the sarcomere takes place.

Slow Twitch Fibers   Another term for type I muscle fibers, fibers that are characterized by a greater amount of capillaries, mitochondria, and myoglobin. These fibers are usually found to have a higher endurance capacity than fast twitch fibers.

Specific Warm-Up   Low-intensity exercise consisting of movements that mimic those that will be included in the more intense exercise that is to follow.

Speed   The ability to move the body in one intended direction as fast as possible.

Speed Strength   The ability of the neuromuscular system to produce the greatest possible force in the shortest possible time.

Spin   Joint motion that depicts the rotation of one joint surface on another. Examples would include the head of the radius rotating on the end of the humerus during pronation and supination of the forearm.

Split-Routine System   A system that incorporates training an individual's body parts with a high volume on separate days.

Stability   The ability of the body to maintain postural equilibrium and support joints during movement.

Stabilization Endurance   The ability of the stabilization mechanisms of the kinetic chain to sustain proper levels of stabilization to allow for prolonged neuromuscular efficiency.

Stabilization Strength   Ability of the stabilizing muscles to provide dynamic joint stabilization and postural equilibrium during functional activities.

Stabilizer   Muscles that support or stabilize the body while the prime movers and the synergists perform the movement patterns.

Starting Strength   The ability to produce high levels of force at the beginning of a movement.

Static Stretching   The process of passively taking a muscle to the point of tension and holding the stretch for a minimum of 30 seconds.

Strength   The ability of the neuromuscular system to produce internal tension to overcome an external load.

Strength Endurance   The ability of the body to repeatedly produce high levels of force for prolonged periods.

Stride Length   The distance covered with each stride.

Stride Rate   The number of strides taken in a given amount of time (or distance).

Stroke Volume (SV)   The amount of blood pumped out of the heart with each contraction.

Structural Efficiency   The structural alignment of the muscular and skeletal systems that allows the body to be balanced in relation to its center of gravity.

Subjective   Information that is provided by a client.

Substrates   The material or substance on which an enzyme acts.

Sucrose   Often referred to as table sugar, it is a molecule made up of glucose and fructose.

Sulcus   A groove in a bone that allows a soft structure to pass through.

Superior   Positioned above a point of reference.

Superset   Set of two exercises that are performed back-to-back, without any rest time between them.

Supination   A triplanar motion that is associated with force production.

Supine   Lying on one's back.

Synarthrosis Joint   A joint without any joint cavity and fibrous connective tissue. Examples would include the sutures of the skull and the symphysis pubis.

Synergist   Muscles that assist prime movers during functional movement patterns.

Synergistic Dominance   **1.** When synergists take over function for a weak or inhibited prime mover. **2.** The neuromuscular phenomenon that occurs when inappropriate muscles take over the function of a weak or inhibited prime mover.

Synovial Joints   Joints that are held together by a joint capsule and ligaments and are most associated with movement in the body.

T

Temporal Lobe   A portion of the cerebral cortex that deals with hearing.

Tendons   Connective tissues that attach muscle to bone and provide an anchor for muscles to produce force.

Tendonitis   An inflammation in a tendon or the tendon covering.

Thoracic Spine   The 12 vertebrae in mid torso that are attached to the rib cage.

Time   The length of time an individual is engaged in a given activity.

Tolerable Upper Intake Level (UL)   The highest average daily nutrient intake level likely to pose no risk of adverse health effects to almost all individuals in a particular life stage and gender group. As intake increases above the UL, the potential risk of adverse health effects increases.

Torque   **1.** The ability of any force to cause rotation around an axis. **2.** A force that produces rotation. Common unit of torque is the newton-meter or Nm.

Training Duration   The timeframe of a workout or the length of time spent in one phase of training.

Training Frequency   The number of training sessions performed during a specified period (usually 1 week).

Training Intensity   An individual's level of effort, compared with their maximal effort, which is usually expressed as a percentage.

Training Plan   The specific outline, created by a fitness professional to meet a client's goals, that details the form of training, length of time, future changes, and specific exercises to be performed.

Training Volume   Amount of physical training performed within a specified period.

Transfer-of-Training Effect   The more similar the exercise is to the actual activity, the greater the carryover into real-life settings.

Transverse Plane   An imaginary bisector that divides the body into top and bottom halves.

Tricuspid Valve   Controls the blood flow from the right atrium to the right ventricle.

Triglycerides   The chemical or substrate form in which most fat exists in food as well as in the body.

Tri-Sets System   A system very similar to supersets, the difference being three exercises back to back to back with little to no rest in between.

Trochanter   Projections protruding from the bone to which muscles, tendons, and ligaments can attach; also known as a condyle, process, tubercle, and epicondyle.

Tubercle   Projections protruding from the bone to which muscles, tendons, and ligaments can attach; also known as a condyle, process, epicondyle, and trochanter.

Type   The type or mode of physical activity that an individual is engaged in.

U

Unipenniform Muscle Fiber   Muscle fibers that are arranged with short, oblique fibers that extend from one side of a long tendon. An example would include the tibialis posterior.

Upper-Extremity Postural Distortion   An individual who exhibits a forward head, rounded shoulder posture.

V

Valsalva Maneuver   A maneuver in which a person tries to exhale forcibly with a closed glottis(windpipe) so that no air exits through the mouth or nose as, for example, in lifting a heavyweight. The Valsalva maneuver impedes the return of venous blood to the heart.

Veins   Vessels that transport blood from the capillaries toward the heart.

Ventilation   The actual process of moving air in and out of the body.

Ventilatory Threshold   The point during graded exercise in which ventilation increases disproportionately to oxygen uptake, signifying a switch from predominately aerobic energy production to anaerobic energy production.

Ventral   Refers to a position on the front or toward the front of the body.

Ventricles   The inferior chamber of the heart that receives blood from its corresponding atrium and, in turn, forces blood into the arteries.

Venules   The very small veins that connect capillaries to the larger veins.

Vertebral Column   A series of irregularly shaped bones called vertebrae that houses the spinal cord.

Vertical Loading   Alternating body parts trained from set to set, starting from the upper extremity and moving to the lower extremity.

$\dot{V}O_{2max}$ The highest rate of oxygen transport and utilization achieved at maximal physical exertion.

W

Weekly Plan   Training plan of specific workouts that spans 1 week and shows which exercises are required each day of the week.

Index

Figures and tables are indicated by f and t following the page number.